# Chemotherapy and Cancer Care

# Chemotherapy and Cancer Care

Editor: Sebastian Young

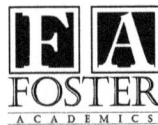

**FA**
**FOSTER**
ACADEMICS

www.fosteracademics.com

www.fosteracademics.com

FA FOSTER
ACADEMICS

Cataloging-in-Publication Data

Chemotherapy and cancer care / edited by Sebastian Young.
    p. cm.
Includes bibliographical references and index.
ISBN 978-1-63242-882-0
    1. Chemotherapy. 2. Cancer--Treatment. 3. Medical care. 4. Cancer--Patients--Hospital care. I. Young, Sebastian.
RM262 .C44 2020
615.58--dc23

Foster Academics,
118-35 Queens Blvd., Suite 400,
Forest Hills, NY 11375, USA

ISBN 978-1-63242-882-0 (Hardback)

# Contents

# Preface

This book has been an outcome of determined endeavour from a group of educationists in the field. The primary objective was to involve a broad spectrum of professionals from diverse cultural background involved in the field for developing new researches. The book not only targets students but also scholars pursuing higher research for further enhancement of the theoretical and practical applications of the subject.

Chemotherapy is a form of cancer treatment, which uses chemotherapeutic agents as part of a standardized regime against cancer. It generally consists of alkylating agents, antimetabolites, cytotoxic antibiotics, anti-microtubule agents and topoisomerase inhibitors. Different cancers are treated using unique combination chemotherapy regimens. Germ cell tumor is treated with bleomycin, etoposide and cisplatin, while colorectal cancer is targeted with folinic acid, 5-fluorouracil and oxaliplatin. Chemotherapeutic drugs can be administered as a part of induction, consolidation, combination, adjuvant and neoadjuvant chemotherapy, among others. It can be given with the aim to cure cancer or to prolong life and reduce symptoms. The efficacy of chemotherapy depends on the type of cancer and its stage. Chemotherapeutic drugs impair mitosis and target fast-dividing cells. They are thus cytotoxic in nature and harm normal cells of the body as well. This leads to several associated side effects, such as myelosuppression, mucositis and alopecia. This book brings forth some of the most innovative concepts and elucidates the unexplored aspects of chemotherapy and cancer cure. The various advancements in oncological medicine are glanced at and their applications as well as ramifications are looked at in detail. It aims to equip students and experts with the advanced topics and upcoming concepts in this area.

It was an honour to edit such a profound book and also a challenging task to compile and examine all the relevant data for accuracy and originality. I wish to acknowledge the efforts of the contributors for submitting such brilliant and diverse chapters in the field and for endlessly working for the completion of the book. Last, but not the least; I thank my family for being a constant source of support in all my research endeavours.

**Editor**

# Digital Expression Profiling Identifies *RUNX2, CDC5L, MDM2, RECQL4,* and *CDK4* as Potential Predictive Biomarkers for Neo-Adjuvant Chemotherapy Response in Paediatric Osteosarcoma

Jeffrey W. Martin[1], Susan Chilton-MacNeill[1], Madhuri Koti[4], Andre J. van Wijnen[2], Jeremy A. Squire[3,5]*, Maria Zielenska[1]

1 Department of Paediatric Laboratory Medicine, Hospital for Sick Children, Toronto, Ontario, Canada, 2 Departments of Orthopedic Surgery and Biochemistry and Molecular Biology, Mayo Clinic, Rochester, Minnesota, United States of America, 3 Department of Pathology and Molecular Medicine, Queen's University, Kingston, Ontario, Canada, 4 Department of Biomedical and Molecular Sciences, Queen's University, Kingston, Ontario, Canada, 5 Departments of Genetics and Pathology, Faculdade de Medicina de Ribeirão Preto - USP, Ribeirão Preto, São Paulo, Brazil

## Abstract

Osteosarcoma is the most common malignancy of bone, and occurs most frequently in children and adolescents. Currently, the most reliable technique for determining a patients' prognosis is measurement of histopathologic tumor necrosis following pre-operative neo-adjuvant chemotherapy. Unfavourable prognosis is indicated by less than 90% estimated necrosis of the tumor. Neither genetic testing nor molecular biomarkers for diagnosis and prognosis have been described for osteosarcomas. We used the novel nanoString mRNA digital expression analysis system to analyse gene expression in 32 patients with sporadic paediatric osteosarcoma. This system used specific molecular barcodes to quantify expression of a set of 17 genes associated with osteosarcoma tumorigenesis. Five genes, from this panel, which encoded the bone differentiation regulator *RUNX2*, the cell cycle regulator *CDC5L*, the *TP53* transcriptional inactivator *MDM2*, the DNA helicase *RECQL4*, and the cyclin-dependent kinase gene *CDK4*, were differentially expressed in tumors that responded poorly to neo-adjuvant chemotherapy. Analysis of the signalling relationships of these genes, as well as other expression markers of osteosarcoma, indicated that gene networks linked to RB1, TP53, PI3K, PTEN/Akt, myc and RECQL4 are associated with osteosarcoma. The discovery of these networks provides a basis for further experimental studies of role of the five genes (*RUNX2, CDC5L, MDM2, RECQL4,* and *CDK4*) in differential response to chemotherapy.

**Editor:** David Loeb, Johns Hopkins University, United States of America

**Funding:** This work was funded by the Canadian Cancer Society through grant CCRI-020247. Additional support was provided by National Institutes of Health grant AR049069 (to AvW). The funders had no role in study design, data collection and analysis, decision to publish, or preparation of the manuscript.

**Competing Interests:** The authors have declared that no competing interests exist.

* E-mail: jsquireinsp@gmail.com

## Introduction

Osteosarcoma is the most common primary malignant bone tumor arising from bone in children and adolescents. The tumor is very rare with an incidence approaching 5 per million per year [1]. Tumors arise from mesenchymal cells predominantly in the metaphyses of the distal femur, proximal tibia, and proximal humerus adjacent to epiphyseal growth plates [2]. In rare cases, osteosarcomas affect the axial skeleton and other non-long bones [1]. Chemotherapy followed by surgical resection is the standard treatment for high-grade osteosarcoma, and the current drug regimen is a combination of high-dose methotrexate, doxorubicin, cisplatin, and ifosfamide.

Histopathologic examination to estimate tumor necrosis following neo-adjuvant pre-operative chemotherapy is currently one of the most reliable tools for response evaluation and prognostication. Unfavorable response, corresponding to a bad prognosis, is indicated by less than 90% estimated necrosis of the tumor following neo-adjuvant chemotherapy [1]. Unlike other paediatric

cancers, there are few consistent genomic translocations, amplifications, or deletions in osteosarcoma that are useful for clinical diagnosis/treatment [3]. Similarly, a large number of gene products have potential for driving oncogenesis or disease progression in osteosarcoma [4]. This complex biology of osteosarcoma has limited the identification of reliable molecular biomarkers for tumor classification or therapeutic targeting.

Definitive diagnosis of osteosarcoma requires the presence of immature osseous matrix around neoplastic cells, which are often osteoblast-like. The predominant epithelial mesenchymal lineages define the tumor subtype based on the main form of extracellular matrix observed: osteoblastic osteosarcoma (osteoid matrix), chondroblastic osteosarcoma (cartilaginous tissue), or fibroblastic osteosarcoma (fibrous tissue). The histological subtype may define specific molecular pathways involved in osteosarcoma development and progression [4]. The high level of genetic and cytogenetic heterogeneity of this tumor, both between patients and within the tumors themselves [5], necessitates specific and personalised treatment approaches to improve outcomes.

Paediatric osteosarcoma represents a challenge to cancer treatment teams and research groups alike, a situation that is contrary to other sarcoma types for which expression signatures exist [6]. In fact, a large proportion of other sarcomas are characterised by a single dominant-acting fusion protein encoded by a disease-specific chromosome translocation, while osteosarcoma cells possess cytogenetically complex karyotypes with no such consistent translocations [7]. Scott et al. used a comparative biology approach to discover molecular subtypes of human osteosarcoma after studying profiles of canine osteosarcoma [8]. RT-PCR- and gene expression microarray-based studies of paediatric osteosarcoma have previously been used to investigate disease-specific expression patterns and signatures [9–12].

Our previous work revealed significant changes in a number of genes involved in tumor suppressive pathways, cell cycle control, and oncogenic mechanisms [10]. In the present study, candidate genes were selected based on our previous work, as well as on the published reports on gene products with potential for involvement in osteosarcoma development. NanoString nCounter Technology, which has been used previously to classify other tumors [13], was used to determine expression levels of RNA from our cohort of 32 osteosarcoma patients. The nanoString Gene Expression Assay is a high-sensitivity, multiplexed method utilizing specific molecular bar codes for the detection of mRNAs that eliminates any enzymatic reactions [14]. An analysis of the interaction of the most prominent biomarkers in this study with some of the other established oncogenic drivers in osteosarcoma was performed to determine which regulatory networks may underlie the varying responses to neo-adjuvant chemotherapy in this cohort.

## Methods

### Ethics Statement

The 32 patient cohort sample used in this study were obtained according to the guidelines and approval of the Sick Kids Hospital Research Ethics Board. Informed written consent to participate in this study was obtained from the patients, or in the case of young children, their next of kin, caretakers, or guardians on their behalf.

### Paediatric Osteosarcoma and Normal Human Osteoblast Samples

Forty sporadic paediatric osteosarcoma tumor samples derived from a cohort of 32 patients were taken from pre-chemotherapeutic biopsies or from surgical resection specimens. All specimens were flash-frozen following the biopsy procedure or surgical resection. All surgical resection specimens had been exposed to the same standard regimen of neo-adjuvant chemotherapy, including methotrexate, doxorubicin, cisplatin, and ifosfamide. For eight patients, the initial diagnostic biopsy samples, which were naïve to neo-adjuvant chemotherapy, and a matched post-chemotherapy resection sample, collected on average 3.8 months after the first sample, were analysed. These eight pairs of RNA samples were used in a subset analysis to calculate the relationships of expression changes that occurred during the neo-adjuvant chemotherapy. Chemotherapy response of <90% necrosis was used to identify those tumors with a bad response following neo-adjuvant chemotherapy, and these values, along with other patient characteristics, are summarised in Table 1. Normal human osteoblasts isolated from surgical bone resections from five healthy individuals were obtained from PromoCell (Heidelberg, Germany)

and combined and run as a single pooled sample. Total RNA was extracted from the tissues using the TRIzol Reagent method according to the manufacturer's protocol (Invitrogen) and quantified using the Bioanalyzer (Agilent Technologies). Total RNA from normal human osteoblasts and osteosarcoma cell lines was retrieved as described previously [11]. All aliquots were diluted to a final concentration of 20 ng/μL.

### nanoString nCounter Assay

The nanoString nCounter gene expression system (nanoString Technologies) was used for expression profiling of the osteosarcomas and normal human osteoblasts. Details of the system are described elsewhere [14]. Briefly, unique multiplexed probes were made with two sequence-specific probes per target mRNA. Two probes were constructed complementary to a 100-base target region. The capture probe comprised a target-specific oligonucleotide coupled to a short sequence linked to biotin. The reporter probe consisted of a second target-specific oligonucleotide linked to a unique chain of dye-labelled RNA segments for detection by the system. Our nCounter code set consisted of 21 probes, including 18 test probes derived from 17 distinct genes (RUNX2 comprised P1 and P2 transcripts) and three control genes (Table S1). Each sample was hybridised in duplicate or triplicate using 100 ng total RNA per reaction, in addition to the capture and reporter probes, as previously described [14].

### Development of Candidate Gene List and nanoString Code Set Design

We selected 17 candidate genes for this study based on published reports describing gene products with the potential for involvement in osteosarcoma development, and based on our own findings (Table 2). The literature we considered, included gene copy number and gene expression microarray experiments, in addition to functional assays of genes, in models of osteosarcoma. In addition we performed pathway analysis using Ingenuity Pathway Analysis (IPA) to delineate overrepresented gene networks in the candidate genes associated with osteosarcoma oncogenesis. IPA employs the Fisher's exact test to determine the relationship between the input dataset and canonical pathways with associated biofunctions (Ingenuity Pathway Analysis system; http://www.ingenuity.com/). Statistically significant overexpression in osteosarcoma tumors relative to normal osteoblasts has been detected previously for RECQL4, RUNX2, and SPP1 [10,15], as is the case for amplification-related overexpression of CDC5L and RUNX2 osteosarcoma specimens [9]. We included probes for each of the two RUNX2 transcript isoforms in the codeset. RUNX2_P1 captures expression of the normal osteoblast-specific version of RUNX2 [16], whereas RUNX2_P2 captures expression of RUNX2 during earlier stages of development. The latter version is also highly expressed in tumors, such as osteosarcomas [10]. Unless otherwise specified as RUNX2 (P1), all of the reported expression of RUNX2 refers to the P2 transcript. Overexpression of the protein products of FOS, MYC, MDM2, CDK4, SPARC, and BCL2L1 have also been associated with osteosarcoma and have well-described tumorigenic potential [17–21]. On the other hand, a high frequency of genetic inactivation and copy number loss in osteosarcoma has been documented for TP53, CDKN2A, RB1, PTEN, and WWOX [22–27]. We included CDKN1A and CDKN1C in our analysis because of their roles in TP53 and RB1-mediated control of cellular proliferation [28]. We selected HMBS, MT-ATP6, and MT-CO1 as housekeeping controls for our experiments because of validation in previous experiments [29–31].

**Table 1.** Clinical characteristics of the 32 patients.

| Parameter | | Number | Percentage |
|---|---|---|---|
| Histopathologic subtype[†] | Osteoblastic | 22 | 69 |
| | Chondroblastic | 4 | 13 |
| | Fibroblastic | 3 | 9 |
| | Mixed[††] | 3 | 9 |
| Gender | Female | 17 | 53 |
| | Male | 15 | 47 |
| Type of sample | Resection | 21 | 66 |
| | Biopsy | 11 | 34 |
| Percent necrosis post-chemotherapy | <90% | 19 | 59 |
| | >90% | 13 | 41 |

[†]All of the tumors were high-grade.
[††]The pathology report described pleomorphic, undifferentiated cells in a tumor comprising cells representing various subtypes.

## Statistical Analysis

All data analysis was performed using the nSolver Analysis Software (nanoString Technologies). Briefly, counts are normalised for all target RNAs in all samples based on the positive control probes to account for differences in hybridisation efficiency and post-hybridisation processing, including purification and immobilisation of complexes. The software calculates the geometric mean of each of the controls for each sample to estimate the overall assay efficiency. Subsequently, mRNA content normalisation was performed using the housekeeping "calibration" genes, *MT-ATP6*, *MT-CO1*, and *HMBS*. Values <0 were blanketed and considered equal to 1 to facilitate downstream statistical analyses. All expression data can be accessed through GEO (Accession Number GSE45275). Following normalization (Table S2A and S2B) and removal of the samples with poor quality control data, the unpaired two-tailed Student's t-test (Table S3) was applied to derive genes that had significant (p<0.05) differential expression in the two groups (25 with poor prognosis and 15 with good prognosis).

## Results

### Correlations of Expression Change with Tumor Response to Chemotherapy

An unsupervised clustering was performed using Cluster 3.0 and Java tree view to determine the aggregation of the 40 RNA samples (in duplicates or triplicates) from the cohort in comparison to normal human osteoblasts and three osteosarcoma cell lines (Figure S1). An unsupervised analysis was repeated using only tumor samples from the cohort. The cluster map (Figure 1) shows the differential expression of the 17-gene probe code set from our nanoString panel, comparing the good to the poor responders. For the eight paired patient samples, only the initial pre-chemotherapy biopsies were used to examine expression levels of the gene set. Tumors with <90% necrosis in response to neo-adjuvant chemotherapy possessed significantly higher expression levels of: *RUNX2*, *CDC5L*, *CDK4*, and *RECQL4;* and significantly reduced levels of *MDM2* (all p≤0.05) (Figure 2).

### Gene Expression Changes Relative to Normal Human Osteoblasts

Using the duplicate measurements for each experiment, expression changes for 32 patient samples were normalised,

averaged, and then ratios relative to normal human osteoblasts were calculated. Statistically significant up-regulated expression in tumors relative to human osteoblasts was detected for *CDKN1C*, *FOS*, *MYC*, *RECQL4*, *RUNX2*, *SPARC*, *SPP1*, and *WWOX*. Down-regulation was observed for *CDKN1A* and *TP53* (Figure S2). Mean expression change and direction relative to normal osteoblasts match our previously published mRNA qRT-PCR analyses for *CDKN1A*, *MYC*, *RUNX2*, and *SPP1* [10].

### Gene Expression Levels Following Exposure to Neo-adjuvant Chemotherapy

For the eight patients with biopsies naïve to chemotherapy and matched resections, it was possible to perform a subset analysis to determine expression changes in resected samples relative to biopsies. mRNA expression was elevated for *BCL2L1* (p<0.05), *CDKN1A* (p<0.05), *MDM2* (p<0.05), *PTEN* (p<0.05), and *WWOX* (p<0.05). No significant differences were seen in the expression levels of *RUNX2*, *CDC5L*, *CDK4*, or *RECQL4*, between biopsy and resection specimens. Of the five genes for which differential expression in tumors was associated with a poor response to chemotherapy, only *MDM2* levels changed after exposure to neo-adjuvant chemotherapy in this subset of eight patients.

**Table 2.** List of experimental genes and control genes assayed.

| | | |
|---|---|---|
| *MYC* | *RB1* | *TP53* |
| *FOS* | *CDKN1C* | *p16INK4* |
| *CDKN1A* | *SPARC* | *RECQL4* |
| *RUNX2 (P1)* | *SPP1* | *PTEN* |
| *RUNX2 (P2)* | *BCL-xL* | *HMBS* (control) |
| *CDC5L* | *MDM2* | *MT-ATP6* (control) |
| *WWOX* | *CDK4* | *MT-CO1* (control) |

Twenty one probes for 17 genes and three controls were assayed for expression in the nanoString code set. Probes for each of the two main promoter regions of *RUNX2* were constructed.

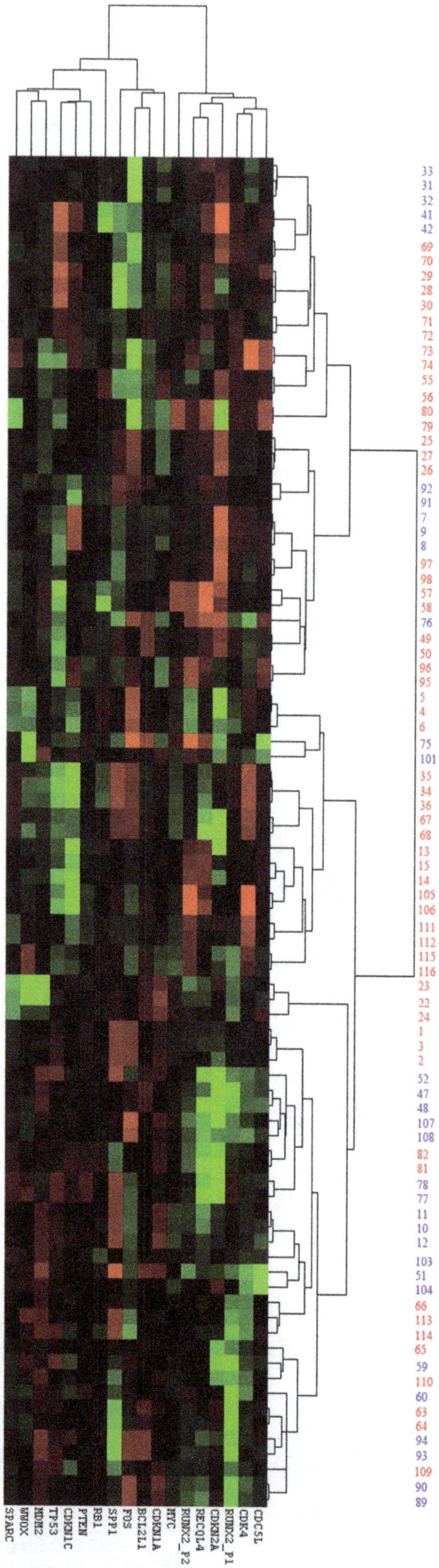


**Figure 1. Cluster map constructed using Cluster 3.0, showing the differential expression of the 17 gene set in osteosarcoma biopsy and resection cases in the cohort.** Patients with >90% tumor necrosis in response to chemotherapy (good response) are shown in blue and those with <90% (poor response) are shown in red. Sample numbers 1–36 were analyzed in triplicates whereas samples 41–116 were analysed in duplicates. Detailed data manipulation for the cohort is presented in Table S2B.

## Pathway-dependent Expression

To investigate the signalling relationship between the 17 selected genes in this study and the 31 candidate osteosarcoma driver genes from a previously published data set [32], standard pathway analysis using IPA software, was performed. Molecular interaction networks explored using IPA tools, allowing a maximum threshold of 35 nodes per network, revealed a total of 15 networks. The top two significant networks are shown in Figures 3A and B. Network 1 included 16 differentially regulated genes (score = 31), with signalling in RB1, TP53, PI3K, PTEN/Akt, MYC, and RECQL4 as the major over-represented gene networks. The interactions between the five-gene signature within signalling network 1 was strong, indicating that there were likely functional interactions of some of the genes with the core cellular regulation of cell cycle control. Network 2 included six genes (score = 8), which are associated with FOS, FAS, NFkB, and ERK1 signalling pathways. These functions are associated with extracellular signalling in the context of bone morphogenesis.

## Discussion

Paediatric osteosarcoma is a rare and complex tumor that has been studied extensively with respect to the genetic alterations that can be present [3]. However, there is still no consistently reliable marker for clinicians to use in prognostication aside from the degree of tumor necrosis in response to chemotherapy, and no targeted therapies exist [33]. Our objective in this study was to characterise a cohort of osteosarcoma tumors using nanoString technology. The nanoString nCounter is a digital expression analysis tool that is increasingly being used to detect and validate molecular signatures distinguishing subgroups of cancers [13]. The efficacy of nanoString molecular bar code analyses relative to traditionally used technologies has been demonstrated by others [34].

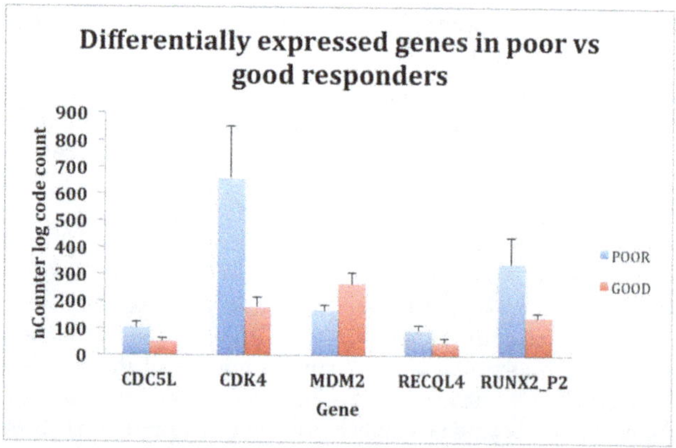


**Figure 2. Mean expression of the most significantly discriminating five genes in the osteosarcoma cohort when poor response (<90% tumor necrosis in response to chemotherapy) was compared to good response (>90% tumor necrosis).** Unpaired Student's t-test was applied to derive the genes that were differentially expressed in the two groups.

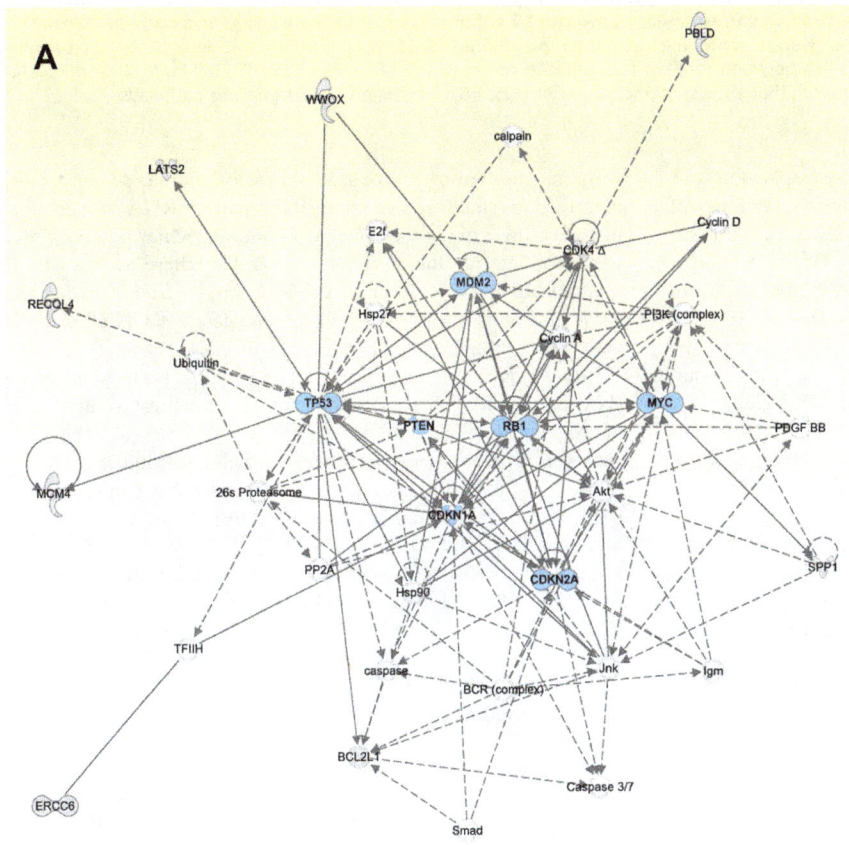

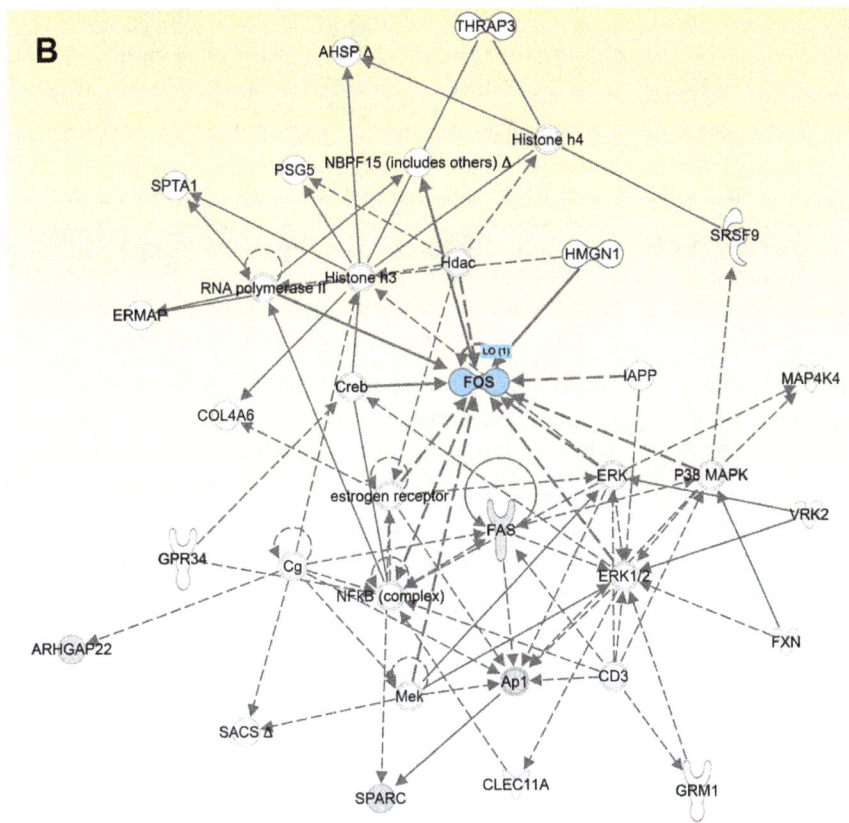

**Figure 3. Gene networks generated by Ingenuity Pathway Analysis using the 17 selected genes in the nanoString code set from this study and 31 candidate osteosarcoma driver genes from a previously published data set** [32]. Panel A depicts the major over-represented network which has molecular relationships between some of the genes in code set and RB1, TP53, PI3K, PTEN/Akt, MYC, and RECQL4 interactions. Panel B depicts the second ranked network that shows interactions with FOS, FAS, NFkB, and ERK1 signalling pathways.

Our nanoString expression analyses closely replicated our previous qRT-PCR analyses of an independent cohort of osteosarcoma specimens. Relative to normal human osteoblasts, we detected up-regulation of CDKN1C, FOS, MYC, RECQL4, RUNX2, SPARC, SPP1, and WWOX, with similar magnitudes of changes for MYC and RUNX2. The initial IPA analysis of our data, combined with that of Kuijjer et al. [32], demonstrates the potential for disruption of the MAPK/ERK signal transduction pathway via up-regulation of FOS, AP-1, and SPARC (Figure 3B). Relative to normal osteoblasts, changes in the network by aberrant expression of these genes would not only interrupt signal transduction through MAPK/ERK, but affect transcription, DNA stability, and apoptosis regulation.

Up-regulation of RUNX2, CDC5L, CDK4, RECQL4 and down-regulation of MDM2 was detected in the tumors that responded poorly to chemotherapy. There was also a statistically significant increase in RECQL4 expression in tumors relative to normal osteoblasts (Figure S2), a finding that corroborates previous studies from our research group [10]. RECQL4 overexpression is associated with elevated genome instability in osteosarcoma [30], and genomic instability may, in turn, contribute to chemoresistance and poor prognosis [35]. This gene encodes a DNA helicase important in DNA replication regulation during G(1) and S phases [36]. Germ-line mutations in RECQL4 are associated with Rothmund-Thomson syndrome, which is linked to the development of several malignancies, including paediatric osteosarcoma [37]. Somatic mutations of RECQL4 have not been detected in sporadic osteosarcomas, but the present study raises the possibility that genetic amplification may be the method by which RECQL4 dysfunction presents in sporadic tumors.

In contrast to RECQL4, there was minimal change in CDC5L or CDK4 expression between tumors and normal human osteoblasts (Figure 2), as was the case in a previous study by our group [10]. Overexpression of CDC5L has been detected in osteosarcoma patient samples and osteosarcoma cell lines alike, and is a probable candidate oncogene within the 6p12-p21 amplicon commonly found in osteosarcomas [9]. CDC5L is an essential component of the spliceosome complex, and elevated CDC5L shortens the G(2)-M cell cycle transition [38]. Furthermore, CDC5L is important in the DNA damage response following exposure to genotoxic agents. It interacts with the checkpoint kinase ATR and is required for activating S-phase checkpoint effectors [39]. The CDK4 protein regulates and promotes cell cycle progression through G1, and elevated levels are common in cancer [40]. CDK4 amplification and overexpression are commonly found in low-grade [41] and dedifferentiated forms of osteosarcoma [21]. CDK4 amplification and overexpression tend to be associated with better prognosis in the rarely occurring low-grade osteosarcomas [42] but is associated with poor prognosis in the majority of osteosarcoma cases. [43]. Expression of MDM2 is known to inhibit TP53 transcriptional activation [55]. Thus, differential expression of CDC5L, MDM2, and CDK4 could contribute to variation in cellular proliferation during osteosarcoma pathogenesis, especially when there is reduced expression of the tumor suppressors RB1 and TP53, or the TP53 target CDKN1A.

These results are also in keeping with a recent report from Kelly et al. [59], who used a similar general experimental approach to identify differentially expressed microRNA associated with chemotherapy response in osteosarcoma. Their study identified a small subset of miRNA and mRNA targets that impacted on some of the same genes and molecular pathways that we identified in this study. For example, there was a strong relationship between some of the gene targets identified in their study and bone morphogenesis proteins such as RUNX2 together with TP53 signaling (Table S4).

Our study also corroborates an expanding body of evidence showing that RUNX2, a transcription factor central to the control of osteoblast differentiation during skeletal development and remodelling, is frequently expressed at high levels in osteosarcoma biopsies [9,24,44,60]. The deregulation of RUNX2 in cancer has been linked to signalling pathways disrupted in tumorigenesis, including RB1 and TP53 [45,46]. RUNX2 is growth suppressive in normal osteoblasts, but can induce proliferation-specific genes if over-expressed [31]. Loss of TP53 increases protein levels of RUNX2 in osteosarcoma cells by post-transcriptional mechanisms Loss of TP53 prevents post-expression of microRNA miR-34c, which directly targets RUNX2 [47]. However, our study indicates that transcriptional mechanisms may also play an important role.

The RUNX2 gene is controlled by two promoters. The P1 promoter is activated at late stages of osteoblast differentiation to elevate RUNX2 levels in support of osteoblast maturation [48]. Strikingly, we noted higher levels of expression of the RUNX2 P2 transcript in tumors which responded poorly to chemotherapy, closely replicating a previous finding from our lab [10]. The P2 promoter contains multiple CpG doublets, and hypomethylation of this promoter may permit expression in mesenchymal stem cells [49]. In addition, RUNX2 expressed from the P2 promoter regulates hypertrophy and proliferation of both chondrocytes and the closely-related immature osteoblasts [50–52]. The human osteosarcoma cell line SAOS-2 has persistently high RUNX2 protein levels, driven by the P2 promoter [53]. Hence, preferential expression of RUNX2 from the 'early-activated' P2 promoter rather than the 'late-activated' P1 promoter in osteosarcomas suggests that osteosarcomas may originate from immature mesenchymal progenitor cells.

The samples in this study consisted of tumor resections both from patients who had been treated with chemotherapy and from pre-chemotherapeutic biopsies. Statistically significant gene expression differences between resections and biopsies existed for the expression levels of CDKN1A, MDM2, BCL2L1, PTEN, and WWOX. CDKN1A is activated in response to activation of the ATM/TP53 DNA damage checkpoint that accommodates double-stranded DNA repair and inhibits cell cycle progression by CDK4 [54], MDM2 is an inhibitor of TP53 [55], BCL2L1 is an anti-apoptotic factor [56], PTEN is a tumor suppressor commonly lost in osteosarcomas [23], and WWOX is a tumor suppressor that inhibits RUNX2 activity [24]. Furthermore, all of these genes encode proteins important for cell cycle regulation. The IPA analysis of the data confirms significant relationships between proteins in the TP53-RB1-centred network of protein interactions that also involve PI3K, PTEN/Akt, MYC, and RECQL4 (Figure 3A). All of the aforementioned genes were more highly expressed in the resections. Our results are consistent with experiments in osteosarcoma cell lines that have shown that drug treatment induces growth arrest and increases levels of CDKN1A, MDM2, and BCL2L1 [57,58].

In conclusion, our results provide preliminary evidence that *RUNX2, CDC5L, MDM2, RECQL4,* and *CDK4* should be further investigated to determine their roles as predictive biomarkers in osteosarcoma, because collectively, their differential expression correlates with poor response to chemotherapy in our cohort.

## Supporting Information

**Figure S1 Cluster map constructed using Cluster 3.0, showing the differential expression of the 16 gene set in osteosarcoma biopsy and resection cases.** Sample numbers 1–36 were analyzed in triplicates whereas, samples 41–116 were analyzed in duplicates. Details of samples are presented in Table S2B. The seven replicates of the three osteosarcoma cell lines and the pooled human osteoblast control used in this comparison cluster to the right as four distinct groupings (C–R). From left to right they are SAOS samples CBAAMLB; MG63 samples GIHQGHP; human osteoblast control samples EDFDEON; and U2OS samples KJLJKSR.

**Figure S2 Expression changes for each of the 32 patient samples were normalized, averaged, and then ratios relative to normal human osteoblast control were calculated.** Statistically significant up-regulated expression in tumors relative to human osteoblasts was detected for *CDKN1C, FOS, MYC, RECQL4, RUNX2, SPARC, SPP1,* and *WWOX.* Down-regulation was observed for *CDKN1A* and *TP53.*

**Table S1 Codeset for expression analysis.**

**Table S2** Table S2A: All nanoString data with normalization applied. Table S2B: Patient nanoString data sets with normalization applied. Patient samples in the first set were analyzed in triplicate, whereas samples in the second and third sets were analyzed in duplicate.

**Table S3 Gene expression levels differentiated groups of tumors.** The unpaired two-tailed Student's t-test was applied to derive genes that had significant ($p < 0.05$) differential expression between the group with poor prognosis (n = 25) and the group with good prognosis (n = 15).

**Table S4 Previously published results show similar pathways of expression deregulation in osteosarcoma.** Genes deregulated in osteosarcoma as identified by Kelly et al. (Additional file 14 Table S5 of reference 59) were functionally related to our experimental genes.

## Acknowledgments

The authors would like to thank Kirsteen Maclean of nanoString technologies for her invaluable help with the cluster analysis and Jennifer Good from Queen's University for her dedication and technical help.

## Author Contributions

Conceived and designed the experiments: MZ JAS AJvW. Performed the experiments: JWM SC-M. Analyzed the data: JWM MK MZ JAS. Contributed reagents/materials/analysis tools: MZ SC-M JAS. Wrote the paper: JWM SC-M MK AJvW MZ JAS.

## References

1. Bielack SS, Kempf-Bielack B, Delling G, Exner GU, Flege S, et al. (2002) Prognostic factors in high-grade osteosarcoma of the extremities or trunk: an analysis of 1,702 patients treated on neoadjuvant cooperative osteosarcoma study group protocols. J Clin Oncol 20(3): 776–790.
2. Cleton-Jansen AM, Anninga JK, Briaire-de Bruijn IH, Romeo S, Oosting J, et al. (2009) Profiling of high-grade central osteosarcoma and its putative progenitor cells identifies tumorigenic pathways. Br J Cancer 101(11): 1909–1918.
3. Martin JW, Squire JA, Zielenska M (2012) The genetics of osteosarcoma. Sarcoma 2012: 627254.
4. Broadhead ML, Clark JC, Myers DE, Dass CR, Choong PF (2011) The molecular pathogenesis of osteosarcoma: a review. Sarcoma 2011: 959248.
5. Selvarajah S, Yoshimoto M, Ludkovski O, Park PC, Bayani J, et al. (2008) Genomic signatures of chromosomal instability and osteosarcoma progression detected by high resolution array CGH and interphase FISH. Cytogenet Genome Res 122(1): 5–15.
6. Chibon F, Lagarde P, Salas S, Perot G, Brouste V, et al. (2010) Validated prediction of clinical outcome in sarcomas and multiple types of cancer on the basis of a gene expression signature related to genome complexity. Nat Med 16(7): 781–787.
7. Helman LJ, Meltzer P (2003) Mechanisms of sarcoma development. Nat Rev Cancer 3(9): 685–694.
8. Scott MC, Sarver AL, Gavin KJ, Thayanithy V, Getzy DM, et al. (2011) Molecular subtypes of osteosarcoma identified by reducing tumor heterogeneity through an interspecies comparative approach. Bone 49(3): 356–367.
9. Lu XY, Lu Y, Zhao YJ, Jaeweon K, Kang J, et al. (2008) Cell cycle regulator gene CDC5L, a potential target for 6p12-p21 amplicon in osteosarcoma. Mol Cancer Res 6(6): 937–946.
10. Sadikovic B, Thorner P, Chilton-Macneill S, Martin JW, Cervigne NK, et al. (2010) Expression analysis of genes associated with human osteosarcoma tumors shows correlation of RUNX2 overexpression with poor response to chemotherapy. BMC Cancer 10: 202.
11. Sadikovic B, Yoshimoto M, Chilton-MacNeill S, Thorner P, Squire JA, et al. (2009) Identification of interactive networks of gene expression associated with osteosarcoma oncogenesis by integrated molecular profiling. Hum Mol Genet 18(11): 1962–1975.
12. Namlos HM, Kresse SH, Muller CR, Henriksen J, Holdhus R, et al. (2012) Global gene expression profiling of human osteosarcomas reveals metastasis-associated chemokine pattern. Sarcoma 2012: 639038.
13. Northcott PA, Shih DJ, Remke M, Cho YJ, Kool M, et al. (2012) Rapid, reliable, and reproducible molecular sub-grouping of clinical medulloblastoma samples. Acta Neuropathol 123(4): 615–626.
14. Geiss GK, Bumgarner RE, Birditt B, Dahl T, Dowidar N, et al. (2008) Direct multiplexed measurement of gene expression with color-coded probe pairs. Nat Biotechnol 26(3): 317–325.
15. Nathan SS, Pereira BP, Zhou YF, Gupta A, Dombrowski C, et al. (2009) Elevated expression of Runx2 as a key parameter in the etiology of osteosarcoma. Mol Biol Rep 36(1): 153–158.
16. Xiao ZS, Thomas R, Hinson TK, Quarles LD (1998) Genomic structure and isoform expression of the mouse, rat and human Cbfa1/Osf2 transcription factor. Gene 214(1–2): 187–197.
17. Dalla-Torre CA, Yoshimoto M, Lee CH, Joshua AM, de Toledo SR, et al. (2006) Effects of THBS3, SPARC and SPP1 expression on biological behavior and survival in patients with osteosarcoma. BMC Cancer 6: 237.
18. Gamberi G, Benassi MS, Bohling T, Ragazzini P, Molendini L, et al. (1998) C-myc and c-fos in human osteosarcoma: prognostic value of mRNA and protein expression. Oncology 55(6): 556–563.
19. Shimizu T, Ishikawa T, Sugihara E, Kuninaka S, Miyamoto T, et al. (2010) c-MYC overexpression with loss of Ink4a/Arf transforms bone marrow stromal cells into osteosarcoma accompanied by loss of adipogenesis. Oncogene 29(42): 5687–5699.
20. Wang ZX, Yang JS, Pan X, Wang JR, Li J, et al. (2010) Functional and biological analysis of Bcl-xL expression in human osteosarcoma. Bone 47(2): 445–454.
21. Yoshida A, Ushiku T, Motoi T, Beppu Y, Fukayama M, et al. (2012) MDM2 and CDK4 immunohistochemical coexpression in high-grade osteosarcoma: correlation with a dedifferentiated subtype. Am J Surg Pathol 36(3): 423–431.
22. Feugeas O, Guriec N, Babin-Boilletot A, Marcellin L, Simon P, et al. (1996) Loss of heterozygosity of the RB gene is a poor prognostic factor in patients with osteosarcoma. J Clin Oncol 14(2): 467–472.
23. Freeman SS, Allen SW, Ganti R, Wu J, Ma J, et al. (2008) Copy number gains in EGFR and copy number losses in PTEN are common events in osteosarcoma tumors. Cancer 113(6): 1453–1461.
24. Kurek KC, Del Mare S, Salah Z, Abdeen S, Sadiq H, et al. (2010) Frequent attenuation of the WWOX tumor suppressor in osteosarcoma is associated with increased tumorigenicity and aberrant RUNX2 expression. Cancer Res 70(13): 5577–5586.
25. Mohseny AB, Tieken C, van der Velden PA, Szuhai K, de Andrea C, et al. (2010) Small deletions but not methylation underlie CDKN2A/p16 loss of

expression in conventional osteosarcoma. Genes Chromosom Cancer 49(12): 1095–1103.

26. Tsuchiya T, Sekine K, Hinohara S, Namiki T, Nobori T, et al. (2000) Analysis of the p16INK4, p14ARF, p15, TP53, and MDM2 genes and their prognostic implications in osteosarcoma and Ewing sarcoma. Cancer Genet Cytogenet 120(2): 91–98.

27. Wunder JS, Gokgoz N, Parkes R, Bull SB, Eskandarian S, et al. (2005) TP53 mutations and outcome in osteosarcoma: a prospective, multicenter study. J Clin Oncol 23(7): 1483–1490.

28. Lapenna S, Giordano A (2009) Cell cycle kinases as therapeutic targets for cancer. Nature Rev 8(7): 547–566.

29. Janssens N, Janicot M, Perera T, Bakker A (2004) Housekeeping genes as internal standards in cancer research. Mol Diagn 8(2): 107–113.

30. Maire G, Yoshimoto M, Chilton-MacNeill S, Thorner PS, Zielenska M, et al. (2009) Recurrent RECQL4 imbalance and increased gene expression levels are associated with structural chromosomal instability in sporadic osteosarcoma. Neoplasia 11(3): 260–268.

31. Teplyuk NM, Galindo M, Teplyuk VI, Pratap J, Young DW, et al. (2008) RUNX2 regulates G protein-coupled signaling pathways to control growth of osteoblast progenitors. J Biol Chem 283(41): 27585–27597.

32. Kuijjer ML, Rydbeck H, Kresse SH, Buddingh EP, Lid AB, et al. (2012) Identification of osteosarcoma driver genes by integrative analysis of copy number and gene expression data. Genes Chromosom Cancer 51(7): 696–706.

33. Clark JC, Dass CR, Choong PF (2008) A review of clinical and molecular prognostic factors in osteosarcoma. J Cancer Res Clin Oncol 134(3): 281–297.

34. Malkov VA, Serikawa KA, Balantac N, Watters J, Geiss G, et al. (2009) Multiplexed measurements of gene signatures in different analytes using the Nanostring nCounter Assay System. BMC Res Notes 2: 80.

35. Turner NC, Reis-Filho JS (2012) Genetic heterogeneity and cancer drug resistance. Lancet Oncol 13(4): e178–185.

36. Thangavel S, Mendoza-Maldonado R, Tissino E, Sidorova JM, Yin J, et al. (2010) Human RECQ1 and RECQ4 helicases play distinct roles in DNA replication initiation. Cell Mol Biol 30(6): 1382–1396.

37. Wang LL, Gannavarapu A, Kozinetz CA, Levy ML, Lewis RA, et al. (2003) Association between osteosarcoma and deleterious mutations in the RECQL4 gene in Rothmund-Thomson syndrome. J Natl Cancer Inst 95(9): 669–674.

38. Bernstein HS, Coughlin SR (1998) A mammalian homolog of fission yeast Cdc5 regulates G2 progression and mitotic entry. J Biol Chem 273(8): 4666–4671.

39. Zhang N, Kaur R, Akhter S, Legerski RJ (2009) Cdc5L interacts with ATR and is required for the S-phase cell-cycle checkpoint. EMBO reports 10(9): 1029–1035.

40. Malumbres M, Barbacid M (2007) Cell cycle kinases in cancer. Curr Opin Genet Dev 17(1): 60–65.

41. Dujardin F, Binh MB, Bouvier C, Gomez-Brouchet A, Larousserie F, et al. (2011) MDM2 and CDK4 immunohistochemistry is a valuable tool in the differential diagnosis of low-grade osteosarcomas and other primary fibro-osseous lesions of the bone. Mod Pathol 24(5): 624–637.

42. Kyriazoglou AI, Vieira J, Dimitriadis E, Arnogiannaki N, Teixeira MR, et al. (2012) 12q amplification defines a subtype of extraskeletal osteosarcoma with good prognosis that is the soft tissue homologue of parosteal osteosarcoma. Cancer Genet 205(6): 332–336.

43. Smida J, Baumhoer D, Rosemann M, Walch A, Bielack S, et al. (2010) Genomic alterations and allelic imbalances are strong prognostic predictors in osteosarcoma. Clin Cancer Res. 16(16): 4256–4267.

44. Won KY, Park HR, Park YK (2009) Prognostic implication of immunohistochemical Runx2 expression in osteosarcoma. Tumori 95(3): 311–316.

45. Lee JS, Thomas DM, Gutierrez G, Carty SA, Yanagawa S, et al. (2006) HES1 cooperates with pRb to activate RUNX2-dependent transcription. J Bone Miner Res 21(6): 921–933.

46. Lengner CJ, Steinman HA, Gagnon J, Smith TW, Henderson JE, et al. (2006) Osteoblast differentiation and skeletal development are regulated by Mdm2-p53 signaling. J Cell Biol 172(6): 909–921.

47. van der Deen M, Taipaleenmaki H, Zhang Y, Teplyuk NM, Gupta A, et al. (2013) MicroRNA-34c inversely couples the biological functions of the Runt-related transcription factor RUNX2 and the tumor suppressor p53 in osteosarcoma. J Biol Chem 288(29): 21307–21319.

48. Liu JC, Lengner CJ, Gaur T, Lou Y, Hussain S, et al. (2011) Runx2 protein expression utilizes the Runx2 P1 promoter to establish osteoprogenitor cell number for normal bone formation. J Biol Chem 286(34): 30057–30070.

49. Kang MI, Kim HS, Jung YC, Kim YH, Hong SJ, et al. (2007) Transitional CpG methylation between promoters and retroelements of tissue-specific genes during human mesenchymal cell differentiation. J Cell Biochem 102(1): 224–239.

50. Lucero CM, Vega OA, Osorio MM, Tapia JC, Antonelli M, et al. (2013) The cancer-related transcription factor Runx2 modulates cell proliferation in human osteosarcoma cell lines. J Cell Physiol 228(4): 714–723.

51. Stein GS, Lian JB, van Wijnen AJ, Stein JL, Montecino M, et al. (2004) Runx2 control of organization, assembly and activity of the regulatory machinery for skeletal gene expression. Oncogene 23(24): 4315–4329.

52. Thomas DM, Johnson SA, Sims NA, Trivett MK, Slavin JL, et al. (2004) Terminal osteoblast differentiation, mediated by runx2 and p27KIP1, is disrupted in osteosarcoma. J Cell Biol 167(5): 925–934.

53. Terry A, Kilbey A, Vaillant F, Stewart M, Jenkins A, et al. (2004) Conservation and expression of an alternative 3′ exon of Runx2 encoding a novel proline-rich C-terminal domain. Gene 336(1): 115–125.

54. Mauro M, Rego MA, Boisvert FM, Esashi F, Cavallo F, et al. (2012) p21 promotes error-free replication-coupled DNA double-strand break repair. Nucleic Acids Res 40(17): 8348–8360.

55. Haupt Y, Maya R, Kazaz A, Oren M (1997) Mdm2 promotes the rapid degradation of p53. Nature 387(6630): 296–299.

56. Brunelle JK, Letai A (2009) Control of mitochondrial apoptosis by the Bcl-2 family. J Cell Sci 122(Pt 4): 437–441.

57. Gallaher BW, Berthold A, Klammt J, Knupfer M, Kratzsch J, et al. (2000) Expression of apoptosis and cell cycle related genes in proliferating and colcemid arrested cells of divergent lineage. Cell Mol Biol 46(1): 79–88.

58. Sato N, Mizumoto K, Maehara N, Kusumoto M, Nishio S, et al. (2000) Enhancement of drug-induced apoptosis by antisense oligodeoxynucleotides targeted against Mdm2 and p21WAF1/CIP1. Anticancer Res 20(2A): 837–842.

59. Kelly AD, Haibe-Kains B, Janeway KA, Hill KE, Howe E, et al. (2013) MicroRNA paraffin-based studies in osteosarcoma reveal reproducible independent prognostic profiles at 14q32. Genome Medicine 5(2): 1–12.

60. Martin JW, Zielenska M, Stein GS, van Wijnen AJ, Squire JA (2011) The Role of RUNX2 in osteosarcoma oncogenesis. Sarcoma 2011: 282745.

# 2

# Treatment Related Impairments in Arm and Shoulder in Patients with Breast Cancer

**Janine T. Hidding**[1,2]*, **Carien H. G. Beurskens**[1], **Philip J. van der Wees**[2], **Hanneke W. M. van Laarhoven**[3], **Maria W. G. Nijhuis-van der Sanden**[2]

**1** Radboud university medical center, Department of Orthopedics, Section of Physical Therapy, Nijmegen, The Netherlands, **2** Radboud university medical center, Scientific Institute for Quality of Healthcare, Nijmegen, The Netherlands, **3** Academic Medical Center, Department of Medical Oncology, University of Amsterdam, Amsterdam, The Netherlands

## Abstract

*Background:* Breast cancer is the most common type of cancer in women in the developed world. As a result of breast cancer treatment, many patients suffer from serious complaints in their arm and shoulder, leading to limitations in activities of daily living and participation. In this systematic literature review we present an overview of the adverse effects of the integrated breast cancer treatment related to impairment in functions and structures in the upper extremity and upper body and limitations in daily activities. Patients at highest risk were defined.

*Methods and Findings:* We conducted a systematic literature search using the databases of PubMed, Embase, CINAHL and Cochrane from 2000 to October 2012, according to the PRISMA guidelines. Included were studies with patients with stage I–III breast cancer, treated with surgery and additional treatments (radiotherapy, chemotherapy and hormonal therapy). The following health outcomes were extracted: reduced joint mobility, reduced muscle strength, pain, lymphedema and limitations in daily activities. Outcomes were divided in within the first 12 months and >12 months post-operatively. Patients treated with ALND are at the highest risk of developing impairments of the arm and shoulder. Reduced ROM and muscle strength, pain, lymphedema and decreased degree of activities in daily living were reported most frequently in relation to ALND. Lumpectomy was related to a decline in the level of activities of daily living. Radiotherapy and hormonal therapy were the main risk factors for pain.

*Conclusions:* Patients treated with ALND require special attention to detect and consequently address impairments in the arm and shoulder. Patients with pain should be monitored carefully, because pain limits the degree of daily activities. Future research has to describe a complete overview of the medical treatment and analyze outcome in relation to the treatment. Utilization of uniform validated measurement instruments has to be encouraged.

**Editor:** Una Macleod, Supportive care, Early Diagnosis and Advanced disease (SEDA) research group, United Kingdom

**Competing Interests:** No authors have any competing interests.

* E-mail: Janine.Hidding@radboudumc.nl

## Introduction

Breast cancer is the most common type of cancer in women in the developed world. Due to new treatment modalities, breast cancer survival has improved over time. However, as a result of breast cancer treatment, many patients suffer from adverse effects and have serious complaints in their arm and shoulder e.g. decreased joint mobility, muscle strength, pain and lymphedema, leading to limitations in activities of daily living and participation in work, sports and leisure activities. [1–3] In a prospective Australian study, 62% of the population still suffered from at least one impairment as a complication of breast cancer treatment and 27% suffered from two to four impairments after six years. [4] Reported variability in onset and severity of upper limb symptoms of patients with breast cancer reported in studies is large [5] and a systematic overview of risk factors related to medical treatment is lacking. This information is of direct clinical relevance, as early physical therapy intervention for these complaints as well as surveillance of patients at risk for developing impairments in daily activities reduces the need for intensive rehabilitation and the associated costs. [6] Based on the misconception that disabilities such as decreased range of motion, pain and lymphedema will resolve over time without intervention, combined with denial of the possible benefits of physical therapy interventions, this has led to the inadequate monitoring of disabilities. [7] To the best of our knowledge, this is the first systematic review with an evidence synthesis on the physical adverse effects of all components of breast cancer treatment, analyzed for each treatment modality, on impairments in the arm and shoulder, leading to limitations in activities that potentially warrant treatment. If the clinician is aware of the risk of adverse effects of the treatment, clinical reasoning regarding surveillance and the early detection of impairments in patients at risk can be applied in a systematic way.

In this article, we present a systematic literature review of the adverse effects of breast cancer treatment in terms of development of constraints in the arm and shoulder in patients with stage I–III breast cancer who underwent curative treatment. We describe the adverse effects for treatment-induced disorders of the musculoskeletal system - classified by International Classification of Functioning, Disability and Health (ICF) domains [8] - and assess the influence of pre-existing comorbidity. More specifically, the following key question is answered in this systematic review: which adverse effects related to breast cancer treatment predict persistent impairments in function and structures of the upper extremities/thorax, e.g. reduced joint mobility, reduced muscle strength, pain, lymphedema and limitations in daily activities?

## Methods

### Study selection criteria

**Search strategy.** We conducted a systematic literature search using the databases of PubMed, Embase, CINAHL and Cochrane. Published studies in English, French and German language were eligible for inclusion. We started with the inclusion of eligible meta-analyses and systematic reviews, and then considered the inclusion of prognostic cohort studies, case-control studies and cross-sectional studies that were not included in published systematic reviews. To minimize bias, only studies with at least 100 patients were included. Studies which had already been included in systematic reviews or meta-analyses were not analyzed separately. To allow for an adequate follow-up and description of late adverse effects, only studies with a follow-up period of at least 3 months were included. When more publications of the same study were published, data were extracted from the most recent publication. As we were merely interested in adverse effects in relation to current medical practice, studies published from January 2000 to October 2012 were included. The search strings are listed in table 1.

**Patients.** Studies on patients with curatively treated breast cancer (Stage I–III) were included.

**Intervention.** Included medical interventions were: surgery (mastectomy, lumpectomy, axillary lymph node dissection [ALND], sentinel node biopsy [SNB], and breast reconstruction) and additional treatments (radiotherapy, chemotherapy and hormonal therapy).

**Outcomes.** The following health outcomes were extracted: impairment in functions and structures in the upper extremity and upper body (reduced joint mobility, reduced muscle strength, pain, and lymphedema), and limitations in daily activities of the upper extremity. Outcomes had to be measured with instruments for which validation studies were published, or for which the authors described validation before initiation of the study.

Description of adverse effects of the medical treatment was divided into effects within the first 12 months and late effects (> 12 months). When outcome measures of severe cases were presented as well, these were presented between brackets in table 2.

### Quality assessment

We evaluated the methodological quality of the included studies to test generalizability and possible bias. Studies were rated using the Oxford Centre for Evidence-Based Medicine, 2011 appraisal sheets and levels of evidence (see table 3) [9]. Two authors (JH + CB) independently scored each item of the appropriate scoring sheet. Disagreements were discussed together or if appropriate in the research group. If the item was well described and its quality was good, a plus (+) was assigned, plus-minus (±) was assigned if the item was incompletely described, and minus (–) was used if the item was not clearly described or not described at all. Five items were used to score systematic reviews leading to a maximum score of 100% (see table 4 and 5). Only systematic reviews including meta-analysis could achieve a full score of 100%. For cohort studies, six items were scored. Since the type of surgical treatment may influence health outcomes, articles describing radiotherapy treatment not taking into account the type of surgical treatment were given no score to the item "Subgroups with different prognosis identified". A full score was assigned to studies assessing the outcome "lymphedema" with measurements of the full arm, using tape measurements to calculate volume, water volumetry, perometry or bio-impedance spectroscopy (BIS). When other methods of multiple tape measurement were used, plus-minus was assigned to "validated outcome" criterion. If the Common Terminology Criteria for Adverse Events (CTCAE) was used as a measurement instrument for lymphedema no score was given, because only one location was measured. Questionnaires on lymphedema were given plus-minus, as these questionnaires led to a higher incidence percentage in relation to volumetric measurements. [10] In selecting studies with a quality score of >50% we aimed at reducing the risk of bias of the included studies resulting in more robust conclusions of our review.

### Synthesis

First, we described detailed characteristics and the main findings of the included systematic reviews, RCTs, and cohort studies, as reported by the authors of the included studies. Second, we assessed adverse effects per impairment and activity limitations for each medical intervention and combination of medical interventions. Adverse effects were assessed for short-term impact (≤ 12 months follow-up) and long-term impact (>12 months follow-up). If a study did not identify which part of the treatment caused

**Table 1.** Search string adverse effects.

| | |
|---|---|
| Pubmed | ((((((("Breast Neoplasms" [Mesh] OR "Breast Neoplasms" OR "breast cancer")) AND (surgery))) AND (((((radiotherapy)) OR (((("Breast Neoplasms/drug therapy" [mesh])) OR ("Antineoplastic Agents" [Mesh]) OR ("chemotherapy" [All Fields]))) OR ("Antineoplastic Agents" [Pharmacological Action])) OR (hormonal therapy)))) AND ((((((((activities)) OR ("Activities of Daily Living" [Mesh]))) OR (range of motion)) OR (("Muscle Strength" [Mesh] OR "Range of Motion, Articular" [Mesh])) OR (muscle strength)) OR (Lymphedema)) OR (pain)) AND (dutch [la] OR english [la] OR german [la] OR french [la]) AND ("2000/01/01" [PDAT] : "3000/12/31" [PDAT]) |
| Cinahl | TI breast cancer AND ((AB "Range of Motion" ) OR (AB "Muscle Strength") OR (AB Lymph*) OR (AB "Activities of Daily Living" ) OR (AB pain)) Limiters: Published Date from: 20000101–20121231 Language English |
| Embase | breast cancer.ti. AND ((activities of daily living.ab.) OR (range of motion.ab.) OR (muscle strength.ab.) OR (muscle strength.ab.) OR (Lymphedema.ab.) OR (pain.ab.)) Limit to (english language and yr ="2000– 2012") |
| Cochrane | Topic 'breast cancer' AND 'adverse effects' |

**Table 2.** Outcome of the studies regarding breast cancer treatment and adverse effects.

| Author/year of publication | Design | Disease stage/treatment/ number of pts included | Number of studies/Dates of inclusion/FU in months (% FU if mentioned) | Measurement instruments in outcome | Main findings |
|---|---|---|---|---|---|
| Hickey et al. 2013 | SR | Concurrent RT + CT vs. sequential n = 107/107/RT then CT vs. CT then RT, n = 117/119 for LE; n = 42/43 for brachial neuropathy | 3 studies: RCT; 3 survival, 2 toxicity/Up till Dec. 2011; 60/135months (FU 74%) | CTCAE/LENT-SOMA | Late toxicity 29% ; **Concurrent vs. sequential RT after CT:** Grade III/IV, in favour of sequencing: atrophy OR = 2.09 (CI = 0.92–4.75); fibrosis OR = 13.77 (CI = 0.77–247.54);LE OR = 2.02 (CI = 0.18 to 22.61). **RT before CT vs. CT before RT:** In favour of RT first: LE OR = 2.11 (CI = 0.67–7.21) ; Brachial neuropathy OR = 3.14 (CI = 0.12–79.39) |
| Moja et al. 2012 | SR | Stage I–III/HER2 pos. BC/ Trastuzumab + CT vs. CT alone(Anthracyclines, Taxanes,Vinorelbine, other CT); CHF n = 5471/4810; LVEF n = 4147/3792 | 8 studies: RCT 8/1996-Feb. 2010/% FU missing/ ≥ 24 months | Cardiac toxicity (CHF, LVEF), other toxicities | **Trastuzumab vs. no trastuzumab:** CHF ↑, cardiac toxicity ↑, LVEF ↓; CHF: trastuzumab administration >6 months OR = 5.11; Cardiac toxicity: trastuzumab before CT OR = 8.42; CT before trastuzumab OR = 11.05; Concurrent CT/trastuzumab OR = 3.90 (overall >6 months OR = 5.12); LVEF ↓ OR = 1.83; < 6 months OR = 0.89; >6 months OR = 2.14. **Trastuzumab before CT:** OR = 1.16. **CT before trastuzumab:** OR = 2.90, Concurrent **CT/trastuzumab:** OR = 1.48 |
| Zhou et al. 2011 | SR | Stage I–IV/Zoledronic acid/ ZOL vs. no ZOL n = 2684/ 2712/Delayed ZOL vs. upfront ZOL n = 119/284 | 4 studies: RCT 4/Up till May 2011 (Art 1. CT [mostly anthracycline] +/− HT; Art 2. Gosselerin + tamoxifen or anastrozole; Art 3/4 adjuvant treatment not specified/% FU missing/ 12–60 months | Not described | **ZOL vs. no ZOL:** ↑ arthralgia (4 studies); ↑ bone pain (2 studies); arthralgia RR = 1.16; bone pain RR = 1.26; muscle pain no differences between groups; complications 0.2–0.8% per item. **Delayed vs. upfront ZOL:** No differences between groups for bone pain/arthralgia; arthralgia RR = 1.28. **Anastrozole alone vs.. tamoxifen alone:** arthralgia 25% vs. 12% ; bone pain (28% vs. 21%) (art 2). **Anastrozole + ZOL vs. tamoxifen + ZOL:** bone pain 35% vs. 25%; arthralgia 24% vs. 18% (art 2) |
| Levangie et al. 2009 | SR | ALND/SNB/RT/Breast cancer vs. non breast cancer n = 1501/ALND vs. SNB vs. none/n = 2353/996/59 | 36 studies: CS 7; CCT 11; prospective 10; retrospective 1; CSS 2; RCT 5/1980–2008/% FU missing/12–126 months | ROM, muscle strength/ grip strength/upper body functions | **ALND vs. SNB or non-affected side:** ROM ↓ flexion, abduction and abduction/ external rotation; OR = 1.02/2.65/9.0*. Muscle strength ↓ grip strength, resistance abduction; OR = 8.82. Pain OR = 3.54 (1.88–6.66). Upper arm activities ↑ limitations compared to non-breast cancer; ↓: ALND OR = 3.18/9.23*. **RT vs. no RT:** OR = 1.32/2.64/4.67* |
| Liu et al. 2009 | SR | SNB vs. SNB + ALND vs. ALND/RT/n = 7135 vs. 1225 vs. 1445. | 17 studies: RCT 5, CCT 12: prospective 9, retrospective 3/SNB vs. SNB + ALND vs. ALND/1993–2008/% FU missing/6–72 months | ROM, Hand-held dynamometer, MPQ, VAS, tape measurement, MASS | **SNB:** *6 months:* LE 3–10%. *12 months:* ROM ↓ 6–31%; RT OR = 2.6; muscle strength ↓ 17–19%; pain 8–36%; LE 6–14%. *24 months:* Pain 8–21%; upper arm activities ↓: RT axilla OR = 2.6. *36 months:*ROM ↓ 0–9%. *60 months* (1 study, SNB): Muscle strength ↓ 11%; pain 9%; LE 7%; axillary RT OR = 2.4; sleep disturbance 9% |
| Tsai et al. 2009 | SR | ALND/SNB/RT/ALND vs. SNB n = 8262/Objective measurements n = 23964 | 98 studies: 10 RCT's, 83 CCT: 40 prospective, 43 retrospective, 5 CSS/ALND vs. no ALND/13 studies/ Radical mastectomy vs. other mastectomy 8 studies/ 1950–2008/% FU missing/ 1–360 months | Tape measurement, BIS, water displacement, self-report | **ALND vs. SNB:** LE RR = 3.07; **ALND vs. no ALND:** LE RR = 3.47; **Radical mastectomy vs. other mastectomy:** LE RR = 3.28; **RT axilla vs. RT no axilla:** LE RR = 2.97 |
| Lee et al. 2008 | SR | Surgery/RT not axilla/ n = 5154/LE risk n = 2416/ ROM ↓ risk n = 476 | 25 studies: RCT 8; CCT24: prospective 17, retrospective 7/1966–2007/% FU missing/7 wks-203 months | ROM, VAS, tape measurement, water displacement, LENT-SOMA, EORTC-QLQ | **ALND vs. SNB:** ROM ↓ 1%–67%; most problems 7–12 months post-surgery; muscle strength ↓ 9%–28%; OR = 4.61; pain 9%–68%; OR = 3.03; LE 0%–34%; OR = 11.67; RT not axilla OR = 1.46; Shoulder complaints: OR = 9.8 |

**Table 2.** Cont.

| Author/year of publication | Design | Disease stage/treatment/ number of pts included | Number of studies/Dates of inclusion/FU in months (% FU if mentioned) | Measurement instruments in outcome | Main findings |
|---|---|---|---|---|---|
| **Ashikaga et al. 2010** | RCT | Stage not described/SNB + ALND vs. SNB (+ ALND in case of positive nodes)/ RT/CT/n = 5611 | 36 months | Abduction ROM, water displacement | **ALND vs. SNB:** *2–3 weeks:* ROM: abduction ↓ : 56% vs. 21%. *6 months:*ROM abduction ↓ : 9% vs. 6%; ALND OR = 1.56; RT axilla OR = 2.48, CT OR = 0.73; LE: 13% vs. 9%. *12 months:*LE: 13% vs. 9%. *36 months:*LE: 14% vs. 8%; ↓ age (+/−50 years) OR = 1.41, dominant affected arm OR = 1.77, RT axilla OR = 3.47 |
| **Andersen et al. 2012** | CCT | Stage not described/Surgery/ RT/CT: CEF vs. CE+T/HT/ n = 2893 | 35/24 months | NPRS, Sensory disturbances in hands and feet | Pain overall 53%; activities: 34% gave up. **CEF vs. CE+T:** Sensory disturbances in both hands: 15% vs. 23%; OR = 1.56. Sensory disturbances in both feet: 18% vs. 32%; OR = 2.00; in younger patients OR = 0.45; ↑ risk of giving up activities OR = 1.59 |
| **Miller et al. 2012** | CCT | Stage not described/ALND vs. SNB/Mastectomy/n = 117 | 29 (3–64) months | Water displacement; perometer; LEFT-BC Questionnaire | **ALND vs. SNB:** LE: 3 vs. 0%; ALND: ↑ subjective symptoms; ↑ Mean weight-adjusted water displacement change |
| **Ozcinar et al. 2012** | CCT | Stage I–II, cT1,2 N0/SNB vs. ALND/RT vs.. RT axilla vs. RT regional LN/n = 221 | (99%); 64 (24–82) months | Tape measurement 10 cm above and below elbow | Lymphedema: *9–12 months:* 25%. *64 months:* 7% (↓ by treatment LE) |
| **Taira et al. 2011** | CCT | ALND level I–III/Mastectomy vs. lumpectomy + RT/n = 196 | FU 97% at 1 months; 96% at 6 months; 95% at 12 months; 80% at 24 months | FACT-G/FACT-B | **Mastectomy vs. lumpectomy + RT:** *1 month (severe):* ROM ↓ 68 (15)% vs. 73 (14)%; muscle strength ↓ 67 (10)% vs. 72 (18)%; pain 75 (18)% vs. 82 (20)%; lymphedema 27 (1)% vs. 41 (7)%; upper arm activities: Lifting ↓ 83 (25)% vs. 88 (20)%; household chores ↓ 61 (4)% vs. 64 (13)%; self-care ↓ 56 (4)% vs. 63 (9)%; physical activities ↓ 73 (19)% vs. 76 (19)%. *1 year (severe):*ROM ↓ 32 (4)% vs. 40 (7)%; muscle strength ↓ 48 (7)% vs. 51 (5)%; pain 60 (12)% vs. 63 (7)%; lymphedema 26 (3)% vs. 48 (11)%; upper arm activities: Lifting ↓ 34 (2)% vs. 39 (3)%; household chores ↓ 28 (4) vs. 33 (1)%; self-care ↓ 16 (0)% vs. 12 (1)%; physical activities ↓ 41 (4)% vs. 39 (4)%. *2 years (severe):*ROM 23 (0)% vs. 30 (4)%; muscle strength ↓ 39 (5)% vs. 56 (7)%; pain 42 (8)% vs. 56 (5)%; lymphedema 33 (10)% vs. 52 (15)%; upper arm activities: Lifting ↓ 20 (1)% vs. 39 (4); household chores ↓ 18 (1)% vs. 21 (3)%; self-care ↓ 10 (0)% vs. 14 (4)%; physical activities: 34 (7)% vs. 31 (5)% |
| **Wernicke et al. 2011** | CCT | stage I–II/ALND vs. SNB/ n = 265 | 119 months | ROM, tape measurement | **ALND vs. SNB:** ROM ↓ ; Lymphedema 35% vs. 5% |
| **Land et al. 2010** | CCT | Node negative invasive BC/ ALND vs. SNB/Mastectomy vs. lumpectomy/n = 747 | 36 months | Questionnaire adapted from DASH | ALND vs. SNB: Upper arm activities ↓ . *6 and 12 months:* ALND group: ↑ arm use avoidance. **Mastectomy vs. lumpectomy (+ ALND):** Lumpectomy: ↑ problems with shoulder/arm function, conducting social and work activities |
| **Yen et al. 2009** | CCT | Stage I–IV/ALND vs. SNB/ Mastectomy vs. lumpectomy/ RT/CT/HT/n = 1338 | 48 months | Telephone interviews: arm functioning related to LE, pain, or tenderness in the arm or hand on the side of surgery | Lymphedema 14% (self-report). ↑ LN removed: 6–10 nodes OR = 4.68; 11–15 nodes OR = 5.61; >16 nodes OR = 10.50 |
| **Bevilacqua et al. 2012** | CoS | Stage II–IIIa/ALND level I–III/ n = 1243 | (84%); 60 months | Tape measurement | Lymphedema 30% at 60 months; curve ↓ increasing after 36 months. Nomogram < 6 months: age, BMI, level of ALND; nomogram >6 months: age, BMI, level of ALND, seroma, early LE |

**Table 2.** Cont.

| Author/year of publication | Design | Disease stage/treatment/ number of pts included | Number of studies/Dates of inclusion/FU in months (% FU if mentioned) | Measurement instruments in outcome | Main findings |
|---|---|---|---|---|---|
| Levy et al. 2012 | CoS | Stages 0-III/ALND/SNB/-/ Mastectomy/lumpectomy/ Breast reconstruction/ n = 115 | >12 months | ROM, MRC-scale, NPRS, perometer, ULDQ, PAQ, BMI | *1 month:* ROM flexion/abduction ↓ 60%; external rotation ↓ 25%. ROM ↓: ALND, ↑ LN removed, mastectomy, stage II, hand dominant side, cording, seroma, BMI ≥25. ROM ↑: ↑ level of PA. *12+ months:*Flexion/abduction 11/10%; external rotation ↓ 5%; muscle strength ↓: 47%; pain 49% (11% moderate); fatigue 43%. ROM ↓: positive LN, mastectomy (flexion), older age (>65 yrs), BMI ≥25. Heavy household chores ↓: feeling stiff OR = 4.60; feeling week OR = 9.67; pain OR = 6.16; LE OR = 4.16; fatigue OR = 9.33; lifting a gallon ↓: feeling week: OR = 6.34; pain: OR = 4.58 |
| Mieog et al. 2012 | CoS | Stage I-III/Tamoxifen vs. exemestane/n = 4724 | 91 months | CTCAEv1 for CTS and MSD | CTS 2%; MSD 43%. **Exemestane vs. Tam:** OR = 9.90 for CTS. Independent risk factors: HT, history of musculoskeletal symptoms, arthralgia, myalgia, osteoarthritis |
| Schmitz et al. 2012 | CoS | Stages I-III+/ALND vs. SNB vs. -/Mastectomy vs. lumpectomy/RT/CT/HT/ n = 287 | (70.7%); 72 months | tape measurement, BIS, DASH, FACT-B+4 | Adverse effects: *6 months:*≥1: 90%; 2-4: 72%; >4: 16%; *12 months:* ≥1: 69%; 2-4: 46%; *18 months:* ≥1: 66%; 2-4: 34%; *72 months:*≥1: 62%; 2-4: 27% |
| Kanematsu et al. 2011 | CoS | Stage 0-IV (1 x IV)/ Aromatase inhibitors/ CT/n = 391 | 40 (9-120) months | CTCAEv4 | Age <55 vs. 55-65 vs. >65 years: Arthralgia 46% vs. 37% vs. 28%; pain frequency ↑: ↓ age at menarche; pain frequency ↓: time since last menstrual period >10 years; HT/CT/disease stage ns |
| Ridner et al. 2011 | CoS | Stages I-IV/ALND/SNB/ RT/n = 138 | 30 months | Perometer, Weight, LBCQ | Lymphedema 20%; BMI ≥30 OR = 3.59; adjusted for ALND as risk factor OR = 4.12; 80% of LE patients heaviness |
| Rief et al. 2011 | CoS | Early stage BC/Mastectomy/ lumpectomy/HT/n = 2160 | 48 months | Symptom Inventory, METs, RAND36, Life Orientation Scale— Revised, MOS, | Pain ↑: pain or depression at baseline, life events first 12 months post-operative, TAM at baseline. Pain ↓: ↑exercise, ↑ years since diagnosis, ↑ education. Pain scores ↑: stage II lumpectomy, and stage I mastectomy |
| Devoogdt et al. 2010 | CoS | Stage 0-IV/ALND/SNB/ n = 267 | (88%); 24 months | FPACQ, MET-hours/ week | Activities: MET's per week *Preoperative:* 269; *3 months:* 244; *6 months:* 246; *12 months:* 258. MET's ↓: ↑ in younger age, being employed, ductal carcinoma |
| Chang & Kim 2010 | CoS | Stage not described/Free flap, Latissimus dorsi flap/ n = 482 | 17 months | missing | Lymphedema 8% pre-existing; 4% ↑ after reconstruction; LE ↓: delayed autologous reconstruction |
| Johnsson et al. 2010 | CoS | Early stage BC/ALND/SNB/ RT breast/chest wall/ regional LN/CT/n = 100 | 10 months | Return to work 25%/5 hours; Li-Sat11; GCQ | Return to work: *6 months:* 66%; *10 months:* 83%. *Return to work ↓:*At 6 months: CT, >30 days of sick leave during the previous 12 months, ↓ satisfaction with current capacity in ADL; at 10 months: RT breast/chest wall/regional LN, ↓ satisfaction with work |
| Kwan et al. 2010 | CoS | Stages I-IV/ALND/SNB/RT/ CT/n = 997 | 21 (1-32) months | CTCAE v.3.0; ICD; lymphedema treatment; compression device | Lymphedema: *12 months:* 10%; *24 months:* 14%. Model 1: ICIDH: African American, ↑ education, each LN removed 4.1% ↑; Model 2: LE treatment: CT; Model 3: Durable medical equipment associated with BC related LE: being obese |
| Norman et al. 2010 | CoS | Stage I-IV/ALND/SNB/RT/ CT/n = 4551 | (86%); 12-60 months | Face to face interview followed by telephone interview | Lymphedema 14%. CT HR = 3.16; Multi-agent CT with anthracycline HR = 3.76 |

**Table 2.** Cont.

| Author/year of publication | Design | Disease stage/treatment/ number of pts included | Number of studies/Dates of inclusion/FU in months (% FU if mentioned) | Measurement instruments in outcome | Main findings |
|---|---|---|---|---|---|
| **Yang et al. 2010** | CoS | ALND/SNB/Mastectomy/ Lumpectomy/Adjuvant treatment/n = 183 | 12 months | MPS, Hawkins' test, supraspinatus test, and Neer's test, PMPS, AWS, tape measurement | **ALND vs. SNB vs. lumpectomy:** Lymphedema 18%; upper arm activities ↓. *At 3 months:*39% vs. 18% vs. 12%; *at 6 months:*40% vs. 12% vs. not described %; *at 12 months:* 44% vs. 19% vs. 18%. Rotator cuff disease 12 months associated with pectoralis tightness and LE at 3 months |
| **Sagen et al. 2009** | CoS | Stage I–III/ALND level I–II/n = 204 | 60 months | VAS, water displacement, EORTC-QLQ-C30, self-generated questionnaire | *At 6 months:*Pain during activities vs. at rest 56% vs. 60% ; lymphedema 7%; upper arm activities: function scores ↓ (from 30 points to 29 points). *At 60 months:*Pain during activities vs. at rest 36% vs. 30% ; lymphedema 13%; physical activity at leisure time at baseline and 6 months predictive for physical functioning at 5 years |
| **Paskett et al. 2007** | CoS | Stage I–III Surgery/ reconstruction/RT/CT/ HT/n = 622 | (93%); 36 months | BMI, self-generated questionnaire, SF12, FACT-B | LE 54%; predictive: tamoxifen |
| **Lundstedt et al. 2012** | CSS | Stage not described/ALND vs. SNB/RT vs. RT SC/n = 814 | 36–96 months | CTCAE | **ALND + RT vs. ALND vs. SNB/no RT:** LE 22% vs. 15 vs. 5%. LE ↑ : RT SC |
| **Sheridan et al. 2012** | CSS | Stage not described/ Surgery/RT/CT/HT/n = 111 | 64 months | S-LANSS, CPAQ, HADS | Pain VAS 32±26. *Pre-operative:* 18%; Risk of chronic pain ↑ OR = 5. *Post-operative:* 36%; 23% intermittent pain; 32% exacerbation by exercise; ↑ chronic pain related to anxiousness, CT |
| **Dahl et al. 2011** | CSS | Stage II–III/Surgery/RT/ n = 337 | 30 months | Self-generated questionnaire, EORTC-QLQ-C30-BR23, FQ, HADS, SF-36 | Pain arm/shoulder 37%; sleep disturbance 30%; ↑ disability pension, depression, anxiety. Sleep disturbance ↑ : arm/ shoulder pain OR = 2.46; LE OR = 2.34; ↓ ROM OR = 2.63 |
| **Nesvold et al. 2011** | CSS | Stage II–III/Surgery/RT/ n = 349 | (56%); 83–113 months | ROM flexion/abduction, tape measurement, KAPS, EORTC-QLQ-BR23, IOC, SF36 | ROM ↓ 33%; pain sign. related to arm-shoulder problems; lymphedema 17%; upper arm activities ↓ 31% |
| **Shamley et al. 2009** | CSS | Stage not described/ALND vs. SNB/Mastectomy vs. lumpectomy/RT/CT/n = 152 | 6–72 months | Polhemus Fastrak™, SPADI | Pain: *0–24 months* 26%; *24–48 months* 43%; *48–72 months* 32%. Upper arm activities: *0–24 months* 26%; *24–48 months* 43%; *48–72 months* 32%. **Affected side vs. unaffected side:** All scapulothoracic movements sign. altered: Right scapulothoracic lateral rotation differences associated with downward movement; left scapulothoracic dysfunction ( ↑ protraction, ↑ posterior tilt, ↓ lateral rotation): CT. Pain and disability associated with scapulothoracic dysfunction; scapulothoracic movements: ↑ difference when left side affected |
| **Park et al. 2008** | CSS | Stage I–III/Mastectomy/RT/CT/ n = 450 | 12–24 months | Tape measurement | Lymphedema 25%; disease stage (OR = 2.58 for stage II; OR = 2.84 for stage III); modified radical mastectomy OR = 7.48; ALND OR = 6.61; axillary RT OR = 6.73; CT; overweight OR = 2.01; non exercise vs. exercise OR = 1.24; not receiving pre-treatment education OR = 2.26; ↓ preventive self-care activities |

**Table 2.** Cont.

| Author/year of publication | Design | Disease stage/treatment/ number of pts included | Number of studies/Dates of inclusion/FU in months (% FU if mentioned) | Measurement instruments in outcome | Main findings |
|---|---|---|---|---|---|
| Ververs et al. 2001 | CSS | Stage not described/ALND/ n = 400 | 3–60 months | Tape measurement, self-generated questionnaire | Muscle strength ↓ in 28%. Pain: comorbidity OR = 3.38. Lymphedema: Objective >2 cm 71%; severe LE 9%; RT SC/axilla OR = 3.57; comorbidity OR = 3.08. Shoulder, neck or back complaints: comorbidity OR = 2.72. Activities: 25–35% daily activities ↓, lifting objects ↓; 14% problems with transportation; 37% gave up hobbies or sports |
| Avraham et al. 2010 | CCS | SNB +/− ALND/Mastectomy/ Tissue expander/n = 316 | 60 months | LBCQ, tape measurement, BMI | **Reconstruction vs.. no reconstruction**: LE: 5% vs. 18% (severe <1% vs.. 4%); (overall 11% objective; 16% subjective). LE ↑: Chest wall RT |
| Mak et al. 2008 | CCS | ALND/n = 202/230 | 42±12/43±14 months | Tape measurement, validated questionnaire | LE ↑: infection: OR = 3.80; ↑ age at surgery OR = 1.06 for each year. Moderate-severe LE: ALND dominant side, medical procedures on hand/arm, ↓ air travel, institution of surgery |

Study design: CCT, clinical controlled trial; Cos, cohort study; CSS, cross sectional study; pts, patients; RCT, randomized controlled trial; SR, systematic review.
Intervention: ALND, axillary lymph node dissection; art, article; CE, cyclophosphamide, epirubicin; CEF, cyclophosphamide, epirubicin and fluorouracil; CT, chemotherapy; FU, follow up; Gy, Grey; HT, hormonal therapy; IMB, internal mammarial boost; IM-MS, internal mammary and medial supraclavicular lymph node chain; IORT, intra operative radiotherapy; LRRT, locoregional radiotherapy corresponding to periclavicular, axillary level 3, and for right-side breast cancers, the internal mammary nodes; LN, lymph node; M, metastasis; N, nodal status; PAB, posterior axillary boost; RT, radiotherapy; SC, supra scapular; SNB, sentinel node biopsy; T, docetaxel; T, tumor; TAM, tamoxifen; vs., versus; wks, weeks; ZOL, Zoledronic Acid.
Measurement instruments: BIS, bio impedance spectroscopy; BMI, body mass index; BSI, Brief Symptom Inventory; CPAQ, Chronic Pain Acceptance Questionnaire; CES-D, center for epidemiologic studies – depression scale; CTCAE, Common Terminology Criteria for Adverse Events ; DASH, disabilities of arm, shoulder and hand; EORTC-QLQ-C30-BR23, European organization for research and treatment of cancer – quality of life questionnaire- breast; FACT-G-B, functional assessment of cancer therapy – general – breast; FLIC, Functional living index – cancer; FQ, fatigue questionnaire; FPACQ, Flemish Physical Activity Computerized Questionnaire; GCQ, general coping questionnaire; HADS, hospital anxiety and depression scale; ICD, international classification of diseases; IOC, impact of cancer scale; KAPS, Kwan's arm problem scale; LANSS, Leeds Assessment of Neuropathic Symptoms and Signs; LBCQ, lymphedema breast cancer questionnaire; LEFT-BC, Lymphedema Evaluation Following Treatment for Breast Cancer; LENT-SOMA, late effects normal tissue – subjective objective management analytic; Li-Sat, life satisfaction; MASS, measure of arm symptoms survey; MET, metabolic equivalent ; MOS, medical outcomes study; MPQ, McGill pain questionnaire; MRC-scale, medical research council scale; MSPQ, Modified Somatic Perception Questionnaire; NPRS, numeric pain rating scale; PAISSR, Psychological Adjustment to Illness Scale-Self-Report; PAQ, physical activity questionnaire; PSI-B, Problem solving inventory-brief; ROM, range of motion; SF-36, short form-36; SPADI, shoulder pain and disability index; ULDQ, upper limb disability questionnaire; v, version; VAS, visual analogue scale; WHR, Waist-Hip ratio.
Outcomes: ADL, activities in daily living; AWS, axillary web syndrome; CHF, cardiac heart failure; CTS, carpal tunnel syndrome; HR, Hazard Ratio; LE, lymphedema; LVEF, left ventricular ejection fraction; ns, non-significant; OR, odds ratio; MPS, myofascial pain syndrome; MSD, musculoskeletal disorders; PA, physical activity; PMPS, Post Mastectomy Pain Syndrome; RR, relative risk; sign, significant; *, data extracted from included studies.

the adverse effects, the study was excluded from the analysis of outcome measures. Third, we assigned a level of evidence for each of the adverse effects related to the common harms of the medical intervention. [9] We anticipated on using a quantitative assessment in a meta-analysis, but due to the heterogeneity of outcome measures, adverse effects, and (combinations of) medical treatment we were unable to pool data from separate studies.

## Results

We identified 804 unique articles, of which 116 were eligible for full-text assessment (see figure 1 for a flow diagram). Of these, 54 studies were excluded because they did not meet the inclusion criteria. Another 23 studies were excluded because they had already been included in one or more systematic reviews(15) or had a quality rating ≤50% (8). Finally, 39 articles were included. In the syntheses 13 articles could not be included because adverse effects were not analyzed separately for each treatment modality.

**Table 3.** Oxford Centre for Evidence-Based Medicine, 2011 Levels of Evidence for common harms (Treatment harms).

| Level 1 | Systematic review of randomized trials, systematic review of nested case-control studies, n-of-1 trial with the patient you are raising the question about, or observational study with dramatic effect |
|---|---|
| Level 2 | Individual randomized trial or (exceptionally) observational study with dramatic effect |
| Level 3 | Non randomized controlled cohort/follow-up study provided there are sufficient numbers to rule out a common harm |
| Level 4 | Case-series, case-control studies or historically controlled studies |
| Level 5 | Mechanism-based reasoning |

**Table 4.** Quality test of methodology of the included systematic reviews based on the critical appraisal sheets of the Centre of Evidence Based Medicine.

| First author/year of publication | Search strategy | Inclusion criteria selection | Quality of the studies | Results homogeneous | Presentation of results | Rating |
|---|---|---|---|---|---|---|
| Hickey et al. 2013[37] | + | + | + | + | + | 100% |
| Moja et al. 2012[14] | + | + | + | +/− | + | 90% |
| Zhou et al. 2011[11] | +/− | + | +/− | + | + | 80% |
| Liu et al. 2009[12] | +/− | + | + | +/− | − | 60% |
| Tsai et al. 2009[1] | +/− | + | +/− | + | + | 80% |
| Lee et al. 2008[15] | + | + | + | +/− | + | 90% |
| Levangie et al. 2008[13] | +/− | + | + | + | − | 70% |

## Methodological quality of the included studies

The methodological quality of the included studies ranged from 60% to 90% for the systematic reviews (see table 4), and from 58% to 100% for prognostic studies and RCTs (see table 5). In four systematic reviews, the search strategy was limited to one database only. [1,11–13] Results in four systematic reviews were not pooled due to the heterogeneity of the data. [11,12,14,15] The majority of the cohort studies presented validated outcome measures, while seven of the 32 studies described outcome by a self-generated and self-validated questionnaire [3,16,17] or performed incomplete measurements. [18–21] In six studies, a description of the outcome was incomplete. [22–27].

## Adverse effects

Table 2 presents a detailed overview of the results of the included studies. Six systematic reviews and 29 cohort studies presented analyses regarding the origin of the adverse effects. Some studies analyzed the relationship of the adverse effects in relation to comorbidity, age or BMI.

In most studies, different subgroups were identified based on surgical treatment. Four studies [17,28–30] focused only on patients that underwent ALND. One systematic review [1] and one cross-sectional study [27] focused on the adverse effects of radiotherapy. The adverse effects of aromatase inhibitors focused on musculoskeletal pain. [11,22,31] Zhou et al. described aromatase inhibitors in combination with zoledronic acids and pain. [11].

Synthesis per outcome measure is summarized and presented in table 6, including levels of evidence.

**Reduction in range of motion (ROM).** Reduced ROM was described in four systematic reviews [1,12,13,15] and six cohort studies. [19,28,32–35] General reduction in ROM was described [12,15,19,28,35] or specified for the shoulder in different directions: abduction, or flexion/abduction and external rotation. [32,33].

Regarding ALND as a medical intervention, one systematic review reported a reduction in ROM in abduction and flexion ranging from 132–175°, which was reported in 1–67% of the patients. [15] Regarding SNB, a second systematic review described a reduction in ROM. [12] Percentages of patients with ROM reduction varied from 6%–31% after 12 months, and reduced to 0%–9% after 24 months. Regarding ALND (directly or after SNB) vs. SNB, change of ROM in the third systematic review was reported in 9%–56% vs. 3%–24% of the patients, or in a mean difference of 1°–20° within 12 months and 8%–20% vs. 0%–4% over 12 months. [13] Odds Ratios (ORs) in the included

studies of this systematic review ranged from 1.02–9.0 for goniometric measurements. [13] One cohort study described a reduced ROM of 21% vs. 56% at 6 months and 6% vs. 9% at 12 months, with an OR of 1.56 at 12 months. [32] Another cohort study reported reduced ROM at six months and > 12 months in a study population in which 71% underwent ALND. Reduction was present in 60% and 11% in flexion/abduction and 25% and 5% in external rotation [33]. ROM reduction was related to ALND, a greater number of lymph nodes removed, cording, seroma, mastectomy, stage II, hand dominance, BMI ≥ 25 and older age (>65 years).

Regarding mastectomy vs. lumpectomy, one systematic review presented an OR of 5.67 for mastectomy as a risk factor for reduced ROM. [15] In one cohort study, ROM reduction was present in 33% of the study population [34]. Mastectomy was indicated as risk factor. Regarding ALND and mastectomy vs. ALND, lumpectomy and radiotherapy reduced ROM was described at one, 12 and 24 months in overall percentages and percentages with severe reduction. Percentages reduced from 68% vs. 73% to 23% vs. 30%. [28]

Regarding radiotherapy vs. no radiotherapy, one systematic review presented ORs of 2.07–12.30, a relative risk (RR) of 4.6 and reduced ROM in 34%–52% vs. 4%–20% of the study population in the included studies. [13] One large cohort study presented an OR of 2.48 for radiotherapy as a risk factor for ROM reduction. [32] Regarding axillary radiotherapy vs. no axillary radiotherapy, the risk of decreased ROM was analyzed in two systematic reviews (RR 2.6; OR 1.67). [1,15] A third systematic review reported changes in joint mobility in 14% vs. 2% of the patients in one included study; ORs in other included studies ranged from 1.70–6.83 for goniometric measurements. Regarding radiotherapy to the axilla and chest vs. radiotherapy to the chest, the same systematic review presented an RR of 1.7 in one included study and reduced ROM in 20%–49% vs. 4%–14% of the study population in other included studies. [13] Regarding chemotherapy vs. no chemotherapy, one large cohort study reported an OR of 0.73 of chemotherapy as a risk factor for ROM reduction. [32].

In synthesizing the results from the included studies, we found level 1 evidence for mastectomy and radiotherapy to the axilla as risk factors for reduced ROM in abduction, flexion and external rotation, and level 2 evidence for ALND and radiotherapy to the chest wall.

**Reduction in muscle strength.** Reduced muscle strength was reported in four systematic reviews [12,13,15,36] and five cohort studies. [17,18,20,33,37].

**Table 5.** Quality test of methodology of the included studies based on the critical appraisal sheets of the Centre of Evidence Based Medicine.

| First author/ year of publication | Study design | Inclusion in common point in the course of disease | Follow up sufficiently long and complete; Number of patients included-analyzed | Outcome criteria objective or based on "subjective judgement" | Subgroups with different prognosis, adjustment for prognostic factors | Results over time | CI stated and narrow | Rating |
|---|---|---|---|---|---|---|---|---|
| Ashikaga et al. 2010[35] | RCT | + | + | + | + | + | + | 100% |
| Andersen et al. 2012[39] | CCT | - | + | + | + | - | + | 67% |
| Miller et al. 2012[44] | CCT | + | - | + | + | - | + | 67% |
| Ozcinar et al. 2012[18] | CCT | + | + | +/- | + | - | - | 58% |
| Taira et al. 2011[28] | CCT | + | + | + | - | +/- | - | 58% |
| Wernicke et al. 2011[19] | CCT | + | + | +/- | + | - | + | 75% |
| Land et al. 2010[3] | CCT | + | + | +/- | + | + | + | 92% |
| Yen et al. 2009[22] | CCT | + | + | - | + | + | + | 83% |
| Bevilacqua et al. 2012[33] | CoS | + | + | + | - | + | + | 83% |
| Levy et al. 2012[29] | CoS | + | + | + | + | + | +/- | 92% |
| Mieog at al. 2012[24] | CoS | + | + | - | + | +/- | + | 75% |
| Schmitz et al. 2012[4] | CoS | + | + | + | + | + | - | 83% |
| Kanematsu et al. 2011[23] | CoS | + | - | - | +/- | + | + | 58% |
| Ridner et al. 2011[45] | CoS | + | + | + | + | + | + | 100% |
| Rief et al. 2011[30] | CoS | + | + | + | +/- | +/- | - | 67% |
| Devoogdt et al. 2010[31] | CoS | + | + | + | + | + | +/- | 92% |
| Chang & Kim 2010[25] | CoS | + | + | + | + | + | - | 83% |
| Johnsson et al. 2010[42] | CoS | + | - | + | + | +/- | + | 75% |
| Kwan et al. 2010[21] | CoS | +/- | - | +/- | + | +/- | + | 58% |
| Norman et al. 2010[26] | CoS | + | + | +/- | + | +/- | + | 83% |
| Yang et al. 2010[46] | CoS | + | + | + | + | + | + | 100% |

**Table 5.** Cont.

| First author/year of publication | Study design | Inclusion in common point in the course of disease | Follow up sufficiently long and complete; Number of patients included-analyzed | Outcome criteria objective or based on "subjective judgement" | Subgroups with different prognosis, adjustment for prognostic factors | Results over time | CI stated and narrow | Rating |
|---|---|---|---|---|---|---|---|---|
| Sagen et al. 2009[40] | CoS | + | − | + | + | + | + | 83% |
| Paskett et al. 2007[16] | CoS | + | + | − | + | + | + | 83% |
| Lundstedt et al. 2012[27] | CSS | − | + | − | + | +/− | + | 58% |
| Sheridan et al. 2012[41] | CSS | − | − | + | + | +/− | + | 58% |
| Dahl et al. 2011[36] | CSS | + | + | + | + | − | + | 83% |
| Nesvold et al. 2011[32] | CSS | − | + | + | + | +/− | − | 58% |
| Shamley et al. 2009[38] | CSS | − | − | + | + | + | + | 67% |
| Park et al. 2008[20] | CSS | + | + | +/− | + | +/− | − | 67% |
| Ververs 2001[17] | CSS | − | − | +/− | + | + | + | 58% |
| Avraham 2010[43] | CCS | − | + | + | + | − | + | 67% |
| Mak et al. 2008[34] | CCS | − | + | + | + | − | + | 67% |

CCS-Case-Control Study; CCT, Clinical Controlled Trial ; CI, confidential interval; CoS, cohort study; CSS, Cross Sectional Study; RCT, Randomized Controlled Trial.

Regarding ALND, one systematic review described reduced muscle strength (OR 3.03) [15]. One cohort study described reduced muscle strength in 28% of the study population [20]. Regarding SNB, a second systematic review reported reduced muscle strength in 17%–19% of the patients after sentinel node biopsy and 11% in the long-term. [12] This systematic review identified patients with young age (<50 years) as a risk factor for muscle strength impairment based on results of one large study comparing ALND vs. SNB. Regarding ALND (directly or after SNB) vs. SNB, a third systematic review reported weakness in 48% vs. 16% of the patients, with loss of abduction strength of 12–15 Nm, loss of grip strength of 12–41 Nm in the included studies and ORs ranging from 5.14–8.82 reported in the included studies. [13].

Regarding lumpectomy and ALND, one systematic review reported reduced muscle strength in9%–28% of the study population. [15] Regarding ALND and mastectomy vs. ALND, lumpectomy and RT reduced muscle strength was described at one, 12 and 24 months. [28] Percentages reduced from 67% vs. 72% to 39% vs. 56% reduced muscle strength. Reductions were larger in the first 12 months compared to later measurements (see table 6).

Regarding chest radiotherapy vs. no radiotherapy, the risk of reduced muscle strength was analyzed in one systematic review. [13] Extracted data from the included studies showed ORs from 1.70–6.83 for radiotherapy as a risk factor for reduced muscle strength and one included study reported reduced muscle strength in 14% vs. 2% of the patients. Regarding axillary radiotherapy vs. radiotherapy to the chest wall, the risk of reduced muscle strength was analyzed in the same systematic review. [13] One included study reported an RR of 1.7; another study showed 59% vs. 40% of the patients with reduced muscle strength. Regarding concurrent radiotherapy and chemotherapy vs. sequential radiotherapy and chemotherapy, a fourth systematic review described the risk of reduced muscle strength by concurrent treatment with an OR of 2.09. [36].

In synthesizing the results of the included studies, we found level 1 evidence for ALND, and concurrent radiotherapy and chemotherapy as risk factors for reduced muscle strength. We found level 2 evidence for SNB, radiotherapy to the chest wall and radiotherapy to the axilla and chest as risk factors for reduced muscle strength.

**Pain.** Pain was described in four systematic reviews [11,12,15,36] and 10 cohort studies. [17,22,28,31,33,35,37–40].

Regarding ALND, one systematic review [15] and one cohort study [38] described pain 12 months post-operative. This systematic review described an OR of 4.61 and percentages of shoulder pain (9%–68%) and breast pain (15%–72%) in the individual studies. [35] The cohort study described pain in 53% of the population. [38] Regarding SNB, a second systematic review reported pain in 8%–36% of the patients within 12 months and 8%–21% at 24 months, analyzing young age (<50 years) as a predictive factor, described in one included study. [12] Regarding ALND (directly or after SNB) vs. SNB, a third systematic review reported pain during motion in one included study in 12% vs. 4% at 12 months and 9% vs. 3% at 19 months and an OR of 3.54 mentioned in another study. [13].

Regarding ALND and mastectomy vs. ALND, lumpectomy and radiotherapy pain was described at 1 month post-operatively, and at 12 and at 24 months. [28] Pain reduced from 75% vs. 82% to 42% vs. 56%. Regarding chest radiotherapy vs. no radiotherapy, one individual study in a systematic review reported at least weekly pain in 26% vs. 4% of patients (OR = 7.10), 6 to 13 years post-operatively. [13] Regarding concurrent radiotherapy and chemo-

```
┌─────────────────────────────┐        ┌─────────────────────────────┐
│ Records identified through   │        │ Records identified through   │
│ PubMed                       │        │ Embase, CINAHL and Cochrane  │
│ (n =773)                     │        │ (n = 170)                    │
└─────────────────────────────┘        └─────────────────────────────┘
               │                                      │
               └──────────────┬───────────────────────┘
                              ▼
                ┌─────────────────────────────┐
                │ Records after duplicates     │
                │ removed                      │
                │ (n = 804)                    │
                └─────────────────────────────┘
                              │
                              │                ┌─────────────────────────────┐
                              ├───────────────▶│ Records excluded based on    │
                              │                │ title                        │
                              ▼                │ (n = 240)                    │
                ┌─────────────────────────────┐└─────────────────────────────┘
                │ Abstracts screened           │
                │ (n = 564)                    │
                └─────────────────────────────┘
                              │
                              ▼
                ┌─────────────────────────────┐┌─────────────────────────────┐
                │ Full-text articles assessed  ││ Full-text articles excluded  │
                │ for eligibility              ││ < 100 pts  n = 18            │
                │ (n = 116)                    ││ Retrospective n = 7          │
                └─────────────────────────────┘│ No match of outcome n = 5    │
                              │                 │ PT Intervention study n = 2  │
                              ├────────────────▶│ Treatment before 2000 n = 18 │
                              │                 │ FU < 3 mo n = 1              │
                              ▼                 │ (n = 54)                     │
                ┌─────────────────────────────┐└─────────────────────────────┘
                │ Studies included in          │
                │ qualitative methodological   │┌─────────────────────────────┐
                │ assessment                   ││ Quality score ≤ 50%          │
                │ (n = 62)                     ││ (n = 23)                     │
                └─────────────────────────────┘└─────────────────────────────┘
                              │                             ▲
                              ├─────────────────────────────┘
                              ▼
                ┌─────────────────────────────┐
                │ Studies included in          │
                │ qualitative and              │
                │ quantitative analysis        │
                │ (n = 39)                     │
                └─────────────────────────────┘
```

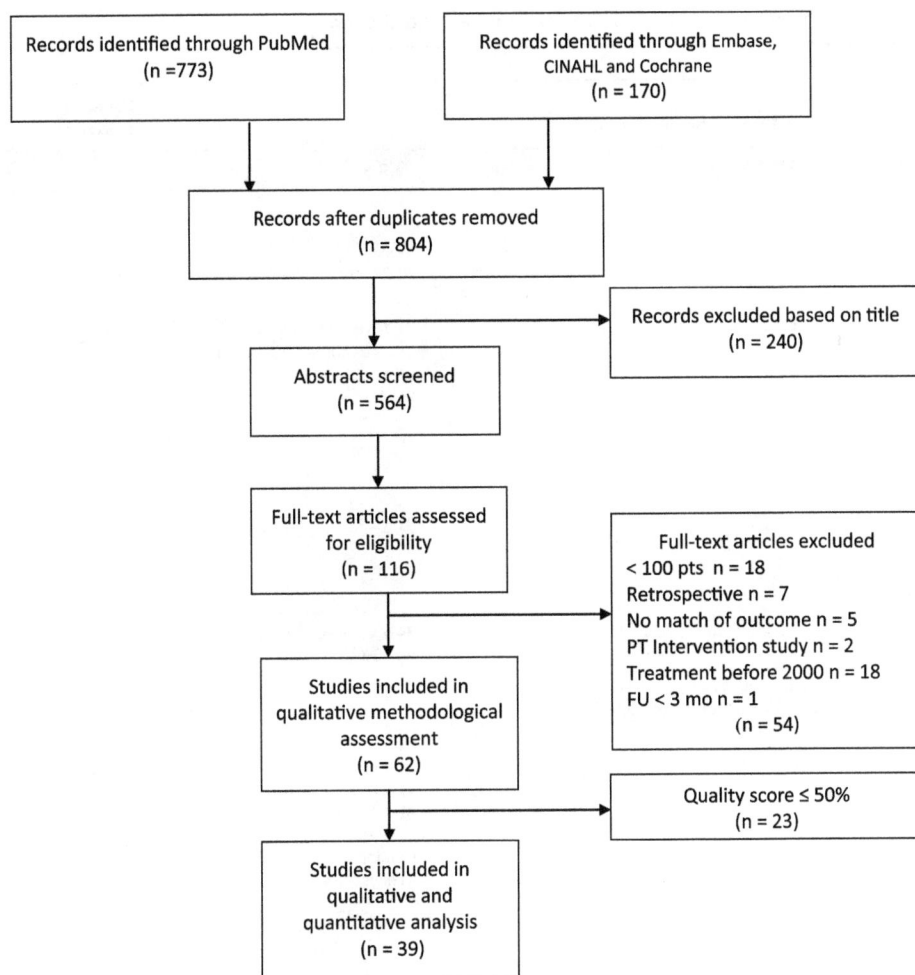

**Figure 1. Flow diagram literature search adverse effects of breast cancer treatment.**

therapy vs. sequential radiotherapy and chemotherapy a fourth systematic review reported the risk of brachial neuropathy (OR 3.14). [36] Regarding chemotherapy vs. no chemotherapy, two cohort studies found chemotherapy to be a risk factor for pain, [38] with a reported OR of 3.00. [40].

Regarding the administration of zoledronic acids vs. no zoledronic acids, one systematic review reported the relative risk (RR) of arthralgia (RR 1.16) and bone pain (RR 1.26). [11] Regarding the upfront administration of zoledronic acids compared to delayed administration, the same systematic review described an increased risk of pain (RR 1.28). Regarding exemestane vs. tamoxifen, one cohort study described an increased risk of carpal tunnel syndrome (OR 9.90). [24] In this study, 43% of the patients had a musculoskeletal disorder and 2% carpal tunnel syndrome. Another cohort study described increased pain incidence by using tamoxifen at baseline and at younger age (< 55 years). [22].

In general, pre-operative pain was a risk factor for post-operative pain (OR 5.17) and prolonged pain. [24,40] Pain was correlated with decreased muscle strength and range of motion, decreased job participation, reduced use of the affected arm in leisure activities and with lifting a gallon of milk or during heavy household chores. [33] At 6 months, pain during daily activities was less than at rest. [31,41] In contrast, one study reported an exacerbation of pain by exercise. [40] Another study reported less

pain during activities compared to rest at six months post-operative and more pain at 60 months. [39] Arm-shoulder pain led to sleep disturbances (OR 3.17). [35].

In conclusion, we found level 1 evidence for ALND, radiotherapy before chemotherapy, and the administration of zoledronic acids (more in case of delayed administration) as risk factors for pain. We found level 2 evidence for SNB and radiotherapy as risk factors for pain.

**Lymphedema.** Lymphedema was described in three systematic reviews [1,12,15] and 20 cohort studies. [4,16–21,23,26–30,32,34,39,42–45] Eight studies reported subjective data based on a lymphedema questionnaire, [16,23,26,28] CTCAE, [21,27] telephone interview, [23,26] or measured only 2 or 3 points of the arm. [18,19].

Regarding ALND, two systematic reviews and five cohort studies described an increased risk of lymphedema. One systematic review described an RR of 3.47. [1] A second systematic review described percentages of pain in the included studies ranging from 0%–34%. [15] Percentages in the cohort studies varied from 13%–30%. [20,29,39] BMI ≥30 as a risk factor for lymphedema was described in one cohort study with an OR of 4.12 [44] and in another cohort study as an increase of 4.1% or HR of 2.61 for each lymph node removed. [26] Regarding SNB, a third systematic review described percentages ranging from 3%–14% in the first 12 months to 7% in the follow-up of 60 months. [12]

**Table 6.** Adverse treatment effects in relation to impairments in upper extremities and thorax.

| Medical intervention | ≤12 months post-surgery %/p value/OR | >12 months post-surgery OR/RR/HR | %/p-value | Level of evidence |
|---|---|---|---|---|
| **Reduction in ROM** | | | | |
| ALND | 1%–67%[15] | | p = 0.0001[19] | level 2 |
| SNB | At 12 months: 6%–31%%[12] | | At 24 months:0%–9%[12] | level 3 |
| SNB + ALND vs. SNB | At 12 months: 24% vs. 24%/9% vs. 3%[13*]; at 6 months: 56% vs. 21%; at 12 months: 9% vs. 6%. OR = 1.56[32] | OR = 1.02/2.65/9.0[13*] | At 18 months: 8% vs. 4%; at >20 months: 20% vs. 0%; at median 30 months 11% vs. 4%[13*] | level 2 |
| Mastectomy vs. lumpectomy | | OR = 5.67 (CI = 1.03–31.16)[15] | | level 1 |
| ALND level I–III + mastectomy vs. ALND level I–III + lumpectomy + RT | At 1 month:68% vs. 73%; at 12 months:32% vs. 40%[28] | | At 24 months:23% vs. 30%[28] | level 3 |
| RT chest wall vs. no RT | | OR = 2.07/6.60/12.30[13*]; RR = 4.6[13]; OR = 2.48[32] | 34% vs. 20%/38% vs. 4%/52% vs. 15%[13*] | level 2 |
| RT axilla vs. no RT | | RR = 2.6 (CI = 1.42–4.03)[1]; OR = 1.67 (CI = 0.98–2.86)[15]; OR = 2.48[35] | | level 1 |
| RT axilla + chest wall vs. RT chest wall | | OR = 2.64/3.37[13*] | 20% vs. 4%/Flexion 39% vs. 4%; 24% vs. 5%/ Abduction 49% vs. 8%; 35% vs. 7%/External rotation 45% vs. 14%; 41% vs. 13%[13*] | level 2 |
| CT vs. no CT | | OR = 0.73, p = 0.003[32] | | level 3 |
| **Reduction in muscle strength** | | | | |
| ALND | | OR = 3.03 (CI = 1.25–7.32)[15] | 28%[20] | level 1 |
| SNB | 17–19%[12] | | At 24 months: 11%[12] | level 2 |
| SNB + ALND vs. SNB | 36% vs. 8%[13] | OR = 8.82[13] | 48% vs. 16% [13] | level 2 |
| ALND + Lumpectomy | 9%–28%[15] | | OR = 4.61 | level 1 |
| ALND level I–III + mastectomy vs. ALND level I–III + lumpectomy + RT | At 1 month:67% vs. 72%; at 12 months:48% vs. 51%[28] | | At 24 months: 39% vs. 56%[28] | level 3 |
| RT chest wall vs. no RT | | OR = 1.70/3.37/6.83[13*] | 14% vs. 2%[13] | level 2 |
| RT axilla + chest vs. RT chest | | RR = 1.7[13] | 59% vs. 40%[13] | level 2 |
| Concurrent RT + CT vs. sequential | | OR = 2.09 (CI = 0.92–4.75)[36] | | level 1 |
| **Pain** | | | | |
| ALND | | OR = 4.61 (CI = 2.01–10.59)[15] | Shoulder pain 9%–68%[15]; Breast pain 15%–72%[14]; 53%[37] | level 1 |
| SNB | 8–36%[12] | | At 24 months:8–21%; at 60 months: SNB 9%[12] | level 2 |
| SNB + ALND vs. SNB | At 12 months: 12% vs. 4%[13] | OR = 3.54 (1.88–6.66)[13] | At 18 months: 9% vs. 3%[13] | level 2 |
| ALND level I–III + mastectomy vs. ALND level I–III + lumpectomy + RT | At 1 month: 75% vs. 82%; at 12 months: 60% vs. 63%[28] | | At 24 months: 42% vs. 56%[28] | level 3 |
| RT vs. no RT | | OR = 7.10[13] | At 6–13 years: weekly pain 26% vs. 4%[13] | level 2 |

**Table 6.** Cont.

| Medical intervention | ≤12 months post-surgery %/p value/OR | >12 months post-surgery OR/RR/HR | %/p-value | Level of evidence |
|---|---|---|---|---|
| RT before CT vs. RT after CT | | Brachial neuropathy: OR = 3.14 (CI = 0.12–79.39)[36] | | level 1 |
| CT vs. no CT | | OR = 3.00 (CI = 1.22–7.40)[40] | | level 3 |
| ZOL vs. no ZOL | | Arthralgia: RR = 1.16 (CI = 1.096–1.232); Bone pain: RR = 1.26 (CI = 1.149–1.376)[11] | | level 1 |
| Delayed ZOL vs. upfront ZOL | | Bone pain: RR = 1.28 (CI = 1.135–1.453)[11] | | level 1 |
| Exemestane vs. Tamoxifen | | OR = 9.90 (CI = 3.52–27.82) for CTS[24] | | level 3 |
| Aromatase inhibitors; CT (with/without taxanes) | | | Age <55 vs. 55–65 vs. >65 yrs: Arthralgia 46% vs. 37% vs. 28%[23]; CTS 2%, MSD 43%[24] | level 3 |
| Lymphedema | | | | |
| ALND | | RR = 3.47[1]; BMI >30: OR = 4.12 (CI = 1.58–10.72)[43] | 0%–34%[15]/25%[20]/each LN removed 4.1% ↑[26]/ HR = 2.61(CI = 1.77–3.84)[26]. At 60 months: 30%[33]/13%[39] | level 1 |
| SNB | At 6 month: 3–10%; at 12 months: 6–14%[12] | | 7%[12] | level 2 |
| SNB + ALND vs. SNB | 13% vs. 9%[35]/3% vs. 0%[44] | RR = 3.07 (no ALND 3.47)[1]/OR = 11.67 (CI = 1.45–93.65)[15]/OR = 6.61 (CI = 1.64–26.57)[18] | 35% vs. 5%[19]/14% vs. 8%[32] | level 1 |
| Mastectomy | | Radical mastectomy vs. other mastectomy RR = 3.28[1]; Modified radical mastectomy OR = 7.48 (CI = 2.38–23.85)[20] | | level 1; level 3 |
| ALND level I–III + mastectomy vs. ALND level I–III + lumpectomy + RT | At 1 month:27% vs. 41%; at 12 months:26% vs. 48%[28] | | At 24 months: 33% vs. 52%[28] | level 3 |
| Reconstruction vs. no reconstruction | | | 5% vs. 18%[42] | level 4 |
| RT axilla vs. RT not axilla | | RR = 2.97[1]/OR = 2.4[12]/OR = 3.57[17] | | level 1 |
| Concurrent vs. sequential RT after CT | | OR = 2.02 (CI = 0.18–22.61)[36] | | level 1 |
| RT before CT vs. RT after CT | | OR = 2.11 (CI = 0.67–7.21)[35] | | level 1 |
| CT vs. no CT | | HR = 1.46 (CI = 1.04–2.04)[26] | | level 3 |
| Reduction in level of activities in daily living | | | | |
| ALND vs. SNB | ↓ arm use: p<0.001[3] | OR = 3.18/9.23[13*] | | level 2 |
| ALND + mastectomy vs. ALND + lumpectomy | shoulder/arm function, social and work activities: p = 0.001[3] | | | level 3 |
| SNB + ALND vs. SNB vs. lumpectomy | At 3 months:39% vs. 18% vs. 12%; at 6 months:40% vs. 12% vs. not described; at 12 months: 44% vs. 19% vs. 18%[46] | | Pain during activities vs. at rest 36% vs. 30%[40]/Daily activities ↓, lifting objects ↓ 25–35%; problems with transportation 14%; gave up hobbies or sports 37%[17] | level 2 |

**Table 6.** Cont.

| Medical intervention | ≤12 months post-surgery %/p value/OR | >12 months post-surgery OR/RR/HR | %/p-value | Level of evidence |
|---|---|---|---|---|
| ALND level I–III + mastectomy vs. ALND level I–III + lumpectomy + RT | At 1 month:Lifting ↓ 83% vs. 88%; household chores 61% vs. 64%; self-care ↓ 56% vs. 63%; physical activities ↓ 73% vs. 76%. At 12 months:Lifting ↓ 34% vs. 39%; household chores ↓ 28 vs. 33%; self-care ↓ 16% vs. 12%; physical activities ↓ 41% vs. 39%[28] | | At 24 month: Lifting ↓ 20% vs. 39%; household chores ↓ 18% vs. 21%; self-care ↓ 10% vs. 14%; physical activities: 34% vs. 31%[28] | level 3 |
| RT chest wall vs. no RT | | OR = 1.32[13] | 29 vs. 4%[13] | level 2 |
| RT axilla + chest wall vs. RT chest wall | | OR = 2.64/4.67[13]* | | level 2 |
| CE+T or CEF | 34%[39] | | | level 3 |

Intervention: ALND, axillary lymph node dissection; CEF, cyclophosphamide, epirubicin and fluorouracil; CE+T, cyclophosphamide, epirubicin + docetaxel; CT, chemotherapy; HT, hormonal therapy; LN, lymph node; MRM, modified radical mastectomy; RM, radical mastectomy; RT, radiotherapy; SC, supraclavicular; SNB, sentinel node biopsy; vs., versus.
Outcomes: CTS, carpal tunnel syndrome; HR, hazard ratio; MSD, musculoskeletal disorder OR, odds ratio; RR, relative risk; ZOL, zoledronic acids; *, data extracted from included studies.

Regarding ALND (directly or after SNB) vs. SNB, two systematic reviews and three cohort studies described lymphedema. One systematic review reported an RR of 3.07 (when compared to no axillary dissection 3.47), [1] while another systematic review reported an OR of 11.67. [15] In the cohort studies, percentages of patients with lymphedema varied from 3%–13% vs. 0%–9% in the first 12 months to 14%–35% vs. 5%–8% in longer follow up. [19,32,43].

Regarding mastectomy, lymphedema was described in one systematic review and one cohort study. The systematic review reported an RR of 3.28, [1] while the cohort study reported an OR of 7.48. [20] Regarding ALND and mastectomy vs. ALND, lumpectomy and radiotherapy lymphedema was described at one month post-operatively, and at 12 and at 24 months. [28] Percentages of patients with lymphedema increased from 27%–41% at one month to 33%–52% at 24 months post-operatively.

Regarding breast reconstruction vs. no reconstruction, one cohort study described lymphedema in 5% vs. 18% of the study population. [42].

Regarding radiotherapy to the chest and axilla vs. radiotherapy to the chest, two systematic reviews and one cohort study described lymphedema. One systematic review described an RR of 2.97, [1] the second an OR of 2.4. [12] The cohort study reported an OR of 3.57. [17] Regarding concurrent radiotherapy and chemotherapy vs. sequential radiotherapy and chemotherapy, one systematic review reported an OR of 2.02. [36] Regarding radiotherapy before chemotherapy vs. radiotherapy after chemotherapy, the same systematic review reported an OR of 2.11.

Regarding chemotherapy vs. no chemotherapy, one cohort study reported a Hazard Ratio (HR) of 1.46. [26] The risk of lymphedema in relation to chemotherapy was investigated in this cohort study in patients with ALND, comparing multi-agent chemotherapy with chemotherapy with anthracyclines. Regarding chemotherapy with radiotherapy vs. chemotherapy without

radiotherapy, HRs in this study varied from 0.30–4.09 vs. 3.78–5.46.

The overall incidence of lymphedema increased over time, except in one study where lymphedema decreased because of decongestive lymphatic therapy. [18] One case control study described the risk of lymphedema due to infection in patients with ALND (OR 3.80). [30] BMI ≥30 as risk factor for lymphedema was described in one systematic review in patients with SNB as weak evidence, not providing data [12] and in two cohort studies (OR 3.59; adjusted for ALND OR = 4.1), [44] while an OR of 2.01 was found for BMI >25. [20] One study followed patients five years after ALND and provided nomograms that indicated a BMI >30 as a risk factor as well. [29] The influence of age on the development of lymphedema was described in one systematic review and four cohort studies, indicating young age (<50 years) [12,16,32] and age >65 years [30] as risk factors and increasing by age in another cohort study. [29].

One study reported that comorbidity led to a higher incidence of lymphedema. [17]

We found level 1 evidence for ALND, radical mastectomy, radiotherapy to the axilla, concurrent radiotherapy and chemotherapy, and radiotherapy before chemotherapy as risk factors for lymphedema.

**Reduction in activities in daily living.** Limitations in activities in daily living were described in two SRs [12,13] and eight cohort studies. [3,17,28,33,38,41,45,46].

Regarding ALND, one cohort study reported decreased degree of daily activities. [17] Regarding ALND vs. SNB one systematic review and one cohort study described an increased risk of problems in performing daily activities. [3,13] ORs were calculated in two included studies in the systematic review (resp. 3.18 and 9.23). [13] Reported ORs for performing different tasks in one of the included studies in the systematic review varied from 2.13–2.34 when stratified by age, with age between 65 and 74 years at most risk and between 40 and 54 years at least risk compared to a non-breast cancer population. Decline in one or more tasks was described in another included study (34% vs. 50%, OR 0.8). One cohort study described the avoidance of normal arm use in cases of ALND compared to SNB (p <0.001). [3] Regarding ALND (directly or after SNB) vs. SNB vs. lumpectomy, one cohort study described a decline of activities in the first year post-operatively in 39%–44% of the patients after ALND, 18%–19% in case of SNB and 12%–19% in case of lumpectomy. [45] Regarding ALND and mastectomy vs. ALND and lumpectomy, one cohort study reported more problems in arm and shoulder function, conducting social activities and work in the lumpectomy group (p<0.001). [3] Regarding ALND and mastectomy vs. ALND, lumpectomy and radiotherapy, daily activities were described at 1 month post-operatively, at 12 and at 24 months in overall percentages and percentages with severe decline in daily activities. [28] Percentages reduced over time, with more problems in the lumpectomy group. Regarding chest wall radiotherapy vs. no radiotherapy, one systematic review reported a decline in daily activities with ORs in three individual studies (resp. 1.32, 8.0 and 10.67) and percentages of 29% vs. 4% in another included study. [13] Regarding radiotherapy to the axilla and chest wall vs. radiotherapy to the chest alone, the same systematic review reported an OR of 2.64 in one included study. Regarding chemotherapy with cyclophosphamide, epirubicin and docetaxel vs. chemotherapy with cyclophosphamide, epirubicin and fluoracil, one cohort study described a higher risk in giving up daily activities (OR 1.59). [38] Overall, 34% of the population in this study showed a decline in the level of daily activities.

Overall, one cross-sectional study described a decline in activities in 31% of the population. [34] One cohort study related radiotherapy to later starting remunerable work. [41] Activity level did not return to the pre-operative level within one year, [46] and at 10 months, 83% of the patients returned to work. [41] Young age as a predictive factor for a reduced number of metabolic equivalents was described in one cohort study. [46] Another cohort study described reduced use of the affected arm in leisure activities and with lifting a gallon of milk or during heavy household chores in relation to pain and feeling weak. [33].

Comorbidity was related to a decreased level of activities in daily living. [17].

We found level 2 evidence for ALND and radiotherapy, especially when the axilla was involved, as risk factors for decreasing the degree of daily activities.

## Discussion

In this systematic review, we showed that breast cancer treatment results in multiple impairments in the arm and shoulder. We analyzed adverse effects for different components of breast cancer treatment and related these to the integrated treatment of breast cancer. Previous systematic reviews, as well as a part of the cohort studies included in this study, merely focused on only a part of the medical treatment and/or outcome measurements, while others only looked at a general level, without distinction between components. By distinguishing between each treatment modality and outcome measurement, we are the first to analyze the risk of each component of breast cancer treatment. We showed that patients treated with ALND are at the highest risk of developing impairments of the arm and shoulder. Reduced ROM and muscle strength, pain, lymphedema and decreased degree of activities in daily living were reported most frequently in relation to ALND. Lumpectomy was related to a decline in the level of activities of daily living. Radiotherapy and hormonal therapy were the main risk factors for pain.

An integrated approach in assessing the adverse effects of distinct breast cancer treatment modalities on impairments in arm and shoulder function is of clinical importance. Recovery from adverse effects can be addressed in multidisciplinary treatment of patients; for example, physical therapy may be suitable for the recovery of ROM, muscle strength, lymphedema and daily activities. In general, we expect that awareness and timely referral are very relevant for patients with impairments interfering with daily activities in early recovery [47]. More attention should be paid to scapular coordination and muscle strength in the early post-operative phase, as these impairments were reported even up to six years post-operatively. [12,13,15,37] We noticed that the included studies focused more on impairments in function than on activities of daily living or participation in remunerable work, hobbies and social activities. In future research, more awareness of these issues is warranted, as performing activities is an important outcome for quality of life. This will further build the body of knowledge for regaining full recovery of activities of patients with breast cancer in a multidisciplinary approach.

Unfortunately, due to the large variety in medical treatments and outcome measures, we could not perform a meta-analysis of our data. This emphasizes the importance of uniform description of treatment, analysis of outcomes, and use of uniform measurement instruments. Validated measurement instruments are important in assessing outcomes of treatments. We found a large variability of instruments, which made it difficult to compare studies and conduct a meta-analysis. This conclusion was also stated by authors of several included systematic reviews in our study [12,13,15]. International consensus regarding measurement instruments and the way of using them should be encouraged.

From our review it became clear that reduced ROM, pain and lymphedema are the most commonly described impairments. ROM decreased, especially in the first month post-operatively. As most systematic reviews presented data only for long-term follow-up after treatment, reductions in the first month were less noticed, but when described in cohort studies significance existed. After 12 months, percentages of patients with reduction in ROM and differences in ROM between the affected and unaffected shoulder were reduced but still existed. Wide variation of percentages shows the variability in defining ROM impairment and the way of measurement.

The incidence of lymphedema increased over time. One study reported a very high incidence of lymphedema after one month. [28] This may be due to real lymphedema or rather seroma or radiotherapy-induced breast infection. [48].

The study of Ozcinar et al. [18] showed that treatment of lymphedema decreased its severity. In general, the reported percentages of patients with lymphedema were higher when lymphedema was measured by a questionnaire. The Norman questionnaire appeared to be sensitive for detection, but not specific, [10] and may be used as an initial tool in detecting lymphedema. Volume is the most important outcome for lymphedema diagnosis and treatment evaluation; therefore, the questionnaire should be followed by tape measurement (calculated to volume) or water volumetry or perometry. Arm volume is also associated with Body Mass Index and body composition. Therefore we advocate to use percentage difference between arms (where A is the affected arm and U is the unaffected arm)

$$\left(\frac{A-U}{U}\right) \times 100$$

or to use the formula for relative volume change (RVC) to determine outcome over time.

$$RVC = \frac{A2/U2}{A1/U1} - 1$$

Activities in daily living and participation are important parameters for quality of life. Limitation in body functions and structures may be restrictive in performing activities and participating in social events. Only one systematic review [13] and six cohort studies [3,17,28,38,41,46] described limitations in activities and only three cohort studies described problems in participation. As half of the patients with breast cancer were of working age, more attention should be paid to daily activities, work capacity, hobbies and sports.

Several limitations to our study should be noted. Our cut-off point with a quality score >50% is to some extent arbitrary and may have resulted in the exclusion of valuable data in our analysis. Main reasons for the low quality scores of excluded studies were issues with subgroup analysis, lack of outcome measures, poor presentation of results and lack of sufficient follow-up. Firstly, we analyzed which articles in our search were included in the systematic reviews. Four systematic reviews were excluded: based on treatment before 2000 or with low quality score. The review with low quality score was narrative and based on retrospective data. We therefore think the exclusion of these studies has avoided bias and contribute to the robustness of our conclusions. Based on the homogeneity of the results our choice seems to be justified. Another point is that, instead of relying on the review synthesis, it would have been a possibility to use existing reviews as sources to identify primary data, which would increase the value of the paper. We choose to follow the recommendations according the Oxford Centre of Evidence-Based Medicine. In this system systematic reviews are one of the factors in evidence classification. If it would have been possible to perform a meta-analysis the original data would have been extracted from the reviews. However, as described, this was not possible. We deemed additional analysis not to be of added value for the purpose of our paper. Therefore we used quality scores to test the credibility of the conclusions of the original authors and used these in the synthesis. Adverse effects of radiotherapy that may influence limitations in arm and shoulder function, such as fibrosis of the skin and sub cutis, were not included in our study. In addition, adverse effects of chemotherapy and target therapy on general cardiopulmonary capacity were not included. Other reported symptoms such as sleep disturbances, weight gain, cardiac function and sensory disturbances have not been reported, as have anxiety and depression, while these problems may influence the capacity of performing daily activities.

## Conclusions

Patients with breast cancer suffer from constraints in arm and shoulder in the first year post-operative and at long-term follow-up. Patients treated with ALND are most at risk for developing impairments of the arm and shoulder. Reduced ROM and muscle strength, pain, lymphedema and decreased degree of activities in daily living were reported most frequently in relation to ALND. Lumpectomy was related to a decline in the level of activities of daily living. Radiotherapy and hormonal therapy were the main risk factors for pain.

An integrated approach in addressing the adverse effects of distinct breast cancer treatment modalities on impairments in arm and shoulder function is of clinical relevance. Patients treated with ALND require special attention to detect and consequently address impairments in the arm and shoulder. Patients with pain should be monitored carefully, because pain limits the degree of daily activities.

## Acknowledgments

We thank the Dutch Society for Lymphology (part of the Royal Dutch Society for Physical Therapy) for funding the publication fee.

## Author Contributions

Conceived and designed the experiments: JTH CHGB PJW HWML MWGN. Analyzed the data: JTH CHGB PJW HWML MWGN. Contributed reagents/materials/analysis tools: JTH CHGB PJW HWML MWGN. Wrote the paper: JTH CHGB PJW HWML MWGN. Search/data extraction carried out by: JTH CHGB. Contributed in analysis: JTH CHGB HWML MWGN. Contributed in synthesis: JTH CHGB PJW HMWL MWGN.

## References

1. Tsai RJ, Dennis LK, Lynch CF, Snetselaar LG, Zamba GK, et al. (2009) The risk of developing arm lymphedema among breast cancer survivors: a meta-analysis of treatment factors. Ann Surg Oncol 16: 1959–1972.
2. Rietman JS, Geertzen JH, Hoekstra HJ, Baas P, Dolsma WV, et al. (2006) Long term treatment related upper limb morbidity and quality of life after sentinel lymph node biopsy for stage I or II breast cancer. Eur J Surg Oncol 32: 148–152.
3. Land SR, Kopec JA, Julian TB, Brown AM, Anderson SJ, et al. (2010) Patient-reported outcomes in sentinel node-negative adjuvant breast cancer patients receiving sentinel-node biopsy or axillary dissection: National Surgical Adjuvant Breast and Bowel Project phase III protocol B-32. J Clin Oncol 28: 3929–3936.
4. Schmitz KH, Prosnitz RG, Schwartz AL, Carver JR (2012) Prospective surveillance and management of cardiac toxicity and health in breast cancer survivors. Cancer 118: 2270–2276.
5. McNeely ML, Campbell K, Ospina M, Rowe BH, Dabbs K, et al. (2010) Exercise interventions for upper-limb dysfunction due to breast cancer treatment. Cochrane Database Syst Rev: CD005211.
6. Stout NL, Pfalzer LA, Springer B, Levy E, McGarvey CL, et al. (2012) Breast cancer-related lymphedema: comparing direct costs of a prospective surveillance model and a traditional model of care. Physical Therapy 92: 152–163.
7. Cheville AL, Tchou J (2007) Barriers to rehabilitation following surgery for primary breast cancer. Journal of surgical oncology 95: 409–418.
8. WHO-FIC website. Available: www.whofic-apn.com/pdf_files/05/ICF.pdf. Accessed 2013 Jun 19.
9. CEBM website. Available: www.cebm.net/index.aspx?o = 5653. Accessed 2012 Feb 15.
10. Hayes S, Speck R, Reimet E, Stark A, Schmitz K (2011) Does the effect of weight lifting on lymphedema following breast cancer differ by diagnostic method: results from a randomized controlled trial. Breast Cancer Res Treat: 227–234.
11. Zhou WB, Zhang PL, Liu XA, Yang T, He W (2011) Innegligible musculoskeletal disorders caused by zoledronic acid in adjuvant breast cancer treatment: a meta-analysis. J Exp Clin Cancer Res 30: 72.
12. Liu CQ, Guo Y, Shi JY, Sheng Y (2009) Late morbidity associated with a tumour-negative sentinel lymph node biopsy in primary breast cancer patients: a systematic review. Eur J Cancer 45: 1560–1568.
13. Levangie PK, Drouin J (2009) Magnitude of late effects of breast cancer treatments on shoulder function: a systematic review. Breast Cancer Res Treat 116: 1–15.
14. Moja L, Tagliabue L, Balduzzi S, Parmelli E, Pistotti V, et al. (2012) Trastuzumab containing regimens for early breast cancer. Cochrane Database Syst Rev.
15. Lee TS, Kilbreath SL, Refshauge KM, Herbert RD, Beith JM (2008) Prognosis of the upper limb following surgery and radiation for breast cancer. Breast Cancer Res Treat 110: 19–37.
16. Paskett ED, Naughton MJ, McCoy TP, Case LD, Abbott JM (2007) The epidemiology of arm and hand swelling in premenopausal breast cancer survivors. Cancer Epidemiol Biomarkers Prev 16: 775–782.

17. Ververs JM, Roumen RM, Vingerhoets AJ, Vreugdenhil G, Coebergh JW, et al. (2001) Risk, severity and predictors of physical and psychological morbidity after axillary lymph node dissection for breast cancer. European journal of cancer 37: 991–999.

18. Ozcinar B, Guler SA, Kocaman N, Ozkan M, Gulluoglu BM, et al. (2012) Breast cancer related lymphedema in patients with different loco-regional treatments. Breast 21: 361–365.

19. Wernicke AG, Goodman RL, Turner BC, Komarnicky LT, Curran WJ, et al. (2011) A 10-year follow-up of treatment outcomes in patients with early stage breast cancer and clinically negative axillary nodes treated with tangential breast irradiation following sentinel lymph node dissection or axillary clearance. Breast Cancer Res Treat 125: 893–902.

20. Park JH, Lee WH, Chung HS (2008) Incidence and risk factors of breast cancer lymphoedema. J Clin Nurs 17: 1450–1459.

21. Kwan ML, Darbinian J, Schmitz KH, Citron R, Partee P, et al. (2010) Risk factors for lymphedema in a prospective breast cancer survivorship study: the Pathways Study. Arch Surg 145: 1055–1063.

22. Kanematsu M, Morimoto M, Honda J, Nagao T, Nakagawa M, et al. (2011) The time since last menstrual period is important as a clinical predictor for non-steroidal aromatase inhibitor-related arthralgia. BMC Cancer 11: 436.

23. Yen TW, Fan X, Sparapani R, Laud PW, Walker AP, et al. (2009) A contemporary, population-based study of lymphedema risk factors in older women with breast cancer. Ann Surg Oncol 16: 979–988.

24. Mieog JS, Morden JP, Bliss JM, Coombes RC, van de Velde CJ, et al. (2012) Carpal tunnel syndrome and musculoskeletal symptoms in postmenopausal women with early breast cancer treated with exemestane or tamoxifen after 2–3 years of tamoxifen: a retrospective analysis of the Intergroup Exemestane Study. Lancet Oncol 13: 420–432.

25. Chang DW, Kim S (2010) Breast reconstruction and lymphedema. Plast Reconstr Surg 125: 19–23.

26. Norman SA, Localio AR, Kallan MJ, Weber AL, Torpey HA, et al. (2010) Risk factors for lymphedema after breast cancer treatment. Cancer Epidemiol Biomarkers Prev 19: 2734–2746.

27. Lundstedt D, Gustafsson M, Steineck G, Alsadius D, Sundberg A, et al. (2012) Long-term symptoms after radiotherapy of supraclavicular lymph nodes in breast cancer patients. Radiother Oncol 103: 155–160.

28. Taira N, Shimozuma K, Shiroiwa T, Ohsumi S, Kuroi K, et al. (2011) Associations among baseline variables, treatment-related factors and health-related quality of life 2 years after breast cancer surgery. Breast Cancer Res Treat 128: 235–247.

29. Bevilacqua JL, Kattan MW, Changhong Y, Koifman S, Mattos IE, et al. (2012) Nomograms for predicting the risk of arm lymphedema after axillary dissection in breast cancer. Ann Surg Oncol 19: 2580–2589.

30. Mak SS, Yeo W, Lee YM, Mo KF, Tse KY, et al. (2008) Predictors of lymphedema in patients with breast cancer undergoing axillary lymph node dissection in Hong Kong. Nurs Res 57: 416–425.

31. Rief W, Bardwell WA, Dimsdale JE, Natarajan L, Flatt SW, et al. (2011) Long-term course of pain in breast cancer survivors: a 4-year longitudinal study. Breast Cancer Res Treat 130: 579–586.

32. Ashikaga T, Krag DN, Land SR, Julian TB, Anderson SJ, et al. (2010) Morbidity results from the NSABP B-32 trial comparing sentinel lymph node dissection versus axillary dissection. J Surg Oncol 102: 111–118.

33. Levy EW, Pfalzer LA, Danoff J, Springer BA, McGarvey C, et al. (2012) Predictors of functional shoulder recovery at 1 and 12 months after breast cancer surgery. Breast Cancer Res Treat 134: 315–324.

34. Nesvold IL, Reinertsen KV, Fossa SD, Dahl AA (2011) The relation between arm/shoulder problems and quality of life in breast cancer survivors: a cross-sectional and longitudinal study. J Cancer Surviv 5: 62–72.

35. Dahl AA, Nesvold IL, Reinertsen KV, Fossa SD (2011) Arm/shoulder problems and insomnia symptoms in breast cancer survivors: cross-sectional, controlled and longitudinal observations. Sleep Med 12: 584–590.

36. Hickey BE, Francis DP, Lehman M (2013) Sequencing of chemotherapy and radiotherapy for early breast cancer. Cochrane Database Syst Rev 4: CD005212.

37. Shamley D, Srinaganathan R, Oskrochi R, Lascurain-Aguirrebena I, Sugden E (2009) Three-dimensional scapulothoracic motion following treatment for breast cancer. Breast Cancer Res Treat 118: 315–322.

38. Andersen KG, Jensen MB, Kehlet H, Gärtner R, Eckhoff L, et al. (2012) Persistent pain, sensory disturbances and functional impairment after adjuvant chemotherapy for breast cancer: cyclophosphamide, epirubicin and fluorouracil compared with docetaxel + epirubicin and cyclophosphamide. Acta Oncol 51: 1036–1044.

39. Sagen A, Kåresen R, Sandvik L, Risberg MA (2009) Changes in arm morbidities and health-related quality of life after breast cancer surgery - a five-year follow-up study. Acta Oncol 48: 1111–1118.

40. Sheridan D, Foo I, O'Shea H, Gillanders D, Williams L, et al. (2012) Long-term follow-up of pain and emotional characteristics of women after surgery for breast cancer. J Pain Symptom Manage 44: 608–614.

41. Johnsson A, Fornander T, Rutqvist LE, Olsson M (2010) Factors influencing return to work: a narrative study of women treated for breast cancer. Eur J Cancer Care (Engl) 19: 317–323.

42. Avraham T, Daluvoy SV, Riedel ER, Cordeiro PG, Van Zee KJ, et al. (2010) Tissue expander breast reconstruction is not associated with an increased risk of lymphedema. Annals of surgical oncology 17: 2926–2932.

43. Miller CL, Specht MC, Skolny MN, Jammallo LS, Horick N, et al. (2012) Sentinel lymph node biopsy at the time of mastectomy does not increase the risk of lymphedema: implications for prophylactic surgery. Breast Cancer Res Treat 135: 781–789.

44. Ridner SH, Dietrich MS, Stewart BR, Armer JM (2011) Body mass index and breast cancer treatment-related lymphedema. Support Care Cancer 19: 853–857.

45. Yang EJ, Park WB, Seo KS, Kim SW, Heo CY, et al. (2010) Longitudinal change of treatment-related upper limb dysfunction and its impact on late dysfunction in breast cancer survivors: a prospective cohort study. J Surg Oncol 101: 84–91.

46. Devoogdt N, Van Kampen M, Geraerts I, Coremans T, Fieuws S, et al. (2010) Physical activity levels after treatment for breast cancer: one-year follow-up. Breast Cancer Res Treat 123: 417–425.

47. Beurskens CHG, Uden van CJT, Strobbe LJA, Oostendorp RAB, Wobbes T (2007) The efficacy of physiotherapy upon shoulder function following axillary dissection in breast cancer, a randomized controlled study. BMC Cancer 166–173.

48. Khan AJ, Arthur D, Vicini F, Beitsch P, Kuerer H, et al. (2012) Six-year analysis of treatment-related toxicities in patients treated with accelerated partial breast irradiation on the American Society of Breast Surgeons MammoSite Breast Brachytherapy registry trial. Ann Surg Oncol 19: 1477–1483.

# 3

# In Situ Quantitative Measurement of HER2mRNA Predicts Benefit from Trastuzumab-Containing Chemotherapy in a Cohort of Metastatic Breast Cancer Patients

**Maria Vassilakopoulou[1]❥, Taiwo Togun[2]❥, Urania Dafni[3], Huan Cheng[1], Jennifer Bordeaux[1], Veronique M. Neumeister[1], Mattheos Bobos[4], George Pentheroudakis[5], Dimosthenis V. Skarlos[6], Dimitrios Pectasides[7], Vassiliki Kotoula[4,8], George Fountzilas[4,9], David L. Rimm[1], Amanda Psyrri[10]***

1 Yale University, School of Medicine, Department of Pathology, New Haven, Connecticut, United States of America, 2 Yale University, School of Public Health, Department of Biostatistics, New Haven, Connecticut, United States of America, 3 Laboratory of Biostatistics, University of Athens School of Nursing, Athens, Greece, 4 Laboratory of Molecular Oncology, Hellenic Foundation for Cancer Research, Aristotle University of Thessaloniki School of Medicine, Thessaloniki, Greece, 5 Department of Medical Oncology, Ioannina University Hospital, Ioannina, Greece, 6 Second Department of Medical Oncology, "Metropolitan" Hospital, Piraeus, Greece, 7 Oncology Section, Second Department of Internal Medicine, "Hippokration" Hospital, Athens, Greece, 8 Department of Pathology, Aristotle University of Thessaloniki School of Medicine, Thessaloniki, Greece, 9 Department of Medical Oncology, "Papageorgiou" Hospital, Aristotle University of Thessaloniki School of Medicine, Thessaloniki, Greece, 10 Division of Oncology, Second Department of Internal Medicine, University of Athens School of Medicine, Attikon University Hospital, Athens, Greece

## Abstract

*Background:* We sought to determine the predictive value of in situ mRNA measurement compared to traditional methods on a cohort of trastuzumab-treated metastatic breast cancer patients.

*Methods:* A tissue microarray composed of 149, classified as HER2-positive, metastatic breast cancers treated with various trastuzumab-containing chemotherapy regimens was constructed. HER2 intracellular domain(ICD), HER2 extracellular domain(ECD) and HER2 mRNA were assessed using AQUA. For HER2 protein evaluation, CB11 was used to measure ICD and SP3 to measure ECD of the HER2 receptor. In addition, HER2 mRNA status was assessed using RNAscope assay ERRB2 probe. Kaplan – Meier estimates were used for depicting time-to-event endpoints. Multivariate Cox regression models with backward elimination were used to assess the performance of markers as predictors of TTP and OS, after adjusting for important covariates.

*Results:* HER2 mRNA was correlated with ICD HER2, as measured by CB11 HER2, with ECD HER2 as measured by SP3 (Pearson's Correlation Coefficient, r = 0.66 and 0.51 respectively) and with FISH HER2 (Spearman's Correlation Coefficient, r = 0.75). All markers, HER2 mRNA, ICD HER2 and ECD HER2, along with FISH HER2, were found prognostic for OS (Log-rank p = 0.007, 0.005, 0.009 and 0.043 respectively), and except for FISH HER2, they were also prognostic for TTP Log-rank p = 0.036, 0.068 and 0.066 respectively) in this trastuzumab- treated cohort. Multivariate analysis showed that in the presence of pre-specified set of prognostic factors, among all biomarkers only ECD HER2, as measured by SP3, is strong prognostic factor for both TTP (HR = 0.54, 95% CI: 0.31–0.93, p = 0.027) and OS (HR = 0.39, 95%CI: 0.22–0.70, p = 0.002).

*Conclusions:* The expression of HER2 ICD and ECD as well as HER2 mRNA levels was significantly associated with TTP and OS in this trastuzumab-treated metastatic cohort. In situ assessment of HER2 mRNA has the potential to identify breast cancer patients who derive benefit from Trastuzumab treatment.

**Editor:** Zoran Culig, Innsbruck Medical University, Austria

**Funding:** This study was supported by the National Cancer Institute. The funders had no role in study design, data collection and analysis, decision to publish, or preparation of the manuscript.

**Competing Interests:** The authors have declared that no competing interests exist.

\* Email: dpsyrri@med.uoa.gr

❥ These authors contributed equally to this work.

## Introduction

In recent years, targeted therapies such as the anti-HER2 humanized monoclonal antibody trastuzumab, have changed the therapeutic landscape in breast cancer. *HER2*, a proto-oncogene encoding HER2 tyrosine kinase receptor, is amplified in 10 to 20% of breast cancers, leading to HER2 protein overexpression and an aggressive tumor phenotype associated with reduced survival and high metastatic potential. The advent of molecular targeting of HER2 receptor with trastuzumab has substantially improved the outcome of breast cancer patients. Although single-agent trastuzumab exerts some antitumor activity, the highest clinical benefit is derived when trastuzumab is combined with chemotherapy [1–5] HER2 testing has become routine practice in every patient with breast cancer since the benefit of trastuzumab is limited to patients with HER-2 positive breast cancer.

Accurate assessment of HER2 status is necessary to recommend therapy for patients who are most likely to benefit from the treatment and minimize unnecessary overtreatment in the setting where potential side effects may occur [6].

Despite the reported and proven benefits of trastuzumab in HER2-overexpressing metastatic breast cancer patients, approximately 50% of them [7] exhibit de novo resistance while the vast majority of patients who initially respond eventually develop acquired resistance within a year [8].

The assessment of HER2 overexpression by two immunohistochemical (IHC) assays and three fluorescent in-situ hybridization (FISH) assays have been approved by the US Food and Drug Administration (FDA) [9–13] However, these methods are suboptimal since up to 33% of patients will not respond to trastuzumab despite their tumors meeting the HER2 prerequisite as determined by these methods [8]. Moreover, recent studies suggest that some patients who are not classified as HER2 positive may benefit from trastuzumab [14]. Differences in methodology

and scoring systems have led to varying results in different studies and patient cohorts, contributing to the debate on the optimal testing method and the role of HER2 as a prognostic and predictive factor. Two independent cooperative group studies reported a less than optimal concordance between locally and centrally performed HER2 assays, as up to 20% of locally performed HER2 assays could not be confirmed by central laboratories [15].

To minimize discrepancies, the American Society of Clinical Oncology (ASCO) and College of American Pathologists (CAP), developed guidelines for optimal laboratory evaluation of HER2 status by modifying the FDA criteria, which had been used in pivotal trastuzumab trials [16]. However, data analysis from the phase III N9831 trial that investigated adjuvant trastuzumab therapy (NCCTG N9831 Clinical Trial Registration. National Institutes of Health Clinical Trials Website. http://clinicaltrials. gov/ct2/show/NCT00005970?term = N9831&rank = 2. Accessed April 18, 2011), showed decrease in the number of patients eligible for trastuzumab therapy when the ASCO/CAP criteria were applied [17]. This analysis showed that the adoption of ASCO/

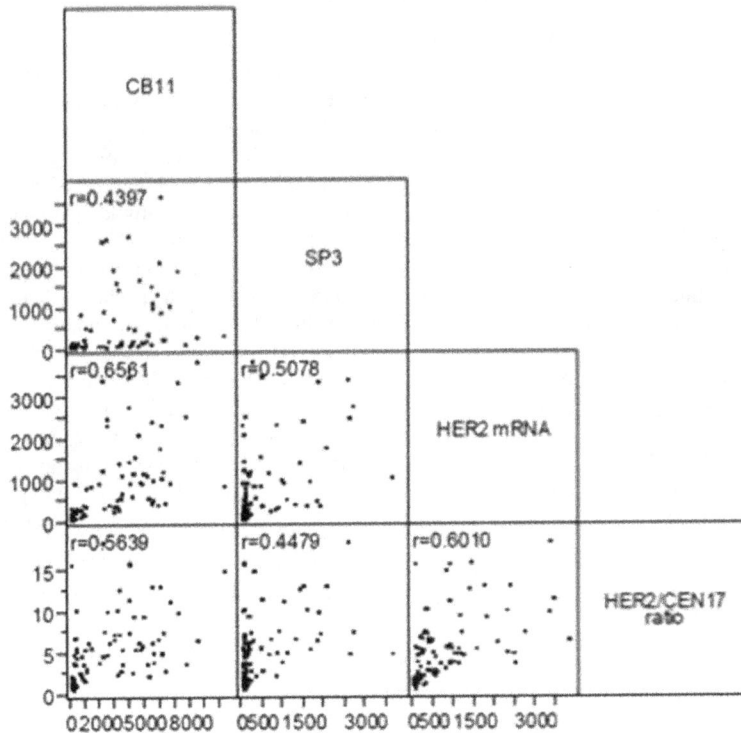

| Variable | by Variable | Spearman ρ | Prob>|ρ| |
| --- | --- | --- | --- |
| SP3 | CB11 | 0.6575 | <.0001* |
| HER2 mRNA | CB11 | 0.8487 | <.0001* |
| HER2 mRNA | SP3 | 0.6210 | <.0001* |
| HER2/CEN17 ratio | CB11 | 0.7116 | <.0001* |
| HER2/CEN17 ratio | SP3 | 0.5196 | <.0001* |
| HER2/CEN17 ratio | HER2 mRNA | 0.7466 | <.0001* |

Pearson's Correlation shown at the upper left corner in each correlation tile

Figure 1. Pearson's Correlation of CB11, SP3, Her2mRNA and FISH.

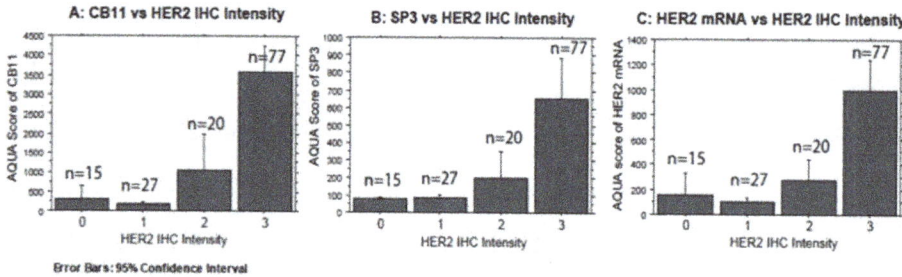

**Figure 2. Comparison of CB11 (A), SP3 (B), Her2mRNA (C) to Her2 IHC.**

CAP criteria may be too restrictive, increasing the "false negative cases" and may disallow up to 4% of patients from receiving anti-HER2 therapy. As a result, ASCO/CAP criteria may exclude patients who would have been eligible for the trastuzumab in the pivotal clinical trials, which led to its approval. Hence, ASCO/CAP has recently revised their guidelines to the original 10% cutpoint [18].

In spite of these changes, efforts to optimize testing methods are ongoing. It has been suggested that HER2 status can be assessed with different approaches as a continuous variable and can be assessed on mRNA level [19]. HER2 gene amplification determined with FISH is strongly associated with elevated mRNA and protein levels and small studies have reported on the concordance of HER2 status by RT-PCR to that by IHC and FISH [20–22]; Two independent studies have reported on the concordance between HER2 Quantitative Reverse Transcription Polymerase Chain Reaction (qRT-PCR) of the Oncotype Dx Test and the FDA-approved IHC/FISH assays and have yielded conflicting results [23,24]. In the first study, a greater than 50% false-negative rate for Oncotype DX RT-PCR for *HER2* assessment was reported. This high false-negative rate of RT-PCR assay highlights the shortcomings of this non-morphologic assay and the importance of standard immunohistological methods in HER2 testing. This result could open the door for a new method of in situ quantitative analysis of HER2 mRNA levels that would reflect more precisely HER2 status by combining quantitative determination of gene expression levels and morphologic assessment.

The aim of this study was to assess HER2- mRNA as a potential predictor of benefit from trastuzumab-based chemotherapy and to correlate it to HER2 protein levels and to FISH by using a combination of automated-quantitative immunofluorescence and a new method of mRNA in situ hybridization marketed as RNAscope.

## Materials and Methods

### Patient cohort

The breast cancer cohort used for this study consists of 149 patients classified as HER2-overexpressing by locally performed IHC at the time of pathological assessment, who were diagnosed in Greece from 1999 through 2006 with metastatic breast cancer. Patients were treated with various Trastuzumab-based combinations for metastatic disease [25,26]. Tissue samples were collected prior to treatment and none of the patients received neoadjuvant therapy. A tissue microarray (TMA) was constructed, composed by histospots of the above cohort. Each clinical case was represented by 2 cores on this TMA (2-fold redundant). All cases were centrally reviewed for HER2 overexpression/amplification by IHC and FISH at the Laboratory of Molecular Oncology, Hellenic Foundation for Cancer Research, Aristotle University of Thessaloniki School of Medicine. Clinical data were comprehensively obtained after review of medical records. Clinicopathologic characteristics of the cohort are found in Table 1. Only patients receiving Trastuzumab as 1st line (n = 130) were included in the

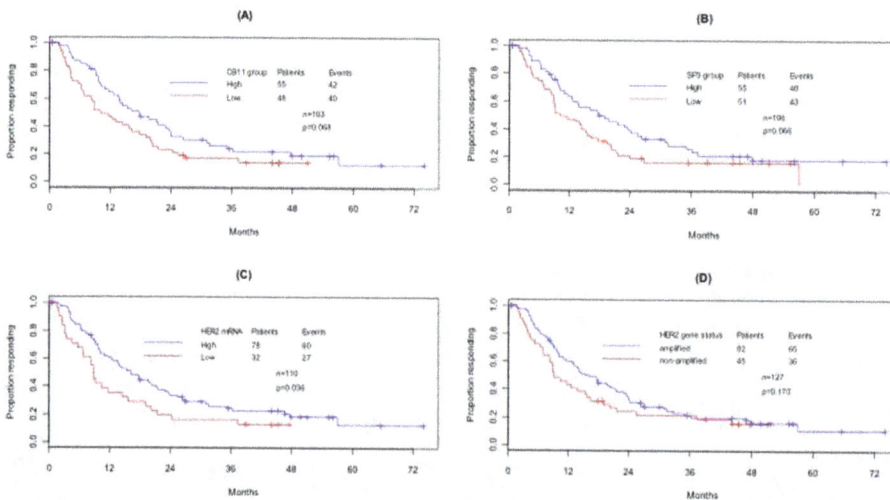

**Figure 3. Time to progression (TTP) by HER2 patient populations, as defined by each biomarker and HER2 gene status (Kaplan-Meier plots).** (A) ICD HER2 as measured by CB11 (high vs. low); (B) ECD HER2 as measured by SP3 (high vs. low); (C) HER2 mRNA (high vs. low); (D) FISH HER2 (amplified vs. non-amplified).

analysis. The translational research protocol was approved by the Bioethics Committee of the Aristotle University of Thessaloniki School of Medicine (Protocol #4283; January 14, 2008) under the general title "Investigation of major mechanisms of resistance to treatment with trastuzumab in patients with metastatic breast cancer". All patients included in the study after 2005 provided written informed consent for the provision of biological material for future research studies, before receiving any treatment. Waiver of consent was obtained from the Bioethics Committee for patients included in the study before 2005.

## RNA in situ hybridization

The RNAscope (Advanced Cell Diagnostics, Inc., Hayward, CA [ACD]) technique of mRNA *in situ* hybridization (ISH) formalin-fixed paraffin embedded (FFPE) tissue has been previously described [27].

Briefly, the assay uses a pool of up to 20 probe pair sets for each mRNA target of interest. Probe pairs bind along an mRNA region and create a unique 28 base-pair sequence recognized by the preAMP which then allows for binding during the subsequent

amplification steps and finally the amplified target is detected by cy5 tyramide & AQUA (Figure S1).

HER2 mRNA status was assessed by in situ hybridization using the RNAscope FFPE assay kit according to the manufacturer's instructions modified for fluorescence detection of transcripts using Cy5-tyramide. In brief, slides with TMA sections were treated with heat and protease digestion followed by hybridization with target probes to *ERBB2 gene (by ACD)*, the housekeeping gene *ubiquitin C (UbC)* as a positive control or the bacterial gene *DapB* as a negative control. *ERBB2 gene* or *UbC* specific hybridization signals were detected with Cy5-tyramide. Sections were then incubated with 0.3% bovine serum albumin (BSA) in 0.1 mol/L of Tris-buffered saline (triethanolamine-buffered saline, pH 8) for 30 minutes at room temperature followed by incubation with a wide-spectrum rabbit anti-cow cytokeratin antibody (Z0622 1:100, DAKO) in BSA/tris-buffered saline for 1 hour at room temperature. The cytokeratin signal was detected with Alexa 546 conjugated goat anti-rabbit (1:100, Molecular Probes) incubated for 1 hour at room temperature. Slides were then mounted using ProlongGold plus 4,6-diamidino-2-phenylindole (DAPI).

**Table 1.** Cohort Description.

| Variables | | Number | % |
|---|---|---|---|
| **Age** | | | |
| | <50 | 39 | 26% |
| | >50 | 110 | 74% |
| **Grade** | | | |
| | 1 | 3 | 2% |
| | 2 | 53 | 36% |
| | 3 | 83 | 56% |
| | Unknown | 10 | 6% |
| **Distant Metastasis** | | | |
| | Yes | 132 | 89% |
| | No | 11 | 7% |
| | Unknown | 6 | 4% |
| **ER** | | | |
| | Positive | 104 | 70% |
| | Negative | 45 | 30% |
| **PR** | | | |
| | Positive | 76 | 51% |
| | Negative | 73 | 49% |
| **HER2** | | | |
| | Positive | 90 | 60% |
| | Negative | 59 | 40% |
| **Trastuzumab** | | | |
| 1st Line | | 130 | |
| | Monotherapy | 4 | 3% |
| | with Anthracycline | 24 | 19% |
| | with Taxane | 102 | 78% |
| 2nd Line + | | 19 | |
| | Monotherapy | 3 | 16% |
| | with Anthracycline | 4 | 21% |
| | with Taxane | 12 | 63% |

## Immunofluorescence staining

In Situ quantitative measurement of biomarkers was done by using the following:

- anti-HER2 mouse monoclonal antibody, clone CB11 (by Biocare) Epitope: Intracellular domain of human HER2 receptor.
- anti-HER2 mouse monoclonal antibody, clone SP3 (by Thermo Fischer) Epitope: Extracellular domain of human c-erbB2.
- ERRB2 probe, for HER2 mRNA (RNAscope assay by ACD), according to the manufacturer's protocol modified for detection with Cy-5 Tyramide.

Each antibody was validated by performing 1) titering, 2) reproducibility assessment on index arrays, and 3) verification of linearity with expression on cell line series, according to a previously described protocol [28]. The immunofluorescence staining was performed by using a standard protocol. In brief, TMA slides were deparaffinized with xylene and rehydrated with ethanol. Antigen retrieval was performed with citrate buffer (pH = 6) at 97°C for 20 minutes. In order to block endogenous peroxidase activity, we used a 2.5% solution of hydroxyl peroxide in methanol, and thereafter slides were incubated with the primary antibody and cytokeratin (Cytokeratin (KRT X) Mouse AE1/AE3/IgG1 M3515 DAKO, Rabbit polyclonal ZO622 DAKO) overnight at 4°C. Each staining was performed by using the Thermo/Fisher Lab Vision autostainer. As secondary antibody we used Alexa 546 conjugated goat antirabbit/mouse (Molecular Probes, Eugene OR) with Mouse/rabbit EnVision reagent (DAKO) and sequentially Cy5-tyramide (Perker Elmer, Life Science, MA). DAPI was used to stain the cell nuclei.

## Quantitative immunofluorescence (QIF)

The AQUA method of QIF has been described elsewhere [29]. This method allows exact and objective measurement of fluorescence intensity within a defined tumor area, as well as within subcellular compartments. Briefly, a series of high-resolution monochromatic images were captured using an Olympus AX-51 epifluorescent microscope based on a previously described algorithm for image collection [29]. According to this algorithm, images were obtained for each sample histospot and for each different fluorescence channel, DAPI (nuclei), Alexa 546 (cytokeratin), or Cy5 (target probe), respectively. A tumor mask was created by binarizing the cytokeratin signal to distinguish stromal from tumor area and target probe expression was quantified only in the tumor. AQUA scores were calculated for a given target within the "tumor mask" by dividing the signal intensity by the area of the "tumor mask" within each histospot. Histospots containing less than 5% tumor, as determined by the percentage of area which was positive for cytokeratin were excluded from the analysis.

## Statistical analysis

Correlation of each biomarker with immunohistochemistry/FISH was assessed by using the Pearson and Spearman's rank correlation coefficient. All biomarkers were treated as binary variables. Dichotomization of CB11 and SP3 was based on the corresponding median AQUA scores (620.41 and 99.42 respectively), whilst the signal-to-noise threshold was used as a cut point for HER2mRNA (<100: negative vs. ≥100 positive). Overall survival (OS) and time to progression (TTP) were the primary endpoints of interest. TTP survival times were calculated in months, from Trastuzumab initiation to the date of disease progression, censoring or last follow-up exam. Survival curves were calculated using the Kaplan-Meier method and differences in survival times between groups were assessed by using the log-rank test. Multivariate Cox regression models were used to assess the performance of each marker and FISH HER2 after adjusting for other important predictors, namely age group (<50 vs. ≥50 years), disease grade (I & II vs. III), status of distant metastasis and ER status. For a simultaneous assessment of all HER2 biomarkers and FISH in the presence of the aforementioned pre-specified set of prognostic factors, multivariate Cox regression models, with backward selection, were also fitted. During the backward elimination process, the possibility of significant interactions between any pair of biomarkers and each biomarker by ER status was also tested. None of these candidates was found statistically significant and hence no interaction terms are included in the final multivariate Cox proportional hazards (PH) models.

Statistical analysis was performed using R Statistical Software (Foundation for Statistical Computing, Vienna, Austria, http://www.r-project.org/).

## Results

### Correlation between HER2 mRNA, HER2- protein and HER2-FISH

The quantitative ISH assay allows for comparison between the HER2 mRNA and protein levels, both of which are quantified on a continuous scale using AQUA on serial TMA sections from the breast cancer cohort. Our cohort demonstrated a positive, linear correlation between HER2 mRNA and protein levels. HER2 mRNA was correlated with ICD HER2, as measured by CB11, with ECD HER2 as measured by SP3 (Pearson's r = 0.66 and 0.51 respectively) and with FISH HER2 (Spearman r = 0.75, Fig. 1).

**Table 2.** TTP analysis: Predictive evaluation of HER2 biomarkers and FISH for given prognostic factors (Cox Proportional Hazards Model).

| | Hazard ratio (HR; 95% CI) | P-value |
|---|---|---|
| SP3 (High vs. Low) | 0.54 (0.31, 0.93) | 0.027 |
| HER2 gene status (amplified vs. non-amplified) | 0.62 (0.35, 1.10) | 0.101 |
| Age group (<50 vs. >=50) | 0.79 (0.46, 1.38) | 0.417 |
| Disease grade (I & II vs. III) | 0.84 (0.51, 1.37) | 0.483 |
| Distant metastasis (no vs. yes) | 0.24 (0.07, 0.80) | 0.020 |
| ER status (negative vs. positive) | 1.96 (1.09, 3.51) | 0.024 |

**Table 3.** OS analysis: Predictive evaluation of HER2 biomarkers and FISH for given prognostic factors (Cox Proportional Hazards Model).

| | Hazard ratio (HR; 95% CI) | P-value |
|---|---|---|
| SP3 (High vs. Low) | 0.39 (0.22, 0.70) | 0.002 |
| Age group (<50 vs. >=50) | 0.91 (0.49, 1.68) | 0.755 |
| Disease grade (I & II vs. III) | 0.56 (0.32, 1.00) | 0.051 |
| Distant metastasis (no vs. yes) | 0.25 (0.06, 1.08) | 0.063 |
| ER status (negative vs. positive) | 1.50 (0.81, 2.77) | 0.196 |

Additionally, HER-2 ICD, ECD and HER2 mRNA AQUA scores showed a significant correlation with immunohistochemistry as centrally tested (Fig. 2A, B and C, respectively).

### Time To Progression (TTP)

Similarly, patients with high HER2 ICD as well as ECD protein expression showed a longer TTP survival compared to patients with low protein expression levels (Log-rank $p = 0.068$ and 0.064 respectively, Fig. 3A and 3B) as determined by the median AQUA score for each marker. Kaplan-Meier analysis showed a longer TTP survival of patients with high HER2 mRNA compared to patients with low HER2 mRNA (Log-rank p $= 0.036$, Fig. 3C) as determined by the detection threshold (the highest noise level measured by DapB as negative control). No significant difference was found between patients with amplified and non-amplified HER2 gene status (Log-rank $p = 0.170$, Fig. 3D).

Cox proportional hazard models fitted for each biomarker separately showed that for given age group, disease grade, status of distant metastasis and ER status, TTP survival is more favorable for HER2 high patients, as defined by the corresponding median AQUA scores. The HR estimated by these models were HR $= 0.52$ (95%CI: 0.31–0.88, $p = 0.014$) for CB11, HR $= 0.46$ (95%CI: 0.27–0.48, $p = 0.004$) for SP3 and HR $= 1.68$ (95%CI: 1.00–2.83, $p = 0.051$) for HER2 mRNA. In a similar model with all pre-specified prognostic factors present, TTP survival was also more favorable for patients with amplified HER2 gene status

($HR = 0.56$, 95%CI: 0.34–0.91, $p = 0.018$).

The multivariate TTP analysis included all biomarkers and FISH HER2 as well as the aforementioned prognostic factors. Applying a backward elimination process, it was found that ECD HER2, as measured by SP3, is the only biomarker that retains its prognostic ability for TTP survival ($HR = 0.54$, 95%CI: 0.31–0.93, $p = 0.027$). FISH HER2 was also marginally significant at $\alpha = 10\%$ (Table 2).

**Overall Survival (OS).** OS was found significantly longer for patients with high HER2 ICD (Log-rank $p = 0.005$, Fig. 4A), high ECD protein expression (Log-rank $p = 0.009$, Fig. 4B), high HER2 mRNA (Log-rank $p = 0.007$, Fig. 4C) and amplified HER2 gene status (Log-rank $p = 0.043$, Fig. 4D).

Separate Cox PH models for each HER2 biomarker and FISH showed that for a given age group, grade of disease, ER status and status of distant metastasis, OS is more favorable for patients with high HER2 ICD ($HR = 0.38$, 95%CI: 0.21–0.68, $p = 0.001$), high HER2 ECD ($HR = 0.39$, 95%CI: 0.22–070, $p = 0.002$), high HER2 mRNA ($HR = 0.46$, 95%CI: 0.26–0.81, $p = 0.007$) and amplified HER2 gene status ($HR = 0.42$, 95%CI: 0.24–0.72, $p = 0.002$).

Multivariate analysis showed that after adjustment for the pre-specified set of prognostic factors, high HER2 ECD protein levels, as measured by SP3, predict better overall survival ($HR = 0.39$, 95%CI: 0.22–070, $p = 0.002$, Table 3). None of the remaining

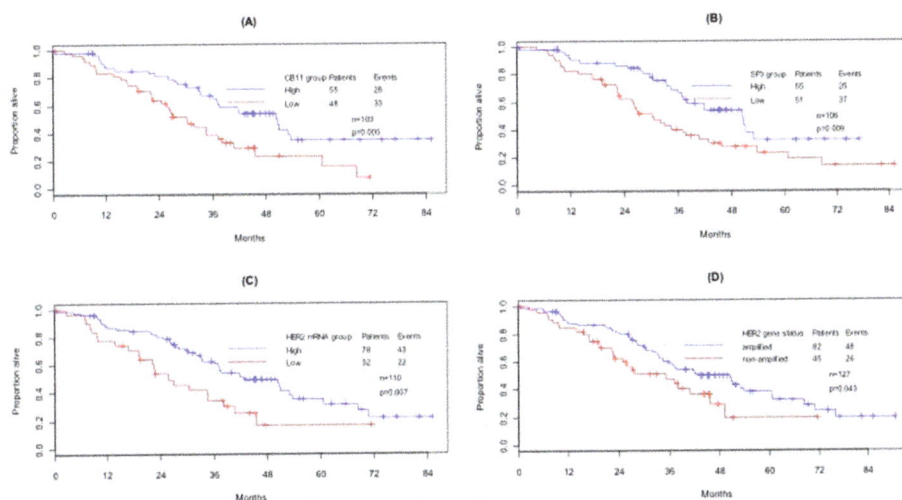

**Figure 4. Overall Survival (OS) by HER2 patient populations, as defined by each biomarker and HER2 gene status (Kaplan-Meier plots).** (A) ICD HER2 as measured by CB11 (high vs. low); (B) ECD HER2 as measured by SP3 (high vs. low); (C) HER2 mRNA (high vs. low); (D) FISH HER2 (amplified vs. non-amplified).

biomarkers was found statistically significant in the multivariate model.

## Discussion

Analyzing biomarkers at the mRNA level for prognostic classification of patients has become popular in recent years. As an example, mRNA analysis is the basis of the FDA-cleared Agendia's MammaPrint test [30] which measures the mRNA level of 70 specific genes in fresh tissue and Genomic Health's popular Oncotype Dx test [31] which uses a RTQ-PCR process to quantify the expression of specific mRNA for 21 cancer genes in FFPE material, both tests for assessing recurrence risk.

It has been previously shown that both HER2 protein overexpression and gene amplification are closely correlated with mRNA levels in formalin-fixed, paraffin-embedded tissue sections, especially when tumour tissue is microdissected [21,32]. The novelty of our study lies on determination of HER2 mRNA levels using a method of quantitative in situ RNA assessment.

The HER2 status is tested on all newly diagnosed breast cancer cases as prognostic factor and predictor for anti-HER2 targeted therapy [33]. The therapeutic response to anti-HER2 treatment can be predicted by HER2 status and is associated with improved outcome in patients with metastatic and operable HER2-positive breast cancers [34–36]. Consistent with these findings, we showed that HER2-protein levels and HER2-m RNA expression are predictors of TTP after trastuzumab-containing chemotherapy in this metastatic breast cancer cohort.

We showed that HER2 ECD as assessed by the SP3 antibody trends to outperform the rest of the HER2 biomarkers and FISH as a predictor for median TTP after trastuzumab therapy. SP3 antibody has been compared to the CB11 antibody (used in the FDA-approved PATHWAY kit-Ventana), Herceptest and FISH and showed a higher discrimination power compared to HercepTest [37–39] while it showed a high concordance with FISH [40].

One possible explanation of our findings may reside in the molecular target of trastuzumab which is the extracellular domain of HER-2 [41] which may be cleaved and shed from the surface of breast cancer cells generating a truncated 95-kd intramembrane protein [42]. This truncated form of HER2 does not possess the extracellular trastuzumab-binding epitope, and its expression has been associated with trastuzumab resistance [43]. Hence, the assessment of the HER2-ECD may be of particular interest and predictive significance as the actual target epitope of trastuzumab.

Our study also shows a significant correlation of HER2-mRNA levels with conventional immunohistochemistry and in situ-hybridization methods as well as FISH. We found that HER2 status by FISH, AQUA HER2-proteins and HER2-mRNA levels are all independent predictor factors for TTP after Trastuzumab-containing chemotherapy in this metastatic cohort. In our study, HER2 mRNA status was assessed by in situ hybridization using the RNAscope FFPE assay in combination with the AQUA method of automated quantitative immunofluorescence. In situ quantitative measurement of both HER2-mRNA and protein; is reproducible, automated method that reduces intra-observer variability. Since the interpretation of HER2 immunostaining and in situ-hybridization may be influenced by laboratory and observer variability, the use of the AQUA automated method in measurement of HER2 protein along with the HER2-mRNA level could improve the diagnostic accuracy of HER2 status,. QISH enables a relatively easy, fast and reproducible quantification of HER2-mRNA expression feasible in routine FFPE tissue.

In summary, our study demonstrates that measurement of HER2-m RNA levels with this novel method has a predictive value for response to Herceptin-based chemotherapy in metastatic breast cancer. Additional studies in prospective cohorts are required to validate these findings with the ultimate goal to build a potential predictive model of trastuzumab therapy and complete the puzzle of HER2 testing optimization.

## Acknowledgments

Portions of this material were presented at the 48th Annual Meeting of the American Society of Clinical Oncology, June 2012.

## Author Contributions

Conceived and designed the experiments: AP GF DLR MV. Performed the experiments: MV VMN. Analyzed the data: MV TT UD DLR AP HC JB MB GP DVS DP VK. Contributed reagents/materials/analysis tools: DLR. Wrote the paper: MV DLR AP. Approved the final version: HC JB MB GP DVS DP VK.

## References

1. Tsang RY, Finn RS (2012) Beyond trastuzumab: novel therapeutic strategies in HER2-positive metastatic breast cancer. Br J Cancer; 106: 6–13.
2. Saini KS, Azim HA Jr, Metzger-Filho O, et al. (2011) Beyond trastuzumab: new treatment options for HER2-positive breast cancer. Breast; 20 Suppl 3: S20–27.
3. Murphy CG, Fornier M (2010) HER2-positive breast cancer: beyond trastuzumab. Oncology (Williston Park); 24: 410–415.
4. Robert N, Leyland-Jones B, Asmar L, et al. Randomized phase III study of trastuzumab, paclitaxel, and carboplatin compared with trastuzumab and paclitaxel in women with HER-2-overexpressing metastatic breast cancer. J Clin Oncol 2006; 24: 2786–2792.
5. Valero V, Forbes J, Pegram MD, et al. (2011) Multicenter phase III randomized trial comparing docetaxel and trastuzumab with docetaxel, carboplatin, and trastuzumab as first-line chemotherapy for patients with HER2-gene-amplified metastatic breast cancer (BCIRG 007 study): two highly active therapeutic regimens. J Clin Oncol; 29: 149–156.
6. Hayes DF, Picard MH (2006) Heart of darkness: the downside of trastuzumab. J Clin Oncol; 24: 4056–4058.
7. Slamon D, Pegram M (2001) Rationale for trastuzumab (Herceptin) in adjuvant breast cancer trials. Semin Oncol; 28: 13–19.
8. Nahta R, Esteva FJ (2006) HER2 therapy: molecular mechanisms of trastuzumab resistance. Breast Cancer Res; 8: 215.
9. Di Leo A, Dowsett M, Horten B, Penault-Llorca F (2002) Current status of HER2 testing. Oncology (Williston Park); 63 Suppl 1: 25–32.
10. Cianciulli AM, Botti C, Coletta AM, et al. (2002) Contribution of fluorescence in situ hybridization to immunohistochemistry for the evaluation of HER-2 in breast cancer. Cancer Genet Cytogenet; 133: 66–71.
11. Pauletti G, Dandekar S, Rong H, et al (2000) Assessment of methods for tissue-based detection of the HER-2/neu alteration in human breast cancer: a direct comparison of fluorescence in situ hybridization and immunohistochemistry. J Clin Oncol; 18: 3651–3664.
12. Perez EA, Roche PC, Jenkins RB, et al. (2002) HER2 testing in patients with breast cancer: poor correlation between weak positivity by immunohistochemistry and gene amplification by fluorescence in situ hybridization. Mayo Clin Proc; 77: 148–154.
13. Hicks DG, Tubbs RR (2005) Assessment of the HER2 status in breast cancer by fluorescence in situ hybridization: a technical review with interpretive guidelines. Hum Pathol; 36: 250–261.
14. Paik S, Kim C, Wolmark N (2008) HER2 status and benefit from adjuvant trastuzumab in breast cancer. N Engl J Med; 358: 1409–1411.
15. Paik S, Bryant J, Tan-Chiu E, et al. (2002) Real-world performance of HER2 testing–National Surgical Adjuvant Breast and Bowel Project experience. J Natl Cancer Inst; 94: 852–854.
16. Wolff AC, Hammond ME, Schwartz JN, et al. (2007) American Society of Clinical Oncology/College of American Pathologists guideline recommendations for human epidermal growth factor receptor 2 testing in breast cancer. J Clin Oncol; 25: 118–145.

17. Perez EA, Dueck AC, McCullough AE, et al. (2012) Predictability of adjuvant trastuzumab benefit in N9831 patients using the ASCO/CAP HER2-positivity criteria. J Natl Cancer Inst; 104: 159–162.

18. Wolff AC, Hammond ME, Hicks DG, et al. (2013) Recommendations for human epidermal growth factor receptor 2 testing in breast cancer: american society of clinical oncology/college of american pathologists clinical practice guideline update. J Clin Oncol; 31: 3997–4013.

19. Thomson TA, Hayes MM, Spinelli JJ, et al. (2001) HER-2/neu in breast cancer: interobserver variability and performance of immunohistochemistry with 4 antibodies compared with fluorescent in situ hybridization. Mod Pathol; 14: 1079–1086.

20. Benohr P, Henkel V, Speer R, et al. (2005) Her-2/neu expression in breast cancer–A comparison of different diagnostic methods. Anticancer Res; 25: 1895–1900.

21. Gjerdrum LM, Sorensen BS, Kjeldsen E, et al. (2004) Real-time quantitative PCR of microdissected paraffin-embedded breast carcinoma: an alternative method for HER-2/neu analysis. J Mol Diagn; 6: 42–51.

22. Slamon DJ, Clark GM, Wong SG, et al. (1987) Human breast cancer: correlation of relapse and survival with amplification of the HER-2/neu oncogene. Science; 235: 177–182.

23. Dvorak L, Dolan M, Fink J, et al. (2013) Correlation between HER2 determined by fluorescence in situ hybridization and reverse transcription-polymerase chain reaction of the oncotype DX test. Appl Immunohistochem Mol Morphol; 21: 196–199.

24. Dabbs DJ, Klein ME, Mohsin SK, et al. (2011) High false-negative rate of HER2 quantitative reverse transcription polymerase chain reaction of the Oncotype DX test: an independent quality assurance study. J Clin Oncol; 29: 4279–4285.

25. Razis E, Bobos M, Kotoula V, et al. (2011) Evaluation of the association of PIK3CA mutations and PTEN loss with efficacy of trastuzumab therapy in metastatic breast cancer. Breast Cancer Res Treat; 128: 447–456.

26. Fountzilas G, Christodoulou C, Bobos M, et al. (2012) Topoisomerase II alpha gene amplification is a favorable prognostic factor in patients with HER2-positive metastatic breast cancer treated with trastuzumab. J Transl Med; 10: 212.

27. Wang F, Flanagan J, Su N, et al. (2012) RNAscope: a novel in situ RNA analysis platform for formalin-fixed, paraffin-embedded tissues. J Mol Diagn; 14: 22–29.

28. Bordeaux J, Welsh A, Agarwal S, et al. (2010) Antibody validation. Biotechniques; 48: 197–209.

29. Camp RL, Chung GG, Rimm DL (2002) Automated subcellular localization and quantification of protein expression in tissue microarrays. Nat Med; 8: 1323–1327.

30. Bogaerts J, Cardoso F, Buyse M, et al. (2006) Gene signature evaluation as a prognostic tool: challenges in the design of the MINDACT trial. Nat Clin Pract Oncol; 3: 540–551.

31. Paik S, Tang G, Shak S, et al. (2006) Gene expression and benefit of chemotherapy in women with node-negative, estrogen receptor-positive breast cancer. J Clin Oncol; 24: 3726–3734.

32. Cronin M, Pho M, Dutta D, et al. (2004) Measurement of gene expression in archival paraffin-embedded tissues: development and performance of a 92-gene reverse transcriptase-polymerase chain reaction assay. Am J Pathol; 164: 35–42.

33. Chia S, Norris B, Speers C, et al. (2008) Human epidermal growth factor receptor 2 overexpression as a prognostic factor in a large tissue microarray series of node-negative breast cancers. J Clin Oncol; 26: 5697–5704.

34. Slamon DJ, Leyland-Jones B, Shak S, et al. (2001) Use of chemotherapy plus a monoclonal antibody against HER2 for metastatic breast cancer that overexpresses HER2. N Engl J Med; 344: 783–792.

35. Vogel CL, Cobleigh MA, Tripathy D, et al. (2002) Efficacy and safety of trastuzumab as a single agent in first-line treatment of HER2-overexpressing metastatic breast cancer. J Clin Oncol; 20: 719–726.

36. Romond EH, Perez EA, Bryant J, et al. (2005) Trastuzumab plus adjuvant chemotherapy for operable HER2-positive breast cancer. N Engl J Med; 353: 1673–1684.

37. Ricardo SA, Milanezi F, Carvalho ST, et al. (2007) HER2 evaluation using the novel rabbit monoclonal antibody SP3 and CISH in tissue microarrays of invasive breast carcinomas. J Clin Pathol; 60: 1001–1005.

38. Nunes CB, Rocha RM, Reis-Filho JS, et al. (2008) Comparative analysis of six different antibodies against Her2 including the novel rabbit monoclonal antibody (SP3) and chromogenic in situ hybridisation in breast carcinomas. J Clin Pathol; 61: 934–938.

39. Dekker TJ, Borg ST, Hooijer GK, et al. (2012) Determining sensitivity and specificity of HER2 testing in breast cancer using a tissue micro-array approach. Breast Cancer Res; 14: R93.

40. Wludarski S (2008) Applied Immunohistochemistry & Molecular Morphology In.; 466–470.

41. Cho HS, Mason K, Ramyar KX, et al. (2003) Structure of the extracellular region of HER2 alone and in complex with the Herceptin Fab. Nature; 421: 756–760.

42. Zabrecky JR, Lam T, McKenzie SJ, Carney W (1991) The extracellular domain of p185/neu is released from the surface of human breast carcinoma cells, SK-BR-3. J Biol Chem; 266: 1716–1720.

43. Scaltriti M, Rojo F, Ocana A, et al. (2007) Expression of p95HER2, a truncated form of the HER2 receptor, and response to anti-HER2 therapies in breast cancer. J Natl Cancer Inst; 99: 628–638.s

# 4

# Chronopharmacology and Mechanism of Antitumor Effect of Erlotinib in Lewis Tumor-Bearing Mice

Peipei Wang[1⟲], Fengmei An[2⟲], Xingjun Zhuang[3], Jiao Liu[1], Liyan Zhao[4], Bin Zhang[1], Liang Liu[1], Pingping Lin[1], Mingchun Li[4]*

1 Department of Pharmacology, Medical College of Qingdao University, Qingdao, China, 2 Hand Surgery Center of the Whole Army, No. 401 Hospital of Chinese People's Liberation Army, Qingdao, China, 3 Department of Oncology, No. 401 Hospital of Chinese People's Liberation Army, Qingdao, China, 4 Department of Pharmacy, No. 401 Hospital of Chinese People's Liberation Army, Qingdao, China

## Abstract

The epidermal growth factor receptor (EGFR), a ubiquitously expressed receptor tyrosine kinase, is recognized as a key mediator of tumorigenesis in many human epithelial tumors. Erlotinib is tyrosine kinase inhibitor approved by FDA for use in oncology. It inhibits the intracellular phosphorylation of tyrosine kinase associated with the EGFR to restrain the development of the tumor. To investigate the antitumor effect of erlotinib at different dosing times and the underlying molecular mechanism via the PI3K/AKT pathway, we established a mouse model of Lewis lung cancer xenografts. The tumor-bearing mice were housed four or five per cage under standardized light-dark cycle conditions (light on at 7:00 AM, 500 Lux, off at 7:00 PM, 0 Lux) with food and water provided ad libitum. The mice were observed for quality of life, their body weight and tumor volume measured, and the tumor growth curves drawn. After being bled, the mice were sacrificed by cervical dislocation. The tumor masses were removed at different time points and weighed. The mRNA expression of EGFR, AKT, Cyclin D1 and CDK-4 were assayed by quantitative real-time PCR (qRT-PCR). Protein expression levels of AKT, P-AKT and Cyclin D1 were determined by Western blot analysis. The results suggest that erlotinib has a significant antitumor effect on xenografts of non-small cell lung cancer in mice, and its efficacy and toxicity is dependent on the time of day of administration. Its molecular mechanism of action might be related to the EGFR-AKT-Cyclin D1-CDK-4 pathway which plays a crucial role in the development of pathology. Therefore, our findings suggest that the time of day of administration of Erlotinib may be a clinically important variable.

**Editor:** Eric M. Mintz, Kent State University, United States of America

**Funding:** The authors have no funding or support to report.

**Competing Interests:** The authors have declared that no competing interests exist.

* Email: lmc401y@163.com

⟲ These authors contributed equally to this work.

## Introduction

Most living organisms exhibit behavioral and physiological rhythms with a period of about 24 h, influenced by environmental factors including light, temperature, water and social interaction and serving to synchronize circadian rhythms to the daily rotation of time [1,2]. Some of these rhythms are controlled by the circadian clock. Recent molecular studies of the circadian clock have revealed that oscillation in the transcription of specific clock genes plays a central role in the generation of 24-h rhythms [3,4]. Studies have shown that the rhythms of cancer cells differ from those of normal cells [5]. Changing the timing of administration along the 24-h time scale can profoundly improve tumor responses to the treatment and overall survival rates and reduce drug toxicities in cancer patients [6,7]. Identification of mechanism involved in the diurnal rhythm of drug susceptibility will help to achieve better chronopharmacotherapy for cancer treatment.

Surgery is the major treatment for most malignant tumors, but recurrence and metastasis often occur after the operations. Systemic chemotherapy can control the recurrence and metastasis effectively, improve the life quality and prolong the survival time of the patients with advance cancers. However, the traditional chemotherapy not only kills tumor cells but also damages the normal cells, resulting in bone marrow suppression, liver and kidney dysfunction, gastrointestinal reactions, decreased immune function and other side effects. Fortunately, this problem can be solved by the molecular targeted drugs. Erlotinib Hydrochloride Tablets (Tarceva) is a new small molecular targeting inhibitor, which inhibits the intracellular phosphorylation of tyrosine kinase associated with the epidermal growth factor receptor (EGFR)[8,9]. It can selectively act on intracellular targets, block EGFR pathway and inhibit the development of tumors, but causes little damage to the normal cells[10,11]. Erlotinib monotherapy is indicated for treating the patients with locally advanced or metastatic non-small cell lung cancer after failure of at least one prior chemotherapy regimen[12]. The most common adverse reactions are rash and diarrhea. Its efficiency can be increased but its toxicity reduced by administering the drugs when they are most effective and/or tolerated. The mechanism may be related to the dosing time-dependent variations in pharmacokinetics, tumor responsiveness, and host immune responsiveness [13]. However, the exact mechanism has not been clarified yet.

Erlotinib inhibits cell growth through down-regulation of EGFR phosphorylation. It elicits the transcription of various genes

**Table 1.** Dose-response effects of erlotinib on tumor growth ($\bar{x}\pm s$, n = 60, N = 240).

| Erlotinib dose (mg·kg$^{-1}$) | Tumor volume growth (cm$^3$) |
|---|---|
| Model | 4274.83 ± 30.57 |
| 15 | 3183.12 ± 33.15[*] |
| 30 | 2183.16 ± 34.74[*△] |
| 60 | 2074.66 ± 29.09[*△] |

[*]$P<0.05$ when compared with the model group, [△]$P<0.05$ when compared with the 15 mg·kg$^{-1}$ group.

through activation of signal transducers and activators of transcription protein. EGFR is overexpressed or constitutively activated in many types of human cancers, associated with a poor prognosis[14]. EGFR activation can be inhibited by small molecule tyrosine kinase inhibitors (TKI), and inhibition of EGFR function has been shown to decrease the growth of several types of human cancer in preclinical researches[15~18]. It has been reported that AKT, CDK-4 (cyclin dependent kinases, CDKs), and Cyclin D1 are the downstream signaling molecules of EGFR[19,20]. Upstream signaling molecules EGFR can stimulate phosphorylation of AKT, activate cellular pathways, and promote tumor cell growth, proliferation, invasion and metastasis[21]. AKT enhances the activity of Cyclin D1 to be combined with CDK-4 to regulate the cell cycle. Both the cell study and the vitro study have proven the overexpression of p-AKT in most human tumor tissues[22]. Therefore, we infer that the mechanism of Erlotinib may be related to EGFR-AKT-CDK4-Cyclin D1 signaling pathway.

The purpose of this paper is to investigate the effects of erlotinib on the inhibition of tumor growth at different dosing times in mice and the underlying mechanism. We aim to find an appropriate time for the chemotherapy to provide the reference to the clinical treatment.

## Materials and Methods

### Animals and Cells

C57BL/6 mice (5 weeks old) were purchased from Vital River Laboratory Animal Technology Co. Ltd. The production license number was SCXK (jing) 2012-0001. The mice were housed four or five per cage under standardized light-dark cycle conditions (light on at 7:00 AM, 500 Lux, off at 7:00 PM, 0 Lux) at $(23\pm1)^{\circ}$C and $(50\pm10)$% humidity with food and water provided ad libitum. This study was carried out in strict accordance with the recommendations in the Guide for the Care and Use of Laboratory Animals of the National Institutes of Health. The experiments were approved by the Committee on the Ethics of Animal Experiments of the No. 401 Hospital of Chinese People's Liberation Army.

Lewis lung cancer cells (ATCC CRL-1642) were provided by Beijing Chuanglian North Carolina Biotechnology Research Institute, and maintained in vitro in high glucose DMEM medium supplemented with 10% heated inactivated fetal bovine serum, 0.5% penicillin, and 0.5% streptomycin at 37°C in a humidified atmosphere with 5% $CO_2$.

### Drugs and Chemicals

Erlotinib Hydrochloride Tablets (150 mg erlotinib in each tablet) were provided by Roche Ltd. Due to their insolubility in water, they were made into suspension with 0.5% sodium carboxymethyl cellulose. FBS, Trypsin enzyme and high glucose DMEM medium were purchased from HyClone. mRNA extraction kit, cDNA extraction kit, RNA amplification kit, primer design and synthesis were provided by Takara. Protein antibody was purchased from Cell Signaling.

### Tumor Model

The growing cells were collected exponentially and the cell density adjusted. 0.2 ml of $1\times10^7$/ml viable tumor cells were inoculated into the subcutaneous of the left hind. Seven days after the tumor cell implantation, the mice were used as tumor-bearing models. They were randomly divided into groups, when the tumors grew to 0.5–1.5 cm$^3$.

### Experiment Design

The experiment was performed in a total of 240 female C57BL/6 tumor-bearing mice and 60 normal mice. The tumor-bearing mice were randomly divided into three treatment groups (15, 30, 60 mg·kg$^{-1}$) and one model group. The mice in the treatment groups were administered successively once a day for twenty days by gavage with 15 mg·kg$^{-1}$, 30 mg·kg$^{-1}$, 60 mg·kg$^{-1}$ of erlotinib suspension, respectively. Those in the model group received the same volume of sodium carboxymethyl cellulose.

We selected the 60 mg·kg$^{-1}$ group to investigate the effects of dosing-times on the anti-tumor effects of erlotinib based on the results of the preliminary experiments. The group was randomly divided into 6 time groups (group 8:00, 12:00, 16:00, 20:00, 24:00, and 04:00). The mice in the 6 time groups were administered successively once a day for twenty days via gavage a single dose of erlotinib (60 mg·kg$^{-1}$) at different circadian times: 8:00, 12:00, 16:00, 20:00, 24:00, and 04:00. Those in the model group received the same volume of sodium carboxymethyl cellulose.

### Determination of Antitumor Effect

Diet, exercise and mental status of the mice were observed during the experiment. Tumor volume was measured with calipers every four days and estimated with the formula: tumor volume (cm$^3$) $= a^2 \times b/2$, where a is the shortest diameter, and b is the longest diameter. The antitumor effect of erlotinib was expressed as the tumor volume change. The tumor growth curves were drawn with the data of tumor volume changes. The mice in the 60 mg/kg group were then sacrificed by cervical dislocation at the corresponding experiment times (8:00, 12:00, 16:00, 20:00, 24:00, and 04:00), and samples of tumor mass were removed at different times and weighed. The tumor inhibition rate was calculated using the formula: tumor inhibition rate (%) = (mean tumor weight of control group - mean tumor weight of experiment group)/mean tumor weight of control group×100%. The tumor masses were immediately stored in liquid nitrogen for the next experiment.

### Histopathology Analysis

Three tumor masses were collected from each group and fixed in 10% formalin over night. The fixed tumor masses were washed with flowing water for at least 8 hours, then cut into 1.5 cm×1.5 cm×0.2–0.3 cm, and dehydrated with 70% ethanol, 80% ethanol, 90% ethanol, and 100% ethanol. The tumor masses were put into xylene solution for 40 min until they became transparent. Then they were put into 56°C–58°C paraffin, dipped into melted solid paraffin, and made into wax blocks after being fixed. The fixed masses were cut into 4–6 μm, and placed in a chamber at 60°C for 15–30 min to remove the interstitial

## Tumor growth

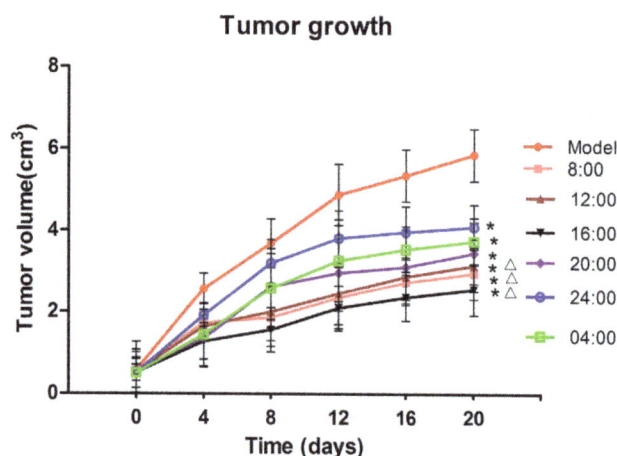

**Figure 1. Influence of dosing times on tumor growth after administration of erlotinib or distilled water on three weeks.** Each value is the mean with SD of ten mice. $^*P<0.05$ when compared with the model group, $^\triangle P<0.05$ when compared with groups 20:00, 24:00, 04:00.

paraffins. Images were obtained with Leica TCS SP5X by hematoxylin-eosin (HE) staining.

## qRT-PCR Analysis

50 mg frozen tissue was immediately transferred into a mortar, into which liquid nitrogen was added, and crushed with pestle to homogenize until powdery. RNAiso Plus was added according to the amount of homogenized tissue. Chloroform was added to the homogenate solution, mixed well, and then centrifuged to separate the solution into three layers. The top liquid layer was removed into a new tube. An isopropanol precipitation was performed to extract the total RNA, which was reversely transcribed into cDNA according to the instruction of PrineScript RT reagent Kit with gDNA Eraser. The expressions of EGFR, AKT1, CDK-4 and CyclinD1 in tumor tissue were detected by qRT-PCR according to the instruction of SYBR PrimeScript RT reagent Kit. GAPDH primer: F: 5′-TGTGTCCGTCGTGGATCTGA-3′, R: 5′-TTG-CTGTTGAAGTCGCAGGAG-3′, 150 bp. EGFR primer: F: 5′-CCTCCACTGTCCAGCTCATTAC-3′, R: 5′-TTCCAGGTA-GTTCATGCCCTTT-3′, 140 bp. AKT1 primer: F: 5′-TGAG-GTTGCCCACACGCTTA-3′, R: 5′-CCCGTTGGCATACTC-

CATGAC-3′, 127 bp. CDK-4 primer: F: 5′-CAGAGCTCTTA-GCCGAGCGTA-3′, R: 5′- GGCACCGACACCAATTTCAG-3′, 87 bp. CyclinD1 primer: F: 5′-TACCGCACAACGCAC-TTTC-3′, R: 5′-AAGGGCTTCAATCTGTTCCTG-3′, 84 bp. Reaction parameters were: 95°C denaturation 30 s, 95°C denaturation 5 s, 55°C annealing 30 s, 72°C extension 30 s, 40 cycles. Each sample was repeated for three times and the mean Ct was calculated. The gene expression was estimated with the formula: $\Delta\Delta Ct$ = (Target gene Ct of experimental group - Reference gene Ct of experimental group) - (Target gene Ct of control group - Reference gene Ct of control group). The relative changes in target gene in different treatment groups were determined by the formula $2^{-\Delta\Delta Ct}$.

## Western-blot Analysis

The frozen tumor masses were transferred into a mortar, into which liquid nitrogen was added, and crushed with pestle to homogenize until powdery. According to the amount of tissue powder, appropriate amount of ice-cold lysis buffer (50 mM Tris–HCl, pH 7.8, 150 mM NaCl, 5 mM EDTA, 0.5% Nonidet P-40, 2 mM PMSF, 1 mM $Na_3VO_4$) was added, and then the homogeneous tissue was cultured on ice for 30 minutes. After the removal of the insoluble materials by centrifugation at 12,000 g for 15 min at 4°C, the resulting supernatants were mixed with an 1/5 volume of 5×sample buffer and boiled at 95°C for 5 min. The protein concentrations in the tumor mass lysates were determined using the BCA protein assay kit (CWBIO, China). The lysate samples were separated on SDS-polyacryl-amide gels electrophoresis, and transferred onto a polyvinylidene difluoride (PVDF) membrane (Millipore, US). The membranes were reacted with antibodies against phosphorylated or nonpho-sphorylated AKT, P-AKT or CyclinD1 (Cell Signaling Technol-ogy, US). Thereafter, specific antigen/antibody complexes were made visible using horseradish peroxidase-conjugated secondary antibodies (Rabbit IgG, Cell Signaling Technology, US) and Immobilon Western Chemiluminescent HRP Substrate (Millipore, US). The images from the immune reaction membrane were digitized. The band intensity of each protein was quantified using NIH Image software.

## Statistical Analysis

All data were represented with mean $(\overline{x})$ ± standard deviation(SD). The statistical significance of the differences among groups was analyzed by one-way ANOVA and SLD (Least-significant difference) with SPSS 17.0. The 5% level of probability was considered to be significant.

## Results

### Dose-response of erlotinib on tumor growth

The effects of various dosages (15, 30, 60 $mg \cdot kg^{-1}$) of erlotinib on tumor growth in tumor-bearing mice gavaged with the drug for twenty days are shown in Table 1. Relative tumor growth was expressed as the tumor volume growth change from the initiation of erlotinib or odium carboxymethyl cellulose treatment. Tumor growth after initiation of erlotinib treatment was significantly suppressed compared with that in the model group given sodium carboxymethyl cellulose ($P<0.05$). The tumor growth of the 30 $mg \cdot kg^{-1}$ and 60 $mg \cdot kg^{-1}$ groups was significantly different from that of the 15 $mg \cdot kg^{-1}$ group. However, no significant difference of tumor growth was found between 30 $mg \cdot kg^{-1}$ and 60 $mg \cdot kg^{-1}$ groups.

**Table 2.** Tumor weight and inhibition rate of each group (n = 10).

| Group | Tumor weight ($\overline{x} \pm s$, g) | Inhibition rate(%) |
|---|---|---|
| Model | 3.93±1.01 | - |
| 8:00 | 2.32±0.68* | 39.58 |
| 12:00 | 2.61±0.54* | 32.03 |
| 16:00 | 1.96±0.77* △ | 48.95 |
| 20:00 | 2.93±0.82* | 23.70 |
| 24:00 | 3.17±0.51 | 17.45 |
| 04:00 | 2.82±0.45* | 26.56 |

$^*P<0.05$ when compared with the model group, $^\triangle P<0.05$ when compared with group 24:00.

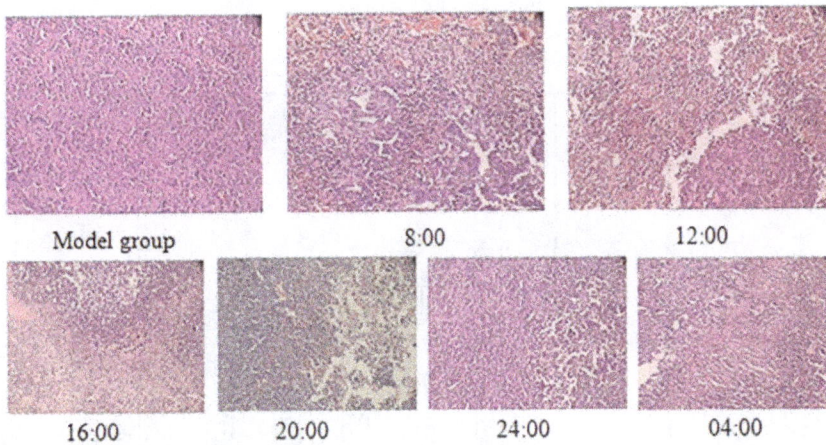

**Figure 2. Microscopic images of pathological observation of tumors formed three weeks after the inoculation of lewis lung carcinoma cells into C57BL/6 mice (HE staining, original magnification ×200).** (Model group): Pathological section from the model group treated with distilled water. The tumor cells were poorly differentiated and arranged tightly, with abundant vessels around them. No obvious tumor cell necrosis could be observed and the boundary was extremely clear. (Groups 8:00, 12:00, 16:00, 20:00): Pathological section from the groups 8:00, 12:00, 16:00 and 20:00 after erlotinib administration. The tumor cells were poorly differentiated and arranged irregularly, with few new vessels around them. Large areas of necrosis, and inflammatory cell infiltration and bleeding were observed. (Groups 24:00 and 04:00): Pathological section from the groups 24:00 and 04:00 given erlotinib at 24:00 and 04:00. Small focal necrosis and inflammatory cell infiltration were observed.

## Influence of dosing times on the antitumor effect of erlotinib

Dosing times showed no significant effect on tumor growth in tumor-bearing mice of the model group (data not shown). Therefore, a mean value from different circadian times was used as the control. The tumor growth after erlotinib treatment (60 mg·kg$^{-1}$) at different times was significantly suppressed in the tumor-bearing mice when compared with that in the model mice given sodium carboxymethyl cellulose ($P<0.05$, Figure 1). Tumor growth in groups 8:00, 12:00, and 16:00 in the light phase was significantly suppressed when compared with that in the dark phase (groups 20:00, 24:00, 04:00), with the effect in group 16:00 being the most effective ($P<0.05$). The tumor weights of group 8:00, 12:00, 16:00, 20:00, 04:00 was significantly suppressed when compared with the model ($P<0.05$, Table 2), and group 16:00 showed the best result.

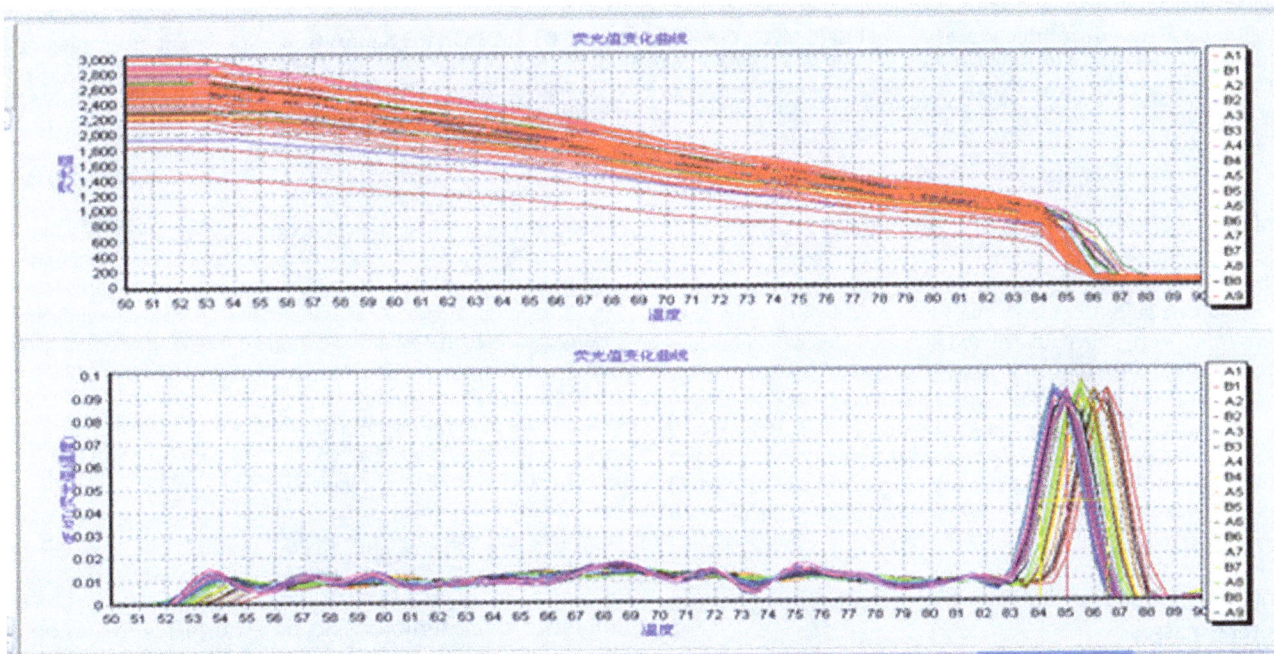

**Figure 3. Dissolution curve of gene expression with qRT-PCR.** There was only one single peak in dissolution curve and it conforms to the annealing temperature. The results of experiment were effective.

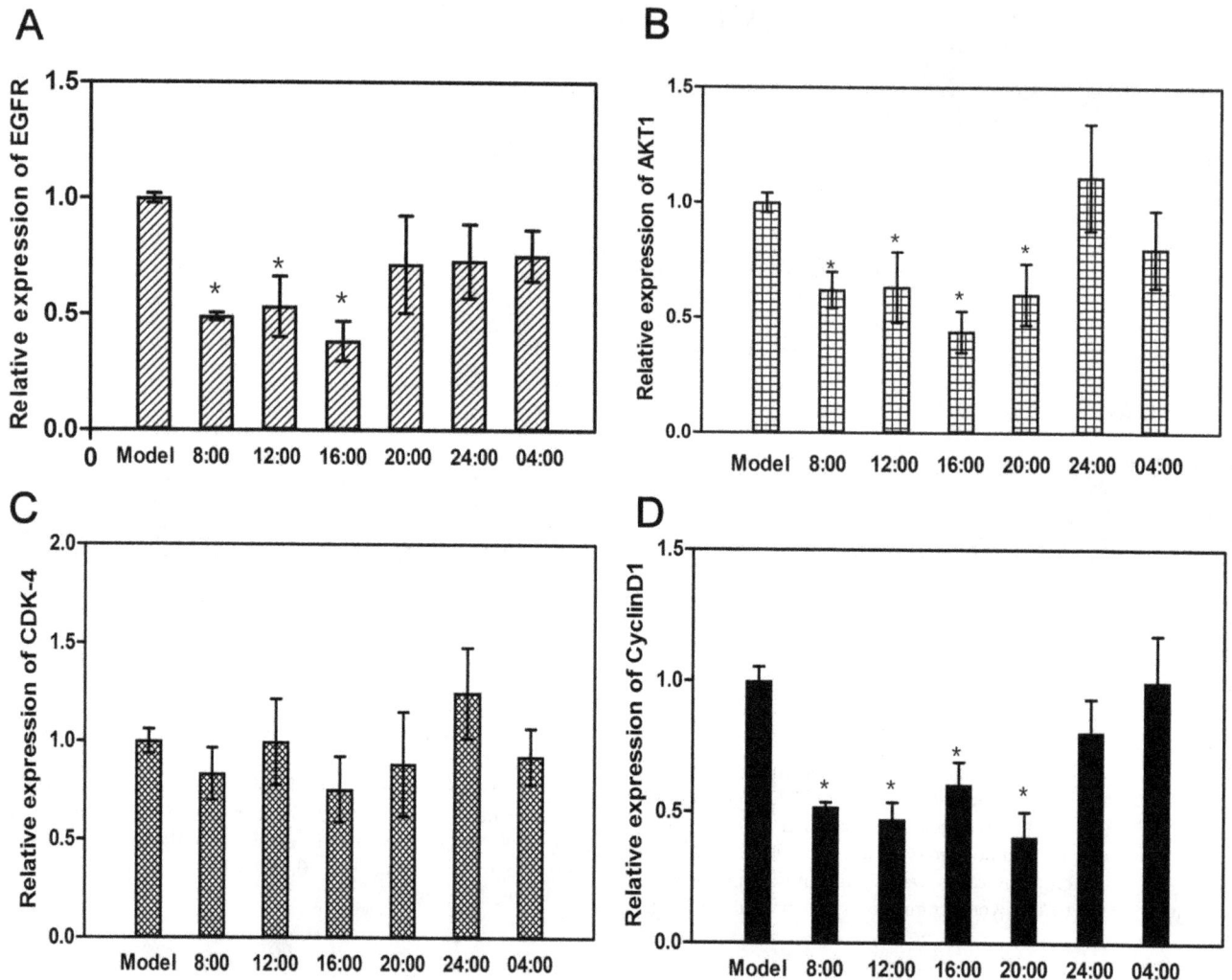

**Figure 4. Relative quantitive expression of EGFR, AKT1, CDK-4, and Cyclin D1 mRNA in the tumors from experiment groups (60 mg/ kg) and model group (distilled water).** Each value is the mean with SD of six mice. (A): The mRNA expression of EGFR in tumors. *$P<0.05$ vs model group. (B): The mRNA expression of AKT1 in tumors. *$P<0.05$ vs model group. (C): The mRNA expression of CDK-4 in tumors. There was no significantly different among these groups. (D): The mRNA expression of Cyclin D1 in tumors. *$P<0.05$ vs model group.

## Influence of dosing times on histopathology

The photographs in Figure 2 show the representative images about sections of tumor tissues, which display significant differences among different time groups. In the model group, the tumor cells were poorly differentiated and arranged closely. No obvious tumor cell necrosis was observed and the boundary was extremely clear. Large areas of necrosis, and inflammatory cell infiltration and bleeding were observed in groups 8:00, 12:00, 16:00, 20:00 and the tumor cells were poorly differentiated and arranged irregularly, with few new vessels around them. In groups 24:00 and 04:00, small focal necrosis and inflammatory cell infiltration were observed.

## Influence of dosing times on the expression of genes in tumor masses

There was only one single peak in the dissolution curve conforming to the annealing temperature (Figure 3), which shows that the results of our experiment were effective. As shown in Figure 4, the expression of EGFR in groups 8:00, 12:00, 16:00 was

significantly lower than that of the model group ($P<0.05$), and that of group 20:00, 24:00, 04:00 had no significant change when compared with the model group ($P>0.05$). The expression of AKT1 in groups 8:00, 12:00, 16:00 and 20:00 was significantly lower than that in the model group ($P<0.05$), the group 16:00 showed the best result ($P<0.05$), and that of groups 24:00 and 04:00 had no significant change when compared with the model group ($P>0.05$). The expression of CDK-4 in all groups was not significantly lower than that in the model group ($P>0.05$). The expression of CyclinD1 in groups 8:00, 12:00, 16:00 and 20:00 was significantly lower when compared with that of the model group ($P<0.05$), and that of groups 24:00 and 04:00 had no significant change when compared with the model group ($P>0.05$).

## Influence of erlotinib dosing time on AKT, P-AKT, and Cyclin D1 protein levels in tumor masses

As shown in Figure 5, the P-AKT protein level in groups 12:00 and 16:00 was significantly lower than that in the model group ($P<0.05$), and it was significantly different between groups 12:00

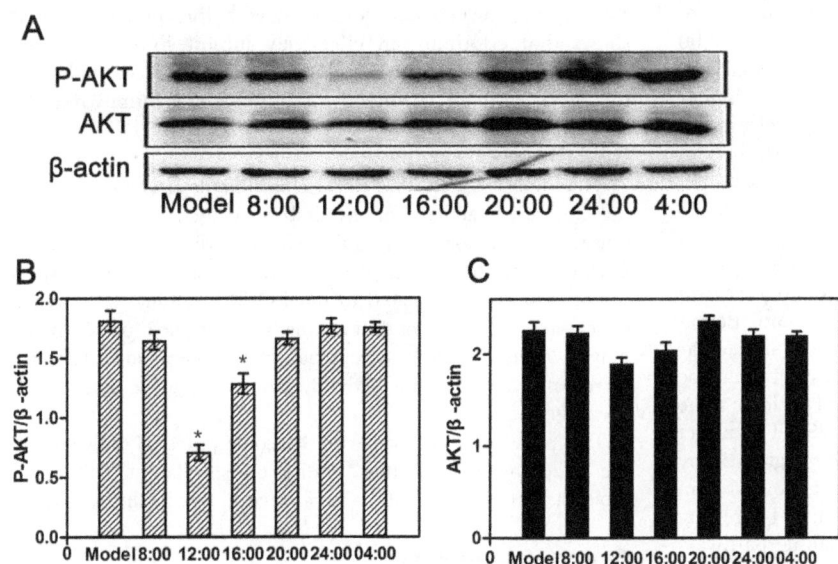

**Figure 5. Influence of dosing times on P-AKT and AKT protein expression (A) or relative P-AKT and AKT protein expression (B and C) in tumor masses after erlotinib (60 mg/kg) administration.** Each value is the mean with SD of six mice. $^*P<0.05$ when compared with the model group.

and 16:00, while the level of AKT remained unchanged ($P>0.05$). As shown in Figure 6, the Cyclin D1 protein level in groups 8:00, 12:00 and 16:00 and 04:00 was significantly lower than that in the model group ($P<0.05$).

## Discussion

Chronochemotherapy, as a new form of chemotherapy, has developed rapidly in the clinical treatment of tumors. It is based on the circadian rhythm of tumor cell synthesis, the related protein

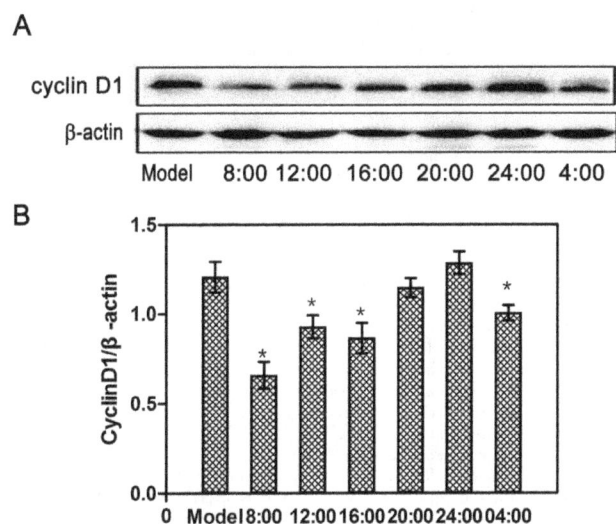

**Figure 6. Influence of dosing times on Cyclin D1 protein expression (A) or relative CyclinD1 protein expression (B) in tumor masses after erlotinib (60 mg/kg) administration.** Each value is the mean with SD of six mice. $^*P<0.05$ when compared with the model group.

factors of drug targets and living organisms themselves. The relationship between the circadian rhythm in drug tolerability and antitumor efficacy constitutes an essential issue for cancer chronotherapy. Studies have shown that chronochemotherapy can significantly prolong the overall survival of cancer patients when compared with conventional chemotherapy and its toxicity can be controlled[23]. Recently, the best times of administration of about 30 drugs have been found, including 5-fluorouracil, methotrexate, vinorelbine, etc [24,25,26]. However, the study on chronopharmacology of molecular targeted drugs has not been reported. As a small molecular-targeted drug, erlotinib has been used for the treatment of advanced NSCLC. Its clinical efficacy has been proved by researches, especially of cancer-related genes and proteins. Erlotinib is effective in treating NSCLC because it can reversibly and competitively inhibits the binding of ATP to the phosphate-binding loop of the ATP site in the intracellular domain of EGFR. By inhibiting the binding of ATP to EGFR, the drug restrains auto-phosphorylation and the activation of downstream signaling pathway further, leading to the inhibition of cell proliferation and inducing apoptosis in NSCLC. Therefore, we chose erlotinib to study, and found that the antitumor effect of erlotinib showed circadian rhythm in our preliminary experiments.

The division, proliferation, and metabolism of cells are related to biological circadian rhythm. Studies[27,28] show that proliferating cells are the most sensitive to anticancer drugs, and DNA synthesis usually peaks between noon and 16:00 and down to the bottom at midnight. Therefore, we selected six hour points, 8:00, 12:00, 16:00 (as the light phase), 20:00, 24:00, 04:00 (as the dark phase), according to the circadian rhythm of DNA synthesis, mouse circadian rhythms and references. Based on the results of dose conversion between human and animals and the preliminary experiments, we selected the doses of 15, 30, and 60 mg·kg$^{-1}$ in our experiment. We investigated the influence of dosing times on the effects of erlotinib to inhibit tumor growth in mice and the underlying mechanism. The results suggested that the antitumor effect of erlotinib showed a significant circadian rhythm with higher levels in the light phase, and the group 16:00 showed the best result. On the contrary, the toxicity of erlotinib showed a significant circadian rhythm with higher levels in the dark phase, especially in the groups 24:00 and 04:00. Generally speaking, the administration of erlotinib in the light phase may be more effective than in the dark phase, which may be related to the different sensitivity of cells to antitumor drugs in different periods.

Until now the mechanism of chronochemotherapy of erlotinib remains unclear. Recent advances identify critical molecular events including that drug metabolism and detoxification controlled by biological rhythms, cell cycle, molecular targets, DNA repair, apoptosis, and angiogenesis. It may be related to drug metabolism, some enzymes of cell cycle or some factors associated with cell signaling pathways[29]. The target of erlotinib is EGFR. Erlotinib inhibits tumor growth by inhibiting EGFR autophosphorylation to block its downstream signal transduction. AKT, CDK-4, and CyclinD1 are the downstream signaling factors of EGFR signaling pathway. Some studies[30] have shown that EGFR plays an important role in angiogenesis, tumor cell metastasis and apoptosis. Based on these findings, we investigated whether the EGFR signaling network was sensitive to the small molecule TKI erlotinib. CyclinD1, G1 phase cyclin, is regulated by growth factors in the cell cycle. It can be combined with CDK4 or CDK6 to form complexes to promote cell proliferation, and lead to tumors when CyclinDl is expressed out of control[31]. In this study, the expression of genes EGFR, AKT, CDK-4, and CyclinD1 and the proteins AKT, p-AKT and CyclinD1 were found to show circadian rhythm on different dosing times. The expressions of these genes or proteins in the light were

significantly lower when compared with the model group. It shows that erlotinib can effectively inhibit EGFR signaling through the AKT pathways. Therefore, we can conclude that the mechanism of chronochemotherapy of erlotinib may be related to the apoptosis pathway mediated by EGFR-AKT-CyclinD1-CDK-4 pathway.

This study suggests that the dosing time-dependent change in the antitumor activity of erlotinib is caused by that in the sensitivity of tumor cells and the circadian rhythm of organisms. Furthermore, the time-dependent changes in the sensitivity of tumor cells may be related to the EGFR signaling pathway. In conclusion, the choice of dosing time based on the diurnal rhythm may help to establish a rational chronotherapeutic strategy, increasing the antitumor activity of the drug in certain clinical situations.

This paper may be not perfect for some practical difficulties in the experiment, so further studies on specific and thorough molecular mechanism will be performed in our further study.

## Acknowledgments

We wish to thank the Department of Pharmacy, Pathology and Laboratory of the NO. 401 Hospital of the PLA for providing us the valuable help. We also wish to thank Yong WANG, Qian SUN, Yongjian SHI, Hui Zhao, Daoyan WANG and Zhaoyan CHEN for their valuable help in our experiment.

## Author Contributions

Conceived and designed the experiments: PW FA ML. Performed the experiments: PW JL BZ PL LL. Analyzed the data: PL XZ LZ. Contributed reagents/materials/analysis tools: ML. Wrote the paper: PL FA ML.

## References

1. Hastings MH, Reddy AB, Maywood ES (2003) A clockwork web: circadian timing in brain and periphery, in health and disease. Nat. Rev. Neurosci 4:649–61.
2. Aschoff J (1963) Comparative physiology: Diurnal rhythms. Annu Rev Physiol 25:581–600.
3. Harbour VL, Weigl Y, Robinson B, Amir S (2013) Comprehensive Mapping of Regional Expression of the Clock Protein PERIOD2 in Rat Forebrain across the 24-h Day. Plos One 8: e76391.
4. Oster H, Baeriswyl S, Van Der Horst GT, Albrecht U (2003) Loss of circadian rhythmicity in aging $mPer1^{-/-}$ $mCry2^{-/-}$ mutant mice. Genes & Development 17:1366–1379.
5. Xian LJ, Jian S, Cao QY, Ye YL, Liu XH, et al. (2002) Circadian Rhythms of DNA Synthesis in Nasopharyngeal Carcinoma Cells. Chronobiol. Int 19 (1):69–76.
6. Hrushesky WJ (1985) Circadian timing of cancer chemotherapy. Science 228:73–75.
7. Ohdo S (2007) Circadian Rhythms in the CNS and Peripheral Clock Disorders: Chronopharmacological Findings on Antitumor Drugs. J Pharmacol Sci 103, 155–158.
8. Herbst RS, Langer CJ (2002) Epidermal growth factor receptors as a target for cancer treatment: the emerging role of IMC-C225 in the treatment of lung,and head and neck cancers. Semin Oncol 29: 27–36.
9. Perez-Soler R (2006) Rash as a surrogate marker for efficacy of epidermal growth factor receptor inhibitors in lung cancer. Clin Lung Cancer 8: S7–S14.
10. Paz-ares L, Sanchez JM, Garcia-Velasco A (2006) A prospective phase II trial of erlotinib in advanced non-small cell lung cell (NSCLC) patients(p) with mutation in the tyrosine kinase (TK) domain of the epidermal growth factor receptor (EGFR). J. Clin Oncol 24: 369–375.
11. Herbst RS, Prager D, Hermann R, Fehrenbacher L, Johnson BE, et al. (2005) TRIBUTE: a phase III trial of erlotinib hydrochloride (OSI-774) combined with carboplatin and paclitaxel chemotherapy in advanced non small cell lung cancer. J Clin Oncol 23(25): 5892–5899.
12. Albanell J, Rojo F, Averbuch S,Feyereislova A, Mascaro JM, et al. (2002) Pharmacodynamic studies of the epidermal growth factor receptor inhibitor ZD1839 in skin from cancer patients: Histopathologic and molecular consequences of receptor inhibition. J Clin Oncol 20:110–124.
13. Smolensky MH, Peppas NA (2007) Chronobiology, drug-delivery, and chronotherapeutics. Adv. Drug Deliv. Rev 59:825–27.
14. Kersemaekers AM, Fleuren GJ, Kenter GG, Van Den Broek LJ, Uljee SM, et al. (1999) Oncogene alterations in carcinomas of the uterine cervix: overexpression of the epidermal growth factor receptor is associated with poor prognosis. Clin Cancer Res 5:577–86.
15. Mendelsohn J (2001) The epidermal growth factor receptor as a target for cancer therapy. Endocr Relat Cancer 8:3–9.
16. Modi S, Seidman AD (2002) An update on epidermal growth factor receptor inhibitors. Curr Oncol Rep 4:47–55.
17. Grunwald V, Hidalgo M (2002) The epidermal growth factor receptor: a new target for anticancer therapy. Curr Probl Cancer 26:109–64.
18. Ritter CA, Arteaga CL (2003) The epidermal growth factor receptor-tyrosine kinase: a promising therapeutic target in solid tumors. Semin Oncol 30:3–11.
19. Darzacq X, Jady BE, Verheggen C, Kiss AM, Bertrand E, et al. (2002) Cajal body-specific small nuclear RNAs: a novel class of 2′-O-methylation and pseudouridylation guide RNAs. EMBO J. 21:2746–2756.
20. Wang XS, Diener K, Jannuzzi D, Trollinger D, Tan TH, et al. (1996) Molecular cloning and characterization of a novel protein kinase with a catalytic domain homologous to mi togen-ctivated protein kinase kinase kinase. J Biol Chem 271: 31607–31611.
21. Xu F, Tian Y, Huang Y, Zhang YY, Guo ZZ, et al (2011) EGFR inhibitous sensitize non-small cell lung cancer cell to TRAIL-induced apoptosis. Chinese Journal of Cancer 30: 701–711.
22. Liu W, Ren H, Ren J, Yin T, Hu B, et al. (2013) The Role of EGFR/PI3K/Akt/cyclinD1 Signaling Pathway in Acquired Middle Ear Cholesteatoma. Mediators of Inflammation Available: http://dx.doi.org/10.1155/2013/651207. Accessed 2013 September 24.
23. Eriguchi M, Levi F, Hisa T, Yanaqie H, Nonaka Y, et al (2003) Chronotherapy for cancer. Biomed Pharmacother (Suppl 1):92.
24. Ohdo S, Inoue K, Yukawa E, Higuchi S, Nakano S, et al. (1997) Chronotoxicity of methotrexate in mice and its relation to circadian rhythm of DNA synthesis and pharmacokinetics. Jpn. J. Pharmacol. 75: 283–290.
25. Filipski E, Amat S, Lemaigre G, Vincenti M, Breillout F, et al. (1999) Relationship between circadian rhythm of vinorelbion toxicity and efficacy in P388-bearing mice. J Pharmacol Exp Ther 289(1):231–235.
26. Patel DM, Jani RH, Patel CN (2011) Design and evaluation of colon targeted modified puldincap delivery of 5-fluorouracil according to circadian rhythm. Int J Pharm Investig 1(3): 172–181.
27. Bjamason GA, Jordan R (2002) Rhythms in Human gastrointestinal Mucosa and Skin. Chronobiol Int 19(1):129–140.

28. Smaaland R, Sothem RB, Laerum OD, Abrahamsen JF (2002) Laerum Rhythms in human bone marrow and blood cells. Chronobiol Int 19(1):101–127.

29. Abolmaali K, Balakrishnan A, Stearns AT, Rounds J, Rhoads DB, et al (2009) Circadian variation in intestinal dihydropyrimidine dehydrogenase(DPD) expression: A potential mechanism for benefits of 5-FU chronochemotherapy. Surgery 146(2):269–273.

30. Wei Q, Sheng L, Shui Y, Hu Q, Nordqren H, et al. (2008) EGFR, HER2, and HER3 Exp ression in Laryngeal Primary Tumors and Corresponding Metastases. Ann Surg Oncol 15 (4): 1193–1201.

31. Morshed K, Skomra D, Korobowicz E, Szymariski M, Polz-Dacewicz M, et al. (2007) An immunohistochemical study of cyclinD1 protein exp ression in laryngeal squamous cell carcinoma. Acta Otolaryngol 127 (7):760–769.

# Expression of Neuron-Specific Enolase in Multiple Myeloma and Implications for Clinical Diagnosis and Treatment

**Haiping Yang[1,2◐], Ruihua Mi[1◐], Qian Wang[1], Xudong Wei[1]\*, Qingsong Yin[1], Lin Chen[1], Xinghu Zhu[1], Yongping Song[1]**

**1** Department of Hematology, Tumor Hospital of Zhengzhou University, Zhengzhou City, China, **2** Department of Hematology, First Affiliated Hospital of Henan University of Science and Technology, Zhengzhou City, China

## Abstract

*Objective:* To determine the expression of neuron-specific enolase (NSE) in patients with multiple myeloma (MM) and to evaluate its clinical value as a tumor marker and, an indicator of disease progression and treatment efficacy.

*Methods:* Using electrochemiluminescence immunoassay (ECLIA), we measured the serum levels of NSE in 47 healthy subjects (control group), 25 patients with small cell lung cancer (lung cancer group), and 52 patients with MM (MM group). For the MM group, serum NSE levels were measured and other disease indicators and related symptoms were monitored before and after chemotherapy. The relationship between NSE expression and other MM-related factors was analyzed. In addition, immunohistochemical staining was performed on bone marrow biopsy specimens from patients with MM.

*Results:* In the control group, serum NSE levels were within the normal range as previously reported, while the lung cancer group and the untreated MM group exhibited NSE levels that were significantly higher relative to the control group ($P < 0.05$). The difference in NSE expression between the lung cancer group and untreated MM group was statistically significant ($P < 0.05$). NSE levels were significantly decreased in MM patients after chemotherapy and were positively correlated with an MM disease index [beta-2 microglobulin ($\beta_2$-MG)]. Changes in NSE were not related to the response rate to chemotherapy but rather were correlated with progression-free survival.

*Conclusions:* Patients with MM may have increased serum NSE levels, and changes in NSE may provide insight into treatment efficacy of chemotherapy and disease progression. Perhaps NSE expression is a viable biomarker for MM and can be a useful reference for the design and adjustment of clinical MM treatment programs.

**Editor:** Maria Fiammetta Romano, Federico II University, Naples, Italy

**Funding:** This study was supported by the National Natural Science Foundation of China (NO. 81170520) and the Henan Department of Health Provincial-Departmental collaboration project (NO. 2011010014). The funders had no role in study design, data collection and analysis, decision to publish, or preparation of the manuscript.

**Competing Interests:** The authors have declared that no competing interests exist.

\* E-mail: xudongwei@zzu.edu.cn

◐ These authors contributed equally to this work.

## Introduction

Multiple myeloma (MM) is a malignant plasma cell disease typified by clonal plasma cells in the bone marrow (plasma cell neoplasms) and is associated with end-organ damage, including bone damage, and the presence of monoclonal protein (M protein) in the serum or urine [1–4]. Treatment efficacy and recurrence can be monitored by measuring the proportion of plasma cells in bone marrow by puncture or biopsy, M protein levels in serum and urine, immune electrophoresis, and the range, number and progression of osteolytic lesions [5]. Also, the levels of blood beta-2 microglobulin ($\beta_2$-MG), albumin, and urine light chain are used to determine therapeutic efficacy and disease progression [6]. The natural disease course of MM ranges widely from a few months to more than 20 years, and the response to treatment is variable. Recently, functional imaging tools, such as F-18 fluorodeoxyglu-cose (FDG) positron emission tomography (PET), have been considered for the assessment of responses [7]. However, application of this technique is quite limited due to the high cost. Therefore, the key to treatment success is to offer patients with an accurate prognosis and to adopt the appropriate treatment strategy after diagnosis.

It is becoming increasingly apparent that the identification of tumor markers is valuable in the diagnosis and treatment of various diseases [1]. Indeed, some markers have become important inference indices for cancer patients. For instance, in lung cancer, tumor markers can aid in the diagnosis of pathological type, stage, metastasis, recurrence, and prognosis. Neuron-specific enolase (NSE) is one of these markers and its application in clinical practice has been gradually increasing in recent years with significant diagnostic value [2–4].

Enolase is an enzyme that catalyzes the decomposition of glycerol in the glycolytic pathway and consists of three subunits ($\alpha$, $\beta$, $\gamma$) and five isozymes ($\alpha\alpha$, $\beta\beta$ $\gamma\gamma$, $\alpha\gamma$, $\beta\gamma$) [3]. The isozymes containing a $\gamma$ subunit are found in neuronal and endocrine tissue, and thus are known as the neuron-specific enolases (NSE). NSE has been implicated in tumorigenesis with neuroendocrine origin. Japanese scholars Jimbo et al. [1] and Nakajima et al. [2] and British scholars Sharma et al. [3] each reported a case where a patient with MM exhibited increased levels of NSE. In China, there are very few reports evaluating NSE levels in MM patients. Zhang et al. [4] reported that patients with MM who had increased NSE levels had a poorer prognosis than those patients with normal NSE levels. Patients with elevated NSE levels exhibited shorter overall survival and decreased progression-free survival. Moreover, although there was no correlation between NSE expression level and age, gender, M protein type, hemoglobin, or serum creatinine, there was a significant correlation between NSE expression and the abundance of myeloma plasma cells and blood $\beta_2$-MG expression level [4]. COX analysis suggested that the levels of NSE and $\beta_2$-MG are two independent prognostic factors that affect the survival of MM. Gao et al. [8] reported that NSE expression was increased in the U266 myeloma cell line and in 67% of MM patients. In addition, NSE expression trended upward as disease severity progressed and the degree of bone destruction increased. In this study, we examined the level of NSE in 52 MM patients before and after chemotherapy. In addition, we monitored the disease condition and efficacy of therapeutic intervention. Taken together, we sought to determine the relationship between NSE and MM, and to evaluate the viability of NSE as a biomarker for the diagnosis, treatment evaluation, and prognosis of MM.

## Patients and Methods

### 1 Subjects

**1.1 Control group.** Forty-seven healthy were included in the control group and underwent physical examination. The group consisted of 29 males and 18 females with a median age of 37 (28–59) years old. ECLIA was used to detect tumor biomarkers in the following systems: respiratory, digestive, genitourinary, endocrine systems, etc. The physical examination included imaging, blood test, biochemistry analysis, infectious disease, immunization, electrocardiogram, and other tests. Those individuals without abnormalities in these tests were enrolled in the healthy control group.

**1.2 Small cell lung cancer group.** Twenty-five patients with small cell lung cancer were included in this group. These patients were hospitalized in the Department of Medical Oncology of our hospital between March 2009 and August 2010. They had clear pathological diagnosis and were composed of 21 males and four females with a median age of 53 (36–80) years old.

**1.3 MM group.** All 52 patients in this group were hospitalized with MM in either our hospital or the First Affiliated Hospital of Henan University of Science and Technology between May 2010 and April 2013, including 26 males and 26 females with a median age of 53 (47–62) years old. Hospitalization examinations were performed to confirm the diagnosis of MM, according to the diagnostic criteria defined in references [5,6]. These included bone marrow biopsy, ECT whole body bone scan (or CT, PET-CT, or other imaging methods), blood count, blood chemistry, blood tumor marker testing, serum protein electrophoresis, and immunofixation electrophoresis.

**1.4 MM treatment programs.** All MM patients were treated with either TD (thalidomide and dexamethasone) or VD

(Velcade plus dexamethasone)-based programs for three courses of chemotherapy, combined with or without mitoxantrone, THP topiramate Star, cyclophosphamide, and etoposide. In patients with elevated NSE levels, 28 adopted the TD-based program (NSE+/T) and six adopted the VD-based program (NSE+/V). In patients with normal NSE levels, 14 adopted the TD program (NSE-/T) and four adopted the VD program (NSE-/V). The difference in choosing either program between the NSE+ and NSE- patient groups was not statistically significant (P = 0.723).

## 2 Research Methods

**Ethics statement.** Informed consent was obtained from all the patients in writing prior to enrollment in the study. This study was performed in strict accordance with the ethical guidelines of the Declaration of Helsinki, and the protocol was approved by the institutional Ethics Committee of Henan Cancer Hospital.

**2.1 Equipment.** Roche Elecsys 2010 (Basel, Switzerland) was used for electrochemiluminescence detection. KDC-2046 low-speed refrigerated centrifuge (Henan, China) was purchased from Anhui Zhongjia Co., Ltd.

**2.2 Reagents.** Reagents specific for ECLIA detection on Roche Elecsys 2010 included NSE detection kit, cleaning fluid (ISE Cleaning Solution), system reagent (Procell), standard solution, and quality control reagent (PreciControl Tumor Marer).

**2.3 NSE detection method.** For ECLIA detection of NSE, four ml of fasting blood was taken from patients in the morning prior to eating and drinking. After coagulation, blood serum was separated at 3000 rpm, and NSE concentration was measured within two hours after separation in strict accordance with the user manual guidelines of the Roche Elecsys 2010 and the NSE electrochemical luminescence detection kit. NSE levels were read automatically on Elecsys 2010. As for detection value criteria, the normal detection range was set from zero to 15 ng/ml, and any values beyond the normal range were considered positive.

In addition, NSE levels were examined by immunohistochemistry in bone marrow biopsy specimens from patients with previously untreated MM. All tissues were fixed in 10% neutral formalin and paraffin-embedded after routine dehydration. Five to six serial sections were prepared with a thickness of four μm. Sections were dewaxed and treated with fresh 3% $H_2O_2$ to block endogenous peroxidase. After rinsing three times with PBS for three min, citric acid antigen retrieval was performed under high pressure. The slices were blocked with normal goat serum for 30 min at room temperature to eliminate nonspecific staining, followed by incubation with primary antibody solution (Abcam, Cambridge, UK) at 4°C overnight. After recovery for 40 min at room temperature, ready-to-use secondary antibody solution (rabbit anti-mouse secondary antibody, Zhongshan Golden Bridge, Beijing, China) was added dropwise to the slices and incubated at room temperature for 40 min followed by three PBS washes for 3 min. DAB reagent was added dropwise to the slices afterwards and developed at room temperature. Slices were observed under a microscope for three to five min to determine the optimal developing time, after which slices were rinsed with tap water, stained with hematoxylin for 90 seconds, differentiated with the hydrochloric acid solution, and treated with saturated aqueous lithium carbonate for blue nuclear staining. Slices were mounted with neutral gum after routine dehydration and observed under a microscope. A positive result was determined by evaluating both staining intensity and positive rates. If the positive rate was less than 10% with weak staining, it was labeled as negative; if the positive rate was greater or equal to 10% with strong brownish-yellow granules, it was labeled as positive.

**Table 1.** Correlation analysis of serum NSE levels and IHC results.

| Patient No. | 1 | 2 | 3 | 4 | 5 | 6 | 7 | 8 | 9 | 10 | 11 | 12 | 13 |
|---|---|---|---|---|---|---|---|---|---|---|---|---|---|
| NSE (ng/ml) | 14.34 | 11.89 | 14.34 | 23.43 | 25.64 | 33.43 | 80.34 | 32.54 | 13.46 | 38.54 | 25.43 | 50.32 | 28.65 |
| IHC result | - | - | - | + | + | + | + | + | + | + | + | + | + |
| Patient No. | 14 | 15 | 16 | 17 | 18 | 19 | 20 | 21 | 22 | 23 | 24 | 25 | 26 |
| NSE (ng/ml) | 22.43 | 12.43 | 14.75 | 24.86 | 24.3 | 38.3 | 9.643 | 14.2 | 12.64 | 40.4 | 26.79 | 49.17 | 29.6 |
| IHC result | - | - | + | + | + | + | - | + | - | + | - | + | + |
| Patient No. | 27 | 28 | 29 | 30 | 31 | 32 | 33 | 34 | 35 | 36 | 37 | 38 | 39 |
| NSE (ng/ml) | 23.77 | 21.48 | 13.64 | 28.96 | 12.54 | 11.65 | 13.87 | 13.26 | 16.88 | 7.23 | 22.76 | 20.21 | 27.82 |
| IHC result | + | + | - | + | - | - | + | - | - | - | + | + | + |
| Patient No. | 40 | 41 | 42 | 43 | 44 | 45 | 46 | 47 | 48 | 49 | 50 | 51 | 52 |
| NSE (ng/ml) | 25.12 | 30.54 | 12.53 | 33.05 | 21.16 | 33.98 | 79.27 | 13.68 | 20.04 | 8.65 | 21.12 | 30.78 | 25.38 |
| IHC result | + | + | - | + | + | + | + | - | + | - | + | + | + |

Note: +, IHC result positive; -, IHC result negative.

Spearman's statistical analysis shows rr = 0.692, p<0.05, indicating that NSE serum levels in MM patients were positively correlated with the IHC results.

**Table 2.** Comparison of serum NSE levels between small cell lung cancer group and control group.

| Indicator(ng/ml) | Group | Cases(n) | Percentile | | | Range | Z | P |
|---|---|---|---|---|---|---|---|---|
| | | | 25th | 50th | 75th | | | |
| NSE | Control | 47 | 8.11 | 9.33 | 10.8 | 5.73–14.40 | 6.937 | P<0.05 |
| | Lung cancer | 25 | 30.86 | 44.6 | 95.85 | 13.91–370.0 | | |

**Table 3.** Comparison of serum NSE levels between MM group and control group.

| Indicator(ng/ml) | Group | Cases(n) | Percentile | | | | Z | P |
| | | | 25th | 50th | 75th | Range | | |
|---|---|---|---|---|---|---|---|---|
| NSE | Control | 47 | 8.11 | 9.33 | 10.8 | 5.73–14.40 | 5.356 | P<0.05 |
| | Lung cancer | 52 | 13.72 | 23.10 | 30.31 | 7.23–880.34 | | |

**Table 4.** Comparison of serum NSE levels between small cell lung cancer group and MM group.

| Indicator(ng/ml) | Group | Cases(n) | Percentile | | | | Z | P |
| | | | 25th | 50th | 75th | Range | | |
|---|---|---|---|---|---|---|---|---|
| NSE | Lung cancer | 25 | 30.86 | 44.6 | 95.85 | 13.91–370.0 | 2.739 | P<0.05 |
| | Lung cancer | 52 | 13.72 | 23.10 | 30.31 | 7.23–880.34 | | |

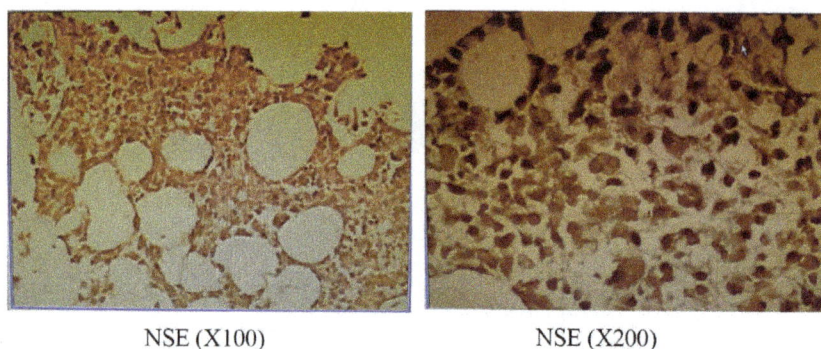

NSE (X100)　　　　　　　　　NSE (X200)

**Figure 1. NSE immunohistochemical results of patients with previously untreated MM.**

We also used reverse transcriptase polymerase chain reaction (RT-PCR) to detect NSE transcript levels in the bone marrow of patients. Two ml bone marrow samples were extracted by bone marrow biopsy from previously untreated MM patients and control healthy subjects. Mononuclear cells were enriched by density gradient centrifugation. Trizol extraction of total RNA was performed followed by PCR (Takara DRR002B). The upstream primer sequence for NSE: 5′-GACTGAGGACACATT-CATTGCTGAC-3′; downstream primer sequence: 5′-CAGCA-CACTGGGATTACGGAAG-3′. Eight μl reaction product together with 2 μl loading buffer was resolved on a 2% agarose ethidium bromide (EB)containing gel by electrophoresis. Results were documented under a UV transmission reflectometer.

### 3 Monitoring of patient condition indices

Prior to each course of chemotherapy, weekly routine preoperative examinations were performed on each patient. These included blood count, liver function, renal function, $\beta_2$-MG, serum NSE, serum protein electrophoresis, immunofixation electrophoresis, serum immunoglobulin (IgG, IgA and IgM) quantification, light chain $(\kappa,\lambda)$ quantification, and bone marrow cell morphology. Meanwhile MM-associated symptoms, such as bone destruction, infection, high viscosity syndrome, anemia, hypercalcemia, and renal damage, were monitored and recorded.

### 4 Statistical analysis

SPSS16.0 software (Armonk, NY, USA) was used for statistical analysis. Because NSE level data in the control group, lung cancer group, and MM group exhibited a skewed distribution, percentiles were chosen for data presentation. Comparisons between the lung cancer group and control group, the MM group and control group, and the lung cancer group and the MM group were

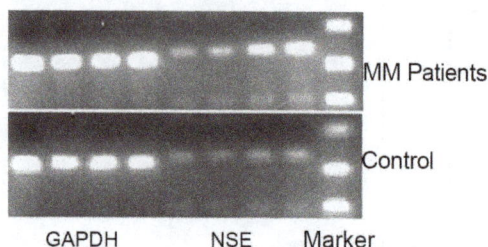

**Figure 2. RT-PCR product electrophoresis for GAPDH (control and NSE) in previously untreated MM patients and controls.**

analyzed by rank-sum test. The correlation between NSE level in MM patients and the amount of the prognostic indicator $\beta_2$-MG was analyzed by Spearman's rank test.

### Results

1

Among the 52 MM patients evaluated, 34 exhibited increased serum NSE levels, accounting for 65.4% of all patients with MM. Spearman's statistical analysis showed r = 0.692, p<0.05 (Table 1), indicating that NSE serum levels in MM patients were positively correlated with IHC results.

### 2 Comparison of serum NSE levels between the control and small cell lung cancer groups (Table 2)

As shown in Table 2, the serum NSE level in the control group all fell within the normal range, whereas the level in lung cancer group were significantly higher at the level of third percentile (P< 0.05).

### 3 Comparison of serum NSE levels between the control and MM groups (Table 3)

As shown in Table 3, NSE serum levels in 18 cases in the MM group were negative. However, at the level of third percentile, NSE levels of the MM group were significantly higher than those of the control group (P<0.05).

### 4 Comparison of serum NSE levels between the small cell lung cancer and MM groups (Table 4)

As shown in Table 4, at the level of third percentile, NSE levels in the small cell lung cancer group were significantly higher than those of the MM group (P<0.05).

5

Immunohistochemistry for NSE in patients with previously untreated MM (Figure 1) reveals clear brownish-yellow granules in cytoplasm with a positive rate of 45%.

6

RT-PCR was used to determine if RNA transcript levels of NSE were elevated in the bone marrow of untreated patients diagnosed with MM. Relative to healthy controls, MM patients exhibited elevated levels of NSE. GAPDH was used as an internal control, and its levels were unchanged between the two groups (Figure 2).

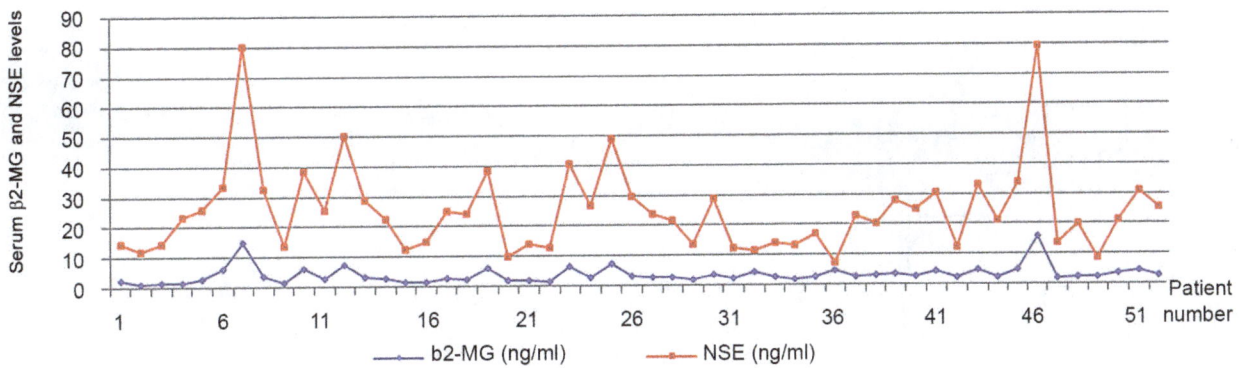

**Figure 3. Correlation between NSE level in patients with previously untreated MM and the amount of the prognostic indicator β2-MG.**

## 7 Correlation between NSE level in patients with previously untreated MM and the amount of the prognostic indicator β2-MG (Figure 3)

According to Spearman's rank test, r = 0.749, P<0.01, there is a significant positive correlation between β2-MG and NSE levels in MM patients.

## 8 Correlation between NSE level and the amount of prognostic indicator β2-MG in MM patients after receiving three courses of chemotherapy (Figure 4)

According to Spearman's rank test, r = 0.618, P<0.01, there is even after chemotherapy a strong positive correlation between β2-MG and NSE levels in MM patients.

## 9 Correlation between NSE level in MM patients and treatment response

After three courses of chemotherapy, the overall response rate (ORR) of the group with elevated NSE levels was 15/28 (53.6%), and three out of 28 patients (10.7%) achieved very good partial response (VGPR). In the group with normal NSE levels, the ORR was 10/14 (71.4%) and two patients (14.3%) achieved VGPR. In the group of patients with elevated NSE levels who adopted the TD-based program (NSE+/T group), the treatment was effective in 15 patients and the ORR was 53.6%. In the group of patients

with elevated NSE levels who adopted the VD-based program (NSE+/V group), the treatment was effective in four patients and the ORR was 66.7%. In the group of patients with normal NSE levels who adopted the TD-based program (NSE-/T group), the treatment was effective in 10 patients and the ORR was 71.4%. In the group of patients with normal NSE levels who adopted the VD-based program (NSE-/V group), all four patients showed effective response. The difference in treatment efficiency between groups with elevated serum NSE levels and the ones with normal NSE levels was not statistically significant (P>0.05).

## 10 Correlation between NSE level in MM patients and progression-free survival (PFS)

The median PFS in patients with elevated and normal serum NSE levels was five months and 13 months, respectively. The difference in PFS was statistically significant (P<0.01) (Figure 5).

## Discussion

To date, there are only a few published studies regarding elevated NSE levels in MM. Jimbo *et al.* [1] reported increased serum NSE level in a 53-year-old female patient diagnosed with IgG-λ type MM with a chest-wall plasmacytoma. Immunostaining of her bone marrow smears and left chest-wall tumor biopsy specimens revealed diffused cytoplasmic NSE staining in the abnormal plasma cells, confirming that myeloma cells can produce

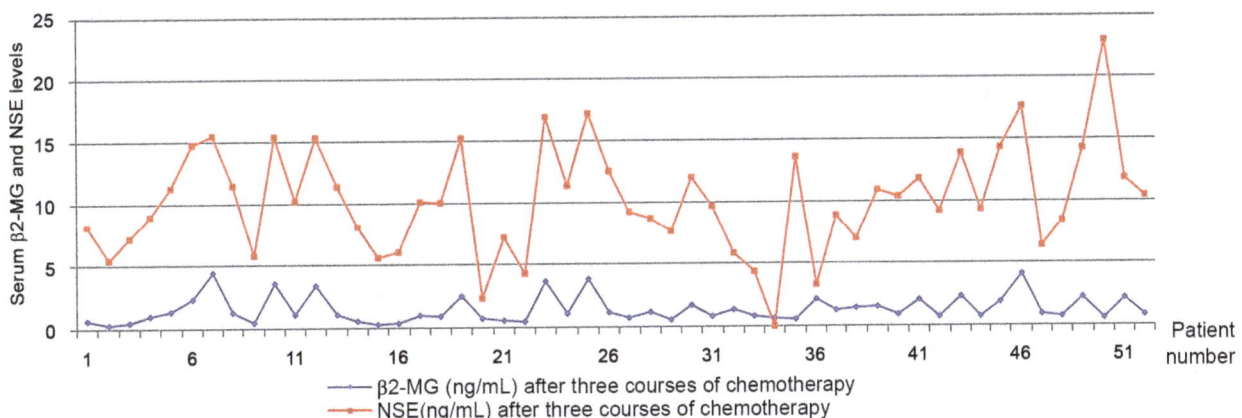

**Figure 4. Correlation between NSE level and the amount of prognostic indicator β2-MG in MM patients after receiving three courses of chemotherapy.**

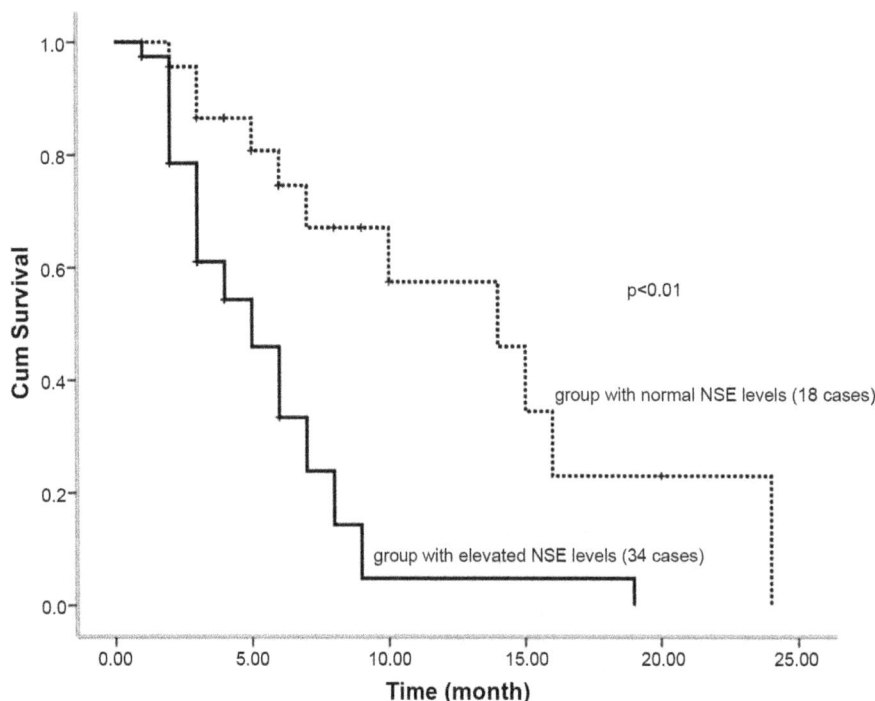

**Figure 5. Correlation between NSE level in MM patients and progression-free survival (PFS).**

NSE. After several cycles of chemotherapy, along with the disappearance of chest-wall plasmacytoma and plasma cells in the bone marrow, her serum NSE level returned to normal. Coincidentally, another Japanese group [2] reported a case of a 68-year-old patient with IgD-λ type MM exhibiting significantly elevated levels of serum NSE. Immunohistochemical staining confirmed NSE expression in myeloma cells. NSE level in this patient was reduced to normal after two cycles of combined interferon-α and vincristine, melphalan, cyclophosphamide, and prednisone (VMCP) chemotherapy. British scholars Sharma *et al.* [3] reported a case of a 75-year-old male patient who was initially hospitalized with sacral pain was diagnosed with prostate cancer. Following chemotherapy, the patient presented with multiple sites of bone pain, hypercalcemia, positive urine for B-J proteins, and elevated serum NSE. Bone marrow biopsy showed atypical plasma cells comprising 20–30% of the nucleated cells. In addition, immunohistochemical staining showed positive staining for CD138, κ light chain, and NSE. The patient was diagnosed with IgG-κ type MM and was treated with cyclophosphamide, thalidomide, and dexamethasone. Moreover, Japanese scholars reported detection of NSE expression in MM cell lines and primary cells by immunohistochemistry and PCR, further confirming the association of NSE expression with MM [9].

In the present study, 34 of the 52 MM patients examined showed elevated NSE levels in the initial detection of NSE. Following chemotherapy, NSE levels exhibited a downward trend. This was particularly true in patients treated with Velcade, a finding consistent with the downward trend of another MM monitoring indicator blood $\beta_2$-MG concentration. There was a significant positive correlation between NSE and $\beta_2$-MG levels. Although no significant correlation was detected, we observed that elevated NSE levels were often present in patients with severe bone pain symptoms or when the symptoms worsened. In contrast, NSE levels were not significantly related to other MM symptoms, such as anemia, hyperviscosity, and hypercalcemia. Consistent with

previous reports, it is important to note that the PFS of patients with elevated NSE levels was significantly shorter than patients with normal levels of NSE. However, the overall survival data was not included for analysis since in all cases the observation time was less than three years, and the tumor burden in patients with disease progression had decreased to some extent after induction of remission therapy. These patients continue to be followed clinically, and the total sample size will continue to expand in order to study the correlation between NSE level and five year overall survival and the impact of different treatment programs on NSE level.

We also observed with the conduct of chemotherapy that MM indices such as proportion of plasma cells and M protein level declined. In parallel, individual NSE levels in each patient also decreased, suggesting that it can be used as an indicator for condition monitoring. The reason for the decline in NSE level with chemotherapy could be that during the process of tumor cell growth, the cell cycle is accelerated and glycolysis is strengthened. NSE is an acidic protease that is involved in glycolysis to catalyze the conversion of β-glycerophosphate into dihydroxy acetone phosphate. Therefore, the upregulation of intracellular NSE in tumor cells leads to increased release of NSE into the blood and results in increased level of serum NSE. Mature plasma cells are the dominant tumor cell type in the majority of myeloma, and the proportion of cells remaining in the cell division cycle is very small [10]. Plasma cell labeling index (PCLI) is a representative of plasma cell DNA synthesis and reflects the progression state of myeloma, and it is an important indicator of prognosis of patients with MM [11]. We speculate that, similar to PCLI, NSE does not primarily reflect the overall myeloma cell load but dynamically reflects the proliferation of myeloma cells. Therefore, NSE levels may become a new prognostic indicator. Importantly, since detection of NSE is simple and relatively inexpensive, NSE may be a more valuable clinical application than PCLI and can be incorporated into the routine examination of neoplastic diseases.

Consistent with previous studies, we found that the level of NSE was significantly higher in patients with untreated small cell lung cancer. It is widely agreed that the NSE level is a reliable indicator for the differential diagnosis of small cell lung cancer and a useful measure for the monitoring of the therapeutic efficacy of radiotherapy and chemotherapy [12–15]. For diagnosis of neuroblastoma, sensitivity of NSE measurements can be up to 90% and have also been used to monitor treatment efficacy and relapse [16]. Increased NSE expression has also been linked to a small number of tumor cell lines, including non-small cell lung cancers, medullary thyroid carcinoma, and pheochromocytoma [17]. Several studies have found that NSE can be used as a sensitive and specific indicator for brain damage, and increases in NSE reflect the size and severity of brain damage [18–19]. An increase in NSE has been found in cerebral ischemia and neuronal injury due to a variety of reasons, such as neonatal asphyxia, pediatric febrile seizures, brain infectious diseases, chronic obstructive pulmonary disease, cerebral infarction, cerebral hemorrhage, systemic lupus erythematosus, Wilson's degeneration, and depression. Bai *et al.* reported that the NSE levels in patients with lymphoma were significantly increased [20]. In addition, increased NSE was seen in patients with extramedullary hemolysis, such as autoimmune hemolytic anemia and paroxysmal nocturnal hemoglobinuria, and can be used as a diagnostic indicator to distinguish *in situ* and extramedullary hemolysis [21].

However, even though there was a multitude of research regarding NSE levels in numerous types of cancer and other disease, there was little data available in the Chinese literature regarding NSE levels in MM. One study by Zhang *et al.* [5] reported that MM patients with increased NSE levels had shorter overall survival, less progression-free survival, and a poorer prognosis than those with normal NSE levels. Consistent with this report, we observed in our study that the PFS of patients with elevated NSE levels was significantly shorter than patients with normal levels of NSE.

Given our data regarding the correlation between NSE level and MM condition changes and in consideration of the above-mentioned studies abroad, we propose that serum NSE levels in patients with multiple myeloma can be increased to varying degrees. NSE levels may not be useful for MM diagnosis or therapeutic evaluation but for the prognosis. However, due to the limited number of cases in this study, confirmation of our conclusions regarding the use of NSE as a prognostic indicator in multiple myeloma will require long-term, large-scale prospective clinical observation.

## Author Contributions

Conceived and designed the experiments: YS XW. Performed the experiments: QW RM HY. Analyzed the data: RM QY LC. Contributed reagents/materials/analysis tools: XZ. Wrote the paper: RM HY.

## References

1. Jimbo J, Sato K, Ikuta K, Inamura J, Hosoki T, et al (2006) A neuron specific enolase-producing multiple myeloma. Rinsho Ketsueki 10: 1381–1386.
2. Nakajima T, Noguchi T, Kumahara Y, Sugihara A, Yamazaki T, et al. (1995) Neuron specific enolase- producing IgD multiple myeloma with high serum amylase activity. Rinsho Ketsueki 36: 359–364.
3. Sharma RA, Wotherspoon AC, Cook G, Morgan GJ, Huddart RA (2006) Neuron-specific enolase expression in multiple myeloma. Lancet Oncol 7: 960.
4. Zhang Y, Hou J, Wei W, Guo Lieping, Shi Haotian, et al. (2012)Serum neuron-specific enolase activity on the prognosis of patients with multiple myeloma. Chinese Journal of Hematology 33:417–419.
5. Zhang Z, Shen T (2007) Diagnosis of blood diseases and treatment standards. 3rd edition, Beijing: Science Press. p232–235.
6. Multiple myeloma working group in China (2008) Multiple myeloma treatment guidelines. Chinese Journal of Internal Medicine 47: 869–872.
7. Bredella MA, Steinbach L, Caputo G, Segall G, Hawkins R (2005) Value of FDG PET in the assessment of patients with multiple myeloma. AJR Am J Roentgenol 184:1199–1204.
8. Gao W, Li H, Li X, Li Bin, He Di, et al. (2012)Expression of NSE in myeloma-related bone diseases. Journal of Chinese General Practice 10: 337–338.
9. Liu Sq, Otsuyama Ki, Ma Z, Abroun S, Shamsasenjan K, et al. (2007) Induction of Multilineage Markers in Human Myeloma Cells and Their Down-Regulation by Interleukin 6. Hematology 85: 49–58.
10. Song S, Chen Y (2004) Williams Hematology. Beijing: People's Health Publishing House. p1342–1368.
11. Zhang Z, Yang T, Hao Y (2003) Hematology. 1st edition. Beijing: People's Health Publishing House. 1341–1359.
12. Ebert W, Muley T, Drings P (1996)Does the assessment of serum markers in patients with lung cancer aid in the clinical decision making process? Anticancer Res 16:2161–2168.

13. Lamy PJ, Grenier J, Kramar A, Pujol JL (2000) Pro-gastrin-releasing peptide, neuron specific enolase and chromogranin A as serum markers of small cell lung cancer. Lung Cancer 29:197–203.
14. Jorgensen LG, Osterlind K, Genolla J, Gomm SA, Hernandez JR, et al. (1996)Serum neuron-specific enolase (S-NSE) and the prognosis in small-cell lung cancer (SCLC): a combined multivariable analysis on data from nine centres. Br J Cancer 74:463–467.
15. Pinson P, Joos G, Watripont P, Brusselle G, Pauwels R (1997) Serum neuron-specific enolase as a tumor marker in the diagnosis and follow-up of small-cell lung cancer. Respiration 64:102–107.
16. Riley RD, Heney D, Jones DR, Sutton AJ, Lambert PC (2004) A systematic review of molecular and biological tumor markers in neuroblastoma. Clin Cancer Res 10:4–12.
17. Zhang Q, Xu J, Wang Y (2005)Expression of human neuron-specific enolase expression in tumor cell lines and its significance. Chinese Journal of Laboratory Medicine 28: 728–731.
18. Bohmer AE, Oses JP, Schmidt AP, Peron CS, Krebs CL, et al. (2011) Neuron-specific enolase, S100B, and glial fibrillary acidic protein levels as outcome predictors in patients with severe traumatic brain injury. Neurosurgery 68:1624–1630.
19. Woertgen C, Rothoerl RD, Wiesmann M, Missler U, Brawanski A (2002) Glial and neuronal serum markers after controlled cortical impact injury in the rat. Acta Neurochir Suppl 81:205–207.
20. Bai Y, Wu D, Liu Y, et al. (2009) The value of serum neuron-specific enolase in the diagnosis of lymphoma. Clinical Hematology 22:379–380.
21. Chen K, Ding B, Zhu J, et al. (2010) NSE expression in the identification of in situ hemolysis and extramedullary hemolysis. Jiangsu Medicine 36:421–422.

# Downregulation of HIPK2 Increases Resistance of Bladder Cancer Cell to Cisplatin by Regulating Wip1

**Jun Lin[1], Qiang Zhang[2], Yi Lu[1], Wenrui Xue[2], Yue Xu[2], Yichen Zhu[1], Xiaopeng Hu[2]***

**1** Department of Urology, Beijing Friendship Hospital Affiliated to Capital Medical University, Beijing, P.R China, **2** Department of Urology, Beijing Chao-Yang Hospital Affiliated to Capital Medical University, Beijing, P.R China

## Abstract

Cisplatin-based combination chemotherapy regimen is a reasonable alternative to cystectomy in advanced/metastatic bladder cancer, but acquisition of cisplatin resistance is common in patients with bladder cancer. Previous studies showed that loss of homeodomain-interacting protein kinase-2 (HIPK2) contributes to cell proliferation and tumorigenesis. However, the role of HIPK2 in regulating chemoresistance of cancer cell is not fully understood. In the present study, we found that HIPK2 mRNA and protein levels are significantly decreased in cisplatin-resistant bladder cancer cell *in vivo* and *in vitro*. Downregulation of HIPK2 increases the cell viability in a dose- and time-dependent manner during cisplatin treatment, whereas overexpression of HIPK2 reduces the cell viability. HIPK2 overexpression partially overcomes cisplatin resistance in RT4-CisR cell. Furthermore, we showed that Wip1 (wild-type p53-induced phosphatase 1) expression is upregulated in RT4-CisR cell compared with RT4 cell, and HIPK2 negatively regulates Wip1 expression in bladder cancer cell. HIPK2 and Wip1 expression is also negatively correlated after cisplatin-based combination chemotherapy *in vivo*. Finally, we demonstrated that overexpression of HIPK2 sensitizes chemoresistant bladder cancer cell to cisplatin by regulating Wip1 expression.

*Conclusions:* These data suggest that HIPK2/Wip1 signaling represents a novel pathway regulating chemoresistance, thus offering a new target for chemotherapy of bladder cancer.

**Editor:** Thomas G. Hofmann, German Cancer Research Center, Germany

**Funding:** The authors have no support or funding to report.

**Competing Interests:** The authors have declared that no competing interests exist.

* E-mail: xiaopenghu@sohu.com

## Introduction

Human bladder cancer is the tenth most common malignancy in women, and the fourth most common in men [1,2]. Pathological studies indicate that bladder cancer comprises two major groups. The most common bladder cancer is urothelial carcinoma (UC) that usually recurs but rarely progress [3,4]. In addition, invasive bladder cancer is more aggressive, and one-half of patients with invasive bladder cancer develop distant metastasis [5,6]. Chemoradiation is a reasonable alternative to cystectomy in advanced/metastatic bladder cancer, but resistance to cancer chemotherapy is a common phenomenon especially in metastatic bladder cancer [7]. However, the advances in chemotherapy for the purpose of bladder cancer treatment have been limited because the underlying mechanisms causing chemoresistance are not known. Revealing the molecular mechanism of chemoresistance is indispensable for developing effective chemotherapeutic agents.

Homeodomain-interacting protein kinase-2 (HIPK2) is a serine/threonine kinase that as been shown to be involved in tumor suppressor [8,9,10]. HIPK2 is activated in response to various types of DNA-damaging agents, such as cisplatin, ultraviolet and roscovitine chemotherapeutic drugs [9]. HIPK2 phosphorylates p53 for specific activation of proapoptotic target genes, including p53AIP1, PIG3, Bax and Noxa and contributes to the regulation of p53-induced apoptosis [11,12,13]. Puca *et al* demonstrated that HIPK2 is an important regulator of p53 activity

in response to a chemotherapeutic drug [14]. HIPK2 is expressed differently in sensitive versus chemoresistant cells in response to different chemotherapeutic drugs (i.e., cisplatin and adriamycin). HIPK2 inhibition suppresses the adriamycin-induced apoptosis in chemoresistant cancer cells, whereas overexpression of HIPK2 triggers apoptosis in chemoresistant cells, associated with induction of p53Ser46-target gene AIP1 [14,15,16]. Lazzari *et al* showed that HIPK2 knockdown induces resistance to different anticancer drugs even by targeting$\Delta$Np63$\alpha$ in p53-null cells [17].

Wild-type p53-induced phosphatase 1 (Wip1) is a p53-inducible serine/threonine phosphatase that switches off DNA damage checkpoint responses by the dephosphorylation of certain proteins, such as p38 mitogen-activated protein kinase, p53, checkpoint kinase 1 and checkpoint kinase 2 [18,19]. Wip1 is targeted by HIPK2 for degradation [20]. Emerging data also indicate that Wip1 is overexpressed in various human tumors, and is associated with chemoresistance [19]. Wang *et al* showed that Wip1 knockdown increases DNA damage signaling and re-sensitizes oral squamous cell carcinoma (SCC) cells to cisplatin [21]. Using xenograft tumor models, they demonstrated that overexpression of Wip1 promotes tumorigenesis and its inhibition improves the tumor response to cisplatin [21]. Oppositely, Goloudina *et al* showed that Wip1 overexpression sensitizes colon cancer cells HCT116 (p53$^{-/-}$) to cisplatin in RUNX2-dependent transcriptional induction of the proapoptotic Bax protein [22]. However,

## A

## B

## C

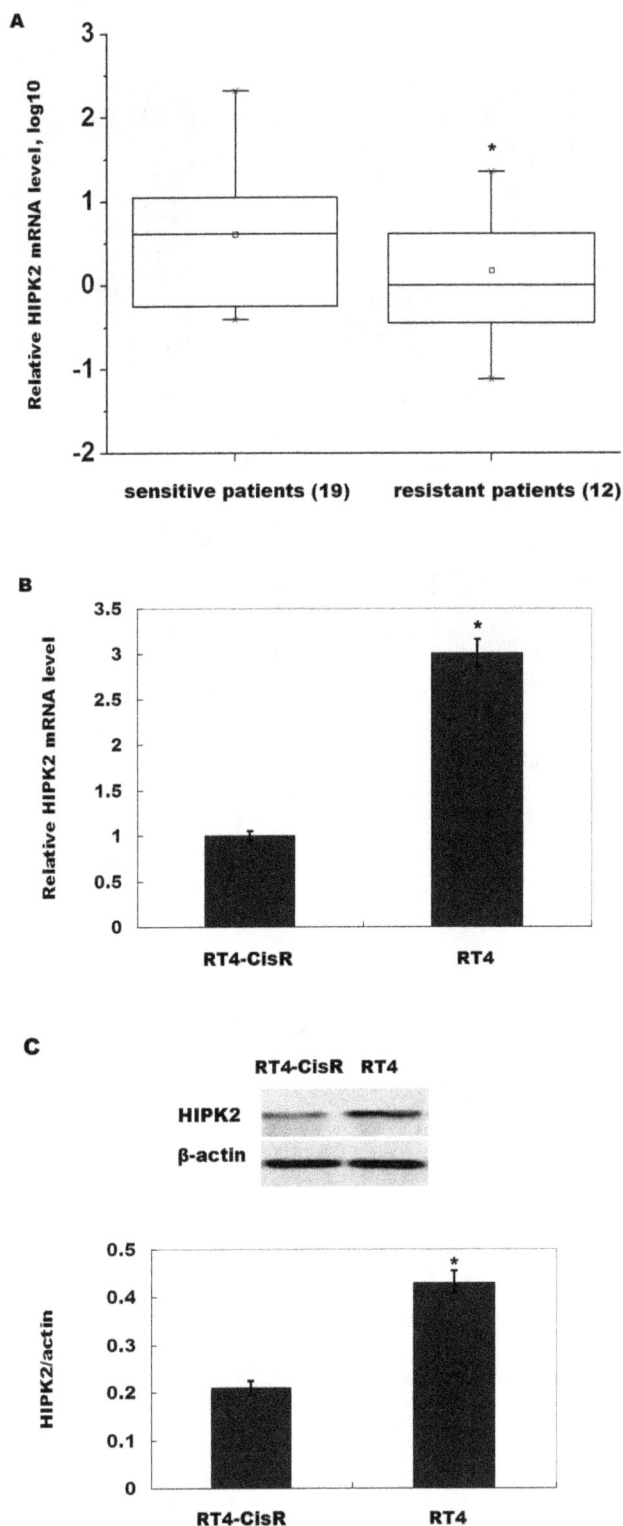

**Figure 1. HIPK2 expression is decreased in chemo-resistant bladder cancer cell.** (A) The analysis of the HIPK2 expression level was performed in blood samples with cisplatin-sensitive patients (n = 19) and cisplatin-resistant patients (n = 12). Total RNA was extracted and subjected to real-time RT-PCR to analyze the relative level of HIPK2 in each sample. Relative expression was calculated and normalized with respect to β-actin mRNA. All data were expressed as fold change relative to a tissue (control, expression = 1). The results were expressed as Log10 ($2^{-\Delta\Delta Ct}$). *$p < 0.05$. (B) The cisplatin-resistant subline RT4-CisR was established by continuous exposure to increasing concentrations

of cisplatin over a time period of 12 months, and HIPK2 levels were analyzed by real-time PCR. Relative HIPK2 levels were calculated with respect to the control. *$p < 0.05$. (C) Western blot analysis of HIPK2 protein level in RT4-CisR and RT4 cells (up). We also showed relative quantification of HIPK2 protein level (bottom, n = 3). *$p < 0.05$.

the role of Wip1 in regulating cisplatin sensitivity of bladder cancer cell is not fully understood.

Based on these findings, we investigated whether HIPK2 regulates chemosensitivity by targeting Wip1 in bladder cancer cell. Here we found that upregulation of HIPK2 inhibits Wip1 expression, which sensitizes chemoresistant bladder cancer cell to cisplatin.

## Materials and Methods

### Cell lines and tissue samples

The protocols used in the study were approved by the Hospital's Protection of Human Subjects Committee. Blood specimens were acquired with written informed consent from the Beijing Friendship Hospital Affiliated to Capital University of Medical Sciences. A total of 31 unresectable/metastatic bladder cancer patients were included in the study, and all the patients received cisplatin-based combination chemotherapy between 12/2011 and 08/2013 (median age 62.3, range 51–80).

Human bladder cancer cell lines with wild type of p53 (RT4 and 253J) were obtained and maintained as recommended by American Type Culture Collection (ATCC, Manassas, VA). The cisplatin-resistant subline RT4-resistance (RT4-CisR) was established by continuous exposure to increasing concentrations of cisplatin over a time period of 12 months, as reported previously [23].

### Real-time PCR

Total RNA was extracted from cells or tissues using Trizol reagent (Invitrogen, Carlsbad, CA), and reverse transcription (RT) reactions were performed according to the manufacturer's protocol. Real-time PCR was performed using a standard protocol from the SYBR Green PCR kit (Toyobo, Osaka, Japan). β-actin were used as references for mRNAs. ΔCt values were normalized to β-actin levels. The $2^{-\Delta\Delta Ct}$ method was used to determine the relative quantitation of gene expression levels. Each sample was analyzed in triplicate.

### Western blot analysis

Western blot analysis to assess HIPK2, Wip1 and β-actin expression was performed as previously described [24]. HIPK2 (ab28507) and Wip1 (ab72000) primary antibodies were purchased from Abcam (Cambridge, MA, USA). The β-actin primary antibodies were purchased from Sigma (MO, USA).

### Cell viability assay

Cells were plated and grown in 96-well plate in 0.1 ml Dulbecco's modified Eagle's medium containing 10% (v/v) fetal calf serum at 37°C for 24 h. Thereafter, the medium was changed and 0.1 ml fresh medium containing indicated drug was added and the cells were incubated for additional 48 h. The number of viable cells was determined by using the 3-(4,5-dimethylthiazol-2-yl)-2,5-diphenyltetrazolium bromide (MTT) assay as described [25].

### RNAi and overexpression

RNAi was performed as described previously [26,27]. The siRNAs used in this study were mixtures of three siRNAs and were

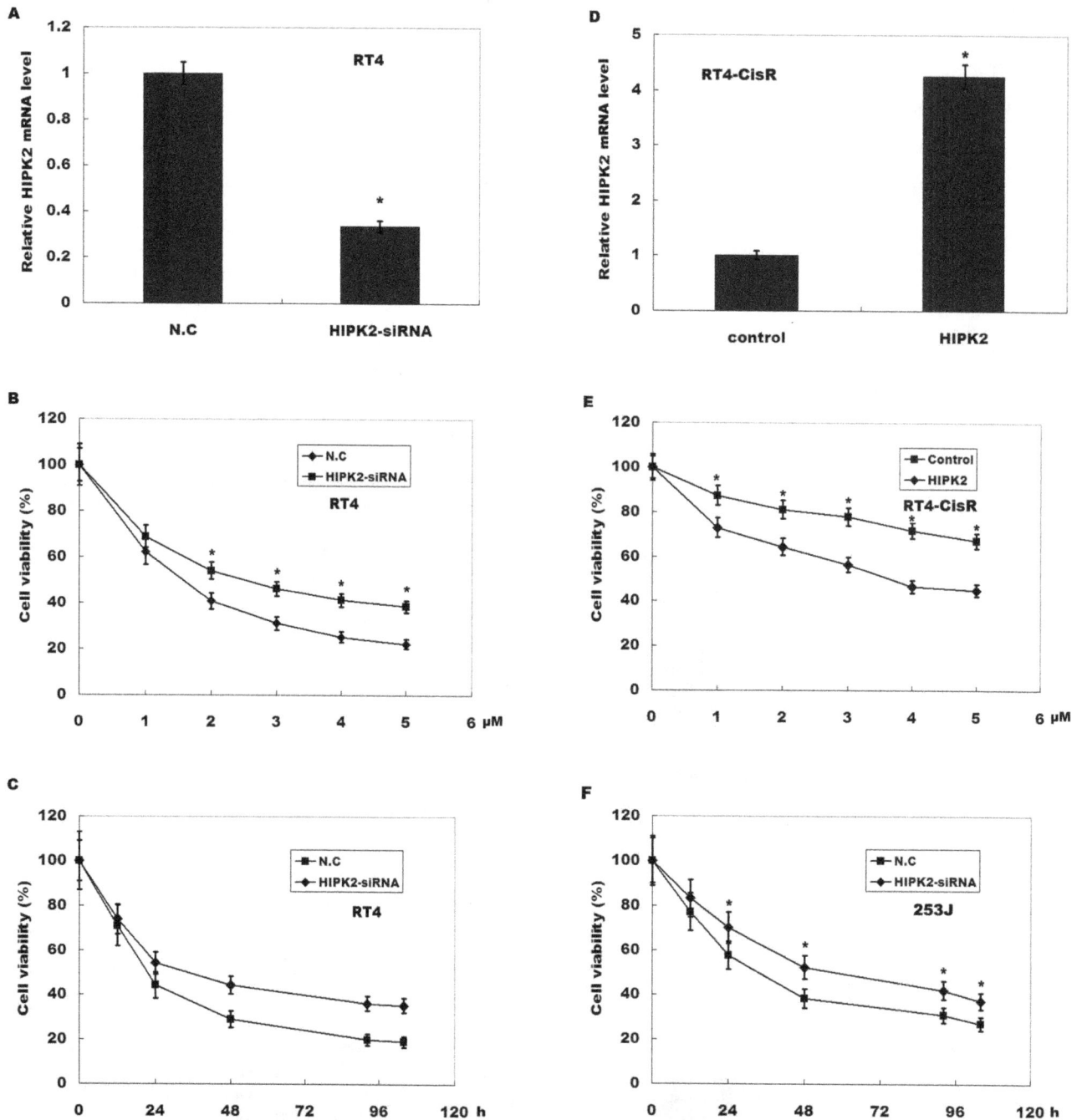

**Figure 2. HIPK2 downregulation increases cell viability during cisplatin treatment in bladder cancer cell.** (A) RT4 cells were transfected with HIPK2-siRNAs and HIPK2 expression level was assayed by real-time PCR. N.C = negative control (scrambled) siRNA. (B) RT4 cells were treated with HIPK2-siRNAs, and cell viability was assayed by using MTT following cisplatin treatment (1 to 6 μM). The results show data from six independent experiments, expressed as the mean ± SD. *$p<0.05$. (C) RT4 cells were treated with HIPK2-siRNAs, and at the indicated time points, cell viability was assayed by using MTT following cisplatin treatment (6 μM). The results show data from six independent experiments, expressed as the mean ± SD. *$p<0.05$. (D) RT4-CisR cells were transfected with pcDNA-HIPK2 and HIPK2 expression level was assayed by real-time PCR. (E) HIPK2 was overexpressed in RT4-CisR cells, and cell viability was assayed by using MTT following cisplatin treatment (1 to 6 μM). The results show data from six independent experiments, expressed as the mean ± SD. *$p<0.05$. (F) 253J cells were treated with HIPK2-siRNAs, and cell viability was assayed by using MTT following cisplatin treatment (6 μM). *$p<0.05$.

purchased from Genepharm (Shanghai, China). pcDNA-HIPK2 and pcDNA-Wip1 were constructed to overexpress HIPK2 or Wip1 by introducing a fragment containing the HIPK2 or Wip1 precursor into pcDNA plasmid.

## Statistical analysis

All data are expressed as mean ± standard deviation (SD) from at least three separate experiments. The differences between groups were analyzed using Student's $t$ test. Differences were deemed statistically significant at $p<0.05$.

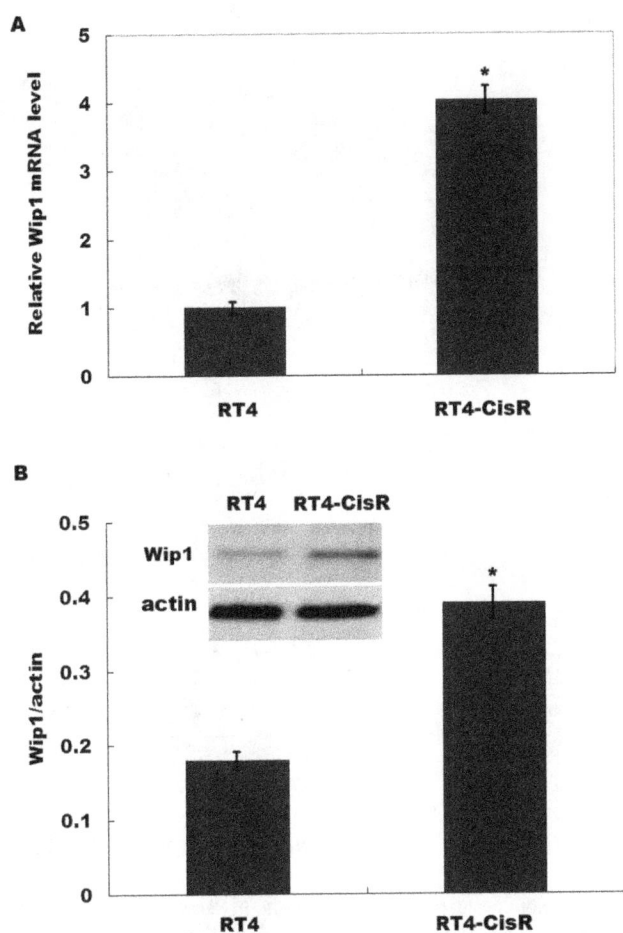

## HIPK2 knockdown increases cell viability during cisplatin treatment in bladder cancer cell

To investigate the role of HIPK2 in cisplatin resistance, separate overexpression and ablation experiments were done using either pcDNA-HIPK2 or HIPK2 siRNA during cisplatin treatment and cell viability was assayed. Figure 2A showed that HIPK2 expression levels were decreased in RT4 cells treated with HIPK2-siRNA. Then RT4 cell were incubated with different concentrations of cisplatin (0, 1, 2, 3, 4, 5 and 6 µM) for 48 h. As shown in Figure 2B, HIPK2 inhibition markedly increases RT4 cell viability compared with negative control (N.C). Expectedly, knockdown of HIPK2 increases RT4 cell viability following cisplatin treatment in time-dependent manner (Figure 2C). In RT4-CisR cells, cisplatin treatment resulted in a modest inhibition of cell viability, whereas overexpression of HIPK2 re-sensitized RT4-CisR cells to cisplatin (Figure 2D and E). Similarly, HIPK2 expression was inhibited in 253J cells after HIPK2-siRNA treatment (Figure S1), and HIPK2 inhibition increases 253J cell viability in time-dependent manner (Figure 2F). These data suggest that HIPK2 increases cisplatin sensitivity of bladder cancer cells.

## HIPK2 negatively regulates Wip1 expression

Previous studies showed that HIPK2 regulates tumor progression and drug resistance via several potential target genes, such as Bax, p53AIP1, Noxa, etc [14]. HIPK2 also plays a critical role in the initiation of double-strand break repair signaling by controlling Wip1 levels in response to ionizing radiation [20]. Recent studies indicate that Wip1 is overexpressed in various human tumors, and is associated with chemoresistance [19]. However, little is known about whether HIPK2 regulates cisplatin resistance by targeting Wip1. We first assayed the expression level of Wip1 in RT4 and RT4-CisR cells. Figure 3A and B showed that Wip1 mRNA and protein levels were significantly upregulated in RT4-CisR compared with RT4 cell. We then assayed whether HIPK2 negatively regulates Wip1 expression. HIPK2 knockdown increased Wip1 expression levels in bladder cancer cell lines (Figure 4A), whereas HIPK2 overexpression remarkably inhibited Wip1 mRNA level in bladder cancer cell lines (Figure 4B). Western blot analysis showed that HIPK2 knockdown increases Wip1 protein level (Figure 4C). *In vivo*, a significant negative correlation is also observed between the HIPK2 levels and the Wip1 levels in patients with bladder cancer after cisplatin-based combination chemotherapy ($r^2 = 0.1507$, $p = 0.0063$, Figure 4D). These data showed that downregulation of HIPK2 results in an increase of Wip1 expression.

## HIPK2 overexpression sensitizes chemoresistant bladder cancer cell to cisplatin by regulating Wip1 expression

We next investigated the role of Wip1 in regulating cell viability during cisplatin treatment. Figure 5A showed that Wip1 overexpression increased cell viability in RT4 cells during cisplatin treatment. HIPK2 inhibits Wip1 expression and decreases cisplatin resistance, and a significant negative correlation is observed between the HIPK2 and the Wip1. We therefore speculated that the role of HIPK2 in regulating cisplatin resistance is mediated by Wip1. Figure 5B showed that HIPK2 inhibition markedly increases RT4 cell viability compared with N.C, whereas Wip1 inhibition in HIPK2-downregulating cells partly reduces cell viability. Similarly, Wip1 inhibition in HIPK2-downregulating cells partly reduces 253J cell viability (Figure 5C). More important, cell viability is decreased by HIPK2 overexpression, whereas Wip1 overexpression increased HIPK2-overexpressing cell viability

**Figure 3. Wip1 expression is upregulated in RT4-CisR cell compared with RT4 cell.** (A and B) Wip1 mRNA and protein expression levels were assayed in RT4 and RT4-CisR cells, respectively. *p<0.05.

## Results

### HIPK2 expression is decreased in chemo-resistant bladder cancer cell

Cisplatin is currently the most effective antitumor agent against advanced bladder cancer. However, resistance to cisplatin-based combination chemotherapy is a common phenomenon especially in metastatic bladder cancer. To clarify the molecular mechanisms underlying cisplatin resistance in bladder cancer, a total of 31 metastatic bladder cancer patients were included, and HIPK2 expression level was assayed after cisplatin-based combination chemotherapy. Figure 1A showed that HIPK2 expression in patients who are chemo-resistant is significantly decreased compared with chemo-sensitive patients. Then we established a cisplatin-resistant subline from the human bladder cancer cell line RT4 (RT4-CisR), and assayed the expression level of HIPK2. As shown in Figure 1B, HIPK2 mRNA levels were lower in RT4-CisR cells compared with RT4 cells. Similarly, HIPK2 protein levels were downregulated in RT4-CisR cells (Figure 1C). These data indicate that downregulation of HIPK2 may be related to cisplatin resistance of bladder cancer cells.

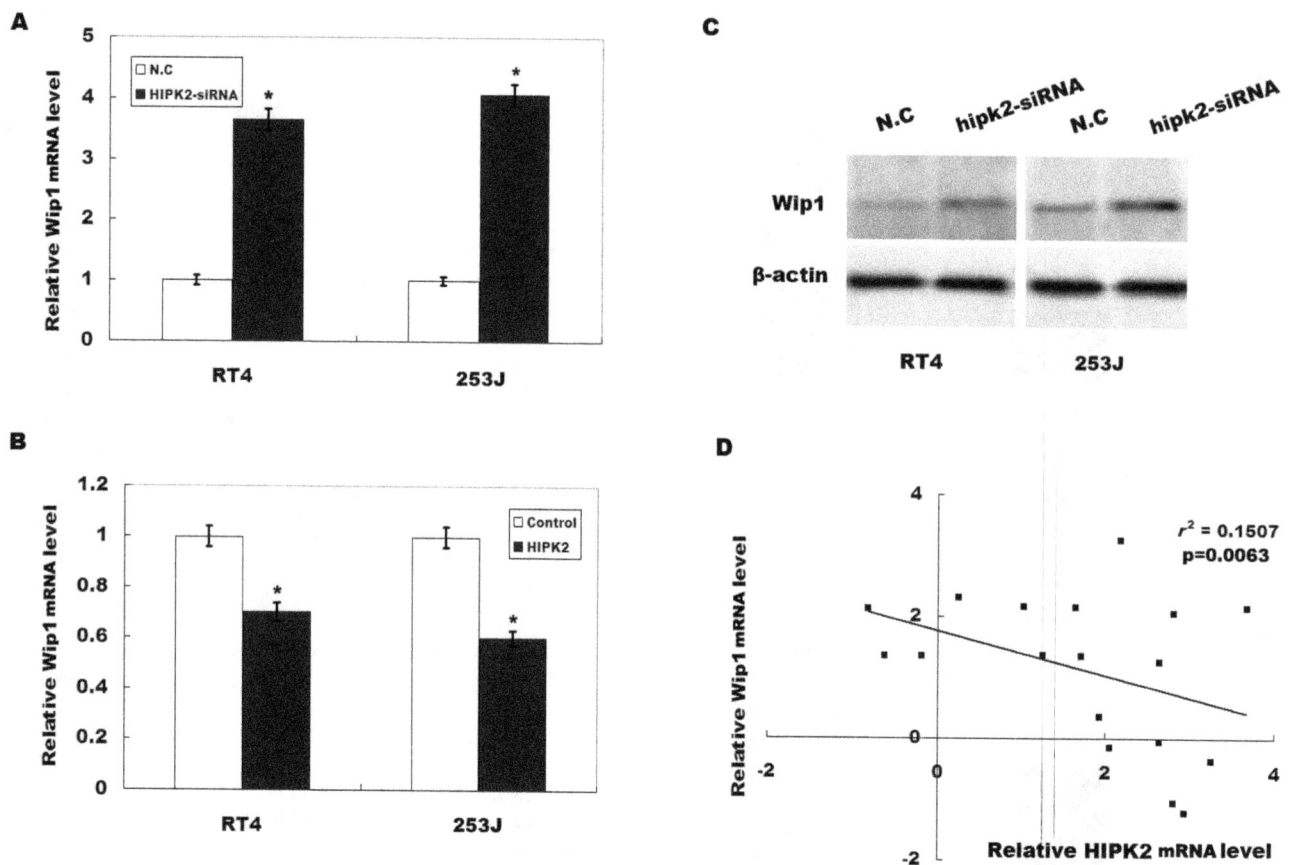

**Figure 4. HIPK2 negatively regulates Wip1 expression.** (A) Wip1 mRNA levels were evaluated by real-time PCR after HIPK2 inhibition in RT4 cells and 253J cells. *$p<0.05$. (B) Relative Wip1 mRNA level after HIPK2 overexpression in RT4 cells and 253J cells. *$p<0.05$. (C) Western blot analysis of Wip1 level after HIPK2 inhibition in RT4 and 253J cells. (D) Negative correlation between the HIPK2 levels and the Wip1 levels in 18 patients with bladder cancer after cisplatin-based combination chemotherapy ($r^2=0.1507$, $p=0.0063$). Relative Wip1 or HIPK2 expression was calculated and normalized with respect to β-actin mRNA. All data were expressed as fold change relative to a tissue (control, expression = 1).

(Figure 5D). These data confirm that HIPK2 overexpression sensitizes chemoresistant bladder cancer cell to cisplatin by regulating Wip1 expression.

## Discussion

Human bladder cancer is one of the most fatal cancers all over the world, and its incidence is increasing in many countries. Besides surgical treatments, systematic chemotherapy, play an important role in bladder cancer treatment especially for patients with advanced and metastatic bladder cancer [28,29]. However, despite a rapid shrinkage in tumor mass following chemotherapeutic cycles, the chemoresistance of cancer cells frequently results in the subsequent recurrence and metastasis of cancer [30,31]. Considering the poor prognosis for patients with bladder cancer, mainly because of late diagnosis and low response to chemotherapy, we attempted to identify predictive markers of therapeutic response and molecular targets to increase sensitivity to treatment.

Our studies provide a rationale for the potential use of HIPK2 transduction to sensitize chemoresistant bladder cancer cells to cisplatin. We showed that HIPK2 expression levels are significantly downregulated in cisplatin-resistant RT4 cell (RT4-CisR) compared with RT4 cell. Downregulation of HIPK2 increases the cisplatin resistance in a dose- and time-dependent manner in RT4 cell, whereas forced expression of HIPK2 reduces the cell viability during cisplatin treatment. Moreover, overexpression of HIPK2

partially overcomes cisplatin resistance in RT4-CisR cell. Previous studies showed that HIPK2 is activated in response to various types of DNA-damaging agents, such as cisplatin, ultraviolet and roscovitine chemotherapeutic drugs [14,32], and is an important regulator of p53 activity in response to a chemotherapeutic drug [11,14]. Overexpression of HIPK2 in p53 wild-type re-sensitizes chemoresistant ovarian cancer cells to chemotherapy by mediating p53 phosphorylation. However, the molecular mechanism of HIPK2 in regulating chemoresistance of cancer cell is not fully understood.

Wip1 is a p53-inducible serine/threonine phosphatase that switches off DNA damage checkpoint responses by the dephosphorylation of certain proteins involved in DNA repair and the cell cycle checkpoint [19]. The Wip1 gene is amplified in many tumor types [33]. Song *et al* showed that Wip1 interacts with and dephosphorylates BAX to suppress BAX-mediated apoptosis in response to γ-irradiation in prostate cancer cells [19]. Radiation-resistant LNCaP cells showed dramatic increases in Wip1 levels and impaired BAX movement to the mitochondria after c-irradiation, and these effects were reverted by a Wip1 inhibitor [19]. Wang *et al* showed that Wip1 is an effective drug target for enhanced cancer therapy [21]. Wip1 inhibition increases DNA damage signaling and resensitizes oral SCC cells to cisplatin. Wip1 upregulation promotes tumorigenesis and its inhbition improves the tumor response to cisplatin. Consistent with above results, we found that expression level of Wip1 is upregulated in RT4-CisR

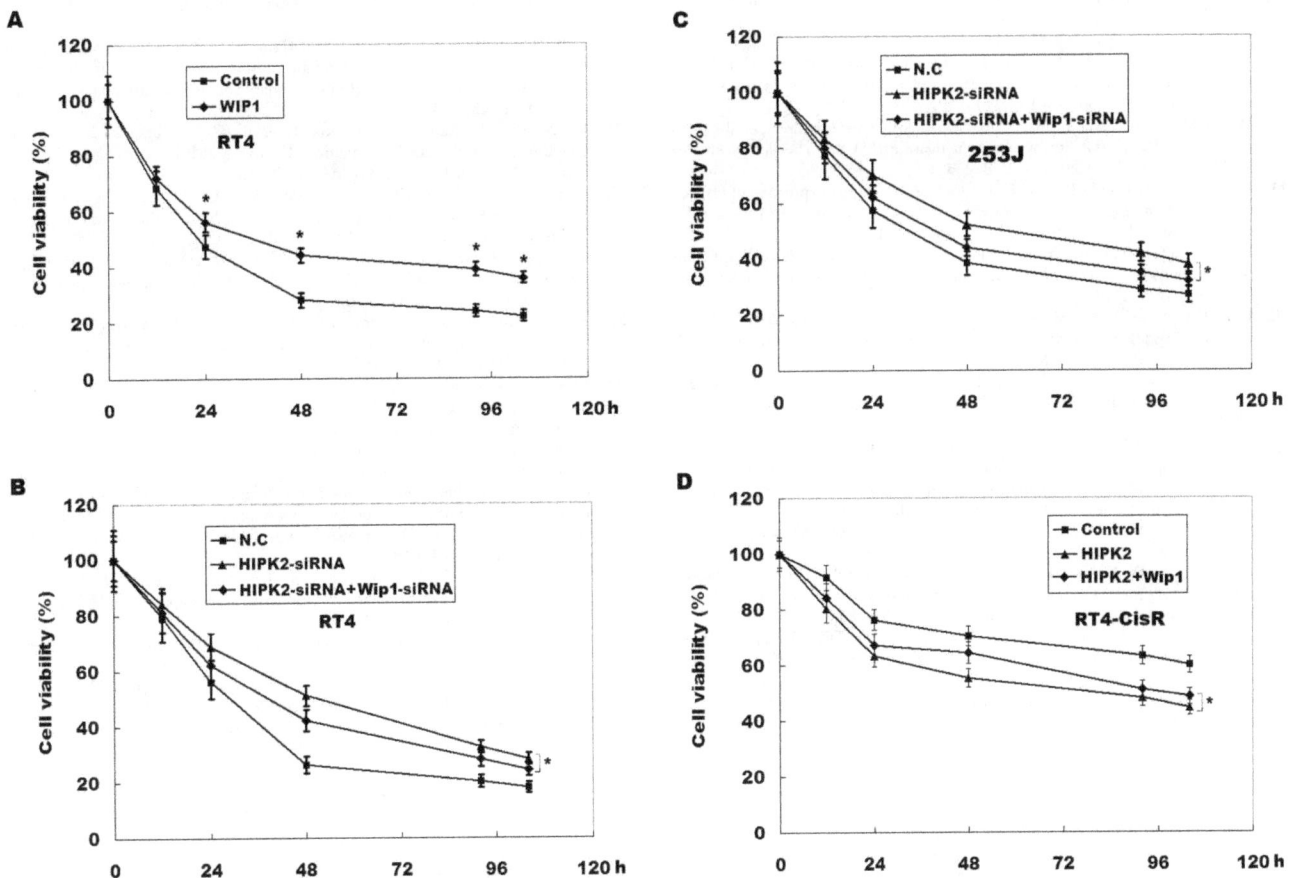

**Figure 5. HIPK2 overexpression sensitizes chemoresistant bladder cancer cell to cisplatin by regulating Wip1 expression.** (A) Wip1 was overexpressed in RT4 cells, and cell viability was assayed by using MTT following cisplatin treatment (6 µM). The results show data from six independent experiments, expressed as the mean ± SD. *$p < 0.05$. (B and C) RT4 and 253J cells were treated with HIPK2-siRNA or HIPK2-siRNA plus Wip1-siRNA, and at the indicated time points, cell viability was assayed by using MTT following cisplatin treatment (6 µM). (D) HIPK2 or HIPK2 plus Wip1 was overexpressed in RT4-CisR cells, and cell viability was assayed by using MTT following cisplatin treatment (6 µM). *$p < 0.05$.

cell compared with RT4 cell, and Wip1 overexpression increases cell viability during cisplatin treatment in RT4 cells. Importantly, we demonstrated that HIPK2 negatively regulates Wip1 expression in bladder cancer cell. HIPK2 and Wip1 expression is also negatively correlated after cisplatin-based combination chemotherapy *in vivo*. Forced expression of HIPK2 sensitizes chemoresistant bladder cancer cell to cisplatin by regulating Wip1 expression. **Conclusion**: These data demonstrated that HIPK2/Wip1 signaling represents a novel pathway regulating

chemoresistance. Thus, this study reveals that HIPK2/Wip1 is an effective drug target for enhanced cancer therapy.

## Author Contributions

Conceived and designed the experiments: XH JL. Performed the experiments: JL QZ YL WX YX YZ. Analyzed the data: YZ XH. Contributed reagents/materials/analysis tools: YL WX YX. Wrote the paper: XH.

## References

1. Cohen SM, Shirai T, Steineck G (2000) Epidemiology and etiology of premalignant and malignant urothelial changes. Scand J Urol Nephrol Suppl: 105–115.
2. Burger M, Catto JW, Dalbagni G, Grossman HB, Herr H, et al. (2013) Epidemiology and risk factors of urothelial bladder cancer. Eur Urol 63: 234–241.
3. Witjes JA, Comperat E, Cowan NC, De Santis M, Gakis G, et al. (2014) EAU Guidelines on Muscle-invasive and Metastatic Bladder Cancer: Summary of the 2013 Guidelines. Eur Urol 65: 778–792.
4. Kirkali Z, Chan T, Manoharan M, Algaba F, Busch C, et al. (2005) Bladder cancer: epidemiology, staging and grading, and diagnosis. Urology 66: 4–34.
5. Pollack A, Zagars GK, Cole CJ, Dinney CP, Swanson DA, et al. (1995) The relationship of local control to distant metastasis in muscle invasive bladder cancer. J Urol 154: 2059-2063; discussion 2063–2054.

6. Said N, Sanchez-Carbayo M, Smith SC, Theodorescu D (2012) RhoGDI2 suppresses lung metastasis in mice by reducing tumor versican expression and macrophage infiltration. J Clin Invest 122: 1503–1518.
7. Chang JS, Lara PN Jr, Pan CX (2012) Progress in personalizing chemotherapy for bladder cancer. Adv Urol 2012: 364919.
8. Wei G, Ku S, Ma GK, Saito S, Tang AA, et al. (2007) HIPK2 represses beta-catenin-mediated transcription, epidermal stem cell expansion, and skin tumorigenesis. Proc Natl Acad Sci U S A 104: 13040–13045.
9. D'Orazi G, Rinaldo C, Soddu S (2012) Updates on HIPK2: a resourceful oncosuppressor for clearing cancer. J Exp Clin Cancer Res 31: 63.
10. Hofmann TG, Glas C, Bitomsky N (2013) HIPK2: A tumour suppressor that controls DNA damage-induced cell fate and cytokinesis. Bioessays 35: 55–64.

11. Puca R, Nardinocchi L, Givol D, D'Orazi G (2010) Regulation of p53 activity by HIPK2: molecular mechanisms and therapeutical implications in human cancer cells. Oncogene 29: 4378–4387.

12. D'Orazi G, Cecchinelli B, Bruno T, Manni I, Higashimoto Y, et al. (2002) Homeodomain-interacting protein kinase-2 phosphorylates p53 at Ser 46 and mediates apoptosis. Nat Cell Biol 4: 11–19.

13. Winter M, Sombroek D, Dauth I, Moehlenbrink J, Scheuermann K, et al. (2008) Control of HIPK2 stability by ubiquitin ligase Siah-1 and checkpoint kinases ATM and ATR. Nat Cell Biol 10: 812–824.

14. Puca R, Nardinocchi L, Pistritto G, D'Orazi G (2008) Overexpression of HIPK2 circumvents the blockade of apoptosis in chemoresistant ovarian cancer cells. Gynecol Oncol 109: 403–410.

15. Hofmann TG, Moller A, Sirma H, Zentgraf H, Taya Y, et al. (2002) Regulation of p53 activity by its interaction with homeodomain-interacting protein kinase-2. Nat Cell Biol 4: 1–10.

16. Rinaldo C, Prodosmo A, Mancini F, Iacovelli S, Sacchi A, et al. (2007) MDM2-regulated degradation of HIPK2 prevents p53Ser46 phosphorylation and DNA damage-induced apoptosis. Mol Cell 25: 739–750.

17. Lazzari C, Prodosmo A, Siepi F, Rinaldo C, Galli F, et al. (2011) HIPK2 phosphorylates DeltaNp63alpha and promotes its degradation in response to DNA damage. Oncogene 30: 4802–4813.

18. Takekawa M, Adachi M, Nakahata A, Nakayama I, Itoh F, et al. (2000) p53-inducible wip1 phosphatase mediates a negative feedback regulation of p38 MAPK-p53 signaling in response to UV radiation. EMBO J 19: 6517–6526.

19. Song JY, Ryu SH, Cho YM, Kim YS, Lee BM, et al. (2013) Wip1 suppresses apoptotic cell death through direct dephosphorylation of BAX in response to gamma-radiation. Cell Death Dis 4: e744.

20. Choi DW, Na W, Kabir MH, Yi E, Kwon S, et al. (2013) WIP1, a homeostatic regulator of the DNA damage response, is targeted by HIPK2 for phosphorylation and degradation. Mol Cell 51: 374–385.

21. Wang L, Mosel AJ, Oakley GG, Peng A (2012) Deficient DNA damage signaling leads to chemoresistance to cisplatin in oral cancer. Mol Cancer Ther 11: 2401–2409.

22. Goloudina AR, Tanoue K, Hammann A, Fourmaux E, Le Guezennec X, et al. (2012) Wip1 promotes RUNX2-dependent apoptosis in p53-negative tumors and protects normal tissues during treatment with anticancer agents. Proc Natl Acad Sci U S A 109: E68–75.

23. Esaki T, Nakano S, Masumoto N, Fujishima H, Niho Y (1996) Schedule-dependent reversion of acquired cisplatin resistance by 5-fluorouracil in a newly established cisplatin-resistant HST-1 human squamous carcinoma cell line. Int J Cancer 65: 479–484.

24. Xu N, Shen C, Luo Y, Xia L, Xue F, et al. (2012) Upregulated miR-130a increases drug resistance by regulating RUNX3 and Wnt signaling in cisplatin-treated HCC cell. Biochem Biophys Res Commun 425: 468–472.

25. Wang F, Li X, Xie X, Zhao L, Chen W (2008) UCA1, a non-protein-coding RNA up-regulated in bladder carcinoma and embryo, influencing cell growth and promoting invasion. FEBS Lett 582: 1919–1927.

26. Yang C, Li X, Wang Y, Zhao L, Chen W (2012) Long non-coding RNA UCA1 regulated cell cycle distribution via CREB through PI3-K dependent pathway in bladder carcinoma cells. Gene 496: 8–16.

27. Yuan G, Regel I, Lian F, Friedrich T, Hitkova I, et al. (2013) WNT6 is a novel target gene of caveolin-1 promoting chemoresistance to epirubicin in human gastric cancer cells. Oncogene 32: 375–387.

28. Juffs HG, Moore MJ, Tannock IF (2002) The role of systemic chemotherapy in the management of muscle-invasive bladder cancer. Lancet Oncol 3: 738–747.

29. Gupta S, Mahipal A (2013) Role of systemic chemotherapy in urothelial urinary bladder cancer. Cancer Control 20: 200–210.

30. Kamat AM, Sethi G, Aggarwal BB (2007) Curcumin potentiates the apoptotic effects of chemotherapeutic agents and cytokines through down-regulation of nuclear factor-kappaB and nuclear factor-kappaB-regulated gene products in IFN-alpha-sensitive and IFN-alpha-resistant human bladder cancer cells. Mol Cancer Ther 6: 1022–1030.

31. Chung J, Kwak C, Jin RJ, Lee CH, Lee KH, et al. (2004) Enhanced chemosensitivity of bladder cancer cells to cisplatin by suppression of clusterin in vitro. Cancer Lett 203: 155–161.

32. Krieghoff-Henning E, Hofmann TG (2008) HIPK2 and cancer cell resistance to therapy. Future Oncol 4: 751–754.

33. Lu X, Nguyen TA, Moon SH, Darlington Y, Sommer M, et al. (2008) The type 2C phosphatase Wip1: an oncogenic regulator of tumor suppressor and DNA damage response pathways. Cancer Metastasis Rev 27: 123–135.

# 7

# S100A8 Contributes to Drug Resistance by Promoting Autophagy in Leukemia Cells

**Minghua Yang[1]\*, Pei Zeng[1], Rui Kang[3], Yan Yu[1], Liangchun Yang[1], Daolin Tang[2,3], Lizhi Cao[1]\***

**1** Department of Pediatrics, Xiangya Hospital, Central South University, Changsha Hunan, China, **2** Department of Infectious Diseases, Xiangya Hospital, Central South University, Changsha, Hunan, China, **3** Department of Surgery, University of Pittsburgh Cancer Institute, Pittsburgh, Pennsylvania, United States of America

## Abstract

Autophagy is a double-edged sword in tumorigenesis and plays an important role in the resistance of cancer cells to chemotherapy. S100A8 is a member of the S100 calcium-binding protein family and plays an important role in the drug resistance of leukemia cells, with the mechanisms largely unknown. Here we report that S100A8 contributes to drug resistance in leukemia by promoting autophagy. S100A8 level was elevated in drug resistance leukemia cell lines relative to the nondrug resistant cell lines. Adriamycin and vincristine increased S100A8 in human leukemia cells, accompanied with upregulation of autophagy. RNA interference-mediated knockdown of S100A8 restored the chemosensitivity of leukemia cells, while overexpression of S100A8 enhanced drug resistance and increased autophagy. S100A8 physically interacted with the autophagy regulator BECN1 and was required for the formation of the BECN1-PI3KC3 complex. In addition, interaction between S100A8 and BECN1 relied upon the autophagic complex ULK1-mAtg13. Furthermore, we discovered that exogenous S100A8 induced autophagy, and RAGE was involved in exogenous S100A8-regulated autophagy. Our data demonstrated that S100A8 is involved in the development of chemoresistance in leukemia cells by regulating autophagy, and suggest that S100A8 may be a novel target for improving leukemia therapy.

**Editor:** Spencer B. Gibson, University of Manitoba, Canada

**Funding:** This work was supported by The National Natural Sciences Foundation of China (81100359 to MY, 30973234 and 31171328 to LC) and a grant from the National Institutes of Health (R01CA160417 to DT). The funders had no role in study design, data collection and analysis, decision to publish, or preparation of the manuscript.

**Competing Interests:** The authors have declared that no competing interests exist.

\* E-mail: yamahua123@163.com (MY); caolizhi318@163.com (LC)

## Introduction

Autophagy is a catabolic process involving the degradation of intracellular aggregated or misfolded proteins, and damaged organelles through lysosomal machinery in response to stress or starvation [1,2]. Deregulation of autophagy is implicated in several human diseases including cancers. Depending on the type of tumor and stage of disease, autophagy induces both tumor cell survival and death during the initiation, progression, maturation and maintenance of cancer [3].

It has been well documented that autophagy plays an important role in the resistance of cancer cells to chemotherapy [4]. Consequently, pharmacological inhibition of autophagy enhances chemotherapeutic drug-induced cytotoxicity and apoptosis in leukemia cells [4–6]. We recently found that damage associated molecular pattern molecules (DAMPs) such as high mobility group box 1 (HMGB1) contribute to chemotherapy resistance though upregulating autophagy in leukemia [7]. S100A8 (also designated MRP8 or calgranulin A) is a member of DAMPs, differentially expressed in a wide variety of cell types and abundant in myeloid cells [8,9]. S100A8 is involved in the progression of various cancers, including leukemia, and induces cell death by functional linkage with Bcl-2 family members [10–14]. We previously found that the expression level of S100A8 correlates with poor clinical outcomes in childhood acute myeloblastic leukemia (AML). Accordingly, knockdown of S100A8 by siRNA-treated myeloid leukemia cells showed sensitization to arsenic trioxide, accompa-

nied with the attenuation of autophagy and disassociation of the BECN1-Bcl-2 complex [14]. The data suggest that S100A8 contributes to chemoresistance *via* regulating the autophagy in leukemia.

In this study, we found that S100A8 enhances drug resistance by upregulating autophagy through promoting the formation of BECN1-PI3KC3 [PI3KC3, phosphatidylinositol 3-kinase class 3] complex, providing a novel potential target for the treatment of leukemia.

## Materials and Methods

### Antibodies and reagents

The antibodies against S100A8 and p62 were obtained from Santa Cruz Biotechnology (Sana Cruz, CA, USA). The antibodies to Actin, BECN1, PI3KC3, C-PARP, ULK1, Bcl-2 and P-ULK1 were from Cell Signaling Technology (Boston, MA, USA). The antibodies to LC3 and TLR-4 were purchased from Abcam (Cambridge, MA, USA). Anti-Atg7 antibody was from Novus (Denver-Littleton, CO, USA). Vincristine (VCR), adriamycin (ADM), rotenone (Rot), thenoyltrifluoroacetone (TTFA), antimycin A (AA), E64D, anti-RAGE antibody and pepstatin were from Sigma (Milpitas, CA, USA). Full-length human S100A8 cDNA (pLPCX-S100A8) was a gift from Dr. RW Stam (Erasmus Medical Center/Sophia Children's Hospital, Netherlands). FITC-Annexin V Apoptosis Detection kit and the Nuclear and Cytoplasmic Protein Extraction kit were purchased form Beyotime Institute of

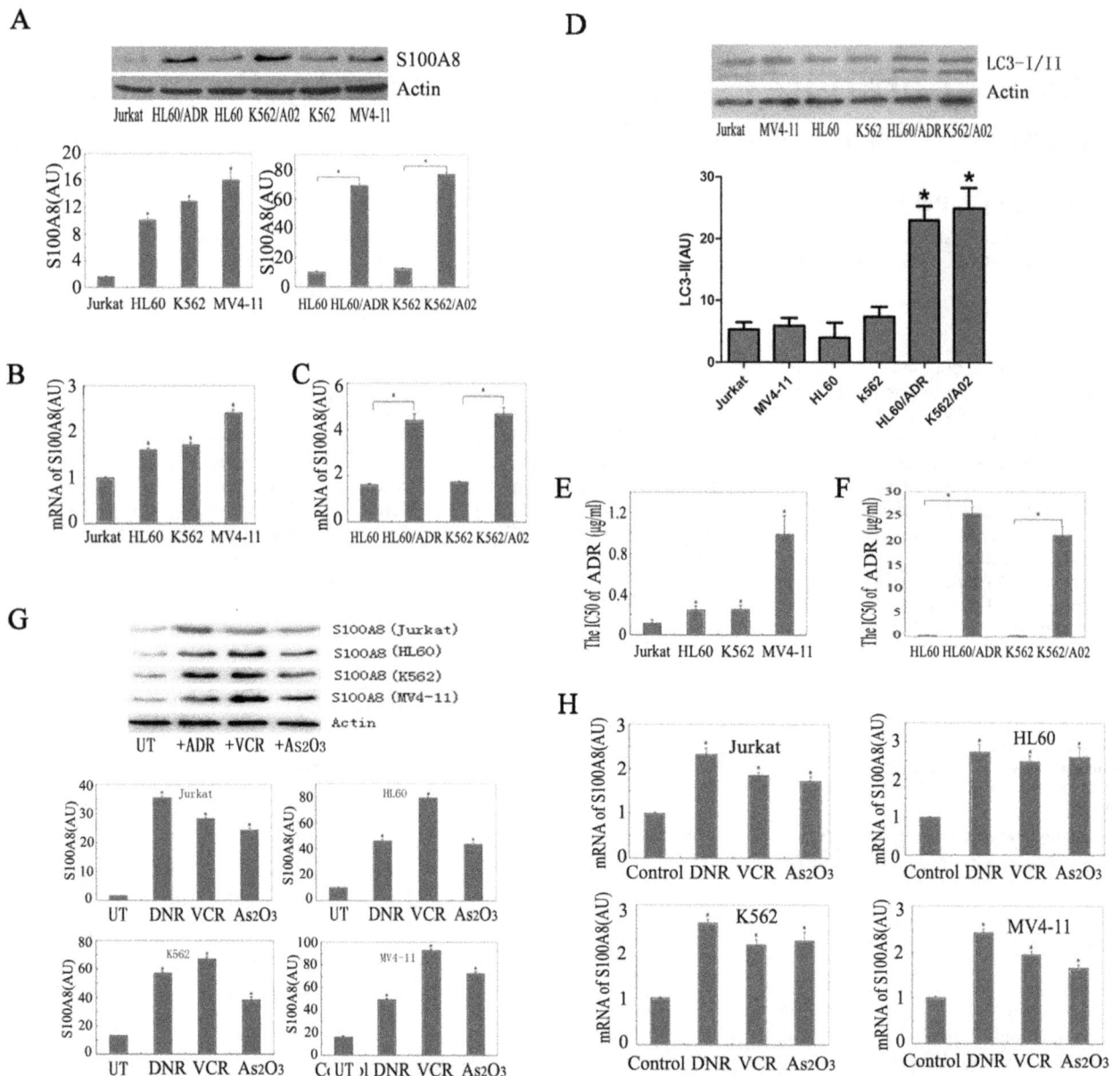

**Figure 1. S100A8 was elevated in drug resistance leukemia cells and chemotherapy agents induced S100A8 expression in leukemia cells.** (A) Protein level of S100A8 was analyzed by Western blotting in Jurkat, HL-60, K562 and MV4-11 cells (n = 3, *P<0.05). (B and C) S100A8 mRNA level in leukemia cells was analyzed by real time RT-PCR (n = 3, *P<0.05 versus Jurkat cells in **B** and *P<0.05 versus HL-60 or K562 in **C**, Jurkat group set as 1). (**D**) Basal LC3-I/II level was analyzed by Western blotting in leukemia cells (n = 3, *P<0.05 *versus* Jurkat cells ). (**E and F**) IC50 levels of adriamycin (ADR) in Jurkat, K562, HL-60, MV-4-11, K562/A02, and HL-60/ADR cells (n = 3, *P<0.05 versus Jurkat cells in **E**, *P<0.05 versus HL-60 or K562 in **F**). (**G**) Jurkat, HL-60, K562 and MV4-11 cells were treated with ADR (1 μg/ml), VCR (1 μg/ml) or As2O3 (5 μM) for 24 hours and S100A8 protein level was analyzed by Western blotting (n = 3, *P<0.05 vs. UT, untreated group). AU, arbitrary unit. (**H**) Jurkat, HL-60, K562 and MV4-11 cells were treated with ADR (1 μg/ml), vincristine (VCR, 1 μg/ml) or arsenic trioxide (As2O3, 5 μM) for 24 hours and S100A8 mRNA level was analyzed by real time RT-PCR (n = 3, *P<0.05 versus control group, control group set as 1).

Biotechnology (Beijing, China). S100A8 protein was obtained from Novus Biologicals. Contaminating LPS was removed by Triton X-114 extraction. LPS content was always below 0.5 ng/mg protein, which did not cause an effect in our assays.

## Cell culture

The human leukemia cell lines, K562 (chronic myeloid leukemia cells), HL-60 (acute myeloid leukemia cells), MV-4-11 (biphenotypic B myelomonocytic leukemia cells), Jurkat (T-cell acute lymphoblastic leukemia cells), and K562/A02 (multidrug resistance K562) were from the American Type Culture Collection; HL-60/ADR (multidrug resistance HL-60) was from the Institute of Hematology & Blood Diseases Hospital of Chinese Academy of Medical Sciences & Peking Union Medical College. Cells were cultured in RPMI-1640 medium supplemented with 10% heat-inactivated FBS and 2 mM glutamine in a humidified incubator with 5% CO2 and 95% air.

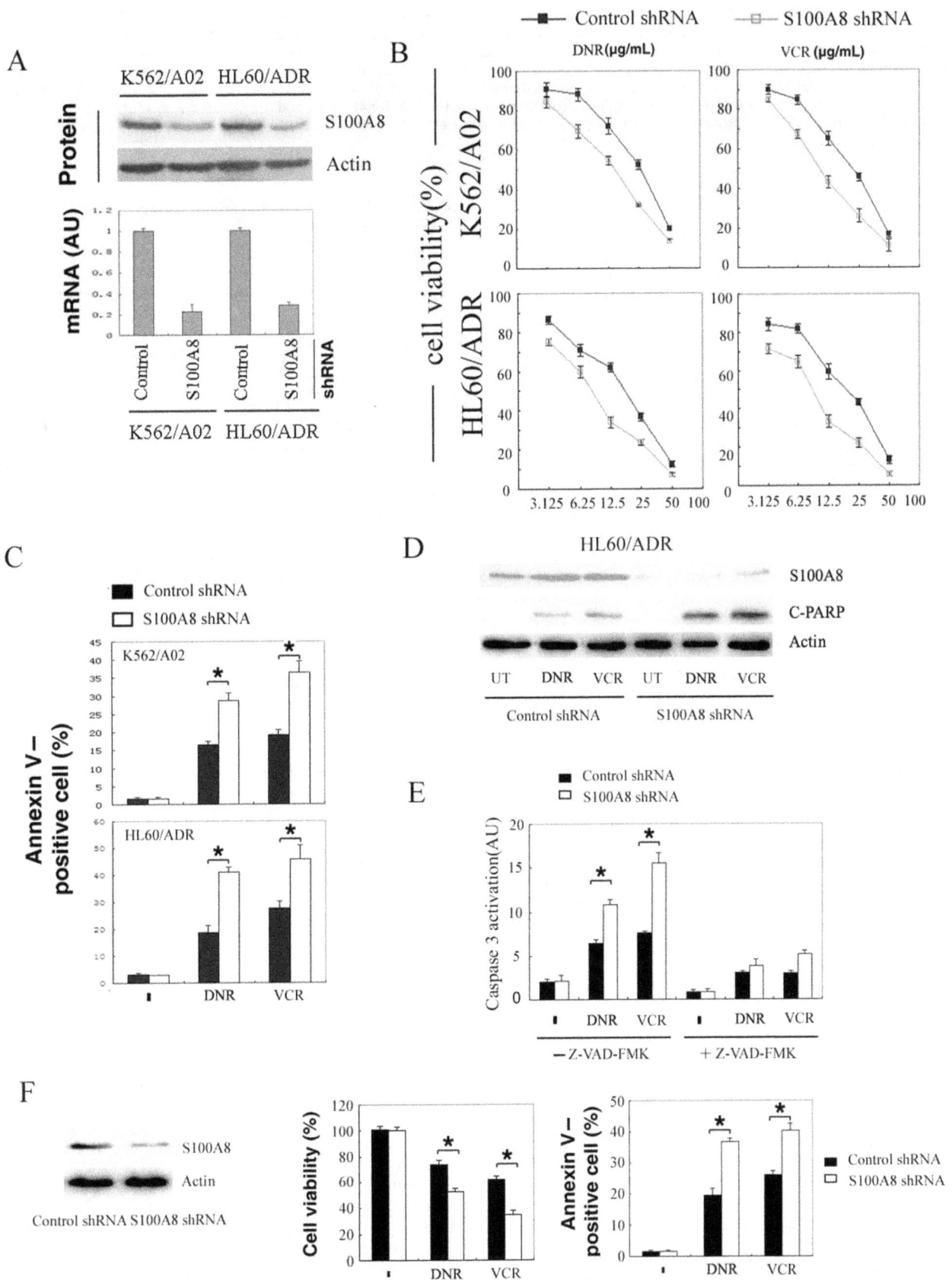

**Figure 2. Suppression of S100A8 sensitized drug resistance leukemia cells to chemotherapy. (A)** HL60/ADR and K562/A02 cells were transfected with control shRNA or S100A8 shRNA for 48 hours. Protein and mRNA level of S100A8 was assayed by Western blot and real time RT-PCR, respectively. **(B)** HL60/ADR and K562/A02 cells were transfected with control shRNA or S100A8 shRNA for 48 hours, then treated with adriamycin

(ADR) and vincristine (VCR) for an additional 24 hours. Cell viability was analyzed by MTT. (**C and D**) HL60/ADR and K562/A02 cells were transfected with control shRNA or S100A8 shRNA for 48 hours, treated with ADR (12.5 μg/mL), VCR (12.5 μg/mL) for additional 24 hours. Apoptosis was analyzed by measuring positive percentage of Annexin V cells via flow cytometry (**C**; n = 3; *$P < 0.05$); cleaved PARP was analyzed by Western blotting (**D**). (**E**) HL60/ADR and K562/A02 cells were transfected with control shRNA or S100A8 shRNA for 48 hours, and then treated with ADR (12.5 μg/mL), VCR (12.5 μg/mL) for additional 24 hours with or without ZVAD-FMK (20 μmol/L). Activation of caspase-3 was analyzed (n = 3; *$P < 0.05$). (**F**) HL60/ADR cells were transfected with control shRNA or S100A8 shRNA (from Gene Pharma, China) for 48 hours and then treated with ADR (12.5 μg/mL), VCR (12.5 μg/mL) for 24 hours. S100A8 protein was determined by Western blot; Cell viability was analyzed by MTT; apoptosis was analyzed by flow cytometry (n = 3; *$P < 0.05$).

## Cell viability assay

Cell viability was assessed by MTT assay. Briefly, leukemia cells were seeded in 96-well plates (4000 cells/well) the day before treatment. Following treatment with ADR for 72 h, 25 μL MTT [3-(4,5-dimethylthiazol-2-yl)- 2,5-diphenyltetrazolium bromide; Sigma] was added to each well and incubated for 3.5 h, followed by the addition of 100 μL of N,Ndimethylformamide (D4551; Sigma). The plates were left at room temperature overnight to allow complete lysis of the cells, and read at 450 nm the following day. Half-maximal inhibitory concentration (IC50) was calculated using MS Excel, as previously described [15].

## Western blot analysis

Cell lysates were prepared with cell lysis buffer [20 mmol/L Tris-HCl, pH 7.5; 150 mmol/L NaCl; 1 mmol/L Na2EDTA; 1 mmol/L EGTA; 1% Triton; 2.5 mmol/L sodium pyrophosphate; 1 mmol/L b-glycerophosphate; 1 mmol/L Na3VO4; 1 mg/mL leupeptin; 1 mmol/L phenylmethylsulfonylfluoride (PMSF); and 1 mmol/L PMSF], and cleared by centrifugation. Total protein concentration was determined with the bicinchoninic acid assay Kit (Bio-Rad). Proteins were resolved on a denaturing 10% SDS-PAGE gel and subsequently transferred to polyvinylidene fluoride membranes *via* semidry transfer. The membrane was blocked with 5% dried milk or 3% bovine serum albumin in Tris-buffered saline and Tween 20 (10 mmol/L Tris, pH 7.5; 100 mmol/L NaCl; and 0.1% Tween20), incubated with primary antibodies, and then with horseradish peroxidase–conjugated secondary antibodies. The signals were visualized by enhanced chemiluminescence.

## Quantitative real-time PCR

Total RNA was extracted using TRIzol (Invitrogen, USA) according to the manufacturer's instructions. Reverse transcription (RT) was performed with 2 μg of total RNA with HiFi-MMLV Enzyme Mix (CWbio, China). Twenty ng cDNA was subjected to real-time quantitative PCR (TaqMan probes) for the evaluation of the relative S100A8 mRNA, with beta actin as an internal control with gene specific primers and fluorogenic probes (S100A8: forward primer 5′- CCTAACCGCTATAAAAGGAG -3′, reverse primer 5′- ATGATGCCCACGGACTTGCC -3, probe 5′ FAM-CCTCTCAGCCCTGCATGTCTCTT -TAMRA 3′; ACTB: forward primer 5′- GGCACCCAGCACAATGAAGA-3, reverse primer 5′-CGTCATACTCCTGCTTGCTG-3′, probe 5′FAM-CTGGAAGGTGGACAGCGAGGC-TAMRA 3′.) in an LightCycler 480 **System** (Roche). Quantification was determined by the standard curve and 2-ΔΔCt methods [15].

## Immunoprecipitation analysis

Cells were lysed at 4°C in ice-cold radioimmunoprecipitation assay lysis buffer (Millipore, Billerica, MA, USA). Cell lysates were cleared by a brief centrifugation (12,000 g, 10 min). Protein concentration in the supernatant was determined by bicinchoninic acid assay. Before immunoprecipitation, equal amounts of proteins were pre-cleared with Protein A or protein G agarose/sepharose

(Millipore) at 4°C for 3 h and subsequently incubated with various irrelevant immunoglobulin-G or specific antibodies (5 μg/ml) in the presence of protein A or G agarose/sepharose beads for 2 h or overnight at 4°C with gently shaking. Following incubation, agarose/sepharose beads were washed extensively with phosphate buffered saline. Proteins were eluted by boiling in 2×SDS sample buffer before SDS–polyacrylamide gel electrophoresis and immunoblot analysis, as previously described [15,16].

## Gene transfection and RNAi

Cells were transfected with S100A8 pLPCX constructs by square-pulse electroporation at 600 V for 2 msec and cultured under selection of neomycin (1 mg/ml; Gibco BRL, USA) and puromycin (10 mg/ml; Sigma) in order to obtain a pure population of transfected cells [13]. Lipofectamine 2000 Transfection Reagent (Invitrogen) was used to transfect S100A8-shRNA, BECN1-shRNA, PI3KC3-shRNA, ULK1-shRNA, RAGE-shRNA, TLR4-shRNA and Atg7 shRNA (Sigma) [16]. As a control experiment, another S100A8-shRNA was obtained from Gene Pharma (Shanghai, China).

## Apoptosis assays

Apoptosis was assessed using the FITC Annexin V Apoptosis Detection kit, which involves staining cells with Annexin V-FITC (a phospholipid-binding protein that binds to disrupted cell membranes) in combination with PI (a vital dye that binds to DNA penetrating into apoptotic cells). Flow cytometric analysis (FACS) was performed to determine the percentage of apoptotic cells (Annexin V$^+$/PI).

## Electron microscopy

Leukemia cells were collected and fixed in 2.5% glutaraldehyde for at least 3 h. Then cells were treated with 2% paraformaldehyde at room temperature for 60 min, 0.1% glutaraldehyde in 0.1 M sodium cacodylate for 2 h, post-fixed with 1% OsO4 for 1.5 h, dehydrated with graded acetone, and embedded in Quetol 812. Ultrathin sections were observed using a Hitachi H7500 electron microscope (Tokyo, Japan) [17].

## Immunofluorescence and confocal microscopy

Cells were collected, fixed and permeabilized with 0.3% triton X-100 for 10 min, incubated with anti-LC3 for 1 h and then FITC-conjugated Anti-LC3A/B antibody (Abcam, ab58610) for 1 h at room temperature. Cell nuclei were stained using ProLong Gold Antifade Reagent with DAPI (Life Technologies). Samples were examined under an Olympus FV1000 confocal microscope. For evaluating tandem fluorescent LC3 puncta, cells were washed with PBS, fixed with 4% paraformaldehyde, mounted with DAPI and viewed under a confocal microscope [17].

## Autophagy assays

To analyze autophagic flux, we monitored the formation of autophagic vesicles by the mRFP–GFP–LC3 method (Invitrogen). Due to the quenching of GFP in the acidic lysosomal environment

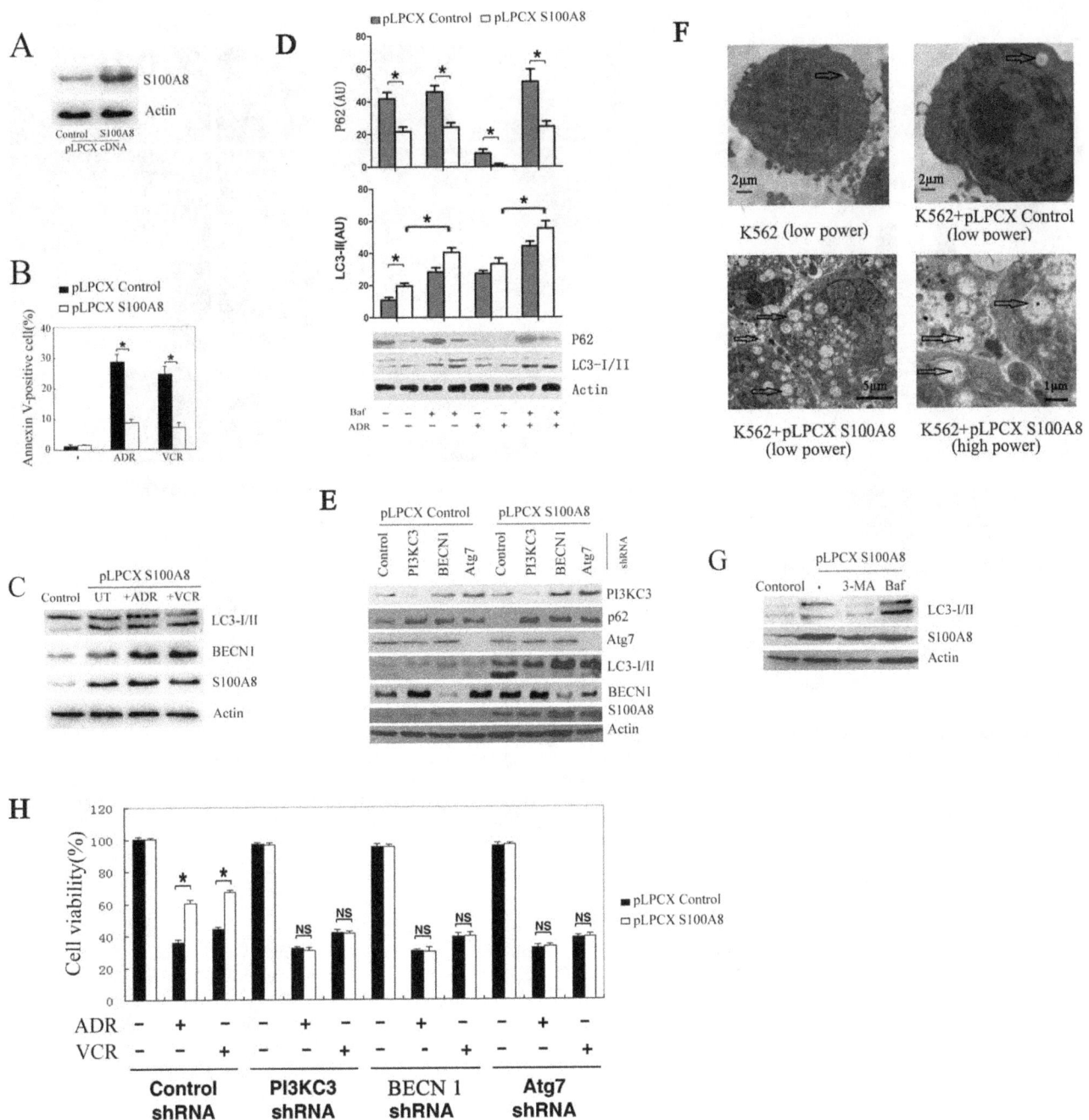

**Figure 3. Overexpression of S100A8 increased the resistance of leukemia cells to chemotherapy.** (A) K562 cells were transfected with control pLPCX or pLPCX-S100A8 plasmids. Protein level of S100A8 was assayed by Western blot. (B) K562 cells transfected with control pLPCX or pLPCX-S100A8 plasmids were treated with ADR (1 µg/mL) or VCR (1 µg/mL) for 24 hours. Apoptosis was analyzed by measuring Annexin V-positive cells with flow cytometry (n = 3; *P<0.05). (C) K562 cells were treated as B, LC3-I/II and BECN1 levels were assayed by Western blot analysis. **UT,** untreated group of K562 cells transfected with S100A8 plasmids. **Control,** K562 cells were transfected with control pLPCX plasmids. (D) K562 cells were transfected with pLPCX control or pLPCX -S100A8 cDNA for 48 hours and then treated with ADR (1 µg/mL) for 24 hours in the presence or absence of bafilomycin A1 (Baf; 100 nmol/L). The protein levels of LC3 and p62 were assayed by Western blot. (E) K562 cells were transfected pLPCX or pLPCX-S100A8 cDNA with or without the indicated shRNA for 48 hours. Protein levels of S100A8, PI3KC3, BECN1, Atg7, LC3, and p62 were assayed by Western blots. (F) K562 cells transfected with control pLPCX or pLPCX-S100A8 cDNA were subjected to TEM analysis. Autophagosomes were highlighted by arrows. (G) K562 cells transfected with PLPCX-S100A8 cDNA were treated with bafilomycin A1 (Baf; 100 nmol/L) or 3-methyladenine (3-MA; 10 mmo/L) for 12 hours. LC3 were assayed by Western blot. **Control,** K562 cells were transfected with control pLPCX. (H) K562 cells transfected the indicated shRNA were treated with ADR (1 µg/mL) and VCR (1 µg/mL) for 24 hours. Cell viability was analyzed by MTT assay (n = 3; *P<0.05). NS, not significant.

[17], we could distinguish the autophagosomes and autolysosomes through detecting both mRFP and GFP signals, followed by only the mRFP signal. K562 cells were transfected with mRFP-GFP-

LC3 expressing pLenti6 lentivirus (Nanjing Mergene Life Science, Nanjing, China). Autophagic flux was determined by evaluating the punctuated pattern of GFP and mRFP (punctae/cell were

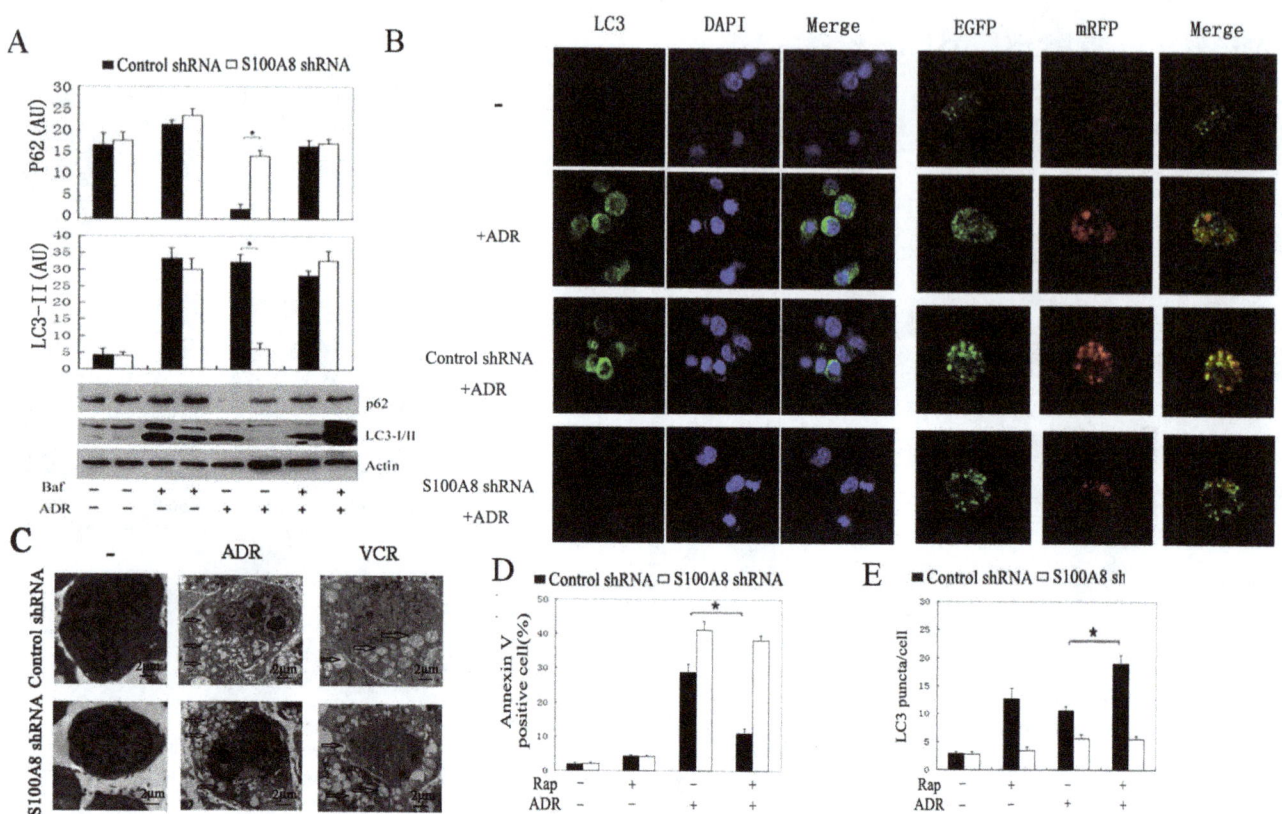

**Figure 4. S100A8 regulated the chemotherapy–induced autophagy in leukemia cells. (A and B)** K562 cells were transfected with control shRNA or S100A8 shRNA for 48 hours and then treated with ADR (1 μg/mL) and VCR (1 μg/mL) for 24 hours in the presence or absence of bafilomycin A1 (Baf; 100 nmol/L). The protein levels of LC3 and p62 were assayed by Western blot (**A**); LC3 puncta were analyzed by LC3 antibody or mRFP–GFP–LC3 (Magnification is 10×60 oil) (**B**) (n = 3; $^*P<0.05$). (**C**) K562 cells were transfected with control shRNA or S100A8 shRNA for 48 hours and then treated with ADR (1 μg/mL) and VCR (1 μg/mL) for 24 hours. Autophagosome-like structures (indicated by the red arrows) were assayed by TEM (n = 3; $^*P<0.05$). Bar = 2 μm. (**D and E**) K562/A02 cells were transfected with control shRNA or S100A8 shRNA for 48 hours. After pretreatment with rapamycin (Rap; 100 nmol/L) for 6 hours, cells were treated with ADR (1 μg/mL) for 24 hours. Apoptosis was analyzed by measuring Annexin V–positive cells with flow cytometry (**D**). Autophagy was analyzed by measuring LC3 puncta formation (**E**; n = 3; $^*P<0.05$).

counted). Fluorescence was analyed on an Olympus (Aartselaar, Belgium) cell imaging station using Cell M software. The protein levels of LC3 and p62 were determined by Western blotting. Transmission electron microscopic (TEM) assessment of autophagosomes-like structures was performed as previously described [7].

### Statistical analysis

All experiments were performed in at least triplicates per group, and data are reported as mean±SEM, unless otherwise indicated. Data were analyzed by 2-tailed Student $t$-test or ANOVA least significant difference test, and P<0.05 was considered significant.

## Results

### S100A8 was overexpressed in drug resistance leukemia cells and anticancer agents increased S100A8 expression in leukemia cells

S100A8 was differentially expressed in different cell lines, with relatively low S100A8 in Jurkat cells. We found that S100A8 protein was significantly increased in the drug resistance leukemia cell line K562/A02, relative to the nondrug resistant cell line K562 (Fig. 1A). Elevated S100A8 protein level was also observed in the drug resistance HL-60/ADR cells compared to HL-60 cells (Fig. 1A). Furthermore, there were relatively high levels of S100A8

mRNAs in HL-60, K562 and MV4-11 cells in comparison to Jurkat cells (Fig. 1B), and significantly increased S100A8 mRNAs in K562/A02 and HL-60/ADR compared with K562 and HL-60, respectively (Fig. 1C). These results showed that drug-resistant leukemia cells overexpress S100A8.

At the same time, we found the basal authophagy level in the drug resistant leukemia cells was higher compared to the non-drug resistant cell lines. We evaluated basal authophagy in leukaemia cells and compared the levels of autophagy with S100A8 expression. Basal authophagy in leukaemia cells was low. Moreover, we found there were no significant difference in levels of LC3-II/LC-I in HL-60, K562 and MV4-11 cells in comparison to Jurkat cells. However, the authophagy level were increased in K562/A02 relative to K562, and HL-60/ADR compared to HL-60 (Fig. 1D).

To explore the functions of S100A8 in drug resistance, we next analyzed the relationship between the IC50 of adriamycin and the expression level of S100A8. Increased expression of S100A8 was correlated with higher IC50 of adriamycin (Fig. 1E). Overexpression of S100A8 in K562/A02 and HL-60/ADR cells was coincident with dramatic increase in IC50 of adriamycin (Fig. 1F), indicating that S100A8 plays an important role in the drug resistance of leukemia cells.

It was reported that chemotherapeutic drugs induce S100A8 in the supernatants of cell cultures [14]. To further determine the

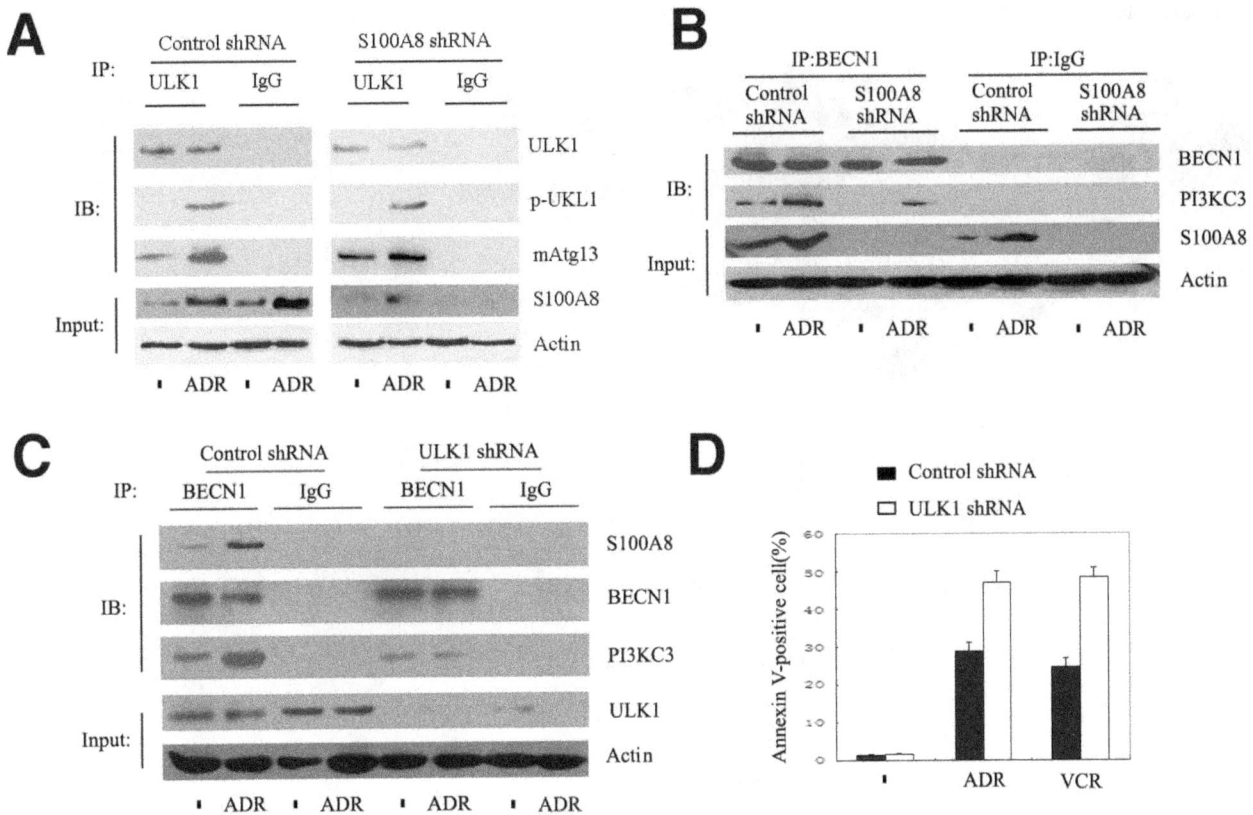

**Figure 5. ULK1-mAtg13 regulated the fomation of S100A8-BECN1 complex formation in leukemia cells. (A-C)** K562 cells were transfected with S100A8 shRNA (A and B) or ULK1 shRNA (C) for 48 hours and then were treated with ADR (1 μg/mL) for 24 hours. Cells were then processed for immunoprecipitation (IP) or Western blotting (IB) as described in Materials and Methods. All data are representative of 3 experiments. **(D)** K562 cells transfected with S100A8 shRNA (A and B) or ULK1 shRNA (C) for 48 hours were treated with ADR (1 μg/mL) or VCR (1 μg/mL) for 24 hours. Apoptosis was analyzed by measuring Annexin V–positive cells with flow cytometry (n = 3; *P<0.05).

potential role of S100A8 in leukemia in response to chemotherapy, we quantified S100A8 of leukemia cells following treatment with vincristine (VCR, 1 μg/ml), adriamycin (ADR, 1 μg/ml), and arsenic trioxide (As2O3, 5 μM), which are widely used for the treatment of hematological malignancies. Treatment of K562, HL-60, Jurkat and MV4-11 cells with VCR, ADR and As2O3 for 24 h led to significant upregulation of S100A8 protein (Fig. 1G) and mRNA (Fig. 1H).

## Suppression of S100A8 rescued the chemotherapy sensitivity in drug resistance leukemia cells

To evaluate whether overexpression of S100A8 results in drug resistance, we knocked down S100A8 by shRNA in HL60/ADR and K562/A02. S100A8 shRNA transfection led to a significant decrease of both S100A8 protein and mRNA in these cells (Fig. 2A). Knockdown of S100A8 significantly sensitized these cells to adriamycin and Vincristine (Fig. 2B), accompanied with high levels of apoptotic cell death (Fig. 2C) and an increase in cleaved PARP1 (Fig. 2D). Moreover, S100A8 knockdown increased the activation of the proapoptotic protein caspase-3 by both adriamycin and Vincristine, which was abolished by addition of the pan-caspase inhibitor Z-VAD-FMK (Fig. 2E). In addition, knockdown of S100A8 in HL60/ADR cells by another S100A8 shRNA from Gene Pharma also increased the sensitivity to DRN- and VCR-induced suppression of cell proliferation and apoptosis (Fig. 2F). These data demonstrated that S100A8 increased the resistance of leukemia cells to cytotoxic agents and knockdown of S100A8 restored the sensitivity of K562/A02 and HL60/ADR cells to adriamycin and vincristine.

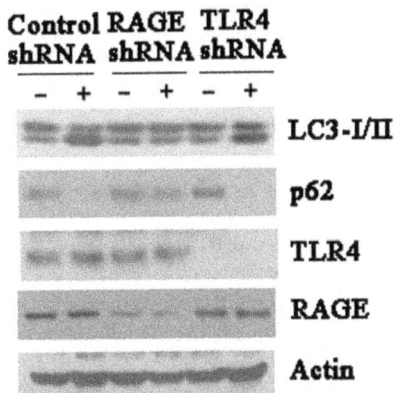

**Figure 6. Exogenous S100A8 regulate autophagy through RAGE receptor.** K562 cells were transfected with control shRNA, RAGE shRNA or TLR4 shRNA for 48 hours, and then treated with S100A8 protein (1 μg/ml) for 24 hours. LC3, p62, RAGE and TLR4 were assayed by Western blot. All data were representatives of 3 independent experiments.

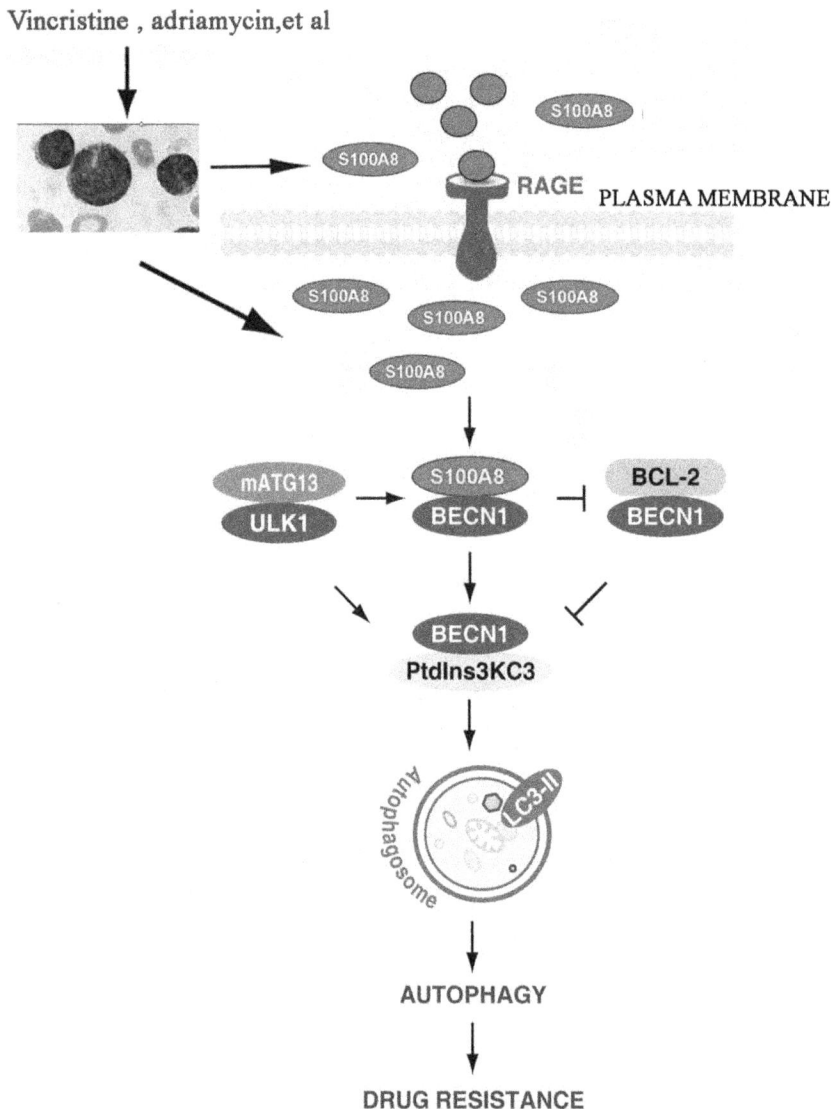

**Figure 7. Scheme of S100A8-mediated autophagy promoting drug resistance in leukemia.** Leukemia is the most common type of cancer occurs in childhood. Vincristine and adriamycin are the commonly used cytotoxic anticancer drugs in the treatment of patients with Leukemia. These drugs increase endogenous mRNA and protein expression of S100A8 in Leukemia cells by an unknown mechanism. Upregulated S100A8 competes with BCL-2 to bind BECN1, which increases the formation of the BECN1-PtdIns3KC3 complex and stimulates autophagosome maturation and autophagy. As an upstream signal, activation of the ULK1-mATG13 complex is required for the interaction between S100A8 and BECN1. Knockdown of S100A8 or inhibition of autophagy increase apoptosis, and reverses drug resistance in leukemia cells. Furthermore, exogenous S100A8 regulates autophagy through the RAGE receptor. Thus S100A8-mediated autophagy is a potential therapeutic target for leukemia.

## Overexpression of S100A8 increases the resistance of leukemia cells to chemotherapy

To further determine the role of S100A8 in leukemia cells after chemotherapy, we transfected K562 leukemia cells with a plasmid containing full-length human S100A8 cDNA (Fig. 3A). Ectopic overexpression of S100A8 in K562 cells promoted resistance to apoptosis induced by adriamycin and vincristine (Fig. 3B). Autophagy and apoptosis can be triggered simultaneously by common upstream signals [18]. During autophagy, microtubule-associated protein light chain 3 (LC3) is processed post-translationally into soluble LC3-I, and subsequently converted to membrane-bound LC3-II, a marker for autophagosome [19]. Overexpression of S100A8 increased LC3-II following treatment with either ADR or VCR in K562 cells (Fig. 3C). Meanwhile, BECN1, which is necessary for the formation of autophagosomes

during the autophagic sequestration process [20], was significantly increased in S100A8 expressing leukemia cells treated with adriamycin or vincristine for 24 h compared with the untreated and control groups (Fig. 3C,D). The polyubiquitin-binding protein SQSTM1/aequestosome 1 (p62) has LC3 binding domains, which target p62 for incorporation into the autophagosomes, thus serving as a selective substrate of autophagy [21]. We found that overexpression of S100A8 increased LC3-II but decreased p62, indicating that p62 degradation is dependent on S100A8-induced autophagy (Fig. 3D,E). Electron microscopy analysis demonstrated that there was increased number of multiple autophagosome-like vacuoles with double-membrane structures in the S100A8 overexpressing cells compared with that of the control group (Fig. 3F).

We further found that increase of S100A8 during anticancer therapy could induce autophagic flux in leukaemia cells. Accumulation of LC3-II was observed in the presence of bafilomycin A1 (an inhibitor of late phase autophagy) in k562 cells both before and after treatment with adriamycin for 24 h compared with the absence of bafilomycin A1 (Fig. 3D). At the same time, overexpression of S100A8 induced autophagic p62 degradation (Fig. 3D).

Bafilomycin A1 increased the induction of LC3-II by S100A8 (Fig 3D), whereas 3-methyladenine, an inhibitor of early-phase autophagy [19], inhibited S100A8-induced LC3-II expression (Fig. 3G). PI3KC3, BECN1 (the mammalian ortholog of yeast Vps30/Atg6), and ATG7 are key regulators of the classical autophagy pathway in mammalian cells [22]. To extend our observation that S100A8 promotes anticancer drug resistance by enhancing autophagy, we knocked down PI3KC3, BECN 1, and Atg7 by shRNA and found that silencing of these genes inhibited LC3-II formation and prevented autophagic p62 degradation in S100A8 overexpressing K562 cells (Fig. 3E). Moreover, downregulation of these genes reversed S100A8-induced protection against chemotherapy (Fig. 3H). These findings indicate that autophagy is required for S100A8-mediated resistance to anticancer agents.

## S100A8 regulates autophagy during chemotherapy in leukemia cells

S100A8 is required for the initiation of As2O3-reduced autophagy in leukemia cells [14]. To further explore the mechanism by which S100A8 regulates autophagy in leukemia cells, we detected LC3-I to LC3-II conversion by immunoblot analysis and LC3 puncta formation by fluorescent imaging analysis. Knockdown of S100A8 inhibited ADR-induced LC3-II (Fig. 4A). LC3 is lipidated and recruited to the autophagosomal membrane following autophagosome formation. Accordingly, accumulation of LC3-II was observed in the presence of bafilomycin A1 (Fig. 4A). Moreover, knockdown of S100A8 inhibited the accumulation of LC3 puncta in leukemia cells as detected by immunofluorenscence with a LC3 antibody (Fig. 4B). In addition, ultrastructural analysis revealed that cells transfected with S100A8 shRNA exhibited fewer autophagosomes during chemotherapy compared with cells transfected with control shRNA (Fig. 4C). To test whether S100A8 influences autophagic flux, we evaluated the expression of p62. Indeed, knockdown of S100A8 inhibited autophagic p62 degradation (Fig. 4A). These findings further support a critical role for S100A8 in the regulation of autophagy in leukemia cells.

Rapamycin induces autophagy by inhibiting the mammalian target of rapamycin complex 1 (mTORC1) [23]. Rapamycin pretreatment prevented ADR from inducing apoptosis in K562/A02 cells (Fig. 4D). However, rapamycin conferred less protection in K562/A02 cells transfected with S100A8 shRNA probably due to diminished autophagic capacity (Fig. 4E). These results suggest that S100A8 is an important regulator of autophagy-mediated leukemia cell survival.

## S100A8 regulates the formation of BECN1–PI3KC3 complex but not ULK1–mAtg13 complex

Mammalian autophagy is a multi-step process including initiation, nucleation, elongation, closure, maturation, and finally degradation or extrusion, and regulated by a core family of ATG proteins [1,24]. To explore the underlying molecular mechanism of S100A8-mediated autophagy, we analyzed the early autophagic signaling event of ULK1 complex formation. ULK1 is essential for autophagy induction and is comprised of a large complex that includes a mammalian homologue of Atg13 (mAtg13). Knockdown of S100A8 did not affect the formation of ULK1-mAtg13 complex and phosphorylation of ULK1 at Ser55 following ADR treatment (Fig. 5A). However, S100A8 knockdown significantly reduced the formation of the BECN1-PI3KC3 complex (Fig. 5B), which mediates vesicle nucleation during autophagy. Consistent with the previous studies [14], S100A8 formed a complex with BECN1 in leukemia cells (Fig. 5C). Moreover, knockdown of ULK1 inhibited the interaction between S100A8 and BECN1 (Fig. 5C) and potentiated anticancer agent-induced cell apoptosis (Fig. 5D). These data suggest that S100A8 is a downstream signaling molecule from the ULK1-mAtg13 complex and facilitates autophagy in leukemia cells by interacting with BECN1.

**RAGE was involved in exogenous S100A8-induced autophagy.** To investigate whether extracellular S100A8 induce autophagy in leukemia cells, we treated K562 cells with 1 μg/ml S100A8 protein for 24 h and detected LC3-I/LC3-II and P62 by immunoblot analysis. We found that S100A8 treatment increased the expression of LC3-II, and decreased the expression of p62. To test the role of RAGE and TLR4 in S100A8-induced autophagy, we knocked down RAGE and TLR4 by shRNA in K562 cells. We found that silencing RAGE inhibited LC3-II formation and prevented autophagic p62 degradation. In contrast, knock down of TLR4 did not influence S100A8-induced autophagic flux. These findings indicate that RAGE is involved in exogenous S100A8-induced autophagy (Fig. 6)

## Discussion

Chemotherapy is the major treatment strategy for nearly all types of childhood leukemia [25,26]; however, drug resistance often renders chemotherapy ineffective and negatively impacts long-term event-free survival [27]. Multidrug resistance results from multiple mechanisms including dysfunctional membrane transport, resistance to apoptosis, and the persistence of stem cell-like leukemia cells. Thus, attenuating drug resistance is a current challenge for the treatment of leukemia.

S100A8 is expressed in a wide variety of cell types and abundant in myeloid cells. Elevated expression of S100A8 has been found in disorders including rheumatoid arthritis, inflammatory bowel disease, and vasculitis [28]. S100A8 and HMGB1 are the ligands of receptor for advanced glycation endproducts (RAGE). RAGE/RAGE ligand interaction is associated with survival of cells expressing this receptor, and is involved in the development and progression of cancer [29]. Inhibition of RAGE interaction with S100p enhanced the anti-tumor activity of conventional chemotherapy in a xenograft model of pancreatic cancer [30]. We previously found that HMGB1-induced autophagy enhances chemotherapy resistance in leukemia cells [16]. It was reported that S100A8 protein balances tumor cell growth and apoptosis in a concentration-dependent manner [31]. Furthermore, variation of S100A8 transcripts has been found in AMLs and correlates with the FAB (French-American-British classification) subtype, or the differentiation of AML [32]. Nevertheless, the role of S100A8 in the pathogenesis of leukemia is unknown.

A number of anticancer therapies, including DNA-damaging chemotherapeutic drugs, induce the accumulation of autophagosomes in tumor cell lines, while pharmacologic inhibition of autophagy or genetic knockdown of phylogenetically conserved autophagy-related genes, such as Atg5 and Atg7, enhanced drug-induced cytotoxicities [33]. The ability to affect chemotherapy sensitivity by regulating autophagy in leukemia cells is a novel function of S100A8 [14]. In this study, we showed that A100A8-mediated autophagy is a significant contributor to drug resistance in leukemia. We found that S100A8 level was elevated in drug resistance leukemia cells relative to the nondrug resistant cells, and vincristine, adriamycin and arsenic trioxide enhanced the expression of S100A8 in human leukemia cells. Further, inhibition of S100A8 or autophagy increased the drug sensitivity of leukemia cells, and knockdown of S100A8 by shRNA increased cell death and suppressed leukemia cell growth. As a member of DAMPs, S100A8 demonstrate an anti-inflammatory, anti-oxidative, and protective effect on cells [34,35]. The expression of S100A8 in AML patients is associated with worse prognosis and a predictor of poor survival [12]. Thus, it is intriguing to propose that release of S100A8 by dying leukemia cells may help process and present leukemia antigens to immune effector cells.

Cancer cells respond to chemotherapy in a variety of ways, ranging from the activation of survival pathways to the initiation of cell death. Increased autophagy is observed in leukemia cells when exposed to chemotherapy drugs [5,36]. In general, autophagy is a "programmed cell survival" mechanism to prevent the accumulation of damaged or unnecessary components, but also functions to facilitate the recycling of these components to sustain homoeostasis. Therefore, autophagy functions as a double-edged sword in cancer development and progression by inducing both tumor cell survival and death. In tumor cells, the role of autophagy may depend on the type of tumors and the stage of tumorigenesis [37]. We found that inhibition of autophagy increases leukemia cell death and reverses S100A8-mediated drug resistance. A systematic study on cells exposed to many compounds showed that no single cytotoxic agent can induce cell death by autophagy [38], supporting the observation that autophagy is mostly a cytoprotective mechanism. Here, we found that knockdown of S100A8

decreased LC3 II formation and p62 degradation, which was associated with a decreased number of membrane-bound autophagosomes, as detected by TEM in leukemia cells.

We previously found that S100A8 interacts with BECN1 and displaces Bcl-2 [14]. In the current study, we found that the ULK1-mAtg13 complex is required for the interaction between S100A8 and BECN1, which promotes BECN1-PI3KC3 complex formation. However, the assembly of the BECN1 complexes is complicated and seems to differ in a cell- or tissue-dependent manner [39]. AMP-activated protein kinase (AMPK) is a key molecular player in energy homeostasis and important for the activation of ULK1 [40]. Further studies are needed to test whether AMPK or other kinases are involved in regulating the interaction between S100A8 and BECN1. Finally, we and found that exogenous S100A8 regulates autophagy through its receptor, RAGE, but not TLR4.

In conclusion, we showed that chemotherapy-induced S100A8 expression in leukemia cells promoted autophagy, which in turn inhibited apoptosis and increased drug resistance, indicating that S100A8 is an important regulator of autophagy. Moreover, suppression of S100A8 expression significantly increased drug sensitivity of leukemia cells, suggesting that S100A8 may be a novel target for leukemia therapy. (Fig 7).

## Author Contributions

Conceived and designed the experiments: MY LC. Performed the experiments: MY PZ RK YY LY DT. Analyzed the data: MY DT LC. Wrote the paper: MY LC.

## References

1. Yang Z, Klionsky DJ (2010) Eaten alive: a history of macroautophagy. Nat Cell Biol 12: 814–822.
2. Kroemer G, Marino G, Levine B (2010) Autophagy and the integrated stress response. Mol Cell 40: 280–293.
3. Helgason GV, Karvela M, Holyoake TL (2011) Kill one bird with two stones: potential efficacy of BCR-ABL and autophagy inhibition in CML. Blood 118: 2035–2043.
4. Zhu S, Cao L, Yu Y, Yang L, Yang M, et al. (2013) Inhibiting autophagy potentiates the anticancer activity of @/IFNalpha in chronic myeloid leukemia cells. Autophagy 9: 317–327.
5. Han W, Sun J, Feng L, Wang K, Li D, et al. (2011) Autophagy inhibition enhances daunorubicin-induced apoptosis in K562 cells. PLoS One 6: e28491.
6. Yu Y, Yang L, Zhao M, Zhu S, Kang R, et al. (2012) Targeting microRNA-30a-mediated autophagy enhances imatinib activity against human chronic myeloid leukemia cells. Leukemia 26: 1752–1760.
7. Liu L, Yang M, Kang R, Wang Z, Zhao Y, et al. (2011) DAMP-mediated autophagy contributes to drug resistance. Autophagy 7: 112–114.
8. Schafer BW, Heizmann CW (1996) The S100 family of EF-hand calcium-binding proteins: functions and pathology. Trends Biochem Sci 21: 134–140.
9. Foell D, Wittkowski H, Vogl T, Roth J (2007) S100 proteins expressed in phagocytes: a novel group of damage-associated molecular pattern molecules. J Leukoc Biol 81: 28–37.
10. Ghavami S, Kerkhoff C, Chazin WJ, Kadkhoda K, Xiao W, et al. (2008) S100A8/9 induces cell death via a novel, RAGE-independent pathway that involves selective release of Smac/DIABLO and Omi/HtrA2. Biochim Biophys Acta 1783: 297–311.
11. Cross SS, Hamdy FC, Deloulme JC, Rehman I (2005) Expression of S100 proteins in normal human tissues and common cancers using tissue microarrays: S100A6, S100A8, S100A9 and S100A11 are all overexpressed in common cancers. Histopathology 46: 256–269.
12. Nicolas E, Ramus C, Berthier S, Arlotto M, Bouamrani A, et al. (2011) Expression of S100A8 in leukemic cells predicts poor survival in de novo AML patients. Leukemia 25: 57–65.
13. Spijkers-Hagelstein JA, Schneider P, Hulleman E, de Boer J, Williams O, et al. (2012) Elevated S100A8/S100A9 expression causes glucocorticoid resistance in MLL-rearranged infant acute lymphoblastic leukemia. Leukemia 26: 1255–1265.
14. Yang L, Yang M, Zhang H, Wang Z, Yu Y, et al. (2012) S100A8-targeting siRNA enhances arsenic trioxide-induced myeloid leukemia cell death by down-regulating autophagy. Int J Mol Med 29: 65–72.
15. Yang MH, Zhao MY, Wang Z, Kang R, He YL, et al. (2011) WAVE1 regulates P-glycoprotein expression via Ezrin in leukemia cells. Leuk Lymphoma 52: 298–309.
16. Liu L, Yang M, Kang R, Wang Z, Zhao Y, et al. (2011) HMGB1-induced autophagy promotes chemotherapy resistance in leukemia cells. Leukemia 25: 23–31.
17. Klionsky DJ, Abdalla FC, Abeliovich H, Abraham RT, Acevedo-Arozena A, et al. (2012) Guidelines for the use and interpretation of assays for monitoring autophagy. Autophagy 8: 445–544.
18. Maiuri MC, Zalckvar E, Kimchi A, Kroemer G (2007) Self-eating and self-killing: crosstalk between autophagy and apoptosis. Nat Rev Mol Cell Biol 8: 741–752.
19. Mizushima N, Yoshimori T, Levine B (2010) Methods in mammalian autophagy research. Cell 140: 313–326.
20. Kihara A, Kabeya Y, Ohsumi Y, Yoshimori T (2001) Beclin-phosphatidylino-sitol 3-kinase complex functions at the trans-Golgi network. EMBO Rep 2: 330–335.
21. Pankiv S, Clausen TH, Lamark T, Brech A, Bruun JA, et al. (2007) p62/SQSTM1 binds directly to Atg8/LC3 to facilitate degradation of ubiquitinated protein aggregates by autophagy. J Biol Chem 282: 24131–24145.
22. Levine B, Kroemer G (2008) Autophagy in the pathogenesis of disease. Cell 132: 27–42.
23. Ravikumar B, Vacher C, Berger Z, Davies JE, Luo S, et al. (2004) Inhibition of mTOR induces autophagy and reduces toxicity of polyglutamine expansions in fly and mouse models of Huntington disease. Nat Genet 36: 585–595.
24. Klionsky DJ, Cregg JM, Dunn WA, Jr., Emr SD, Sakai Y, et al. (2003) A unified nomenclature for yeast autophagy-related genes. Dev Cell 5: 539–545.
25. Pui CH, Robison LL, Look AT (2008) Acute lymphoblastic leukaemia. Lancet 371: 1030–1043.
26. Rubnitz JE, Inaba H (2012) Childhood acute myeloid leukaemia. Br J Haematol 159: 259–276.
27. Norgaard JM, Olesen LH, Hokland P (2004) Changing picture of cellular drug resistance in human leukemia. Crit Rev Oncol Hematol 50: 39–49.
28. Nacken W, Roth J, Sorg C, Kerkhoff C (2003) S100A9/S100A8: Myeloid representatives of the S100 protein family as prominent players in innate immunity. Microsc Res Tech 60: 569–580.
29. Chavakis T, Bierhaus A, Nawroth PP (2004) RAGE (receptor for advanced glycation end products): a central player in the inflammatory response. Microbes Infect 6: 1219–1225.

30. Arumugam T, Ramachandran V, Logsdon CD (2006) Effect of cromolyn on S100P interactions with RAGE and pancreatic cancer growth and invasion in mouse models. J Natl Cancer Inst 98: 1806–1818.

31. Ghavami S, Rashedi I, Dattilo BM, Eshraghi M, Chazin WJ, et al. (2008) S100A8/A9 at low concentration promotes tumor cell growth via RAGE ligation and MAP kinase-dependent pathway. J Leukoc Biol 83: 1484–1492.

32. Cui JW, Wang J, He K, Jin BF, Wang HX, et al. (2004) Proteomic analysis of human acute leukemia cells: insight into their classification. Clin Cancer Res 10: 6887–6896.

33. Eisenberg-Lerner A, Bialik S, Simon HU, Kimchi A (2009) Life and death partners: apoptosis, autophagy and the cross-talk between them. Cell Death Differ 16: 966–975.

34. Sun Y, Lu Y, Engeland CG, Gordon SC, Sroussi HY (2013) The anti-oxidative, anti-inflammatory, and protective effect of S100A8 in endotoxemic mice. Mol Immunol 53: 443–449.

35. Yonekawa K, Neidhart M, Altwegg LA, Wyss CA, Corti R, et al. (2011) Myeloid related proteins activate Toll-like receptor 4 in human acute coronary syndromes. Atherosclerosis 218: 486–492.

36. Evangelisti C, Ricci F, Tazzari P, Tabellini G, Battistelli M, et al. (2011) Targeted inhibition of mTORC1 and mTORC2 by active-site mTOR inhibitors has cytotoxic effects in T-cell acute lymphoblastic leukemia. Leukemia 25: 781–791.

37. Dikic I, Johansen T, Kirkin V (2010) Selective autophagy in cancer development and therapy. Cancer Res 70: 3431–3434.

38. Shen S, Kepp O, Michaud M, Martins I, Minoux H, et al. (2011) Association and dissociation of autophagy, apoptosis and necrosis by systematic chemical study. Oncogene 30: 4544–4556.

39. Kang R, Zeh HJ, Lotze MT, Tang D (2011) The Beclin 1 network regulates autophagy and apoptosis. Cell Death Differ 18: 571–580.

40. Kim J, Kundu M, Viollet B, Guan KL (2011) AMPK and mTOR regulate autophagy through direct phosphorylation of Ulk1. Nat Cell Biol 13: 132–141.

# 8

# Current Status of Cancer Care for Young Patients with Nasopharyngeal Carcinoma

**Marlinda Adham**[1,9], **Sharon D. Stoker**[6,9], **Maarten A. Wildeman**[6,9], **Lisnawati Rachmadi**[2], **Soehartati Gondhowiardjo**[3], **Djumhana Atmakusumah**[4], **Djayadiman Gatot**[5], **Renske Fles**[6], **Astrid E. Greijer**[7], **Bambang Hermani**[1], **Jaap M. Middeldorp**[7], **I. Bing Tan**[6,8,10]*

1 Ear, Nose and Throat, University of Indonesia, Dr. Cipto Mangunkusumo hospital, Jakarta, Indonesia, 2 Anatomy-Pathology, University of Indonesia, Dr. Cipto Mangunkusumo hospital, Jakarta, Indonesia, 3 Radiotherapy, University of Indonesia, Dr. Cipto Mangunkusumo hospital, Jakarta, Indonesia, 4 Haematology-Medical Oncology Internal Medicine, University of Indonesia, Dr. Cipto Mangunkusumo hospital, Jakarta, Indonesia, 5 Medical Oncology Pediatric Department, University of Indonesia, Dr. Cipto Mangunkusumo hospital, Jakarta, Indonesia, 6 Department of Head and Neck Oncology and Surgery, The Netherlands Cancer Institute, Amsterdam, The Netherlands, 7 Department of Pathology, VU University Medical Center, Amsterdam, The Netherlands, 8 Ear, Nose and Throat Department, Gadjah Mada University, Yogyakarta, Indonesia, 9 Department of Otorhinolaryngology, Academic Medical Centre, Amsterdam, The Netherlands, 10 Department of Oral and Maxillofacial Surgery, Academic Medical Centre, Amsterdam, The Netherlands

## Abstract

*Background:* Nasopharyngeal carcinoma (NPC) is endemic in Indonesia and 20% of the patients are diagnosed before the age of 31. This study evaluates presentation and treatment outcome of young patients in Jakarta, in a tertiary referral centre.

*Methods:* Forty-nine patients under the age of 31, diagnosed with NPC between July 2004 and January 2007, were evaluated. Baseline data included histological type, stage of disease and presenting symptoms. We intended to follow all patients after diagnosis to reveal treatment outcome and overall survival (OS).

*Results:* All but two patients had advanced stage disease (94%), 7 (14%) had distant metastasis. The median interval between start of complaints and diagnosis was 9 months. Forty-two patients were planned for curative intent treatment. Eleven patients (26%) never started treatment, 2 patients did not complete treatment and 3 patients did not return after finishing treatment. Four patients died before radiation could start. Three patients died within 4 months after treatment. Nine patients (21%) had a complete response. Due to the high number of patients who were lost to follow-up (LFU), OS was analyzed as follows: a best-case (patients censored at last contact) and a worst-case scenario (assuming that patients who did not finish treatment or had disease at last contact would have died). The 2-year OS for patients without distant metastases was 39–71%.

*Conclusion:* Treatment outcome for young patients with NPC in this institute was poor. Improvement can be achieved when NPC is diagnosed at an earlier stage and when there is better treatment compliance.

**Editor:** Maria G. Masucci, Karolinska Institutet, Sweden

**Funding:** This study was sponsored by a grant of the Dutch Cancer Society, project number KWF-VUmc IN2006-21. The funders had no role in study design, data collection and analysis, decision to publish, or preparation of the manuscript.

**Competing Interests:** The authors have declared that no competing interests exist.

* Email: l.tan@nki.nl

⑨ These authors contributed equally to this work.

## Introduction

The incidence of nasopharyngeal carcinoma (NPC) in Indonesia is estimated to be 6:100.000, meaning that every month at least 1000 patients are diagnosed. Probably related to better diagnostics and improved awareness this number increases every year [1]. In Jakarta 20% of the patients are diagnosed before the age of 31 [1]. A study conducted in Yogyakarta, revealed a 3-year overall survival of 30% for adults with NPC, compared to 80% in literature [2,3]. The current study reveals the presentation and treatment outcome of young patients in Jakarta, in a tertiary referral centre.

NPC in young patients differs in certain aspects from adults. The percentage of non-keratinizing undifferentiated carcinoma is higher, and the association with Epstein-Barr virus (EBV) is stronger [1,4–6]. Young patients have more advanced disease at diagnosis and distant metastases are more frequently seen [4–9]. This might be caused by the undifferentiated state of the tumor, which is prone to develop distant metastasis [4,6–7]. Another hypothesis is the late recognition of complaints belonging to NPC in young patients, since early symptoms of NPC are non-specific and can look like ordinary upper airway infections, which are common in children.

Treatment for young patients generally follows the guidelines established for adults; radiotherapy on the nasopharynx and cervical nodal levels, usually combined with chemotherapy [4]. Despite the advanced stage at presentation, survival of young patients does not differ from adults. Several retrospective trials have proven the benefit of additional chemotherapy in juveniles [4,9–12]. Five-year disease-free survival varies between 45–77% and 5-year overall survival is 52–77% [5,7–12]. Recently, Buehren et al. published more promising results by adding adjuvant interferon beta after standard (chemo-) radiotherapy. This resulted in an event-free survival rate of 92.4% after a median follow-up of 30 months and an overall survival of 97.1% [7,13].

All these results are derived from top-end hospitals and some are in clinical trial settings. Here we present a prospective observational study on routine treatment results of young patients with NPC at a top end hospital in Jakarta. We will describe the tumor characteristics and complaints at presentation, the given treatment and the treatment outcome.

## Methods

### Patients

This was a prospective cohort study. All patients diagnosed with NPC between July 2004 and January 2007 at the Rumah Sakit Cipto Mangunkusumo (RSCM), a university hospital in Jakarta, were eligible for inclusion. Patients were included if they were below the age of 31 at diagnosis and had histological proven NPC. In this period 228 patients were diagnosed with NPC, and 49 patients met the inclusion criteria of age and histological confirmed NPC. Ethical approval was obtained at the Ethical committee of the Faculty of Medicine of the university of Indonesia. All patients or their parents/ legal guardian signed informed consent. To get more insight in the specific problems of patients at young age, the patients were divided into two groups, i.e. ≤15 years and >15–30 years.

Baseline information consisted of patient demographics, including the type of insurance. Jakarta has three types of insurances; jamkesmas (poor people), askes (civil servants) and patients who pay health care out of the pocket or have private insurance (self-finance) [14–15]. We hypothesized that type of insurance would have an impact on treatment outcome.

### Presentation and Diagnosis

Information on symptoms was gathered from the clinical medical record. Symptoms were scored for presence at diagnosis and duration till diagnosis. The histological diagnosis was made according to the World Health Organization (WHO) classification, WHO type 1; keratinizing squamous cell carcinoma, WHO type 2; non-keratinizing squamous cell carcinoma, WHO type 3; undifferentiated carcinoma. The extent of disease was determined by clinical examination using rigid or flexible nasopharyngoscopy, Computed Tomography (CT)-scan of the head and neck region, chest radiography, ultrasonography of the abdomen and a bone scan. Tumor stage was classified according to the 2002 criteria of the 6th American Joint Committee on Cancer (AJCC).

### Treatment

Due to the waiting time to radiation, different schedules were used. Three different radiation schedules were used; conventional fractionated schedule (daily fraction of 2 Gy, total 33–35 fractions); hyper fractionated schedule (2 fractions/ day of 1.2 Gy with 6 hours in between, total dose 81.6 Gy); accelerated

hyper fractionated schedule (daily fraction of 1.8 Gy in the first 4 weeks, followed by 2 weeks of daily 1 fraction of 1.8 Gy and a surdosage to macroscopic tumor of 1.5 Gy with 6 hours in between, total 72 Gy). All schedules could be completed in 6–7 weeks. Neo-adjuvant chemotherapy consisted of intravenous cisplatin 100 mg/m2/day on day 1, and 5-fluoro-uracil 1000 mg/m2/day on day 1–5, every 3 weeks for 3–4 courses. Concurrent chemotherapy consisted of intravenous cisplatin 40 mg/m2 weekly during radiotherapy.

Patients with distant metastasis received palliative chemotherapy; cisplatin 100 mg/m2/day on day 1 and, 5-fluoro-urasil 1000 mg/m2/day on day 1–4. The number of courses depended on the clinical condition. Palliative radiotherapy was given on bone metastasis.

### Follow-up

Patients were scheduled for routine follow-up at the outpatient clinic. Treatment response measurements were planned 8 to 12 weeks after treatment, by physical examination, nasopharyngoscopy and CT-scan. The follow-up schedule proceeds with 3 monthly visits during the first 2 years after radiotherapy.

### Statistics

To test for association between age and tumor stage at diagnosis, linear-by-linear test was used. For symptoms at diagnosis two scales were constructed: the number of complaints at diagnosis and the maximum duration to diagnosis. For patient's missing data on symptom duration, the median duration was imputed. Associations between these two scales and both age (as a continuous variable) and AJCC stage were tested using linear-by-linear tests.

Association between age and diagnosis-to-treatment interval (DTI) and overall-radiotherapy-treatment time (OTT) was assessed by Spearman correlation test. The Statistical Package for the Social Sciences, version 20 was used for analysis. P-values less than 0.05 were considered as significant.

Kaplan-Meier analyzed overall survival. Survival time was defined as the time between the date of diagnosis till the date of death. Stratification was done by M stage, and M0 was further stratified by age (0–15 and 16–30). For comparison between the 0–15 and the 16–30 age group a log rank test was used.

## Results

### Patients

Forty-nine patients were included. The median age was 21 and ranged between 3–30 years. WHO type 3 was the histological type in 46 patients (94%) and 3 patients (6%) had WHO type 1. The mean follow-up period for the patients without distant metastasis at diagnosis was 18 months and for patients with distant metastasis 7 months.

### Stage of disease at presentation

T-stage was dominated by advanced stage (66%). Lymph node metastasis was seen in 96% of the patients (table 1). Ninety-four per cent had advanced stage of disease. Seven patients (14%) had distant metastasis at diagnosis. All had metastases to the bone. In addition, two patients had lung metastasis and one of these had also liver metastasis. No association was found between age and stage of disease at presentation (linear-by-linear p = 0.85).

### Symptoms at diagnosis

Information on presenting symptoms at diagnosis was available for 41 patients (table 2). The median number of complaints at

**Table 1.** Patient & tumor characteristics.

| | | 0–15 Year | 16–30 Year |
|---|---|---|---|
| | | n = 14 | n = 35 |
| **AGE AT DIAGNOSIS** | | | |
| | Median | 11 | 26 |
| | (Range) | (3–15) | (16–30) |
| **GENDER** | | Number (percentage) | Number (percentage) |
| | Male | 10 (71) | 18 (51) |
| | Female | 4 (29) | 17 (49) |
| **INSURANCE** | | | |
| | Jamkesmas | 14 (100) | 27 (77) |
| | Askes | 0 (0) | 2 (6) |
| | Self Finance | 0 (0) | 4 (11) |
| | Missing | | 2 (6) |
| **TUMOR** | | | |
| T | T1 | 0 (0) | 2 (6) |
| | T2a | 0 (0) | 2 (6) |
| | T2b | 4 (29) | 9 (26) |
| | T3 | 5 (36) | 8 (23) |
| | T4 | 5 (36) | 14 (40) |
| N | N0 | 0 (0) | 2 (6) |
| | N1 | 0 (0) | 7 (20) |
| | N2 | 3 (21) | 7 (20) |
| | N3a | 8 (57) | 15 (43) |
| | N3b | 3 (21) | 4 (11) |
| M | M0 | 12 (86) | 30 (86) |
| | M1 | 2 (14) | 5 (14) |
| **STAGE** | 2b | 0 (0) | 3 (9) |
| | 3 | 3 (21) | 4 (11) |
| | 4a | 0 (7) | 9 (26) |
| | 4b | 9 (64) | 14 (40) |
| | 4c | 2 (14) | 5 (14) |

diagnosis was 5 (range 2–10). The median interval to diagnosis was 9 months (range 1–36 months). A neck mass was mentioned in 93% of the patients at diagnosis, more than 50% of the patients (21/40) had bilateral neck masses.

No associations (linear-by-linear) were detected between either age and the number of complains at diagnosis (p = 0.41) or the duration to diagnosis (p = 0.79). Also no associations were found between the stage of disease at diagnosis and the number of complaints (p = 0.25) and interval to diagnosis (p = 0.29).

## Treatment

Forty-two patients could be planned for treatment with curative intent. For 22 patients data was available on given radiotherapy treatment (table 3). The median interval between diagnosis and radiotherapy was 110 days (28–690 days). Patients in the 16–30 age group had to wait longer than the younger patients (130 vs. 77 days), although no association with age was found (Spearman correlation p = 0.99).

For 18 patients data on the overall radiotherapy treatment time (OTT) was available. The median OTT was 55 days (range 38–160), no association with age was found (spearman correlation

p = 0.41). Since almost all patients had jamkesmas insurance, no association between the insurance type and the DTI or OTT could be found.

## Treatment outcome and follow-up

Directly after diagnosis 11 patients (26%) did not return to the hospital. Two patients stopped therapy during treatment, and directly after therapy 3 patients never returned to the hospital. Despite several attempts to contact these 16 patients, no information on their health status could be retrieved. Four patients died before radiation treatment could start. Figure 1 shows the chart-flow.

Accordingly, for 22 patients the effect of treatment could be studied. Three patients died within 4 months after radiotherapy, before response was assessed. For three patients survival data was available, but no data on therapy response; one died 19 months after neo-adjuvant chemotherapy (unknown if he finished radiation treatment), one was alive 30 months after radiation and clinical suspect for distant metastases, and one died 65 months after radiation (reason unknown).

**Table 2.** Complaints at diagnosis and interval between first appearance and diagnosis.

| | 0–15 Year | 16–30 Year | | 0–15 Year | 16–30 Year |
|---|---|---|---|---|---|
| | n = 10 (100%) | n = 31 (100%) | Duration of symptom in months | | |
| **NECK MASS** | | | | | |
| Yes | 10 (100) | 28 (90) | Median | 11 | 9 |
| No | 0 (0) | 2 (6) | Range | 5–18 | 2–36 |
| Missing | | 1 (3) | | | |
| **NASAL CONGESTION** | | | | | |
| Yes | 8 (80) | 23 (74) | Median | 4 | 3 |
| No | 2 (20) | 8 (26) | Range | 1–18 | 1–12 |
| | | | Missing | | 1 |
| **EPISTAXIS** | | | | | |
| Yes | 7 (70) | 17 (55) | Median | 4 | 2 |
| No | 3 (30) | 14 (45) | Range | 1–18 | 1–12 |
| | | | Missing | | 1 |
| **POST NASAL DRIP** | | | | | |
| Yes | 4 (40) | 10 (32) | Median | 7 | 10 |
| No | 6 (60) | 17 (55) | Range | 4–10 | 3–12 |
| Missing | | 4 (13) | Missing | 2 | 4 |
| **DIPLOPIA** | | | | | |
| Yes | 3 (30) | 9 (29) | Median | 1 | 3 |
| No | 7 (70) | 22 (71) | Range | 0.5–5 | 0.25–7 |
| **DEAFNESS** | | | | | |
| Yes | 7 (70) | 21 (68) | Median | 1 | 1 |
| No | 3 (30) | 10 (32) | Range | 1–2 | 1–2 |
| | | | Missing | | 1 |
| **TINNITUS** | | | | | |
| Yes | 5 (50) | 17 (54) | Median | 3 | 3 |
| No | 5 (50) | 14 (45) | Range | 2–12 | 1–24 |
| | | | Missing | | 2 |
| **EAR PAIN** | | | | | |
| Yes | 2 (20) | 7 (23) | Median | 2 | 1.5 |
| No | 6 (60) | 20 (65) | Range | 2–2 | 0.03–12 |
| Missing | 2 (20) | 4 (13) | Missing | 1 | 3 |
| **OTORRHEA** | | | | | |
| Yes | 0 (0) | 3 (10) | Median | | 6 |
| No | 9 (90) | 22 (71) | Range | | 6–12 |
| Missing | 1 (10) | 6 (19) | | | |
| **CEPHALGIA** | | | | | |
| Yes | 5 (50) | 21 (68) | Median | 6 | 3 |
| No | 5 (50) | 10 (32) | Range | 1–12 | 1–36 |
| | | | Missing | | 2 |
| **NERVE PARALYSIS** | | | | | |
| Yes | 2 (20) | 5 (16) | Median | 5.5 | 1 |
| No | 7 (70) | 25 (81) | Range | 5–6 | 1–5 |
| Missing | 1 (10) | 1 (3) | Missing | | 1 |

Nine patients underwent examination 2–3 months after treatment, one patient had the examination 1 month after treatment and six patients had examination later than 3 months after therapy. Complete response was seen in 9 of these 16 patients, partial response in 5 patients and progressive disease in 2 patients.

**Table 3.** Radiotherapy treatment.

|  | 0–15 Year | 16–30 Year |
|---|---|---|
| **DIAGNOSIS TO RADIOTHERAPY IN DAYS** | n = 7 | n = 15 |
| Median | 77 | 130 |
| (Range) | (28–690) | (34–320) |
| **RADIOTHERAPY DURATION IN DAYS OVERALL** | n = 4 | n = 14 |
| Median | 55 | 56 |
| (Range) | (50–160) | (38–77) |

## Overall survival

The number of patients who were lost to follow-up (LFU) in this study was high. Despite multiple attempts to contact them or their family, it was not possible to minimize the missing data. The assumption that the risk to death was equally distributed between patients who were LFU and patients who were still in the study is not likely. This is based on the fact that some patients never started treatment, stopped during treatment or had disease at the last date of follow-up. Therefore we made two Kaplan-Meier curves, representing a best-case scenario and a worst-case scenario. The best-case scenario is a regular Kaplan-Meier curve, wherein all patients are censored on the last date of follow-up. For the worst-case scenario; for patients without distant metastasis, all patients who did not return to the hospital before starting treatment (n = 11), before finishing treatment (n = 2), or who had disease at last moment of contact (n = 6) were assumed to be death at the last date of contact; for patients with distant metastasis at diagnosis, the last date of contact was set as the date of death. A realistic overall survival curve will be positioned between these two Kaplan-Meier curves.

The 2-year overall survival for patients without distant metastasis at diagnosis was 39–71% (worst- and best-case scenario, respectively). The 2-year survival for patients with distant metastasis at diagnosis was 0% (table 4). Overall survival, analyzed in the best-case scenario was significantly poorer for the younger patients (log rank p = 0.021). In the worst-case scenario this was not significant (log rank p = 0.142)(figure 2 and 3).

Overall survival was tested on association with stage of disease, symptoms at diagnosis, waiting time for radiotherapy and treatment duration. No significant results were found. It was not possible to test for association with insurance, since the group of patients with other insurance than jamkesmas was too small.

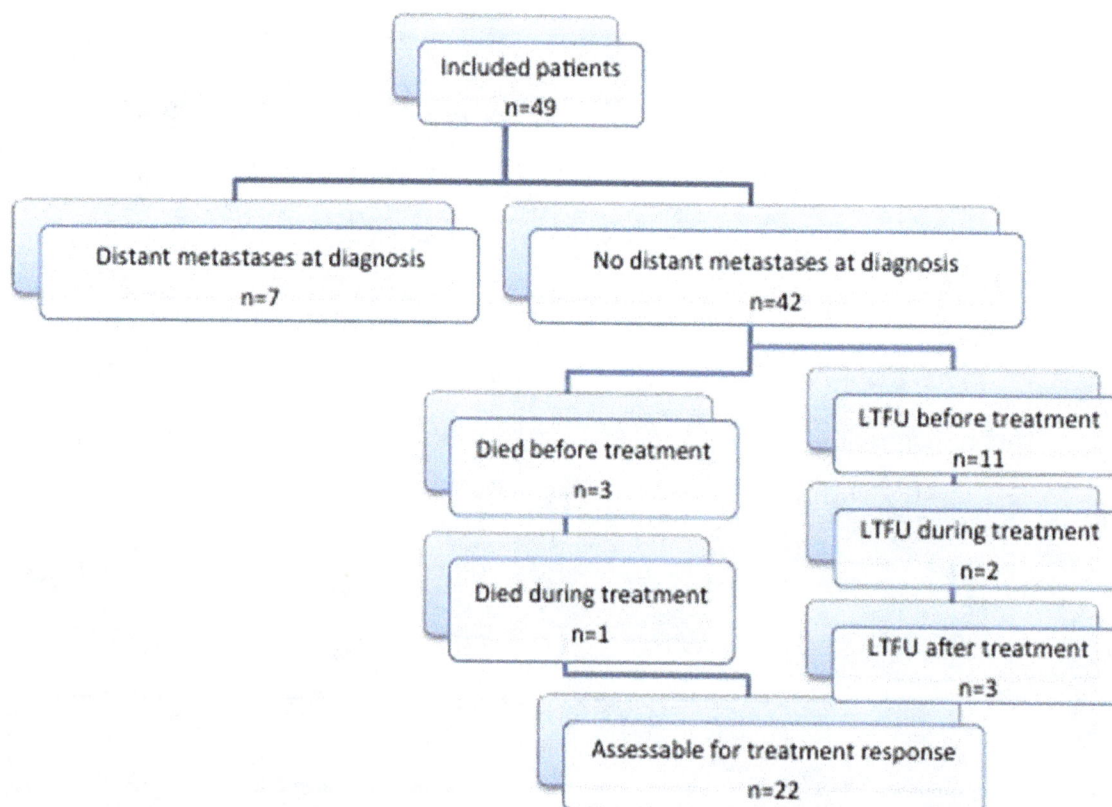

**Figure 1. Patient overview.** LTFU = lost to follow-up.

**Table 4.** Overall survival.

| | 6 months | | 2 years | | 5 years | |
|---|---|---|---|---|---|---|
| | Worst-case scenario | Best-case scenario | Worst-case scenario | Best-case scenario | Worst-case scenario | Best-case scenario |
| 0–15 year (M0, n = 12) | 58% | 78% | 20% | 50% | 0% | 0% |
| 16–30 year (M0, n = 30) | 60% | 91% | 46% | 79% | 23% | 52% |
| 0–30 year (M0, n = 42) | 60% | 87% | 39% | 71% | 16% | 38% |
| Distant metastasis (n = 7) | 43% | 83% | 0% | 0% | 0% | 0% |

## Discussion

Cancer is the leading cause of death worldwide [16–17]. The distribution of cancer mortality shifts towards the low- and middle-income countries. Currently, 70% of cancer deaths occur in these countries and this burden increases every year [16–18]. Their health-care systems are not prepared for the number of patients.

Unlike high-income countries, where cancer survival improves due to better treatment facilities and enhanced protocols, low-income countries lack facilities and medication. Funding for research and solutions aiming to resolve these limitations is hardly available. The gap in treatment results between high-income and low-income countries is therefore widening [17]. Major improvement

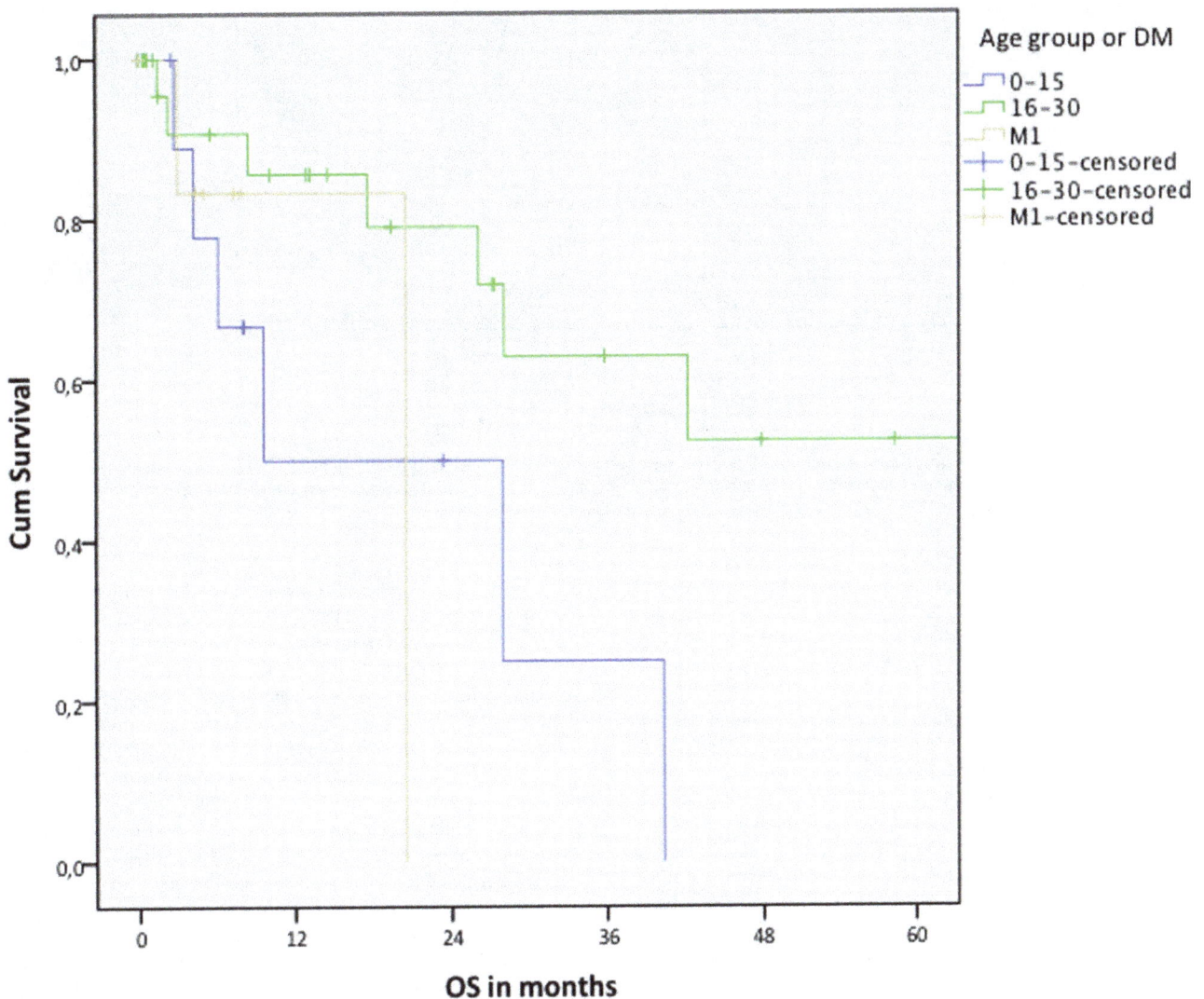

**Figure 2. Overall survival: best-case scenario.** All patients who were lost to follow up were censored at the moment of last contact (Log rank is p = 0.021, when comparing patients without distant metastasis: 0–15 vs. 16–30 year). DM = distant metastasis at diagnosis; OS = overall survival.

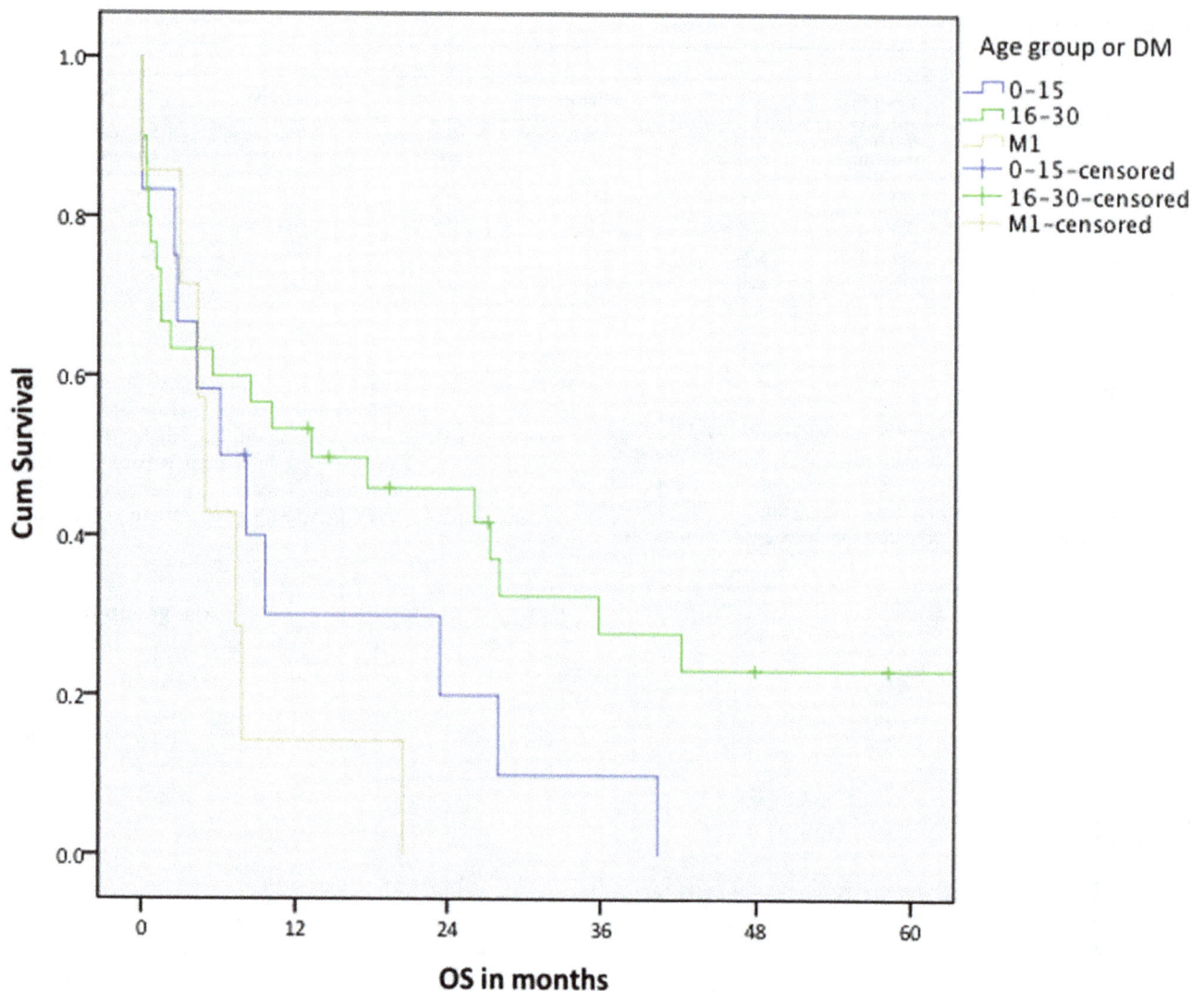

**Figure 3. Overall survival: worst-case scenario.** All patients who were lost to follow up before treatment (n = 11) or during treatment (n = 2), or who had disease at last moment of follow up (n = 6) are assumed to be death (Log rank p = 0. 142, when comparing patients without distant metastasis: 0–15 vs. 16–30 year). DM = distant metastasis at diagnosis; OS = overall survival.

in the health care systems is needed. Although many authors have emphasized this, solid data on the actual problems are lacking. This study reveals some of the current problems in the treatment of NPC in Jakarta, a major referral hospital and one of the top end hospitals in Indonesia.

Cancer care for young patients with NPC in Jakarta is poor compared to international literature. In literature, 1–4% of the young patients with NPC have distant metastasis at initial diagnosis [4–5]. In this study 14% of the patients presented with distant metastasis. Two years after diagnosis many patients were lost to follow-up, only 47 per cent of them were still in the study (23/49). Ten out of these 23 patients had already died at this point. The 5-year overall survival for patients without distant metastasis lies between 16–38%, compared to 52–77% in the literature [4–5,7–13]. These results might be caused by the late stage of presentation at the hospital, insufficient treatment (compliance) and poor follow-up.

Advanced stage of disease at diagnosis was seen in 94% of the patients. Since stage of disease is strongly associated with prognosis, this partly accounts for the poor survival. Advanced

stage at diagnosis is related to a long interval to diagnosis [19]. In our study the mean interval from start of complaints till diagnosis was 9 months, which is long compared to the 4 to 8 months found in China [19], India [12] and Turkey [5]. This long interval can be caused both by patient's or doctor's delay. Early stage symptoms of NPC look like an ordinary inflammatory upper airway infection. In our young patient group, the early stage symptoms are not mentioned as complaints with the longest duration. Apparently, the early symptoms are not evidently present or do not trigger patients to seek medical help. The latter explanation might be plausible in this patient group, due to the non-specificity of the complaints and the frequency of upper airway complaints in the young population.

Neck masses, a late stage symptom, were present in 93 per cent of our patients at diagnosis. In almost all patients this complaint existed with the longest interval to diagnosis. One should assume that when a neck mass is present, a patient (or parent) should make effort to consult a doctor. Instead, a time interval of 9.5 months was found before definitive diagnosis. It seems that patients (and probably doctors) are not aware of the probability for NPC involvement in young patients with an unexplained neck mass.

Patient's delay to diagnosis can also be caused by the long distance to health care facilities or limited financial resources of patients, 84% had poor men's insurance. Besides, we know by experience that many patients first seek medical help in the alternative circuit. Even when NPC is diagnosed some patients prefer alternative therapy above conventional. We cannot confirm this by our study results, but eleven patients did not return to the hospital after diagnosis. Unfortunately, we could not retrieve the reason for not returning. More public awareness about the symptoms of NPC and need for early treatment with (chemo-) radiotherapy can contribute to an earlier consultation of the doctor and better compliance to the advised therapy. Previous studies have already shown the effectiveness of public awareness campaigns in breast and cervical cancer [20].

As mentioned before, the doctor can also cause the delay to diagnosis; when doctors do not recognize the symptoms as related to cancer or when they are not aware of the high probability of NPC. Earlier research revealed that the knowledge of general practitioners (GP's) on NPC in Indonesia was insufficient [21]. A sequel study showed that after teaching there was a great improvement of knowledge [22]. More educational programs can improve early diagnosis. Furthermore, with the increasing awareness of NPC's associated with Epstein-Barr virus (EBV) infection and the availability of tests with EBV-related tumor markers which can be performed by the GPs, improvement in earlier diagnosis is within reach [1,23–25].

Another result of this study was the insufficiency of the treatment itself. The median interval between diagnosis and radiotherapy was almost 4 months. This is partly caused by the insurance system. Almost all patients had jamkesmas insurance. Hereby, approval is needed for every investigation and treatment, which takes valuable time. Another key reason for the long interval to treatment is shortage in capacity of radiotherapy facilities. In 2008, 35 radiotherapy devices were available for a population of 229 million. A substantial number of these devices are out of order on a regular base, resulting in 0.13 accelerators per million inhabitants [26]. This is not enough. For comparison, in Europe 2–5.5 accelerators are available per one million inhabitants [27]. We assumed that the patient's type of insurance would have a strong impact on all parameters, unfortunately no statistical analysis could be performed due to the small group who had other insurance than Jamkesmas. The presented results do emphasize the low financial resources of this patient group and the need for improvement of the national health care system.

The long waiting time, the neo-adjuvant chemotherapy to overcome the waiting time and the treatment of radiation (with or without concurrent chemotherapy) has impact on patient's physical status. In this study three patients died before treatment could start, one patient died during neo-adjuvant treatment and another four patients died directly after treatment, accordingly 19% died soon after diagnosis. This percentage might be an underestimation, since directly after diagnosis 11 patients were lost to follow-up. These patients did not get treatment, so it is assumable that some of them also would have died. The results are comparable to a recent study of adults with NPC, conducted in Yogyakarta, here 13% of the patients died before radiotherapy started and 29% died before treatment response could be assessed

[2]. Studies involving preservation or improving the patient's physical performance status during the waiting time and during treatment might be of great value to lower the mortality. Suggestions are other treatment modalities, like photodynamic therapy to overcome the waiting time, or protocols to observe and improve the nutritional status [28]

The overall treatment time of radiotherapy was 55 days. Optimally, a total dose of 66 to 70 Gray should be given in 33–35 fractions in a maximum of 47 days. For each day by which radiotherapy treatment is extended, effective dose is lost, and the success rate declines rapidly [29–30]. The long overall treatment time is therefore most probably also a reason for the poor complete response percentage.

Another problem that we encountered was the lack of data management and poor follow-up. This made it impossible to compare the different treatment protocols and made statistical analysis difficult. In general the lack of proper data management causes a lack of essential feedback for doctors, which results in the absence of a learning curve and current insight in problems in cancer care in general. Besides, poor follow-up results in late recognition of recurrent disease, which immediately affects the patient's health and chances of survival. A digital data management system may result in better insights in clinical performance and stimulate the treatment learning curve [31].

## Conclusions

This is the first study presenting the treatment results of young patients with NPC in Indonesia, where 20% of the patients are diagnosed before the age of 31. Comparable, poor treatment outcome has been found in an independent study among adults with NPC in Yogyakarta, and it is assumable that other low and middle-income countries are coping with similar problems in handling NPC patients [2,28]. The study revealed serious weaknesses at different levels in diagnosis and treatment. The current changes in the insurance system of Indonesia, aiming to provide health care for every one, will put even more pressure on the health care facilities. Therefore it is likely that the problems might get bigger.

Establishing more radiotherapy facilities would be the best step to solve a big part of the problems. However, even when financial resources are not the limiting factor, it will take a decade to built new bunkers and educate doctors and nurses to accomplish this. In the meanwhile the focus should be to treat people who can have treatment in a proper way. Earlier diagnosis, better treatment compliance and improved follow-up are the key points to accomplish this. More public, medical and patient awareness for these key points might be one of the answers.

## Acknowledgments

We thank Judi N.A. van Diessen, radiation oncologist in The Netherlands Cancer Institute, for her comments and suggestions on the manuscript.

## Author Contributions

Conceived and designed the experiments: MA SG DA DG AG BH JM IT. Performed the experiments: MA SS MW LR SG DA DG BH IT RF. Analyzed the data: MA SS. Contributed reagents/materials/analysis tools: MA SS MW LR SG DA DG IT RF. Wrote the paper: MA SS.

## References

1. Adham M, Kurniawan AN, Muhtadi AI, Roezin A, Hermani B, et al. (2012) Nasopharyngeal carcinoma in Indonesia: epidemiology, incidence, signs, and symptoms at presentation. Chin J Cancer 31: 185–96

2. Wildeman MA, Fles R, Herdini C, Indrasari RS, Vincent AD, et al. (2013) Primary Treatment Results of Nasopharyngeal Carcinoma (NPC) in Yogyakarta, Indonesia. PLoS One 8: e63706.

3.  Lee AW, Lin JC, Ng WT (2012) Current management of nasopharyngeal cancer. Semin Radiat Oncol 22: 233–44.

4.  Ayan I, Kaytan E, Ayan N (2004) Childhood nasopharyngeal carcinoma: from biology to treatment. Lancet Oncol 4: 13–21.

5.  Ayan I, Altun M (1996) Nasopharyngeal carcinoma in children: retrospective review of 50 patients. Int J Radiat Oncol Biol Phys 35: 485–492.

6.  Wei WI, Sham JS (2005) Nasopharyngeal carcinoma. Lancet 365: 2041–2054.

7.  Mertens R, Granzen B, Lassay L, Bucksy P, Hundgen M, et al. (2005) Treatment of nasopharyngeal carcinoma in children and adolescents: definitive results of a multicenter study (NPC-91-GPOH). Cancer 104: 1083–1089.

8.  Downing NL, Wolden S, Wong P, Petrik DW, Hara W, Le QT (2009) Comparison of treatment results between adult and juvenile nasopharyngeal carcinoma. Int J Radiat Oncol Biol Phys 75: 1064–1070.

9.  Ozyar E, Selek U, Laskar S, Uzel O, Anacak Y, et al. (2006) Treatment results of 165 pediatric patients with non-metastatic nasopharyngeal carcinoma: a Rare Cancer Network study. Radiother Oncol 81: 39–46.

10.  Wolden SL, Steinherz PG, Kraus DH, Zelefsky MJ, Pfister DG, Wollner N (2000) mproved long-term survival with combined modality therapy for pediatric nasopharynx cancer. Int J Radiat Oncol Biol Phys 46: 859–864.

11.  Cheuk DK, Billups CA, Martin MG, Roland CR, Ribeiro RC, et al. (2011) Prognostic factors and long-term outcomes of childhood nasopharyngeal carcinoma. Cancer 117: 197–206.

12.  Laskar S, Sanghavi V, Muckaden MA, Ghosh S, Bhalla V, et al. (2004) Nasopharyngeal carcinoma in children: ten years' experience at the Tata Memorial Hospital, Mumbai. Int J Radiat Oncol Biol Phys 58: 189–195.

13.  Buehrlen M, Zwaan CM, Granzen B, Lassay L, Deutz P, et al. (2012) Multimodal treatment, including interferon beta, of nasopharyngeal carcinoma in children and young adults: Preliminary results from the prospective, multicenter study NPC-2003-GPOH/DCOG. Cancer 118: 4892–4900.

14.  Satriana S, Schmitt V (2012) Social protection assessment based national dialogue: Towards a nationally defined social protection floor in Indonesia/International Labour Organization. Jakarta, Indonesia.

15.  Tangcharoensathien V, Patcharanarumol W, Ir P, Aljunid SM, Mukti AG, et al. (2011) Health-financing reforms in southeast Asia: challenges in achieving universal coverage. Lancet 377: 863–873.

16.  Ferlay J, Shin HR, Bray F, Forman D, Mathers C, et al. (2010) Estimates of worldwide burden of cancer in 2008: GLOBOCAN 2008. Int J Cancer 127: 2893–2917.

17.  Farmer P, Frenk J, Knaul FM, Shulman LN, Alleyne, et al. (2010) Expansion of cancer care and control in countries of low and middle income: a call to action. Lancet 376: 1186–1193.

18.  Kimman M, Norman R, Jan S, Kingston D, Woodward M (2012) The burden of cancer in member countries of the Association of Southeast Asian Nations (ASEAN). Asian Pac J Cancer Prev 13: 411–420.

19.  Lee AW, Foo W, Law SC, Poon YF, Sze WM, et al. (1997) Nasopharyngeal carcinoma: presenting symptoms and duration before diagnosis. Hong Kong Med J 3: 355–361.

20.  Devi BC, Tang TS, Corbex M (2007) Reducing by half the percentage of late-stage presentation for breast and cervix cancer over 4 years: a pilot study of clinical downstaging in Sarawak, Malaysia. Ann Oncol 18: 1172–1176.

21.  Fles R, Wildeman MA, Sulistiono B, Haryana SM, Tan IB (2010) Knowledge of general practitioners about nasopharyngeal cancer at the Puskesmas in Yogyakarta, Indonesia. BMC Med Educ 10: 81.

22.  Wildeman MA, Fles R, Adham M, Mayangsari ID, Luirink I, et al. (2012) Short-term effect of different teaching methods on nasopharyngeal carcinoma for general practitioners in Jakarta, Indonesia. PLoS One 7: e32756.

23.  Hutajulu SH (2012) Clinical, Virological and Host Epigenetic Markers for Early Identification of Nasopharyngeal Carcinoma in High Risk Populations in Indonesia. PhD Thesis.

24.  Ho KY, Lee KW, Chai CY, Kuo WR, Wang HM, Chien CY (2008) Early recognition of nasopharyngeal cancer in adults with only otitis media with effusion. J Otolaryngol Head Neck Surg 37: 362–365.

25.  Ji MF, Yu YL, Cheng WM, Zong YS, Ng PS et al (2011) Detection of Stage I nasopharyngeal carcinoma by serologic screening and clinical examination. Chin J Cancer 30: 120–123.

26.  Gondhowiardjo S, Prajogi G, Sekarutami S (2008) History and growth of radiation oncology in Indonesia. Biomed Imaging Interv J 4: e42.

27.  Slotman BJ, Cottier B, Bentzen SM, Heeren G, Lievens Y, van den Bogaert W (2005) Overview of national guidelines for infrastructure and staffing of radiotherapy. ESTRO-QUARTS: work package 1. Radiother Oncol 75: 349–354.

28.  Stoker SD, Wildeman MA, Fles R, Indrasari SR, Herdini C, et al. (2014) A prospective study: current problems in radiotherapy for nasopharyngeal carcinoma in yogyakarta, indonesia. PLoS One 23: e85959.

29.  Akimoto T, Mitsuhashi N, Hayakawa K, Sukarai H, Murata O, et al. (1997) Split-course accelerated hyperfractionation radiotherapy for advanced head and neck cancer: influence of split time and overall treatment time on local control. Jpn J Clin Oncol 27: 240–243.

30.  Platek ME, McCloskey SA, Cruz M, Burke MS, Reid ME, et al. (2012) Quantification of the effect of treatment duration on local-regional failure after definitive concurrent chemotherapy and intensity-modulated radiation therapy for squamous cell carcinoma of the head and neck. Head Neck 35: 684–8.

31.  Wildeman MA, Zandbergen J, Vincent A, Herdini C, Middeldorp JM, et al. (2011) Can an online clinical data management service help in improving data collection and data quality in a developing country setting? Trials 12: 190.

# 9

# The Synergistic *In Vitro and In Vivo* Antitumor Effect of Combination Therapy with Salinomycin and 5-Fluorouracil against Hepatocellular Carcinoma

Fan Wang[1ᴼ], Weiqi Dai[1ᴼ], Yugang Wang[2], Miao Shen[1], Kan Chen[1], Ping Cheng[1], Yan Zhang[1], Chengfen Wang[1], Jingjing Li[1], Yuanyuan Zheng[1], Jie Lu[1], Jing Yang[1], Rong Zhu[3], Huawei Zhang[4], Yingqun Zhou[1], Ling Xu[2]*, Chuanyong Guo[1]*

1 Department of Gastroenterology, Shanghai Tenth People's Hospital, Tongji University of Medicine, Shanghai, PR China, 2 Department of Gastroenterology, Shanghai Tongren Hospital, Jiaotong University of Medicine, Shanghai, PR China, 3 Department of Gastroenterology, Clinical Medicine of Shanghai Tenth People's Hospital, Nanjing Medical University, Shanghai, PR China, 4 Department of Gastroenterology, The First Hospital Affiliated to Suzhou University, Suzhou, PR China

## Abstract

Hepatocellular carcinoma (HCC) is one of the few cancers in which a continuous increase in incidence has been observed over several years. Drug resistance is a major problem in the treatment of HCC. In the present study, we used salinomycin (Sal) and 5-fluorouracil (5-FU) combination therapy on HCC cell lines Huh7, LM3 and SMMC-7721 and nude mice subcutaneously tumor model to study whether Sal could increase the sensitivity of hepatoma cells to the traditional chemotherapeutic agent such as 5-FU. The combination of Sal and 5-FU resulted in a synergistic antitumor effect against liver tumors both *in vitro and in vivo*. Sal reversed the 5-FU-induced increase in CD133(+) EPCAM(+) cells, epithelial-mesenchymal transition and activation of the Wnt/β-catenin signaling pathway. The combination of Sal and 5-FU may provide us with a new approach to reverse drug resistant for the treatment of patients with HCC.

**Editor:** Yu-Jia Chang, Taipei Medicine University, Taiwan

**Funding:** This research was funded by National Nature Science Foundation of China (No. 81302788). The funders had no role in study design, data collection and analysis, decision to publish, or preparation of the manuscript.

**Competing Interests:** The authors have declared that no competing interests exist.

* E-mail: guochuanyong@hotmail.com (CG); xuling606@sina.com (LX)

ᴼ These authors contributed equally to this work.

## Introduction

Hepatocellular carcinoma (HCC) is one of the few cancers in which a continuous increase in incidence has been observed over several years [1]. According to the Barcelona Clinic Liver Cancer (BCLC) diagnostic and treatment strategy, chemotherapy is the best option for advanced stage tumors or HCC with extrahepatic diseases [2]. However, multidrug resistance has been identified as a major factor in the poor prognosis of patients suffering from advanced staged HCC. In recent years, investigations have focused on the factors contributing to drug resistance in HCC and possible approaches towards overcoming this therapeutic challenge have aroused interest in many researchers.

To date, more than 100 drugs are used to treat HCC. The chemotherapeutic drug 5-fluorouracil (5-FU), is effective against various types of cancer, including colorectal [3], breast [4], stomach and gullet cancer [5], it is also the optimal drug for the treatment of HCC [6]. However, the rapid development of acquired resistance to 5-FU has limited its clinical usage [7–9]. As the traditional chemotherapeutic agent available for the treatment of advanced HCC, 5-FU monotherapy is not very effective and is associated with multiple adverse events and drug resistance.

The recent emergence of the cancer stem cells (CSCs) concept suggests why treatment with chemotherapy such as 5-FU may often seem to be initially successful, but eventually results in not only a failure to eradicate the tumor, but also possible tumor relapse [10,11]. Commonly used anticancer drugs such as 5-FU are effective against HCC by targeting the rapidly proliferating and differentiating HCC cells which constitute the bulk of the tumor. These therapies may spare CSCs, allowing for regeneration of the tumor [12,13]. Recently, a robotic high-throughput screening approach was used to evaluate approximately 16,000 compounds from chemical libraries for activity against human breast CSCs, and only salinomycin (Sal) which was originally used to kill bacteria, fungi, and parasites, markedly and selectively reduced the viability of breast CSCs [14]. Then, Tang et al. [15] demonstrated that Sal is an effective inhibitor of osteosarcoma stem cells, Kusunoki et al. [16] reported that Sal had an inhibitory effect on the properties of endometrial CSCs. In our previous studies [17,18] we showed that Sal could down-regulate the proportion of CD133+ cell subpopulations which have stem cell properties in HCC and pancreatic cancer.

Based on the idea that cancer cells at different degrees of differentiation are targeted by 5-FU and Sal, we combined Sal and 5-FU to determine whether this combination could increase HCC sensitivity to 5-FU and eradicate HCC cells. The possible mechanisms of this effect were also investigated.

## Materials and Methods

### 2.1 Cell Lines and Cultures

The HCC cell lines Huh7, LM3 and SMMC-7721 were purchased from the Chinese Academy of Sciences Committee Type Culture Collection Cell Bank. The three cell lines were cultured in high glucose Dulbecco's modified Eagle's medium (DMEM-h; Thermo, China) supplemented with 10% fetal bovine serum, 100 U/ml penicillin, and 100 μg/ml streptomycin in a humidified incubator at 37°C in 5% $CO_2$.

### 2.2 Drugs and Antibodies

5-FU and Sal were purchased from Sigma Aldrich (St. Louis, MO, USA). A stock solution of 25 mg/ml 5-FU and 25 mM Sal which prepared using dimethyl sulfoxide (DMSO) were stored in the dark at −20°C. The final 5-FU and Sal concentrations used in the experiments were prepared from the stock solutions by dilution in DMEM-h. The antibodies CD133 (Miltenyi, Germany) and EPCAM (eBioscience, USA) were used for flow cytometric analysis, β-actin(Santa Cruz, CA, USA), E-cadherin (Abcam, USA), vimentin (Abcam, USA), p-GSK-3β-Tyr216(Santa Cruz, CA, USA), p-β-catenin (Cell Signaling Technology, USA) and active β-catenin (Cell Signaling Technology, USA) for Western blotting, active β-catenin (Cell Signaling Technology, USA) for immunofluorescence, CD133 (Bioss, China), EPCAM (eBioscience, USA), E-cadherin (Abcam, USA), vimentin (Abcam, USA) and active β-catenin (Cell Signaling Technology, USA) for immunohistochemistry.

### 2.3 Cell Viability

The HCC cell lines Huh7, LM3 and SMMC-7721were plated in 96-well plates (100 μl media per well). One day after seeding, 5-FU (0 ug/ml, 2 ug/ml, 4 ug/ml, 8 ug/ml, 16 ug/ml) and Sal (0 μM, 2 μM, 4 μM, 8 μM, 16 μM) were added in five replicates to each cell population. Cell viability was measured after 24 h, 48 h and 72 h using the MTT assay and a microplate reader at 490 nm. A calibration curve was prepared using the data obtained from wells that contained a known number of viable cells.

### 2.4 Combination Analysis

To evaluate the pharmacological interactions of the different combinations of drugs, we used the method of Chou et al [19]. Briefly, synergism, additivity or antagonism in the different combinations was calculated on the basis of the multiple drug effect equation and quantitated by the combination index (CI), where $CI = 1$ indicates that the two drugs have additive effects, $CI < 1$ indicates more than additive effects ("synergism") and $CI > 1$ indicates less than additive effects ("antagonism"). The CI was calculated based on: $CI = (D)1/(Dx)1+(D)2/(Dx)2+(D)1(D)2/(Dx)1(Dx)2$, where $(Dx)1$ and $(Dx)2$ are the doses of drug 1 and drug 2, alone, inhibiting 'x%', whereas $(D1)$ is the dose of drug 1 in combination, and $(D2)$ the dose of drug 2 in combination that gives the experimentally observed 'x' inhibition. Because our aim was to achieve maximal effect of the drugs tested on cancer cells, a mean CI was calculated from data points with fraction affected (Fa) $>0.5$. Fa$<0.5$ indicated lower growth inhibition and a large fraction of the cell population indicated growth. Fa$<0.5$ was therefore considered irrelevant. Furthermore, we evaluated the drug dose in a synergistic combination. This was designated as the dose reduction index (DRI): $(DRI)1 = (Dx)1/(D)1$ and $(DRI)2 = (Dx)2/(D)2$ where DRI$>1$, which showed that combinations could result in reduced drug doses compared with the doses for each drug alone. Classical isobolograms were also constructed by plotting drugs concentrations (alone and in combination) that inhibits 50%, 60%, 70% HCC cell viability. First, the concentrations of 5-FU and Sal required to produce a defined single-agent effect, when used as single agents, are placed on the $x$ and $y$ axes in a two-coordinate plot, corresponding to ($C_{5-FU}$, 0) and (0, $C_{Sal}$), respectively. The line connecting these two points is the line of additivity. Second, the concentrations of the two drugs used in combination to provide the same effect, denoted as ($C_{5-FU}$, $C_{Sal}$), are placed in the same plot. Synergy, additivity, or antagonism are indicated when ($C_{5-FU}$, $C_{Sal}$) is located below, on, or above the line, respectively.

### 2.5 Flow Cytometric Analysis

Analysis of apoptosis: Huh7, LM3 and SMMC-7721 cells were plated in 6-well plates. After 48 h, control cells, 5-FU-treated cells (8 ug/ml,) Sal-treated cells (4 uM) and 5-FU plus Sal treated cells were collected, washed twice in cold PBS, mixed in 100 ml of binding buffer, and incubated at room temperature for 15 min with an annexin-V/PI (BD Biosciences) double staining solution. Stained cells were analyzed by flow cytometry and the percentage of apoptotic cells was calculated using ModFitLT software (Verity Software House).

Analysis of CD133(+) EPCAM(+) cells: Huh7 cells were plated (100,000 cells per well) in six-well plates. After 48 h, cells from the control group, the 5-FU group, the Sal group and the 5-FU plus Sal group were collected, and washed twice in cold phosphate buffered saline (PBS). Dissociated cells were stained with PE (phycoerythrin)-conjugated CD133 antibody and FITC (fluorescein isothiocyanate)-conjugated EPCAM antibody, and then co-incubated for 30 min at 4°C. Mouse IgG1-phycoerythrin was used as an isotype control antibody. Dead cells were eliminated with 7-aminoactinomycin D. The labeled cells were analyzed by the BD FACSVantage system (BD Biosciences, San Jose, CA, USA) in accordance with the manufacturer's protocols. Gating was implemented on the basis of negative control staining profiles.

### 2.6 Colony/Sphere Formation Assays

Huh7 cells treated with DMSO vehicle, 5-FU, Sal and Sal plus 5-FU were resuspended as single cells in 1.2% agar (Sigma-Aldrich, St. Louis, MO, USA) and diluted with ddH2O. This was overlaid on a base of 0.6% agar diluted with ddH2O. Both the top and base layers were mixed with DMEM-h and 20% FBS. After 10 days, the number of colonies which developed within each well were counted and photographed under a microscope using an inverted digital camera.

### 2.7 Animal Experiments

Animal experiments were performed on 6-week-old male nude mice (athymic, BALB/C nu/nu). A high standard of ethics was applied in carrying out the investigations. The mice were housed in a standard animal laboratory with free access to water and food. They were kept under constant environmental conditions with a 12-hour light-dark cycle. All operations were performed under aseptic conditions. All procedures were approved by the Animal Care and Use Committee of Shanghai Tongji University. The animal experiment permit number is SYXK (Shanghai) 2011-0111.

### 2.8 Treatments in Mouse Xenograft Models

Huh7 ($5 \times 10^6$ cells) in 100 μl DMEM-h and 100 μl Matrigel (Becton Dickinson, Bedford, MA, USA) were injected subcutaneously into each mouse. When the tumor volume was approximately 100 mm$^3$, the animals were randomly divided into four groups (saline, 5-FU, Sal and Sal plus 5-FU), and intraperitoneally injected with test reagents or saline daily for 4 weeks.

## 2.9 Anticancer Drug In vivo Analysis

Data were evaluated using the National Cancer Institute guidelines for assessment of anticancer drug effects in subcutaneously growing human tumor xenografts [20–22]. The anti-tumor effect was observed by measuring tumor diameter in the test animals twice per week, and tumor volume (TV) was calculated as: $TV = 1/2 \times a \times b^2$ (a, b denote the long and short diameters, respectively). Relative tumor volume (RTV) was calculated based on the measured results: $RTV = Vt/V_0$ ($V_0$: the tumor volume at initial administration, Vt: the tumor volume at each time measurement). Anti-tumor activity was evaluated by the relative tumor growth rate $T/C$ (%) = $TRTV/CRTV \times 100$%, (TRTV: treatment group RTV; CRTV: negative control group RTV). Then tumor weight was used to evaluate the efficacy of the drugs. Following administration, the animals were killed, and the tumor block was dissected and weighed. The tumor weight evaluation formula: tumor growth inhibition rate = (the average tumor weight in the administration group - the average tumor weight in the negative control group)/the average tumor weight in the negative control group × 100%.

## 2.10 Immunofluorescence

Huh7 cells treated with DMSO vehicle, 5-FU, Sal or Sal plus 5-FU were planted on poly-L-lysine coated glass coverslips, fixed with cold acetone for 1 h, and permeabilized in 0.5% Triton X-100 (Sigma-Aldrich) for 10 min. The cells were blocked with bovine serum albumin (BSA) in PBS and incubated with primary antibodies (anti-active β-catenin) overnight at 4°C. The following morning, the slides were washed with PBS and incubated with appropriate fluorescein isothiocyanate-conjugated secondary antibody for 1 h. The cells were washed and incubated with DAPI (Invitrogen, Carlsbad, CA, USA) for nuclear staining, washed and mounted with propyl gallate under glass coverslips. The slides were visualized with a scanning laser microscope (Zeiss 710, Germany).

## 2.11 Immunohistochemistry

Tumor tissues from the control group, 5-FU-treated group, Sal-treated group, and 5-FU plus Sal-treated group were analyzed by immunohistochemistry. Sections (4 μm thick) from paraffin-embedded tumors were deparaffinized and rehydrated using xylene and ethanol, respectively, and immersed in 3% hydrogen peroxide solution for 10 min to block endogenous peroxidases. Sections were boiled for 30 min in 10 mM citrate buffer solution (pH 6.0) for antigen exposure. Slides were incubated for 45 min with 5% BSA and incubated overnight at 4°C with the primary antibodies against CD133, EPCAM, E-cadherin, vimentin and active β-catenin. These specimens were incubated for 45 min at 37°C with the appropriate peroxidase-conjugated secondary antibody and visualized using the Real Envision Detection Kit (Gene Tech Shanghai Company Limited, China) following the manufacturer's instructions.

## 2.12 Reverse Transcription-Polymerase Chain Reaction (RT-PCR) and Real-time PCR

Total RNA was extracted and first-strand cDNA was synthesized using the Omniscript RT kit (QIAGEN, Gaithersburg, MD, USA), with 2000 ng RNA (per 20 μl reaction) and oligo (dT) primers. cDNA was used in real-time PCR reactions to analyze E-cadherin, vimentin, and β-actin expression. Primers used in the PCR reactions are listed in **Table 1**. PCR reactions were amplified for 40 cycles. Each cycle consisted of denaturation for 1 min at 94°C, annealing for 1 min at 60°C, and polymerization for 2 min at 72°C. PCR products were quantified using the Molecular Analyst software (Bio-Rad, Hercules, CA, USA). The ratio of each gene *vs* β-actin was calculated by standardizing the ratio of each control to the unit value.

## 2.13 Western Blot Assays

Sample proteins were electrophoretically separated on a 10% polyacrylamide gel at 80 volts. The proteins were transferred to a polyvinylidene difluoride membrane. Membranes were blocked for 60 min with a 5% (v/v) milk solution prepared in PBS. The membranes were incubated overnight at 4°C with 1:500 dilutions of the primary antibodies (against E-cadherin, vimentin, p-GSK-3β (Tyr216), p-β-catenin, active-β-catenin and β-actin). Membranes were washed three times for 5 min each with Tween 20 (1:1000) in PBS and incubated for 45 min with the appropriate peroxidase-conjugated secondary antibody (1:1000 in PBS). Membranes were washed three times with Tween 20-PBS, for 10 min each, and were developed using the Odyssey Two-color Infrared Laser Imaging System (Li-Cor, Lincoln, NE, USA). The signal generated by β-actin was used as an internal control.

## 2.14 Statistical Analyses

SPSS 17.0 software (IBM, Armonk, NY, USA) was used for statistical analyses. Experiments were repeated at least three times. Unless otherwise stated, data are expressed as the mean ± standard deviation. The real-time PCR data were 2-$\triangle\triangle$Ct transformed before analysis and were analyzed using analysis of variance (ANOVA). The results of MTT assay, flow cytometric analysis, colony/sphere formation assay, tumor volume and weight analysis, and western blots were analyzed using ANOVA. If the result of the ANOVA was significant ($p < 0.05$ versus control), pairwise comparisons between the groups were performed using a post hoc test (S-N-K procedure). In all cases, $p < 0.05$ was considered statistically significant.

# Results

## 3.1 Single Drug Treatment with 5-FU or Sal

To test the effects of 5-FU on growth of HCC cells, HCC cell lines Huh7, LM3 and SMMC-7721 were treated with increasing concentrations of 5-FU (0, 2, 4, 8 and 16 ug/ml) for 24 h, 48 h and 72 h. As shown in **Fig. 1A**, cell growth was inhibited by 5-FU in a dose- and time-dependent manner. We subsequently evaluated the effect of Sal (0, 2, 4, 8 and 16 μM) for 24 h, 48 h and 72 h on cell growth, and found that Sal was effective in inhibiting cell growth of all cell lines tested (**Fig. 1B**). These results indicate that 5-FU or Sal was an effective inhibitor of HCC cell growth as a single agent. Subsequent studies were undertaken to examine if the cells treated with Sal combined with 5-FU were more sensitive to the cytotoxic effect of 5-FU.

## 3.2 Combination Treatment with Sal and 5-FU

The effect of Sal combined with 5-FU on cell viability was investigated using the MTT assay. For these studies, HCC cell lines Huh7, LM3 and SMMC-7721 were treated with 5-FU (0, 2, 4, 8, and 16 ug/ml), Sal (0, 2, 4, 8, and 16 μM), or Sal plus 5-FU for 48 h. Viable cells were evaluated using the MTT assay. Treatment of HCC cells with 5-FU plus Sal for 48 h resulted in a decrease in cell viability which was greater than either 5-FU or Sal alone (**Table 2**). Fraction affected (Fa) values (indicating the fraction of cells inhibited after drug exposure) were obtained after

**Table 1.** Real-time PCR Primer Sequences.

| Gene | | Primer sequence (5'→3') |
|---|---|---|
| E-cadherin | Forward | ATTTTTCCCTCGACACCCGAT |
| | Reverse | TCCCAGGCGTAGACCAAGA |
| Vimentin | Forward | AGTCCACTGAGTACCGGAGAC |
| | Reverse | CATTTCACGCATCTGGCGTTC |
| β-actin | Forward | CTGGAACGGTGAAGGTGACA |
| | Reverse | AAGGGACTTCCTGTAACAATGCA |

exposure of the cells to a series of drug concentrations. To indicate the effects at different Fa values, the CI (combination index) and DRI (dose reduction index) values were calculated for each Fa. **Fig. 2A** shows the Fa-CI plots illustrating the effects of Sal and 5-FU at different fixed drug ratios, and demonstrates synergism (CI<1) at Fa>0.5 for HCC cell lines Huh7, LM3 and SMMC-7721. As expected, synergism corresponding to CI<1 always yielded a favorable DRI (>1) for both drugs. The Fa-DRI plots are shown in **Fig. 2B**, and indicate that chemotherapeutic doses of 5-FU may be significantly reduced for combinations with Sal that are synergistic at Fa>0.5. Classical isobolograms were shown in Fig. 2C, we can see that ($C_{5\text{-}FU}$, $C_{Sal}$) is located below the line (synergy) at $IC_{60}$, $IC_{70}$ for HCC cell lines Huh7, LM3 and SMMC-7721. At last the combination effect of Sal and 5-FU on apoptosis effects were evaluated by flow cytometric analysis. The results (Fig. 2D) showed that combination therapy increased apoptosis of HCC cell lines Huh7, LM3 and SMMC-7721 significantly.

To explore the effects of the combination of 5-FU and Sal *in vivo*, we established mouse xenograft models using Huh7 cells. Saline, 5-FU (8 mg/kg) [23], Sal (4 mg/kg) [17] and 5-FU (8 mg/kg) plus Sal (4 mg/kg) were used for the *in vivo* experiments. There were six mice of each group. Dynamic observations of the anti-tumor effects of the test substances were carried out for 4 weeks. It can be seen in **Fig. 2E** that the subcutaneous tumor volume (we choose two representative mice in each group) was reduced in the combination therapy group compared to the other three groups. HE staining (**Fig. 2F**) showed the area of apoptosis and necrosis induced by drugs in tumor tissue of treatment group. Details of the evaluation criteria and methods are shown in the Materials and Methods section. The anti-tumor effect was observed by measuring tumor diameter in the test animals twice per week, and the tumor growth curve is shown in **Fig. 2G**. The result showed that tumor growth rate in the combination therapy group was slower

than that in the other three groups. The relative tumor proliferation rate $V_{Treatment}/V_{Control}$ (**Fig. 2H**) in the combination therapy group was slower (*$p<0.05$) than that in the other three groups. Tumor weight was calculated to evaluate drug efficacy and is shown in **Fig. 2I**. The tumor blocks in the combination therapy group weighed lighter (*$p<0.05$) than those in the other three groups. Tumor growth inhibition rate (**Fig. 2R**) was greater in the combination therapy (*$p<0.05$). These findings suggested that 5-FU combined with Sal was effective and tolerable as a novel therapeutic modality for HCC.

## 3.3 Effects of 5-FU, Sal and their Combination on the Cancer Stem Cell Properties of HCC Cells

EpCAM and CD133 have been used as cancer stem cells (CSCs) markers in HCC. Research has shown that both EpCAM and CD133 surface markers were more representative for CSC s in HCC Huh7 cells [24]. We performed flow cytometry to determine the effects of 5-FU and Sal on the proportion of HCC cells with the CD133(+) EPCAM(+) antigenic phenotype (**Fig. 3A**). Treatment with 5-FU increased the proportion of the CD133(+) EPCAM(+) cell subpopulation from 27.77±4.72% (vehicle-treated controls) to 53.5±3.17% (*$p<0.05$). In contrast, treatment with Sal reduced this proportion from 27.77±4.72% (vehicle-treated controls) to 6±1.70% (*$p<0.05$). There was a significant decrease in the CD133(+) EPCAM(+) cell subpopulation in the 5-FU plus Sal combination therapy group compared with 5-FU monotherapy (26.73±8.27% *vs* 53.57±3.17, *$p<0.05$). We know that cancer stem cells have a strong proliferative ability, thus, colony-forming assays (**Fig. 3B**) were performed to measure the proliferative ability of single cancer cells. Huh7 cells were treated with DMSO vehicle, 5-FU (44 ug/ml), Sal (2 μM) and Sal plus 5-FU for 96 h. In all cases, colonies were visible after 10 days. The number of colonies increased in the 5-FU treatment group (8.25±0.25 colonies/high power field (HPF)), and decreased in the Sal treatment group (1.83±0.29 colonies/HPF), relative to vehicle-treated controls (4.75±0.05 colonies/HPF) (*$p<0.05$). The number of colonies was significantly lower in the Sal plus 5-FU combination group (4.42±0.29 colonies/HPF) compared with the 5-FU treatment group (8.25±0.25 colonies/HPF) (*$p<0.05$).

Finally, the expression of CD133 and EPCAM (**Fig. 3C**) were evaluated in the tumors of mouse xenograft models by immuno-histochemistry (200×). The expression of CD133 was increased in the 5-FU group compared with the saline group. In contrast, Sal treatment reduced the expression of CD133 compared with the saline group, and 5-FU combined with Sal reduced the proportion of CD133 compared with the 5-FU treatment group. Similar results were obtained for the expression of EPCAM.

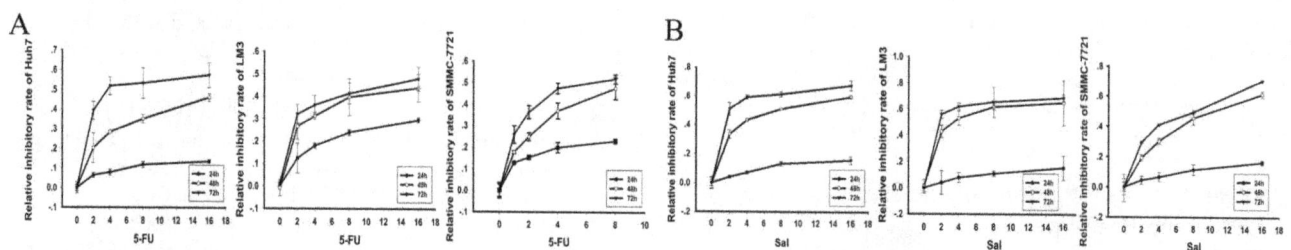

**Figure 1. Growth inhibition curves for HCC cell lines Huh7, LM3, and SMMC-7721.** 5-FU (A) and Sal (B) inhibit HCC cell proliferation. Huh7, LM3, and SMMC-7721 ($5\times10^4$ cells/ml) were treated with Sal and 5-FU for various times (24, 36, and 48 h). Cell viability was determined using the MTT assay. The data show that Sal and 5-FU exposure reduced Huh7, LM3, and SMMC-7721 cell viability in a dose- and time-dependent manner.

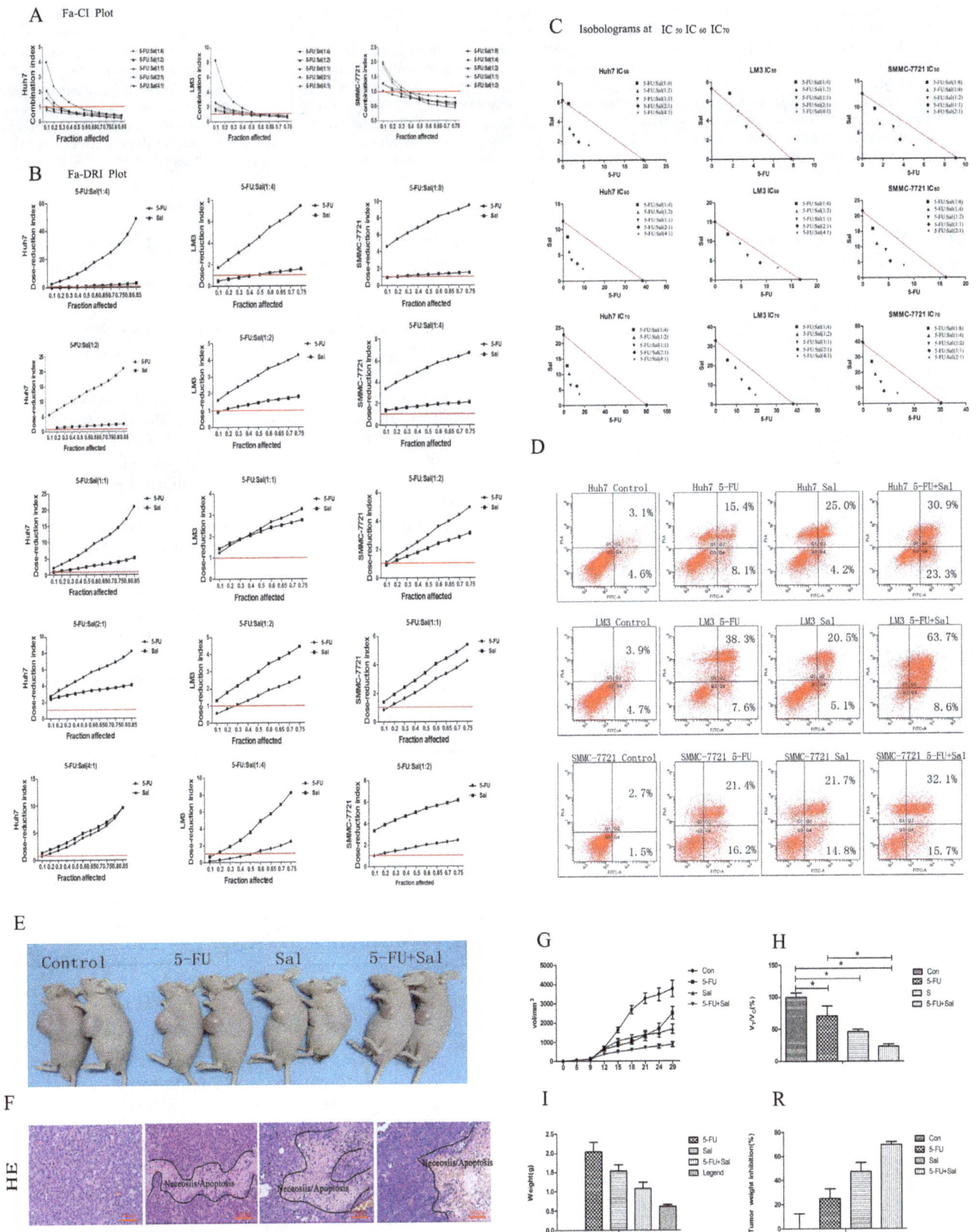

**Figure 2. Combination treatment with 5-FU and Sal.** (A–D) Illustrative Fa-CI and Fa-DRI plots for the combination of 5-FU and Sal using different fixed drug ratios. (A) CI values were calculated from each Fa for HCC cell lines Huh7, LM3, and SMMC-7721. Average synergism (CI<1) at Fa> 0.5 for all three HCC lines. (B) DRI values were calculated from each Fa for HCC cell lines Huh7, LM3, and SMMC-7721. The 5-FU and Sal chemotherapeutic doses may be significantly reduced (DRI>1) for combinations that are synergistic at Fa>0.5 for all three HCC lines. (C) Isobologram analysis at $IC_{50}$, $IC_{60}$ and $IC_{70}$ for the combinations of HCC cell lines Huh7, LM3, and SMMC-7721. The results indicates synergy, additivity or antagonism

when the points are located below, on or above the line, respectively. We can see that $(C_{5-FU}, C_{Sal})$ is located below the line (synergy) at $IC_{60}$, $IC_{70}$ for HCC cell lines Huh7, LM3 and SMMC-7721. (D) The combination effect of Sal and 5-FU on apoptosis effects were evaluated by flow cytometric analysis. The results showed that combination therapy increased apoptosis of HCC cell lines Huh7, LM3 and SMMC-7721 significantly. (E–R) Combination treatments in the *in vivo* models (E) Subcutaneous tumor volume following combination therapy was reduced compared to that of the other three groups (two representative mice in each group). (F) HE staining showed the area of apoptosis and necrosis induced by drugs in tumor tissue of treatment group. (G) The tumor growth curve showed that tumor growth rate following combination therapy was slower than that of the other three groups. (H) The relative tumor proliferation rate, $V_{Treatment}/V_{Control}$, showed that proliferation rate of the combination therapy group was slower than that of the other three groups. (**p<0.05**)s. (I) In the combination therapy group, tumor blocks weighed lighter than those of the other three groups (**p<0.05**). (R) The tumor growth inhibition rate indicated that the combination therapy significantly inhibited tumor growth than the other three groups (**p<0.05**).

## 3.4 Sal Altered Epithelial-Mesenchymal Transition (EMT) Induced by 5-FU

Many laboratories have shown that EMT can endow cells with stem cell-like characteristics [25], and similar results have been found in hepatoma cells [26]. Emerging evidence has associated chemo-resistance with acquisition of EMT which is involved in acquired resistance to 5-FU [27]. To determine whether Sal altered the EMT process induced by 5-FU, we evaluated EMT in Huh7 cells treated with vehicle control, 5-FU, Sal and Sal plus 5-FU. Following treatment with 5-FU, Huh7 cellular morphology was converted to a diffuse fibroblast-like morphology, characteristic of EMT, as compared with untreated cells. Cells treated with Sal were round and cells in the combination treatment group were rounder than those in the 5-FU group (**Fig. 4A**). In order to further investigate EMT in Huh7 cells, we examined the more common markers of EMT, using Real time-PCR and western blot. The data showed that 5-FU induced EMT in Huh7 cells by down-regulation of E-cadherin and up-regulation of vimentin expression. In contrast to 5-FU, Sal inhibited EMT by upregulating the expression of E-cadherin and down-regulating the expression of vimentin. In addition, 5-FU combined with Sal demonstrated that

Sal altered EMT induced by 5-FU (**Fig. 4B, *p<0.05**). Similar results were observed in tumors in mouse xenograft models by immunehistochemistry (200×) (**Fig. 4C**).

## 3.5 Sal Blocks the Wnt-β-catenin Pathway

Wnt/beta-catenin signaling contributes to the activation of tumorigenic liver progenitor cells [28,29]. and EMT [30,31]. β-catenin is a key component of the Wnt/β-catenin signaling pathway. In canonical Wnt signaling pathways, Gsk-3β is the upstream adjustment factor of β-catenin and can compose a complex with APC and axin to phosphorylation β-catenin, leading to β-catenin degradation. Here we examined the protein expression of p-GSK-3β(Tyr216) which is the active GSK-3β, p-β-catenin which is the inactive β-catenin and active β-catenin *in vitro* and *in vivo* by western-blot (Fig. 5A). Compared to 5-FU group, p-GSK-3β (Tyr216) expression of Sal group and combination therapy group were significantly up-regulated and we found the similar changes in p-β-catenin protein. Decreased expression of active β-catenin protein were also observed in Sal group and combination therapy group in comparison with 5-FU alone group. In addition to examining the change of protein expression of

**Table 2.** Relative inhibitory by 5-FU, Sal and their combination for HCC cell lines.

| Huh7 | 5-FU(0 μg/ml) | 5-FU(2 μg/ml) | 5-FU(4 μg/ml) | 5-FU(8 μg/ml) | 5-FU(16 μg/ml) |
|---|---|---|---|---|---|
| Sal(0 μM) | 0±0.027 | 0.203±0.077 | 0.282±0.050 | 0.351±0.022 | 0.461±0.019 |
| Sal(2 μM) | 0.335±0.027 | 0.485±0.069 | 0.510±0.029 | 0.559±0.051 | 0.591±0.082 |
| Sal(4 μM) | 0.433±0.079 | 0.549±0.014 | 0.568±0.078 | 0.622±0.063 | 0.714±0.037 |
| Sal(8 μM) | 0.509±0.061 | 0.582±0.163 | 0.629±0.094 | 0.674±0.044 | 0.738±0.029 |
| Sal(16 μM) | 0.597±0.009 | 0.649±0.102 | 0.747±0.101 | 0.775±0.029 | 0.873±0.072 |
| **LM3** | **5-FU(0 μg/ml)** | **5-FU(2 μg/ml)** | **5-FU(4 μg/ml)** | **5-FU(8 μg/ml)** | **5-FU(16 μg/ml)** |
| Sal(0 μM) | 0±0.005 | 0.292±0.056 | 0.462±0.015 | 0.518±0.082 | 0.568±0.060 |
| Sal(2 μM) | 0.320±0.048 | 0.423±0.030 | 0.451±0.154 | 0.495±0.043 | 0.596±0.009 |
| Sal(4 μM) | 0.420±0.054 | 0.508±0.088 | 0.531±0.018 | 0.607±0.018 | 0.660±0.015 |
| Sal(8 μM) | 0.520±0.022 | 0.527±0.013 | 0.582±0.072 | 0.628±0.054 | 0.688±0.015 |
| Sal(16 μM) | 0.603±0.173 | 0.636±0.047 | 0.645±0.078 | 0.680±0.072 | 0.736±0.025 |
| **SMMC-7721** | **5-FU(0 μg/ml** | **5-FU(1 μg/ml)** | **5-FU(2 μg/ml)** | **5-FU(4 μg/mlg)** | **5-FU(8 μg/ml)** |
| Sal(0 μM) | −0.001±0.008 | 0.178±0.006 | 0.248±0.018 | 0.369±0.038 | 0.475±0.050 |
| Sal(2 μM) | 0.193±0.021 | 0.223±0.087 | 0.336±0.105 | 0.452±0.116 | 0.552±0.124 |
| Sal(4 μM) | 0.303±0.019 | 0.397±0.049 | 0.432±0.061 | 0.539±0.029 | 0.600±0.014 |
| Sal(8 μM) | 0.453±0.042 | 0.460±0.086 | 0.524±0.050 | 0.572±0.011 | 0.690±0.028 |
| Sal(16 μM) | 0.478±0.021 | 0.553±0.067 | 0.601±0.038 | 0.673±0.060 | 0.721±0.036 |

Cells were exposed to a concentration range of 5-FU, Sal and their combination for 48 h.
Values (relative inhibitory) are means ± standard error of the mean (SE) for 3–5 experiments.

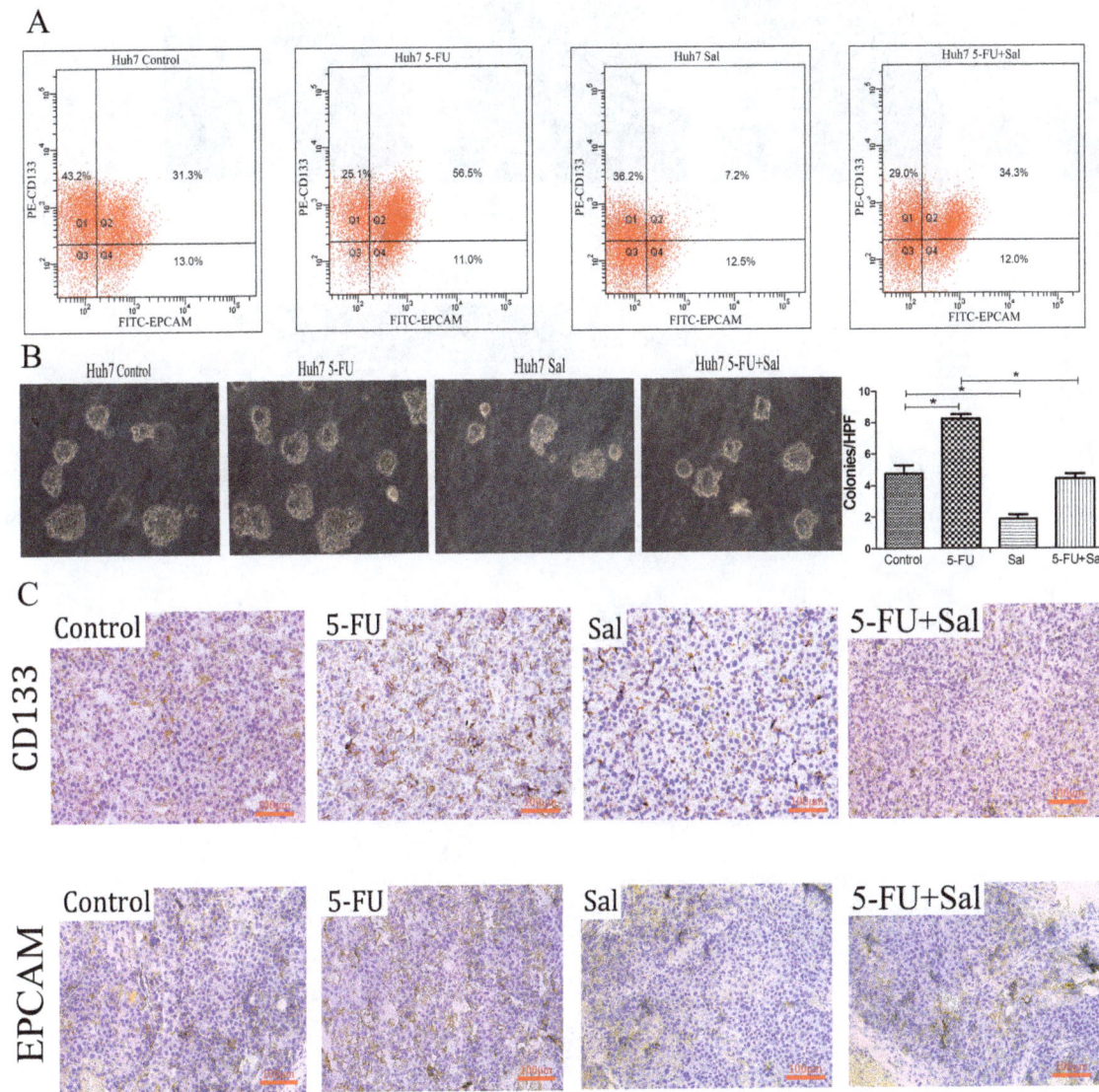

**Figure 3. Effects of 5-FU, Sal and their combination on cancer stem cell properties in HCC cells.** (A) Flow cytometry assays showed that treatment with 5-FU increased the proportion of the CD133+ EPCAM+ Huh7 cell subpopulation compared with the control group. In contrast, treatment with Sal reduced this proportion compared with the control group. 5-FU combined with Sal reduced this proportion compared with the 5-FU group (*$p<0.05$). (B) Colony-forming assays were performed to measure the proliferative ability of single cancer cells. The number of colonies increased in the 5-FU treatment group compared with the control group, decreased in the Sal treatment group compared with the control group. The number of colonies was significantly lower in the Sal plus 5-FU combination group compared with the 5-FU treatment group (*$p<0.05$). (C) Immunohistochemistry indicates CD133+ and EPCAM+ expression in the tumors of mouse xenograft models. (Magnification is 200×).

avtive β-catenin, the changes in active β-catenin localization were also obversed following treatment with 5-FU, Sal, and Sal plus 5-FU by indirect immunofluorescence detection in Huh7 cells (Fig. 5B). In the control condition, active β-catenin was present in the cytomembrane and cytoplasm. However, in the 5-FU treated group, active β-catenin preferentially accumulated in the nuclear and perinuclear region which promoted the activation of Wnt/β-catenin signaling pathway. In contrast, in the cells treated with Sal, active β-catenin was preferentially accumulated in the cytomembrane and down-regulated expression which meant translocation of active β-catenin to the nucleus was blocked. Interestingly, treatment with 5-FU and Sal showed decreased accumulation of active β-catenin in the nuclear area compared with the 5-FU group. We also observed comparable results following immuno-

histochemical analysis of tumors in mouse xenograft models (Fig. 5C).

## Discussion

Once diagnosed with HCC, only 30–40% of patients are deemed eligible for curative treatment, including surgical resection, liver transplantation, and chemoembolization. Most patients will receive some form of chemotherapy in the hope of prolonging life. Emerging data has indicated that HCC CSCs are resistant to conventional chemotherapy such as 5-FU. Targeting CSCs therapeutically is likely to be challenging, because both bulk tumor cells and CSCs must be eliminated, potentially demanding combination drug therapies. Sal, an antibiotic used to kill bacteria, fungi and parasites, has recently been shown to selectively deplete

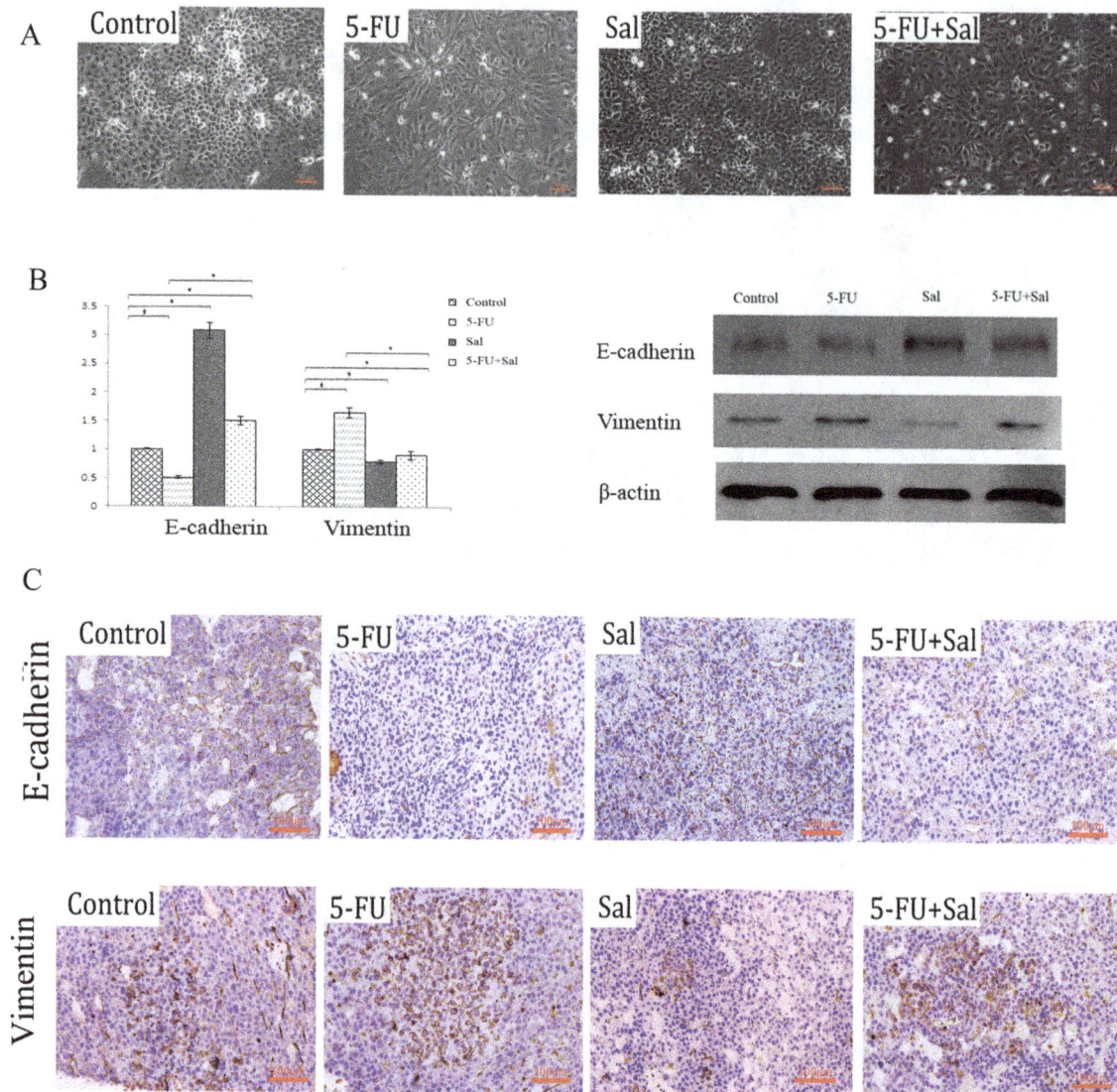

**Figure 4. Effect of 5-FU, Sal, and 5-FU combined with Sal on the epithelial-mesenchymal transition (EMT)-related process.** (A) Morphological changes after the indicated treatment in Huh7 cells (Magnification 200×). (B) Real-time PCR was performed to examine mRNA expression of EMT-related genes (E-cadherin, vimentin) (*$p < 0.05$). Western blot was performed to examine protein expression of EMT-related genes (E-cadherin, vimentin). (C) Immunohistochemistry indicates E-cadherin and vimentin expression in the tumors of mouse xenograft models (Magnification 200×).

human breast cancer stem cells [14] and colorectal cancer stem cells [22]. In previous experiments we found that Sal down-regulated the CD133+ cell subpopulation in HCC cells [17]. Taking into account the characteristics of Sal, in this study we used three HCC cell lines and a nude mouse subcutaneous tumor model to determine if the combination of 5-FU and Sal could enhance the sensitivity of HCC cells to conventional chemotherapy such as 5-FU. We found that combination therapy with Sal and 5-FU had a synergistic antitumor effect against liver tumors both *in vitro* and *in vivo*.

We next explored whether Sal affected drug resistance induced by 5-FU. The cell surface markers, CD133 and EPCAM, are frequently used to identify CSCs in various tumors, including HCC [32,33]. In addition, research [24] has shown that the CD133(+) EpCAM(+) phenotype is precisely represented by CSCs in Huh7 cells. In our study, the results showed that Sal combined with 5-FU decreased the proportion of CD133(+) EpCAM(+)

which were increased in the 5-FU alone group of Huh7 cells. Sal combined with 5-FU also inhibited the expression of CD133 and EPCAM respectively in subcutaneous tumor tissue of nude mice. Another observed effect of treatment on HCC CSCs was decreased clonogenicity. These effects may be due to Sal combined with 5-FU reducing the proportion of CD133(+) EpCAM(+) cell subpopulations within Huh7 cells, suggesting that inhibition of tumorigenic/proliferative ability of HCC CSCs by Sal was associated with sensitization of HCC cells to 5-FU.

Many laboratories have shown that EMT is related to chemotherapy drug resistance as it can endow cells with stem cell-like characteristics [34–36], and similar results were obtained with hepatoma cells [37,38]. In the present study, we found that 5-FU induced Huh7 cells to mesenchymal-like cancers *in vitro* and *in vivo*, by reducing E-cadherin and increasing vimentin expression, however, treatment with Sal plus 5-FU could reverse EMT induced by 5-FU.

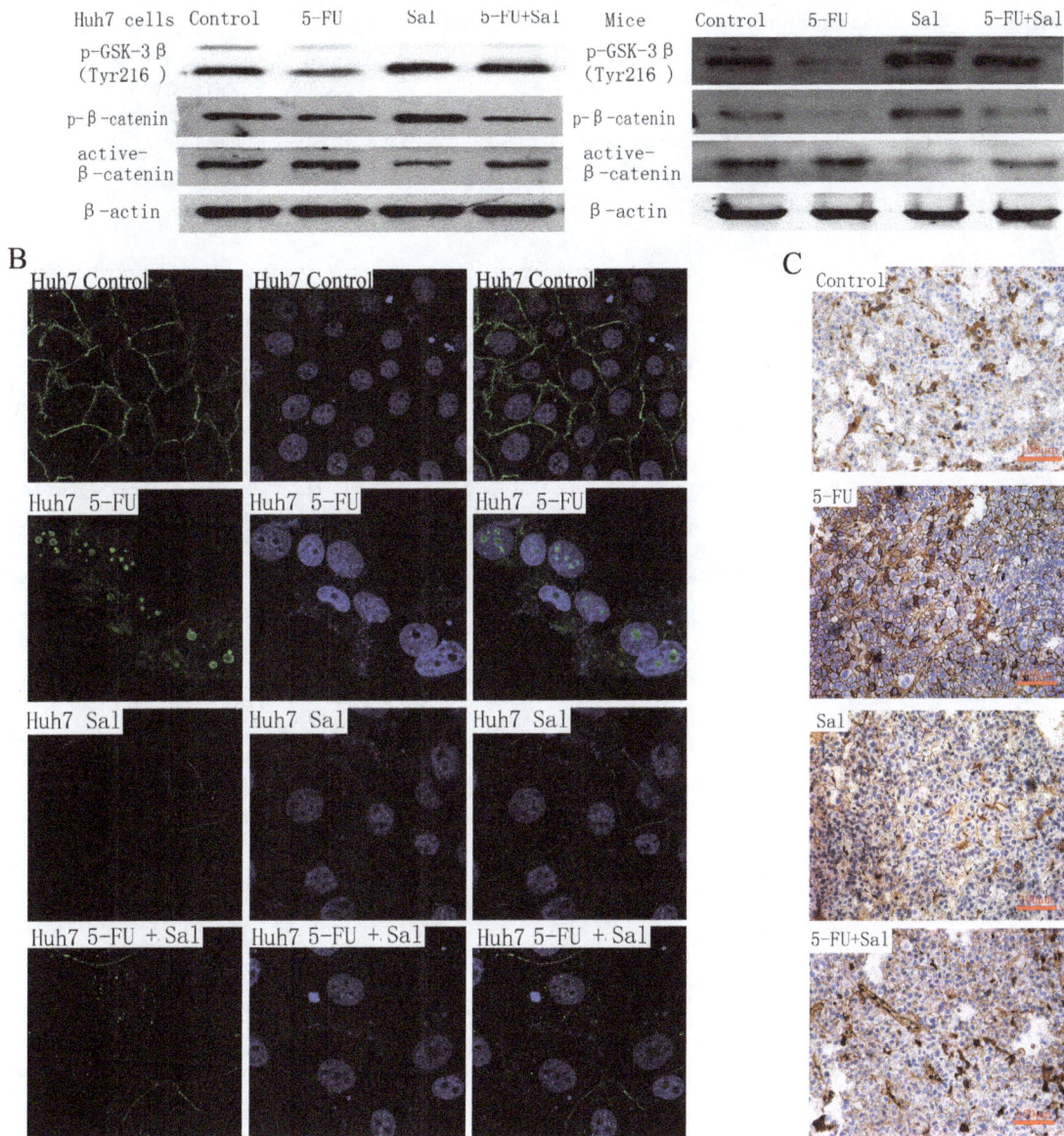

**Figure 5. Translocation of β-catenin.** (A) The protein expression of p-GSK-3β (Tyr 216) which is active-GSK-3β, p-β-catenin which is inactive β-catenin and active-β-catenin were detected by western-blot in vitro and in vivo. Compared to 5-FU group, p-GSK-3β (Tyr216) expression of Sal group and combination therapy group were significantly up-regulated and we found the similar changes in p-β-catenin protein. Decreased expression of active β-catenin protein were observed in Sal group and combination therapy group compared to 5-FU alone group. (B) Changes in cellular localization of active β-catenin cellular localization was evaluated by indirect immunofluorescence. Immunofluorescence were labeled of active β-catenin in Huh7 cells (untreated, treated with 5-FU, Sal and Sal plus 5-FU) for 48 h. Nuclei were stained with DAPI, and regions were merged to assess signal colocalization. Magnification is 630×. In the control condition, active β-catenin is present in the cytomembrane and cytoplasm. In the 5-FU treated groups, active β-catenin preferentially accumulates in the nuclear and perinuclear region. In contrast, cells treated with Sal showed preferential localization of active β-catenin in cytomembrane, altering the translocation of active β-catenin to the nucleus. Cells treated with the combination of 5-FU and Sal showed decreased accumulation of β-catenin in the nuclear and perinuclear region compared with the 5-FU treated groups. (C) Immunohistochemistry indicates similar results for β-catenin in the tumors of mouse xenograft models. Magnification is 200×.

Studies have shown that dysregulation of the Wnt/β-catenin signaling pathway is involved in cancer chemoresistance [39], contributes to the induction of EMT [40] and promotes stem cell maintenance [41]. The classical Wnt signaling pathway is mediated by β-catenin, and accumulated nuclear localization of active β-catenin increases resistance to 5-FU in HCC cells. In the present study, our results demonstrated that Sal alone and Sal combined with 5-FU down-regated the expression of active β-catenin by down-regating p-GSK-3β (Tyr216) which is active

GSK-3β and induced preferential periplasmic membrane localization of active β-catenin in comparison with 5-FU alone, The result indicated combination therapy revised the activation of Wnt/β-catenin signaling pathway induced by 5-FU.

In conclusion, our current findings show that Sal potentiates the antitumor effects of 5-FU by down-regulating CSCs in HCC cells. Strategies to modulate EMT by blocking the translocation of active β-catenin to the nucleus might play a role in the down-regulation of CSCs. In addition to 5-FU, there are many drug resistance processes caused by CSCs enrichment such as those involved in resistance to cisplatin [42] and cyclophosphamide [43]. This study provides us with a new approach to reverse drug resistant for the treatment of patients with HCC.

## Acknowledgments

Preparation of the manuscript was done with the assistance of BioScience Writers LLC, Houston, TX, USA.

## Author Contributions

Conceived and designed the experiments: CG LX FW. Performed the experiments: FW WD YW MS KC PC Y. Zhang CW J. Li Y. Zheng. Analyzed the data: J. Lu JY RZ HZ Y. Zhou. Contributed reagents/materials/analysis tools: FW CG. Wrote the paper: FW WD.

## References

1. Siegel R, Naishadham D, Jemal A (2013) Cancer statistics, 2013. CA Cancer J Clin 63(1): 11–30.

2. Ikeda M, Okusaka T, Ueno H, Morizane C, Kojima Y, et al. (2008) Predictive factors of outcome and tumor response to systemic chemotherapy in patients with metastatic hepatocellular carcinoma. Jpn J Clin Oncol 38(10): 675–82.

3. Macdonald JS, Astrow AB (2001) Adjuvant therapy of colon cancer. Semin Oncol 28(1): 30–40.

4. Martin M, Pienkowski T, Mackey J, Pawlicki M, Guastalla JP, et al. (2005) Adjuvant docetaxel for node-positive breast cancer. N Engl J Med 352(22): 2302–13.

5. Macdonald JS, Smalley SR, Benedetti J, Hundahl SA, Estes NC, et al. (2001) Chemoradiotherapy after surgery compared with surgery alone for adenocarcinoma of the stomach or gastroesophageal junction. N Engl J Med 345(10): 725–30.

6. Lin DY, Lin SM, Liaw YF (1997) Non-surgical treatment of hepatocellular carcinoma. J Gastroenterol Hepatol 12(9–10): S319–28.

7. Yoo BK, Gredler R, Vozhilla N, Su ZZ, Chen D, et al. (2009) Identification of genes conferring resistance to 5-fluorouracil. Proc Natl Acad Sci U S A 106(31): 12938–43.

8. Jin J, Huang M, Wei HL, Liu GT (2002) Mechanism of 5-fluorouracil required resistance in human hepatocellular carcinoma cell line Bel(7402). World J Gastroenterol 8(6): 1029–34.

9. Haraguchi N, Ishii H, Mimori K, Tanaka F, Ohkuma M, et al. (2010) CD13 is a therapeutic target in human liver cancer stem cells. J Clin Invest 120(9): 3326–39.

10. Dean M, Fojo T, Bates S (2005) Tumour stem cells and drug resistance. Nat Rev Cancer 5(4): 275–84.

11. Huntly BJ, Gilliland DG (2005) Cancer biology: summing up cancer stem cells. Nature 435(7046): 1169–70.

12. Terpstra W, Ploemacher RE, Prins A, van Lom K, Pouwels K, et al. (1996) Fluorouracil selectively spares acute myeloid leukemia cells with long-term growth abilities in immunodeficient mice and in culture. Blood 88(6): 1944–50.

13. Collura A, Marisa L, Trojan D, Buhard O, Lagrange A, et al. (2013) Extensive characterization of sphere models established from colorectal cancer cell lines. Cell Mol Life Sci 70(4): 729–42.

14. Gupta PB, Onder TT, Jiang G, Tao K, Kuperwasser C, et al. (2009). Identification of selective inhibitors of cancer stem cells by high-throughput screening. Cell 138(4): 645–59.

15. Tang QL, Zhao ZQ, Li JC, Liang Y, Yin JQ, et al. (2011) Salinomycin inhibits osteosarcoma by targeting its tumor stem cells. Cancer Lett 311(1): 113–21.

16. Kusunoki S, Kato K, Tabu K, Inagaki T, Okabe H, et al. (2013). The inhibitory effect of salinomycin on the proliferation, migration and invasion of human endometrial cancer stem-like cells. Gynecol Oncol 129(3): 598–05.

17. Wang F, He L, Dai WQ, Xu YP, Wu D, et al. (2012). Salinomycin inhibits proliferation and induces apoptosis of human hepatocellular carcinoma cells in vitro and in vivo. PLoS One 7(12): p. e50638.

18. He L, Wang F, Dai WQ, Wu D, Lin CL, et al. (2013) Mechanism of action of salinomycin on growth and migration in pancreatic cancer cell lines. Pancreatology 13(1): 72–78.

19. Chou, T C. (2006) Theoretical basis, experimental design, and computerized simulation of synergism and antagonism in drug combination studies. Pharmacol Rev, 58(3): p. 621–81.

20. Workman P, Aboagye EO, Balkwill F, Balmain A, Bruder G, et al. (2010) Guidelines for the welfare and use of animals in cancer research. Br J Cancer 102(11): 1555–77.

21. Kelland LR (2004) Of mice and men: values and liabilities of the athymic nude mouse model in anticancer drug development. Eur J Cancer 40(6): 827–36.

22. Voskoglou-Nomikos T, Pater JL, Seymour L. (2003) Seymour, Clinical predictive value of the in vitro cell line, human xenograft, and mouse allograft preclinical cancer models. Clin Cancer Res 9(11): 4227–39.

23. Miyake M, Anai S, Fujimoto K, Ohnishi S, Kuwada M, et al. (2012), 5-fluorouracil enhances the antitumor effect of sorafenib and sunitinib in a xenograft model of human renal cell carcinoma. Oncol Lett 3(6): 1195–02.

24. Chen Y, Yu D, Zhang H, He H, Zhang C, et al. (2012), CD133(+) EpCAM(+) phenotype possesses more characteristics of tumor initiating cells in hepatocellular carcinoma Huh7 cells. Int J Biol Sci. 8(7): 992–04.

25. Zhang W, Feng M, Zheng G, Chen Y, Wang X, et al. (2012) Chemoresistance to 5-fluorouracil induces epithelial-mesenchymal transition via up-regulation of Snail in MCF7 human breast cancer cells. Biochem Biophys Res Commun 417(2): 679–85.

26. Uchibori K, Kasamatsu A, Sunaga M, Yokota S, Sakurada T, et al. (2012) Establishment and characterization of two 5-fluorouracil-resistant hepatocellular carcinoma cell lines. Int J Oncol 40(4): p. 1005–10.

27. Tanahashi T, Osada S, Yamada A, Kato J, Yawata K, et al. (2013) Extracellular signal-regulated kinase and Akt activation play a critical role in the process of hepatocyte growth factor-induced epithelial-mesenchymal transition. Int J Oncol 42(2): 556–64.

28. Yang W, Yan HX, Chen L, Liu Q, He YQ, et al. (2008) Wnt/beta-catenin signaling contributes to activation of normal and tumorigenic liver progenitor cells. Cancer Res 68(11): 4287–95.

29. Wagner RT, Xu X, Yi F, Merrill BJ, Cooney AJ. (2010) Canonical Wnt/beta-catenin regulation of liver receptor homolog-1 mediates pluripotency gene expression. Stem Cells 28(10): 1794–04.

30. Yang L, Lin C, Liu ZR. (2006) P68 RNA helicase mediates PDGF-induced epithelial mesenchymal transition by displacing Axin from beta-catenin. Cell 127(1): 139–55.

31. Li X, Xu Y, Chen Y, Chen S, Jia X, et al. (2013) SOX2 promotes tumor metastasis by stimulating epithelial-to-mesenchymal transition via regulation of WNT/beta-catenin signal network. Cancer Lett 336(2): p. 379–89.

32. Tanahashi T, Osada S, Yamada A, Kato J, Yawata K, et al. (2013) CD133 silencing inhibits stemness properties and enhances chemoradiosensitivity in CD133-positive liver cancer stem cells. Int J Mol Med 31(2): 315–24.

33. Sun YF, Xu Y, Yang XR, Guo W, Zhang X, et al. (2013) Circulating stem cell-like epithelial cell adhesion molecule-positive tumor cells indicate poor prognosis of hepatocellular carcinoma after curative resection. Hepatology 57(4): 1458–68.

34. Mani SA, Guo W, Liao MJ, Eaton EN, Ayyanan A, et al. (2008) The epithelial-mesenchymal transition generates cells with properties of stem cells. Cell 133(4): 704–15.

35. Morel AP, Lièvre M, Thomas C, Hinkal G, Ansieau S, et al. (2008) Generation of breast cancer stem cells through epithelial-mesenchymal transition. PLoS One 3(8): p. e2888.

36. Santisteban M, Reiman JM, Asiedu MK, Behrens MD, Nassar A, et al. (2009) Immune-induced epithelial to mesenchymal transition in vivo generates breast cancer stem cells. Cancer Res 69(7): 2887–95.

37. Dang H, Ding W, Emerson D, Rountree CB (2011) Snail1 induces epithelial-to-mesenchymal transition and tumor initiating stem cell characteristics. BMC Cancer 11: 396.

38. Na DC, Lee JE, Yoo JE, Oh BK, Choi GH, et al. (2011) Invasion and EMT-associated genes are up-regulated in B viral hepatocellular carcinoma with high expression of CD133-human and cell culture study. Exp Mol Pathol 90(1): 66–73.

39. Noda T, Nagano H, Takemasa I, Yoshioka S, Murakami M, et al. (2009) Activation of Wnt/beta- catenin signalling pathway induces chemoresistance to interferon-alpha/5- fluorouracil combination therapy for hepatocellular carcinoma. Br J Cancer 100(10): 1647–58.

40. Yook JI, Li XY, Ota I, Hu C, Kim HS, et al. (2006). A Wnt-Axin2-GSK3beta cascade regulates Snail1 activity in breast cancer cells. Nat Cell Biol 8(12): 1398–06.

41. Yang W, Yan HX, Chen L, Liu Q, He YQ, et al. (2008) Wnt/beta-catenin signaling contributes to activation of normal and tumorigenic liver progenitor cell. Cancer Res 68(11): 4287–95.

42. Zhang Y, Wang Z, Yu J, Shi Jz, Wang C, et al. (2012) Cancer stem-like cells contribute to cisplatin resistance and progression in bladder cancer. Cancer Lett 322(N): 70–77.

43. Dylla SJ, Beviglia L, Park IK, Chartier C, Raval J, et al. (2008) Colorectal cancer stem cells are enriched in xenogeneic tumors following chemotherapy. PLoS One 3(6): e2428.

# 10

# *In Vivo* Near-Infrared Fluorescence Imaging of Apoptosis using Histone H1-Targeting Peptide Probe after Anti-Cancer Treatment with Cisplatin and Cetuximab for Early Decision on Tumor Response

**Hyun-Kyung Jung[1,2], Kai Wang[3], Min Kyu Jung[4], In-San Kim[1,2], Byung-Heon Lee[1,2]***

**1** Department of Biochemistry and Cell Biology and School of Medicine, Kyungpook National University, Daegu, Korea, **2** BK21 Plus KNU Biomedical Convergence Program, Department of Biomedical Science, Graduate School, Kyungpook National University, Daegu, Korea, **3** Department of Plastic Surgery, Henan Provincial People's Hospital, Zhengzhou, Henan, China, **4** Department of Internal Medicine, School of Medicine, Kyungpook National University, Daegu, Korea

## Abstract

Early decision on tumor response after anti-cancer treatment is still an unmet medical need. Here we investigated whether *in vivo* imaging of apoptosis using linear and cyclic (disulfide-bonded) form of ApoPep-1, a peptide that recognizes histone H1 exposed on apoptotic cells, at an early stage after treatment could predict tumor response to the treatment later. Treatment of stomach tumor cells with cistplatin or cetuximab alone induced apoptosis, while combination of cisplatin plus cetuximab more efficiently induced apoptosis, as detected by binding with linear and cyclic form of ApoPep-1. However, the differences between the single agent and combination treatment were more remarkable as detected with the cyclic form compared to the linear form. In tumor-bearing mice, apoptosis imaging was performed 1 week and 2 weeks after the initiation of treatment, while tumor volumes and weights were measured 3 weeks after the treatment. *In vivo* fluorescence imaging signals obtained by the uptake of ApoPep-1 to tumor was most remarkable in the group injected with cyclic form of ApoPep-1 at 1 week after combined treatment with cisplatin plus cetuximab. Correlation analysis revealed that imaging signals by cyclic ApoPep-1 at 1 week after treatment with cisplatin plus cetuximab in combination were most closely related with tumor volume changes ($r^2 = 0.934$). These results demonstrate that *in vivo* apoptosis imaging using Apopep-1, especially cyclic ApoPep-1, is a sensitive and predictive tool for early decision on stomach tumor response after anti-cancer treatment.

**Editor:** Subhash Gautam, Henry Ford Health System, United States of America

**Funding:** This study was supported by a grant from the national R&D Program for Cancer Control, Ministry of Health & Welfare, Republic of Korea (0720550-2 to Byung-Heon Lee) and a grant NRF-2012M2A2A7035589 (to Byung-Heon Lee) through the National Research Foundation of Korea. The funders had no role in study design, data collection and analysis, decision to publish, or preparation of the manuscript.

**Competing Interests:** The authors have declared that no competing interests exist.

\* Email: leebh@knu.ac.kr

## Introduction

Gastric cancer is the second leading cause of cancer death worldwide [1]. Single-agent chemotherapy for advanced gastric cancer includes capecitabine or 5-fluorouracil, while combination therapy includes cisplatin plus 5-fluorouracil or cisplatin plus capecitabine [2]. Unfortunately, gastric cancer has shown low responsibility to chemotherapy. The response rate of advanced gastric cancer ranges from 10–30% for single-agent therapy and 30–60% for combined chemotherapy [2]. In addition, molecular targeted drugs such as cetuximab (anti-epidermal growth factor receptor antibody) and trastuzumab (anti-Her2 receptor antibody) have been used in combination with chemotherapy, resulting in diverse response rates [3–5]. In the light of these low response rates, monitoring and early decision of stomach tumor response after treatment with anti-cancer drugs is therefore very important in the management of cancer therapy.

Traditionally, decision on tumor response has been performed by measuring the changes in tumor size using computed tomography (CT). Such a tumor size-based decision on tumor response, however, is usually possible at two months after the start of treatment. According to the guidelines of Response Evaluation Criteria in Solid Tumors (RECIST), when there is at least 30% reduction in tumor size, the treatment is considered as a partial response, while when there is a 20% or greater increase in tumor size, it is defined as a progressive disease [6]. To reduce the consuming of time and cost for an anti-tumor therapy, it is required to make the go/no-go decision on the therapy earlier than the current method based on tumor size measurement by CT.

Measuring the uptake of $^{18}$F-fluorodeoxyglucose ($^{18}$F-FDG) by tumor using positron emission tomography (PET) imaging has enabled us to make an earlier decision on tumor response after anti-tumor therapy than size-based CT imaging. $^{18}$F-FDG uptake of tumor tissue is decreased by the reduction in the metabolism and burden of tumor cells after chemotherapy. However, it is known that the uptake of $^{18}$F-FDG mainly depends on histopathological types of gastric cancer. For example, Signet-ring cell carcinoma and mucinous adenocarcinoma uptake [18]F-FDG at low levels due to low levels of GLUT-1 transporter [7,8]. These features make decision on gastric cancer response by [18]F-FDG uptake limited. In addition, some types of tumor, such as breast cancer, show metabolic flare, a temporary increase of [18]F-FDG uptake after chemotherapy, which is difficult to discriminate it from tumor relapse [9].

When tumor cells are treated with chemotherapy and molecular targeted drugs, they generally die of apoptosis [10–12]. Apoptotic cell death appears to occur before anatomical change or reduction in tumor size [13,14]. In this regards, imaging of apoptosis would enable us to decide whether tumor is responsive to a treatment at an earlier stage than does imaging of size reduction. Moreover, apoptosis directly represents tumor cell death, while [18]F-FDG uptake represents tumor metabolism and thus indirectly represents tumor cell death. Apoptotic cells put signatures or biomarkers on their surface, such as phosphatidylserine and histone H1, that are little or absent on the surface of healthy cells [15–17]. Apoptosis imaging probes such as annexin V and dipicoyl zinc amide that bind to phosphatidylserine have been exploited for monitoring tumor cell apoptosis in vivo [15–17].

We have previously identified ApoPep-1 that recognized apoptotic and necrotic cells through binding to histone H1 on the surface of apoptotic cells and in the nucleus of necrotic cells, respectively [18]. ApoPep-1 has been shown to be accumulated at tumor after treatment with doxorubicin [18]. Also, it has been used for imaging myocardial cell death at an early stage after myocardial infarction for the assessment of long-term heart function [19]. For therapeutic purposes, ApoPep-1 has been employed as a targeting moiety to enhance drug and T cell delivery to tumor after induction of apoptosis by chemotherapy [20,21]. In this study, we examined whether in vivo imaging signals of apoptosis obtained by the uptake of linear and cyclic (disulfide-bonded) form of ApoPep-1 at an early stage after treatment are correlated with changes in tumor volume later and are able to make an early decision on tumor response possible.

## Materials and Methods

### Synthesis and fluorescence labeling of peptides

Linear (CQRPPR) or cyclic (CQRPPRC, cyclization via disulfide bonding at amino and carboxy termini) form of ApoPep-1 peptides were synthesized and purified using high-performance liquid chromatography (HPLC) to >90% purity by Peptron Inc. (Daejeon, Korea.). Peptides were labeled with FPR675 near-infrared (NIR) fluorescence dye (Bioacts Inc., Incheon, Korea.)

### In vitro binding of peptides to apoptotic cells

SNU16 human stomach cancer cell line was purchased from KCLB (Seoul, Korea). To induce apoptosis, cells were treated with cisplatin (300 ng/ml), cetuximab (200 µg/ml), and cisplatin (300 ng/ml) plus cetuximab (200 µg/ml) in combination for 24 h. The concentrations of cisplatin and cetuximab were chosen according to the previous reports [22,23]. After treatment, cells were incubated with 10 µM of fluorescein isothiocyanate (FITC)-conjugated linear or cyclic form of ApoPep-1 at 4°C for 1 h. As control, cells were stained with Alexa488-conjugated annexin V (Life technologies, Carlsbad, CA) for 15 min at RT. Percentages of fluorescent (peptide-bound or annexin V-bound) cells were measured by flow cytometry.

### Anti-tumor treatment of mice and tumor size measurement

All animal experiments were performed in compliance with institutional guidelines and according to the animal protocol approved by the guideline of the Institutional Animal Care and Use Committee (IACUC) of Kyungpook National University (permission No. KNU 2012-15).

Eight-week old female athymic (nu/nu) Balb/c mice were purchased from Orient laboratories (Seongnam, Korea) and were housed under specific-pathogen-free conditions with laboratory chow and water ad libitum. Stomach tumor xenografts were established by subcutaneously injecting 1 x 10^7 SNU-16 cells in 100 µl saline into the right flank. Tumors were allowed to reach 50–60 mm^3 of volume before randomization and initiation of treatment. Treatment of tumor-bearing mice with cisplatin and cetuximab was conducted according to a previously described protocol [24]. Mice were divided into four treatment groups (n = 6 per group) and treated for two weeks: 1) saline control; 2) cisplatin (5 mg/kg, intraperitoneal (i.p.) injection, once per week for total two injections); 3) cetuximab (1.5 mg/kg, i.p., twice per week for total four injections); 4) cisplatin (5 mg/kg, i.p., once per week for total two injections) plus cetuximab (1.5 mg/kg, i.p., twice per week for total four injections). One round of treatment includes the injection of cisplatin at day 1 per week and cetuximab at day 1 and day 4 per week. Changes in tumor size were measured over three weeks. Diameters of tumor were measured with automatic caliper. Tumor volumes were calculated using the formula: volume = (length x width x height)/2, where length, width, and height means the longest dimension, shorter dimension parallel to the mouse body, and diameter of tumor perpendicular to the length and width, respectively. Tumor weights were measured after isolation of tumor mass.

### In vivo NIR fluorescence imaging of tumor apoptosis

In vivo NIR fluorescence imaging was performed after the first and second round of treatment. Each treatment group (n = 6) was divided into two subgroups (n = 3) for imaging with linear and cyclic form of ApoPep-1, respectively. Linear and cyclic form of FPR675–labeled ApoPep-1 (1.45 mg/kg and 1.54 mg/kg, respectively; equivalent to 800 nmol/kg for each peptide) was injected through the tail vein into mice. At 90 min after administration, mice were anesthetized and subjected to imaging. NIR fluorescence (typically, between 650 and 1100 nm) is favored for in vivo optical imaging because of its low tissue absorption and deep tissue penetration properties [25]. The excitation/emission wavelength of the FPR675 dye used in this study was 675/698 nm. Images were taken using the eXplore Optix optical imaging system (ART Inc., Montreal, Canada). This time-domain tomography system has been shown to be more sensitive with higher detection depth and spatial resolution than a continuous wave planar imaging system [26]. The acquisition time for a whole-body scanning was 15 min per mouse. Fluorescence intensity at region of interest (ROI) was measured using a analysis software provided by the manufacturer (ART Inc.).

### Histologic analysis of apoptosis

After in vivo imaging, mice were euthanized and the tumors were removed and frozen quickly in O.C.T. embedding medium (Sakura Finetechnical, Tokyo, Japan). Tissues were cut into 6 µm sections and stained with DAPI (4′,6-diamidino-2-phenylindole) for nucleus counterstaining. Terminal deoxy-nucleotidyl transferase-mediated dUTP nick-end labeling (TUNEL) staining was conducted using Apoptag Red In Situ Apoptosis Detection kit according to the instructions provided by the manufacturer (Millipore, Billerica, MA). Tissue sections were observed under a fluorescence microscope (Carl Zeiss, Jena, Germany).

## Correlation analysis between fluorescence intensity and tumor volume

At 3 weeks after treatment (endpoint of experiments), tumor volumes were measured and tumors were isolated for the weight measurement. The correlation between NIR fluorescence intensity and tumor volume was evaluated by the linear regression analysis using the Graphpad software.

## Stability of peptides in the serum

Peptide stability in the serum was examined as previously described [27]. Blood from mice was collected and allowed to clot, and then serum was obtained by centrifugation at 4°C twice followed by filtration (0.22 μm pore). Peptide (100 μg in 50 μl of PBS) was incubated with 50 μl of filtered serum at 37°C for the indicated time period. The incubated samples were diluted 100-fold and fractionated by C18 reverse phase FPLC with linear gradient of acetonitrile (Vydac protein and peptide C18, 0.1% trifluoroacetate in water for equilibration, and 0.1% trifluoroacetate in acetonitrile for elution). To confirm the identity of the peak from the profiles of C18 reverse phase FPLC, each peak was collected, vacuum dried, and analyzed by mass spectrometry (MS) using an MALDI-TOF mass spectrometer (Life Technologies, Carlsbad, CA).

## Statistical analysis

The statistical significance of differences between experimental and control groups was analyzed using one-way analysis of variance (ANOVA).

## Results

### In vitro detection of apoptosis of stomach tumor cells using ApoPep-1 after treatment with cisplatin and cetuximab

To examine the detection of apoptosis by ApoPep-1, stomach tumor cells were treated with cisplatin, cetuximab, and cisplatin plus cetuximab and then incubated with linear and cyclic form of ApoPep-1. Cyclic form of ApoPep-1 (CQRPPRC) was prepared by adding cysteine residue at the carboxy terminal of linear form

of ApoPep-1 (CQRPPR) and cyclization through disulfide bonding. The percentages of apoptotic cells detected by the linear form of ApoPep-1 were approximately 28%, 25%, and 34% after treatment with cisplatin, cetuximab, and cisplatin plus cetuximab, respectively (Figure 1A). The percentages of apoptotic cells detected by the cyclic form of ApoPep-1 were approximately 56%, 49%, and 78% after treatment with cisplatin, cetuximab, and cisplatin plus cetuximab, respectively (Figure 1B). The percentages of apoptotic cells detected by annexin V were approximately 43%, 40%, and 45% after treatment with cisplatin, cetuximab, and cisplatin plus cetuximab, respectively (Figure 1C). These results show that the combined treatment of cisplatin and cetuximab induces apoptosis of stomach tumor cells at higher levels than the treatment of cisplatin or cetuximab alone does. Also, these results suggest that the cyclic form of ApoPep-1 more sensitively detects apoptosis of stomach tumor cells than the linear form of ApoPep-1 or annexin V does.

### In vivo imaging of apoptosis of stomach tumor using ApoPep-1 in response to cisplatin and cetuximab

To examine in vivo detection and imaging of apoptosis of stomach tumor using ApoPep-1, we measured the fluorescence intensity at tumor by the accumulation of NIR fluorescence dye labeled-ApoPep-1 to tumor tissue after the first and second round of treatment (equivalent to one week and two weeks after the initiation of treatment, respectively). Quantification of fluorescence intensity at tumor site by either linear or cyclic form of ApoPep-1 showed that the intensities were significantly higher in groups treated with cisplatin, cetuximab, and cisplatin plus cetuximab, compared to untreated control group, after the first or second round of treatment (Figure 2A, 2B). Fluorescence intensities by linear ApoPep-1 were higher in the group treated with cisplatin plus cetuximab compared to the group treated with cisplatin alone ($p<0.05$ and $p<0.05$ after the first and second round of treatment, respectively, Figure 2A) and cetuximab alone ($p<0.01$ and not significant after the first and second round of treatment, respectively, Figure 2A). Notably, fluorescence intensities at tumor site by cyclic ApoPep-1 were remarkably higher in the group treated with cisplatin plus cetuximab compared to the group treated with cisplatin alone ($p<0.01$ and $p<0.01$ after the first and second round of treatment, respectively, Figure 2B) and cetuximab alone ($p<0.001$ and $p<0.01$ after the first and second round of treatment, respectively, Figure 2B). Representative whole body

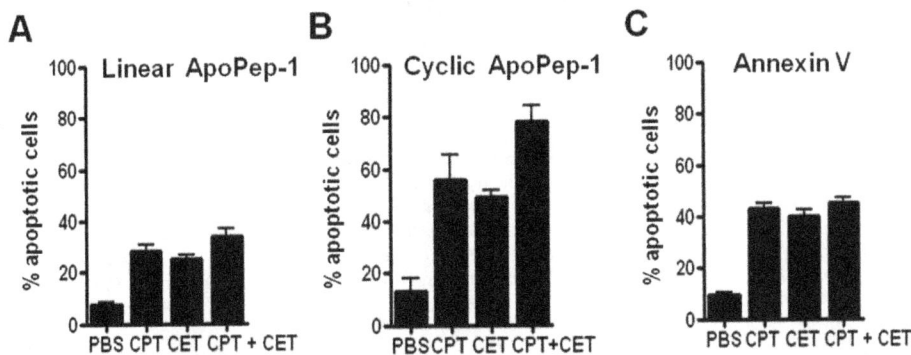

**Figure 1.** *In vitro* **detection of apoptosis.** Cells were incubated with cisplatin (300 ng/ml), cetuximab (200 μg/ml), and cisplatin (300 ng/ml) plus cetuximab (200 μg/ml) in combination for 24 h. Cells were harvested and incubated with FITC-labeled ApoPep-1 at 4°C for 1 h or with annexin V at room temperature for 15 min. Data represent percentages of apoptotic cells as measured by flow cytometry. (A-C) Percentages of apoptotic cells detected by linear form of ApoPep-1, cyclic form of ApoPep-1, and annexin V, respectively. PBS, phosphate-buffered saline; CPT, cisplatin; CET, cetuximab; CPT+CET, cisplatin plus cetuximab.

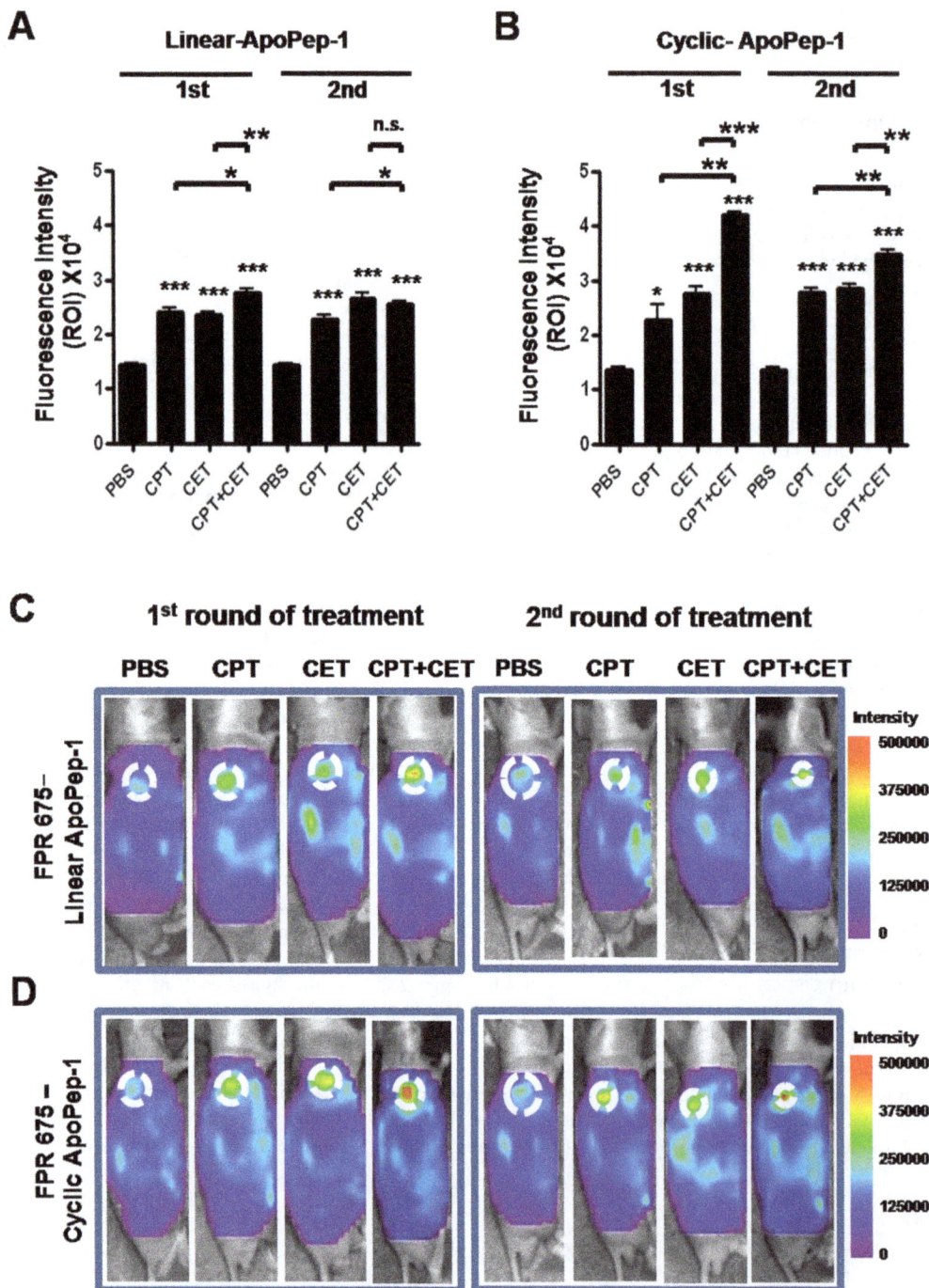

**Figure 2. Monitoring of tumor response by *in vivo* imaging of apoptosis.** SNU-16 stomach tumor-bearing mice were treated with cisplatin, cetuximab, and cisplatin plus cetuximab. After the first and second round of treatment, linear or cyclic form of FPR675 NIR fluorescence dye-labeled ApoPep-1 was intravenously injected into mice. *In vivo* NIR fluorescence images were taken at 90 min after administration. (A) (B) Quantification of NIR fluorescence signal intensity of the region of interest (ROI) in groups injected with linear and cyclic ApoPep-1. Bars represent the signal intensity at ROI obtained from three individual mice (mean ± S.D.). Asterisks represent statistical significance compared to PBS. Asterisks on brackets represent significance in difference between the two groups. * $p<0.05$, ** $p<0.01$, and *** $p<0.001$ by one-way ANOVA ($n=3$ per group). (C) (D) Representative NIR fluorescence images by the uptake of linear and cyclic ApoPep-1 to tumor were shown. Scale bars represent normalized fluorescence intensity. Circles represent the ROI.

fluorescence images by linear and cyclic form of ApoPep-1 were shown (Figure 2C, 2D, respectively). Little background fluorescence signals were observed in other organs, including the liver and lung (Figure 2C, 2D).

## Measurement of tumor volumes and weights after anti-tumor treatment with cisplatin and cetuximab

To examine anti-tumor growth effect of cisplatin or cetuximab alone and in combination, tumor volumes and weights after

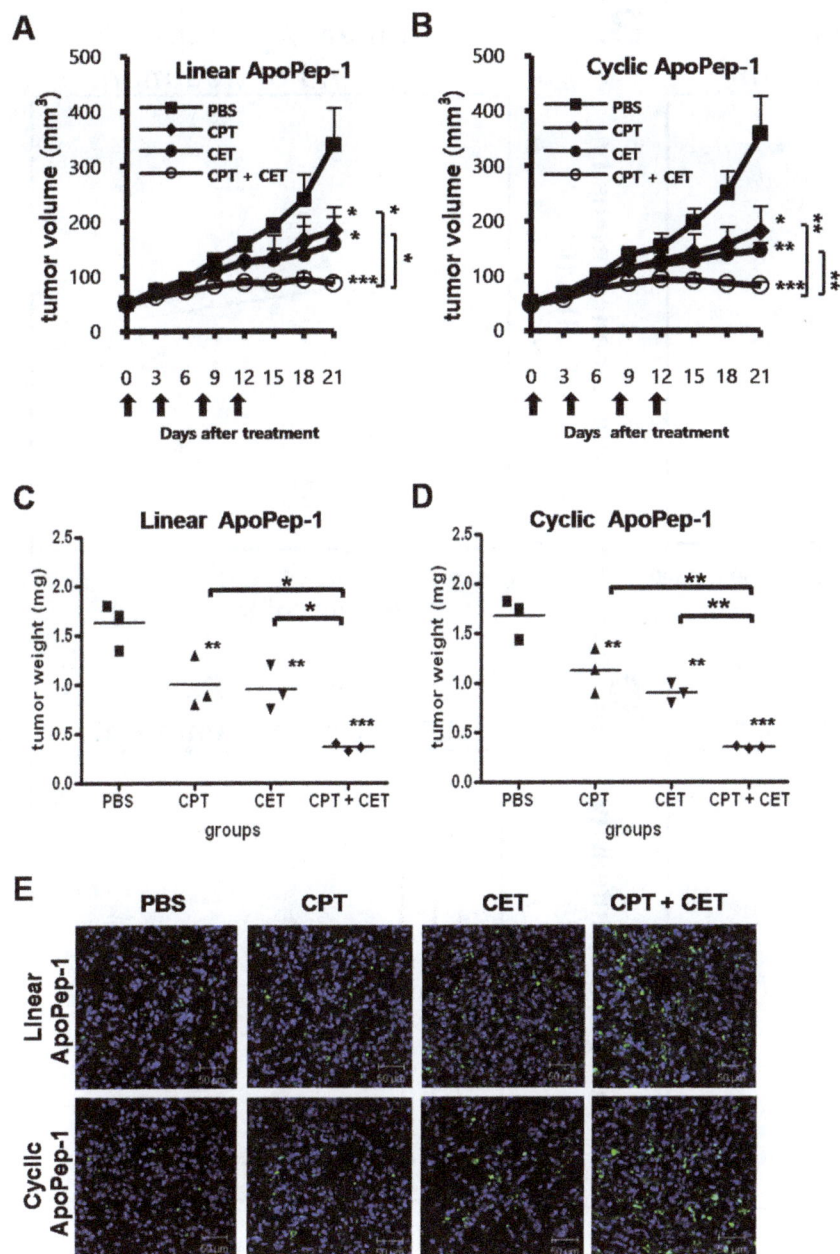

**Figure 3. Changes of tumor volumes and weights in response to therapy.** SNU-16 stomach tumor-bearing mice that were analyzed for imaging signals after the first and second round of treatment were maintained for the measurement of tumor size. (A) (B) Measurement of tumor volumes at 3 weeks after treatment. (C) (D) Measurement of weights of isolated tumor mass at 3 weeks after treatment. * $p < 0.05$, ** $p < 0.01$, and *** $p < 0.001$ by one-way ANOVA. Arrows represent the time points of treatment. Asterisks represent statistical significance compared to PBS. Asterisks on brackets represent significance in difference between the two groups. (E) TUNEL staining of tumor tissues. Green, apoptotic cells; Blue, nucleus. PBS, phosphate-buffered saline; CPT, cisplatin; CET, cetuximab; CPT+CET, cisplatin plus cetuximab. Scale bars represent 50 μm.

treatment were measured. Treatment with cisplatin, cetuximab, and cisplatin plus cetuximab reduced tumor volumes, compared to untreated control, in the linear ApoPep-1 group ($p < 0.05$, $p < 0.05$, and $p < 0.001$, respectively, Figure 3 A) and in the cyclic ApoPep-1 group ($p < 0.05$, $p < 0.01$, and $p < 0.001$, respectively, Figure 3B). Combined treatment of cisplatin and cetuximab more efficiently reduced tumor volumes, compared to treatment with cisplatin or cetuximab alone, in the linear ApoPep-1 group ($p < 0.05$ and $p < 0.05$, respectively, Figure 3 A) and in the cyclic ApoPep-1 group ($p < 0.01$ and $p < 0.01$, respectively, Figure 3B).

Similar pattern of changes in tumor weights after treatment with cisplatin, cetuximab, and cisplatin plus cetuximab compared to untreated control were observed in the linear ApoPep-1 group ($p < 0.01$, $p < 0.01$, and $p < 0.001$, respectively, Figure 3C) and in the cyclic ApoPep-1 group ($p < 0.01$, $p < 0.01$, and $p < 0.001$, respectively, Figure 3D). Treatment with cisplatin plus cetuximab more efficiently reduced tumor weights, compared to treatment with cisplatin or cetuximab alone, in the linear ApoPep-1 group ($p < 0.05$ and $p < 0.05$, respectively, Figure 3C) and in the cyclic ApoPep-1 group ($p < 0.01$ and $p < 0.01$, respectively, Figure 3D).

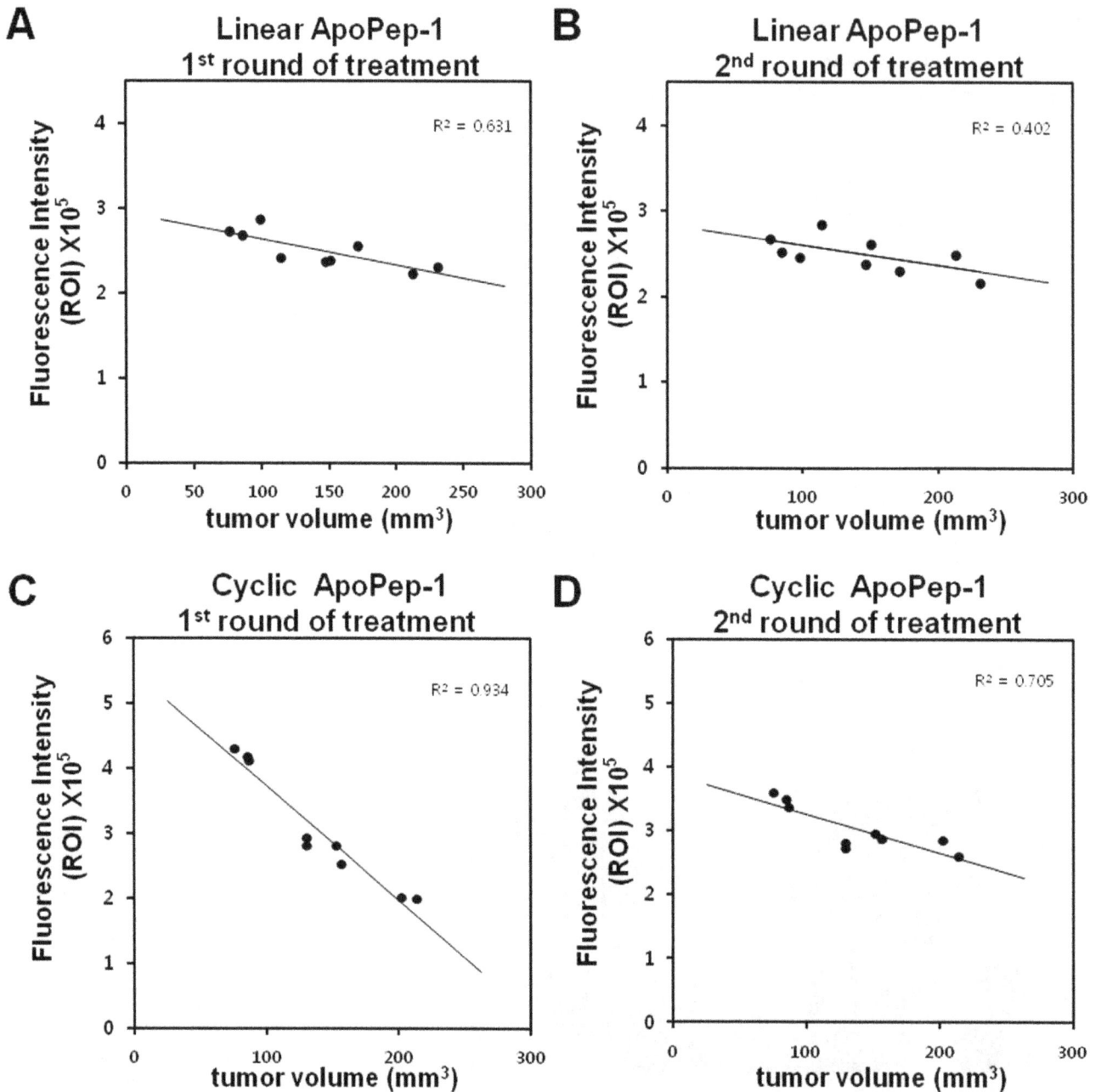

**Figure 4. Linear regression analysis of correlation between tumor volume and fluorescence intensity.** Data represent correlation between NIR fluorescence intensities obtained in Figure 2A and 2B and tumor volumes obtained in Figure 3A and 3B. (A) (B) Correlation between fluorescence intensities obtained by linear ApoPep-1 after the first and second round of treatment and tumor volumes. (C) (D) Correlation between fluorescence intensities obtained by cyclic ApoPep-1 after the first and second round of treatment and tumor volumes.

The levels of reduction in tumor volumes and weights after the treatment between groups injected with linear and cyclic form of ApoPep-1 were similar, and there were no differences in tumor volumes between those two groups at the time of imaging. Higher levels of apoptosis after treatment with cisplatin plus cetuximab in combination, compared to cisplatin or cetuximab alone, was further demonstrated by the TUNEL staining of the tumor tissues (Figure 3E).

## Correlation between fluorescence intensity and tumor volume

We examined the correlation between the fluorescence intensity of *in vivo* imaging of apoptosis after the first and second round of treatment (equivalent to one week and two weeks after the initiation of treatment, respectively) and tumor volume later (at 3 weeks after the initiation of treatment). The fluorescence intensities of images taken by cyclic ApoPep-1 after the first round of treatment were inversely correlated with tumor volumes with the strongest agreement (correlation coefficient $r^2 = 0.934$, Figure 4C),

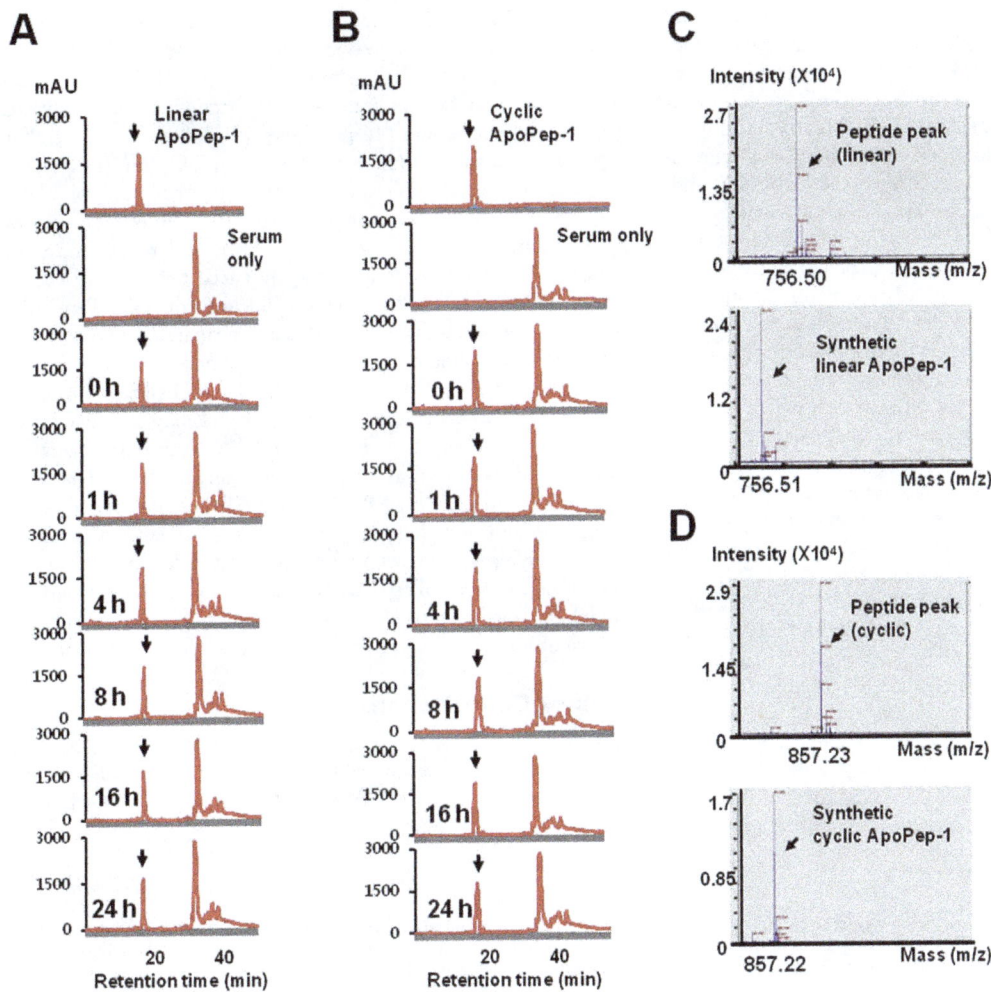

**Figure 5. Stability of linear and cyclic ApoPep-1 in the serum.** Linear and cyclic ApoPep-1 peptides were incubated with mouse serum at 37°C for the indicated time periods. (A) (B) Linear and cyclic form of ApoPpep-1 samples and mouse serum were fractionated by C18 reverse-phase FPLC. Y axis represents the absorbance unit at 215 nm. Each peptide peak was indicated by an arrow and separable from serum peaks. (C) (D) MS spectrum of the linear and cyclic peptide peak collected from 24 h FPLC fraction and synthetic linear and cyclic ApoPep-1.

compared to those taken by cyclic ApoPep-1 after the second round of treatment ($r^2 = 0.705$, Figure 4D) and by linear ApoPep-1 after the first ($r^2 = 0.631$, Figure 4A) and second round of treatment ($r^2 = 0.402$, Figure 4B).

### Stability of linear and cyclic ApoPep-1 in the serum

We examined whether higher levels of imaging signals by the cyclic ApoPep-1 compared to those of the linear ApoPep-1 was due to the difference in serum stability of peptides. After incubation of the linear and cyclic form of ApoPep-1 with mouse serum up to 24 h, the amount of the peptide remaining in the serum was analyzed. The peptide peak was separable from nonspecific peaks of serum and the amount of linear and cyclic form of peptide remaining in the serum, as calculated by peak area, was not significantly changed up to 24 h (Figure 5A and 5B, respectively). MS analysis of each peptide peak confirmed the identity of the linear (Figure 5C) and cyclic (Figure 5D) form of ApoPep-1. These results suggest that both the linear and cyclic forms of ApoPep-1 are stable in the serum up to 24 h with no difference in stability within the incubation time period.

### Discussion

Here we showed that the *in vivo* imaging of apoptosis by the uptake of ApoPep-1 to tumor at an earlier stage (one week after treatment) could predict the stomach tumor response and subsequent reduction in tumor volume at a later stage (three weeks after treatment). In addition, the cyclic form of ApoPep-1 showed higher levels of *in vitro* binding to apoptotic cells and *in vivo* imaging signals and more remarkable difference between cisplatin or cetuximab alone and cisplatin plus cetuximab in combination than the linear form of ApoPep-1 did (more sensitive detection). The intensities of imaging signals taken by the cyclic ApoPep-1 after the first round of treatment showed closer correlation with changes in tumor volume than did those by linear ApoPep-1 (more specific detection). These results indicate that the imaging of apoptosis using the cyclic ApoPep-1 could be a useful tool for an earlier decision of stomach tumor response after anti-cancer treatment than currently available tool based on the tumor size measurement by CT scan.

Apoptosis imaging probes that recognize different biomarkers have been labeled with diverse imaging moieties and exploited for monitoring of tumor response after anti-cancer treatment. For example, fluorescence dye-labeled annexin V was given into colon tumor-bearing mice after one week of cetuximab treatment and showed a peak accumulation at 24 h after intravenous administration, which was associated with a decrease of epidermal growth factor uptake and activation of caspase-3 [28]. $^3$H-labeled butyl-2-methyl-malonic acid that binds to anionic phospholipid was given into colon tumor-bearing mice at 24 h after chemotherapy and was accumulated at tumor by 2 h after injection, which was accompanied with a decrease of tumor weights [29]. Fluorescence dye-labeled caspase activity-based peptide probe was given into mice bearing colon tumor at 12 h after treatment with Apomab to induce apoptosis, which in turn showed fluorescence signals at 50 min after injection [30]. $^{124}$I-labeled phosphatidylserine antibody was injected into mice bearing prostate tumor 24 h after treatment with chemotherapy or radiotherapy, in which images were taken 48 h after antibody injection and showed increased uptake of the antibody at tumor and inverse correlation between antibody uptake and the change in tumor volume ($r^2 = 0.85$) [13]. Compared to the previous reports, our results suggest that ApoPep-1 is a promising probe in terms of fast uptake rate (2 h) and close correlation with tumor volume change ($r^2 = 0.934$).

A cyclic form of a peptide is generally more stable against degradation by protease and more selective in target binding than its linear form [31]. A cyclic form of RGD peptide, for example, shows improved stability against pH changes [32]. Clinical trials as a potential angiogenesis inhibitor are undergoing with cyclic form of RGD peptide [31]. In some cases, however, linear form of a peptide showed better binding activity and imaging signals [31]. In the present study, we compared linear and cyclic form of ApoPep-1 to see which form shows better activity in detecting apoptosis.

We found that cyclic form of ApoPep-1 was more sensitive in binding and detecting apoptotic cells than its linear form. Why did the cyclic form of ApoPep-1 show better *in vitro* binding and *in vivo* detection activity on apoptotic cells? We examined the stability of peptides in the serum. It has been previously described that ApoPep-1 was stable up to 2 h in the serum [33]. In this study, we extended the incubation time period and found that both the linear and cyclic form of ApoPep-1 were stable in the presence of serum until 24 h. This suggests that the difference in serum stability does not contribute to the enhanced targeting activity of the cyclic form of ApoPep-1 over the linear form of ApoPep-1. An alternative explanation may be that the formation of constrained structure by disulfide bonding may lead to more favorable binding to apoptotic cells by the cyclic ApoPep-1 over its linear form.

In addition to fluorescence dyes, ApoPep-1 may be labeled with radioisotopes, such as $^{123}$I, $^{18}$F, and $^{68}$Ga, through chemical linkers and be used as a probe for single photon emission computed tomography (SPECT) or PET imaging. As a future direction, PET imaging of apoptosis using $^{18}$F-labeled linear or cyclic ApoPep-1 remains to be investigated for monitoring of tumor response. ApoPep-1-based imaging of apoptosis would be useful in consideration of therapeutic strategies in clinics and contribute to the development of new anti-cancer therapeutics.

## Author Contributions

Conceived and designed the experiments: ISK BHL. Performed the experiments: HKJ BHL. Analyzed the data: HKJ BHL. Contributed reagents/materials/analysis tools: KW MKJ. Contributed to the writing of the manuscript: HKJ BHL.

## References

1. Lozano R, Naghavi M, Foreman K, Lim S, Shibuya K, et al. (2012) Global and regional mortality from 235 causes of death for 20 age groups in 1990 and 2010: a systematic analysis for the Global Burden of Disease Study 2010. Lancet 380: 2095–2128.
2. Sastre J, Garcia-Saenz JA, Diaz-Rubio E (2006) Chemotherapy for gastric cancer. World J Gastroenterol 12: 204–213.
3. Lordick F, Kang YK, Chung HC, Salman P, Oh SC, et al. (2013) Capecitabine and cisplatin with or without cetuximab for patients with previously untreated advanced gastric cancer (EXPAND): a randomised, open-label phase 3 trial. Lancet Oncol 14: 490–499.
4. Bang YJ, Van Cutsem E, Feyereislova A, Chung HC, Shen L, et al. (2010) Trastuzumab in combination with chemotherapy versus chemotherapy alone for treatment of HER2-positive advanced gastric or gastro-oesophageal junction cancer (ToGA): a phase 3, open-label, randomised controlled trial. Lancet 376: 687–697.
5. Casadei R, Rega D, Pinto C, Monari F, Ricci C, et al. (2009) Treatment of advanced gastric cancer with cetuximab plus chemotherapy followed by surgery. Report of a case. Tumori 95: 811–814.
6. Padhani AR, Ollivier L (2001) The RECIST (Response Evaluation Criteria in Solid Tumors) criteria: implications for diagnostic radiologists. Br J Radiol 74: 983–986.
7. Yoshioka T, Yamaguchi K, Kubota K, Saginoya T, Yamazaki T, et al. (2003) Evaluation of 18F-FDG PET in patients with advanced, metastatic, or recurrent gastric cancer. J Nucl Med 44: 690–699.
8. Alakus H, Batur M, Schmidt M, Drebber U, Baldus SE, et al. (2010) Variable 18F-fluorodeoxyglucose uptake in gastric cancer is associated with different levels of GLUT-1 expression. Nucl Med Commun 31: 532–538.
9. Tu DG, Yao WJ, Chang TW, Chiu NT, Chen YH (2009) Flare phenomenon in positron emission tomography in a case of breast cancer—a pitfall of positron emission tomography imaging interpretation. Clin Imaging 33: 468–470.
10. Barry MA, Behnke CA, Eastman A (1990) Activation of programmed cell death (apoptosis) by cisplatin, other anticancer drugs, toxins and hyperthermia. Biochem Pharmacol 40: 2353–2362.
11. Dive C, Hickman JA (1991) Drug-target interactions: only the first step in the commitment to a programmed cell death? Br J Cancer 64: 192–196.
12. Amezcua CA, Lu JJ, Felix JC, Stanczyk FZ, Zheng W (2000) Apoptosis may be an early event of progestin therapy for endometrial hyperplasia. Gynecol Oncol 79: 169–176.
13. Stafford JH, Hao G, Best AM, Sun X, Thorpe PE (2013) Highly Specific PET Imaging of Prostate Tumors in Mice with an Iodine-124-Labeled Antibody Fragment That Targets Phosphatidylserine. PLoS One 8: e84864.
14. Belhocine T, Steinmetz N, Hustinx R, Bartsch P, Jerusalem G, et al. (2002) Increased uptake of the apoptosis-imaging agent (99 m)Tc recombinant human Annexin V in human tumors after one course of chemotherapy as a predictor of tumor response and patient prognosis. Clin Cancer Res 8: 2766–2774.
15. Smith BA, Smith BD (2012) Biomarkers and molecular probes for cell death imaging and targeted therapeutics. Bioconjug Chem 23: 1989–2006.
16. Blankenberg FG, Strauss HW (2012) Recent advances in the molecular imaging of programmed cell death: part I—pathophysiology and radiotracers. J Nucl Med 53: 1659–1662.
17. Blankenberg FG, Norfray JF (2011) Multimodality molecular imaging of apoptosis in oncology. AJR Am J Roentgenol 197: 308–317.
18. Wang K, Purushotham S, Lee JY, Na MH, Park H, et al. (2010) In vivo imaging of tumor apoptosis using histone H1-targeting peptide. J Control Release 148: 283–291.
19. Acharya B, Wang K, Kim IS, Kang W, Moon C, et al. (2013) In vivo imaging of myocardial cell death using a peptide probe and assessment of long-term heart function. J Control Release 172: 367–373.
20. He X, Bonaparte N, Kim S, Acharya B, Lee JY, et al. (2012) Enhanced delivery of T cells to tumor after chemotherapy using membrane-anchored, apoptosis-targeted peptide. J Control Release 162: 521–528.
21. Wang K, Na MH, Hoffman AS, Shim G, Han SE, et al. (2011) In situ dose amplification by apoptosis-targeted drug delivery. J Control Release.
22. Choi CH, Cha YJ, An CS, Kim KJ, Kim KC, et al. (2004) Molecular mechanisms of heptaplatin effective against cisplatin-resistant cancer cell lines: less involvement of metallothionein. Cancer Cell Int 4: 6.
23. Yun J, Song SH, Park J, Kim HP, Yoon YK, et al. (2012) Gene silencing of EREG mediated by DNA methylation and histone modification in human gastric cancers. Lab Invest 92: 1033–1044.
24. Steiner P, Joynes C, Bassi R, Wang S, Tonra JR, et al. (2007) Tumor growth inhibition with cetuximab and chemotherapy in non-small cell lung cancer xenografts expressing wild-type and mutated epidermal growth factor receptor. Clin Cancer Res 13: 1540–1551.
25. Konig K (2000) Multiphoton microscopy in life sciences. J Microsc 200: 83–104.
26. Keren S, Gheysens O, Levin CS, Gambhir SS (2008) A comparison between a time domain and continuous wave small animal optical imaging system. IEEE Trans Med Imaging 27: 58–63.
27. Yoo SA, Bae DG, Ryoo JW, Kim HR, Park GS, et al. (2005) Arginine-rich anti-vascular endothelial growth factor (anti-VEGF) hexapeptide inhibits collagen-induced arthritis and VEGF-stimulated productions of TNF-alpha and IL-6 by human monocytes. J Immunol 174: 5846–5855.

28. Manning HC, Merchant NB, Foutch AC, Virostko JM, Wyatt SK, et al. (2008) Molecular imaging of therapeutic response to epidermal growth factor receptor blockade in colorectal cancer. Clin Cancer Res 14: 7413–7422.

29. Grimberg H, Levin G, Shirvan A, Cohen A, Yogev-Falach M, et al. (2009) Monitoring of tumor response to chemotherapy in vivo by a novel small-molecule detector of apoptosis. Apoptosis 14: 257–267.

30. Edgington LE, Berger AB, Blum G, Albrow VE, Paulick MG, et al. (2009) Noninvasive optical imaging of apoptosis by caspase-targeted activity-based probes. Nat Med 15: 967–973.

31. Roxin A, Zheng G (2012) Flexible or fixed: a comparative review of linear and cyclic cancer-targeting peptides. Future Med Chem 4: 1601–1618.

32. Bogdanowich-Knipp SJ, Chakrabarti S, Williams TD, Dillman RK, Siahaan TJ (1999) Solution stability of linear vs. cyclic RGD peptides. J Pept Res 53: 530–541.

33. He X, Na MH, Kim JS, Lee GY, Park JY, et al. (2011) A Novel Peptide Probe for Imaging and Targeted Delivery of Liposomal Doxorubicin to Lung Tumor. Mol Pharm.

# 11

# Clinical Predictive Models for Chemotherapy-Induced Febrile Neutropenia in Breast Cancer Patients: A Validation Study

**Kai Chen[1]⑨, Xiaolan Zhang[1]⑨, Heran Deng[1]⑨, Liling Zhu[1], Fengxi Su[1], Weijuan Jia[1]\*, Xiaogeng Deng[2]\***

1 Breast Tumor Center, Sun Yat-sen Memorial Hospital, Sun Yat-sen University, Guangzhou, P.R. China, 2 Department of Pediatric Surgery, Sun Yat-sen Memorial Hospital, Sun Yat-sen University, Guangzhou, P.R. China

## Abstract

*Background:* Predictive models for febrile neutropenia (FN) would be informative for physicians in clinical decision making. This study aims to validate a predictive model (Jenkin's model) that comprises pretreatment hematological parameters in early-stage breast cancer patients.

*Patients and Methods:* A total of 428 breast cancer patients who received neoadjuvant/adjuvant chemotherapy without any prophylactic use of colony-stimulating factor were included. Pretreatment absolute neutrophil counts (ANC) and absolute lymphocyte counts (ALC) were used by the Jenkin's model to assess the risk of FN. In addition, we modified the threshold of Jenkin's model and generated Model-A and B. We also developed Model-C by incorporating the absolute monocyte count (AMC) as a predictor into Model-A. The rates of FN in the 1st chemotherapy cycle were calculated. A valid model should be able to significantly identify high-risk subgroup of patients with FN rate >20%.

*Results:* Jenkin's model (Predicted as high-risk when ANC$\leq$3.1\*10^9/L;ALC$\leq$1.5\*10^9/L) did not identify any subgroups with significantly high risk (>20%) of FN in our population, even if we used different thresholds in Model-A(ANC$\leq$4.4\*10^9/L;ALC$\leq$2.1\*10^9/L) or B(ANC$\leq$3.8\*10^9/L;ALC$\leq$1.8\*10^9/L). However, with AMC added as an additional predictor, Model-C(ANC$\leq$4.4\*10^9/L;ALC$\leq$2.1\*10^9/L; AMC$\leq$0.28\*10^9/L) identified a subgroup of patients with a significantly high risk of FN (23.1%).

*Conclusions:* In our population, Jenkin's model, cannot accurately identify patients with a significant risk of FN. The threshold should be changed and the AMC should be incorporated as a predictor, to have excellent predictive ability.

**Editor:** Burton B. Yang, University of Toronto, Canada

**Funding:** This work was supported by the National Natural Science Foundation of China (Grant No. 81172524/H1622 and 81372817/ H1622). The funders had no role in study design, data collection and analysis, decision to publish, or preparation of the manuscript.

**Competing Interests:** The authors have declared that no competing interests exist.

\* Email: jiaweijuan@aliyun.com (WJ); dengxiaogeng@aliyun.com (XD)

⑨ These authors contributed equally to this work.

## Introduction

Febrile neutropenia (FN) is one of the most common complications in breast cancer patients treated with chemotherapy. Approximately 25–40% of treatment-naïve patients develop FN [1]. FN may predispose patients to life-threatening infection and/or broad-spectrum antibiotic use, prolonged hospitalization, treatment delay or dose reductions[2]. Therefore, prophylactic use of colony stimulating-factor (CSF) in selected patients is critical. Many guidelines recommend that the decision to use CSF prophylactically should depend on the risk of FN with the chemotherapy regimens[3–8], which have been categorized into high-risk (>20%), intermediate-risk (10–20%) and low-risk (< 20%) regimens of FN.

Although the chemotherapy regimen is the most critical external reason for FN in breast cancer patients, it should not be ignored that even for those patients receiving dose-dense chemotherapy regimens, 30–50% of them will not experience FN

[9–11]. Therefore, internal reasons exist that may account for FN. Advanced or metastatic disease, age, comorbidity status, history of some chronic diseases, liver function and renal function have all been reported to be associated with FN[12–17]. These factors, however, are not a direct reflection of the granulocyte reservoir or the stem cell pool of the bone marrow. Therefore, pretreatment hematological parameters, such as white blood cell count[18], platelet count[19], absolute neutrophil count (ANC) [20,21], absolute lymphocyte count (ALC) [22,23] or absolute monocyte count (AMC) [16,19,24], are hypothesized to reflect, to some extent, the patient's predisposition to FN. Jenkins et al. developed a model using pretreatment ANC and ALC in breast cancer patients receiving CEF (5-fluorouracil, epirubicin and cyclophosphamide) chemotherapy[20]. They categorized patients into five subgroups based on different combinations of quintiles of ANC and ALC values [20,21]. Group V (ANC$\leq$3.1$\times$10^9/L & ALC$\leq$1.5$\times$10^9/L) was defined as a high-risk subgroup in their studies

**Table 1.** Patients features of the included patients.

| Items | n | FN n | FN % | no-FN n | no-FN % | P |
|---|---|---|---|---|---|---|
| Age (yrs, Mean±std) | 47.3±9.8 | 45.9±9.3 | | 47.5±9.9 | | NS |
| BMI (Mean±std) | 23.2±4.0 | 22.7±3.8 | | 23.3±4.0 | | NS |
| BSA (m^2 Mean±std) | 1.6±0.2 | 1.52±0.2 | | 1.56±0.2 | | NS |
| Hypertension history | | | | | | <0.05 |
| No | 386 | 54 | 14 | 332 | 86 | |
| Yes | 41 | 1 | 2 | 40 | 98 | |
| Diabetes history | | | | | | NS |
| No | 411 | 53 | 13 | 358 | 87 | |
| Yes | 17 | 2 | 12 | 15 | 88 | |
| Menopausal status | | | | | | NS |
| Pre/peri-menopausal status | 276 | 38 | 14 | 238 | 86 | |
| Post menopausal status | 146 | 15 | 10 | 131 | 90 | |
| T-stage | | | | | | NS |
| T1 | 196 | 22 | 11 | 174 | 89 | |
| T2 | 214 | 31 | 14 | 183 | 86 | |
| T3 | 12 | 2 | 17 | 10 | 83 | |
| N-stage | | | | | | <0.05 |
| N0 | 277 | 28 | 10 | 249 | 90 | |
| N1 | 95 | 17 | 18 | 78 | 82 | |
| N2 | 32 | 4 | 13 | 28 | 88 | |
| N3 | 22 | 6 | 27 | 16 | 73 | |
| Pathology subtype | | | | | | NS |
| IDC | 376 | 15 | 4 | 361 | 96 | |
| ILC | 7 | 1 | 14 | 6 | 86 | |
| IDC+ILC | 12 | 1 | 8 | 11 | 92 | |
| Others | 33 | 2 | 6 | 31 | 94 | |
| ER status | | | | | | NS |
| Negative | 81 | 12 | 15 | 69 | 85 | |
| Positive | 340 | 43 | 13 | 297 | 87 | |
| PR status | | | | | | NS |
| Negative | 121 | 12 | 10 | 109 | 90 | |
| Positive | 301 | 43 | 14 | 258 | 86 | |
| HER2 | | | | | | <0.05 |
| Negative | 292 | 34 | 12 | 258 | 88 | |

**Table 1.** Cont.

| Items | n | FN | | no-FN | | P |
|---|---|---|---|---|---|---|
| | | n | % | n | % | |
| Intermediate | 31 | 1 | 3 | 30 | 97 | |
| Positive | 104 | 20 | 19 | 84 | 81 | |
| Ki67 | | | | | | NS |
| Negative | 101 | 11 | 11 | 90 | 89 | |
| Positive | 303 | 39 | 13 | 264 | 87 | |
| Neoadjuvant chemotherapy | | | | | | <0.05 |
| No | 98 | 20 | 20 | 78 | 80 | |
| Yes | 328 | 35 | 11 | 293 | 89 | |
| Blood type | | | | | | NS |
| A | 120 | 12 | 10 | 108 | 90 | |
| B | 108 | 20 | 19 | 88 | 81 | |
| O | 172 | 20 | 12 | 152 | 88 | |
| AB | 22 | 2 | 9 | 20 | 91 | |
| Chemotherapy regimens? | | | | | | <0.01 |
| CMF | 18 | 0 | 0 | 18 | 100 | |
| CEF | 21 | 1 | 5 | 20 | 95 | |
| EC | 22 | 5 | 23 | 17 | 77 | |
| TC | 53 | 1 | 2 | 52 | 98 | |
| DC | 29 | 2 | 7 | 27 | 93 | |
| TEC | 16 | 3 | 19 | 13 | 81 | |
| DEC | 43 | 14 | 33 | 29 | 67 | |
| ET | 78 | 11 | 14 | 67 | 86 | |
| ED | 62 | 17 | 27 | 45 | 73 | |
| Others | 7 | 1 | 14 | 6 | 86 | |
| Chemotherapy regimens with different risk of FN? | | | | | | <0.01 |
| Low | 222 | 9 | 4 | 213 | 96 | |
| Intermediate | 101 | 15 | 15 | 86 | 85 | |
| High | 105 | 31 | 30 | 74 | 70 | |

BMI, body mass index. BSA, body surface area ER, estrogen receptor; PR, progesterone receptor; HER2, human epidermal growth factor receptor 2; FN, febrile neutropenia.?High risk regimen(DEC, DE); Intermediate risk regimen (TEC,ET OTHERS); ?C, Cyclophosphomide;M, Methotrexate; E, epirubicin; F, 5-Fluorouracil; T, Paclitaxel; D, Docetaxel;Others included regimens contained herceptins cisplatin, or nolvelbine; NS, non-significant;

**Table 2.** Pretreatment WBC, ANC and ALC values in our population are comparable to Jenkins study.

| Items | 2009 Dataset in Jenkin's study | | Our dataset | | | | | |
|---|---|---|---|---|---|---|---|---|
| | Mean±SD (10^9/L) | Normal range (10^9/L) | Mean±SD (10^9/L) | Normal range (10^9/L) | Median (10^9/L) | Range (10^9/L) | Median (10^9/L) | Range (10^9/L) |
| WBC | 6.96±1.82 | 3.60–11.00 | 6.70±2.00 | 4.00–10.00 | 6.90 | 3.80–19.5 | 6.46 | 2.39–13.47 |
| ANC | 4.32±1.48 | 1.80–7.50 | 4.30±1.80 | 2.00–7.50 | 4.30 | 1.60–17.9 | 3.93 | 0.35–12.47 |
| ALC | 2.02±0.64 | 1.50–4.00 | 1.90±0.60 | 0.80–4.00 | 1.90 | 0.30–4.4 | 1.82 | 0.07–4.63 |

with an FN risk higher than 20%. Their model has been externally validated in breast cancer patients receiving the TAC (docetaxel, adriamycin and cyclophosphamide) regimen, which showed a high risk of FN ($>$20%) [21].

The aims of this study are 1) to evaluate whether the pretreatment hematological parameters are predictive of FN and 2) to validate Jenkin's predictive model in our population.

## Methods

### Patients and Data Collection

We searched our database for early-stage breast cancer patients who received neoadjuvant/adjuvant chemotherapy between 2005 and 2013 at our Sun Yat-sen Memorial Hospital. Exclusion criteria include 1) stage IV breast cancer, 2) history of other cancers, 3) essential data unavailable, 4) history of anemia or other hematological disorders, 5) the first chemotherapy cycle was not administered at our hospital, and 6) prophylactic use of CSF. A total of 428 patients were finally identified and included. All of the included patients received breast-conserving surgery or mastectomy when appropriate. FN was defined as a temperature $>$38.5°C and an ANC$<$0.5$\times$10$^9$/L or$<$1.0$\times$10$^9$/L and expected to fall below 0.5$\times$10$^9$/L. In the current study, we only focused on FN occurring in the 1$^{st}$ cycle of chemotherapy. Based on the policy of our institution, we did not administer prophylactic CSF for chemotherapy in early-stage breast cancer patients, except for those who received dose-dense regimens. Clinicopathological features of the patients and the results of the hematological tests were extracted from the medical records. For patients with no FN events recorded in our database, we performed telephone interviews for confirmation. This study was approved by the Institutional Review Broad of Sun Yat-sen Memorial Hospital. Written informed consents were obtained from the included patients.

### Chemotherapy

The chemotherapy regimens were employed as follows: CMF, cyclophosphamide + methotrexate+5-fluouracil; EC, epirubicin + cyclophosphamide; TC, paclitaxel + cyclophosphamide; DC, docetaxel + cyclophosphamide; CEF, cyclophosphamide + epirubicin+5-fluouracil; ET, epirubicin + paclitaxel; TEC, epirubicin + paclitaxel+ cyclophosphamide; ED, epirubicin + docetaxel; and DEC, epirubicin + docetaxel + cyclophosphamide. Patients were required to have whole blood counts measured at baseline, as well as on the 7$^{th}$, 9$^{th}$ and 14$^{th}$ days of each chemotherapy cycle, and the results and/or any febrile events were reported to their physician. CSF (filgrastim 5 mcg/kg until post-nadir ANC recovery) was employed for ANC $<$1.0$\times$10$^9$/L at the 7$^{th}$ or 9$^{th}$ day of each cycle. Antibiotics were employed at any time when FN occurred. No prophylactic antibiotics were used before treatment.

### Statistical Consideration

For the comparison of FN rates in patients with different pathological features, Fisher's exact test/chi-squared test and the Mann-Whitney U test were used for categorical and continuous variables, respectively. The Mann-Whitney U test was also used in univariate analysis to screen the pretreatment blood count variables for independent risk factors of FN.

In the Jenkin's model, patients were classified into five subgroups (Group I–V) based on their ANC and ALC values [21,25]. To validate the Jenkin's model, we calculated the FN rate of each subgroup (Table 1). The model was considered valid if the actual rate of FN in the predicted high-risk group (Group V) was higher than 20% and the FN rates among subgroups were of

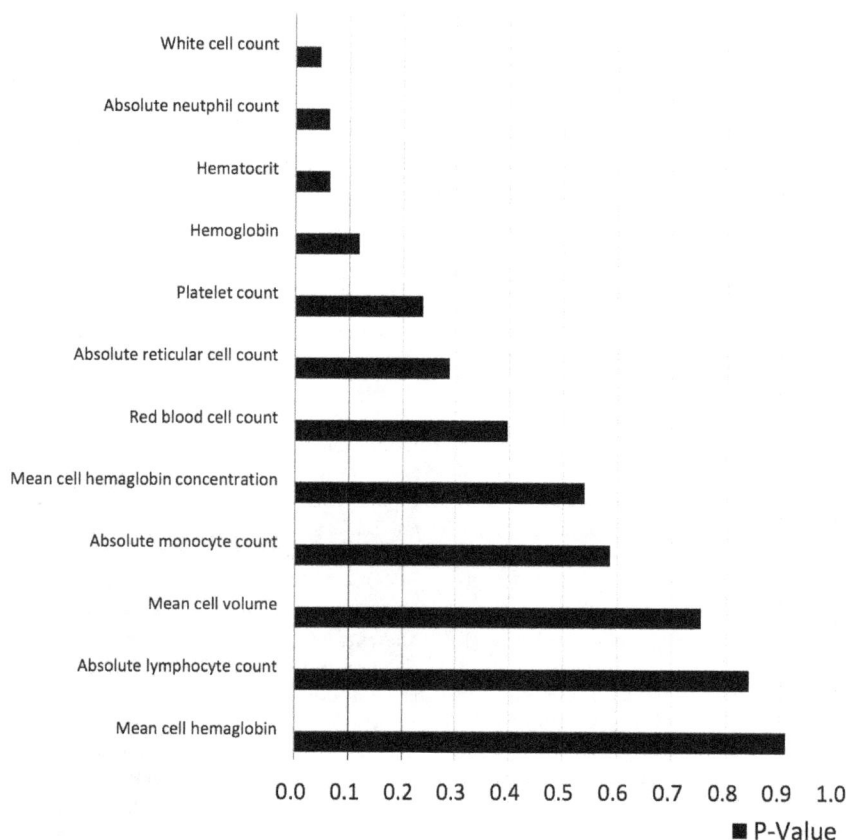

**Figure 1. Univariate analysis of predictive hematological factors for FN.** Mann-Whitney U test was used as a univariate analysis and the P-value was shown. White cell count, absolute neutrophil count and hematocrit with P-value less than 0.1 was incorporated into multivariate analysis.

statistical significance. In addition, we modified Jenkin's model by combining the five subgroups into two subgroups (low-risk and high-risk). The modified Jenkin's models A and B (referred to as Model-A and Model-B hereafter) were generated as follows:

**Model-A.** Group I and II as a low-risk subgroup; Group III, IV and V as a high-risk subgroup.

**Model-B.** Group I, II and III as a low-risk subgroup; Group IV and V as a high-risk subgroup.

To improve the performance of Model-A, we incorporated the AMC value as one of the predictors and generated Model-C. Patients in the high-risk subgroup of Model-A were classified as high-risk in Model-C when their AMC values were lower than a specific threshold. To determine the optimal threshold of AMC for Model-C, we used ROC curves and calculated the corresponding AUC and P values when a different threshold of AMC was used. The AMC value that enabled the AUC and P value of Model-C to reach a significant level was used as the threshold of AMC. Multivariate analysis was performed using logistic regression. All tests of significance were two tailed. Statistical analyses were carried out using SPSS v18.0 (Chicago, IL, USA).

## Results

### Clinicopathological Features

The clinicopathological features and hematological test results of the 428 patients are summarized in Table 1 and Figure 1. The mean and median pretreatment WBC, ANC and ALC values of our population are comparable to those in Jenkin's studies (Table 2). Fifty-five patients (12.8%) developed FN during the 1st cycle of chemotherapy. The median and mean ANC nadir in FN patients was $0.06 \times 10^9$/L and $0.20 \times 10^9$/L, respectively.

### Univariate Analysis of Clinicopathological Factors and Pretreatment Hematological Parameters

History of hypertension (P<0.05), N stage (P<0.05), Her2 status (P<0.05), neoadjuvant chemotherapy (P<0.05), white cell count (P<0.05) and chemotherapy regimens (P<0.01) were significantly associated with FN. Hematocrit (P = 0.06) and ANC (P = 0.06) were marginally significant in predicting FN. The FN rates of different regimens are shown in Figure 2. DEC and ED were classified as high-risk regimens (>20%), whereas TEC, ET and others (carboplatin- and/or trastuzumab-based regimens) were classified as intermediate-risk regimens (10–20%). CMF, CEF, EC, ET, TC and DC regimens were classified as low risk (<10%).

### Validation of Jenkin's Model

Jenkin's model classified patients into five subgroups. The number of patients distributed in these subgroups in our dataset is similar to that reported by Jenkin et al. in 2009[20] and 2012[21] (see Figure S1 and Table S1). Based on Jenkin's model, the FN rates were not significantly different among the five subgroups in our patients, and none of them had an FN rate higher than 20% (Table 3). Model-A, rather than Model-B, could identify patients with a significantly higher FN rate (17.2% vs. 9.7, P<0.05), but did not reach the 20% high-risk threshold.

Therefore, we investigated whether incorporating the AMC value could improve the performance. As shown in Figure 3a, the performance of Model-A can reach a plateau with AUC≈0.58–

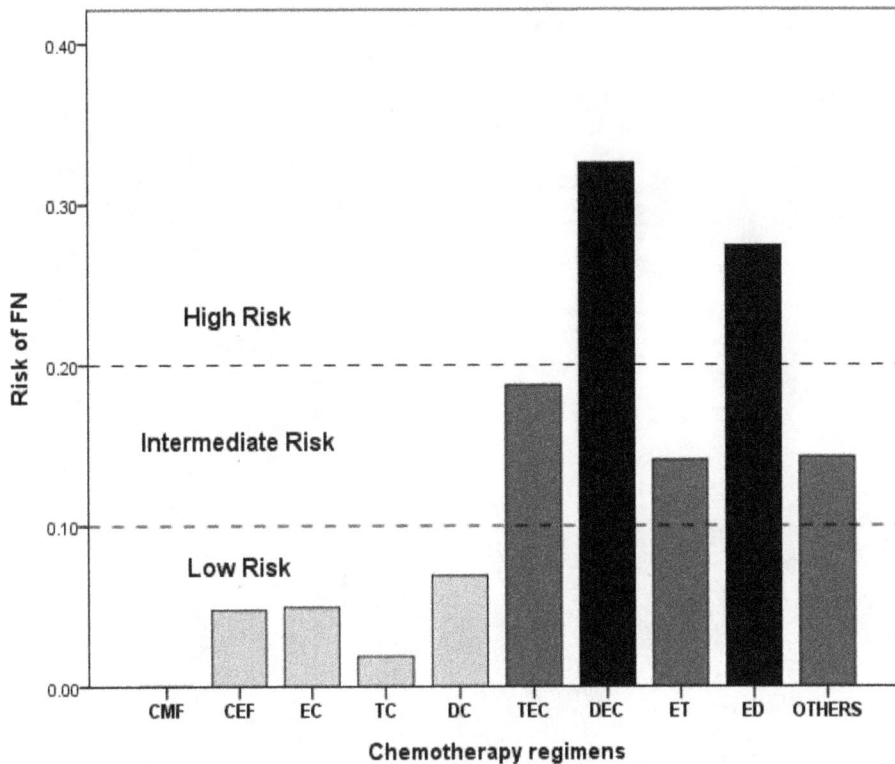

**Figure 2. FN rate in patients receiving different chemotherapy regimens.** Chemotherapy regimens were catagorized into high-, intermediate- or low-risk regimens based on their probability of having FN events.

0.60 and P≈0.05 for an AMC threshold value$>$0.28$\times$10$^9$/L. By contrast, the performance of Model-B could not be improved regardless of the AMC value used (Figure 3b). Therefore, the optimal threshold of AMC to be used should be 0.28$\times$10$^9$/L, and a new model (Model-C) was generated based on Model-A:

**Model-C.** High-risk subgroup: ANC$\leq$4.4$\times$10$^9$/L, ALC$\leq$2.1$\times$10$^9$/L and AMC$\leq$0.28$\times$10$^9$/L.

Low-risk subgroup: Patients do not fulfill the criteria for inclusion in the high-risk subgroup.

The high-risk subgroup in Model-C demonstrated a significantly higher FN rate compared with the low-risk subgroup (23.1% vs. 10.1%; P$<$0.01). The sensitivity, specificity, false-negative rate, false-positive rate, positive predictive value and negative predictive value were 38.2%, 81.2%, 61.8%, 18.8%, 23.1% and 89.1%, respectively.

## Multivariate Analysis

Clinicopathological factors and pretreatment hematological factors that were shown to be associated with FN in the univariate analysis, together with the chemotherapy regimen (classified as low-, intermediate- and high-risk) and Model-C (low-risk vs. high-risk subgroup), were included in logistic regression as the multivariate analysis. The chemotherapy regimen (intermediate-vs. low-risk regimen (HR $=$ 3.51; P$<$0.01; 95% CI: 1.45–8.53); high- vs. low-risk regimen (HR $=$ 9.48; P$<$0.01; 95% CI: 4.26–21.1)) and the Model-C subgroup (high- vs. low-risk group; HR $=$ 2.77; P$<$0.01; 95% CI: 1.42–5.37) are the only two independent predictors for FN.

## Discussion

### Chemotherapy Regimens and FN

Assessing the risk of FN would be informative for physicians in clinical decision making before chemotherapy. The regimens and dosage are the major considerations when evaluating the risk of FN. The estimated risk of FN from each regimen suggested by the current guidelines was limited by the specific populations, study methods and different clinical scenarios. For example, the CMF (cyclophosphamide, methotrexate, fluorouracil) regimen is classified as a low-risk ($<$10%) or intermediate-risk (10–20%) regimen in the EORTC [3] or NCCN [5] guidelines, respectively. Hence, we assessed the FN rate in different chemotherapy regimens in our population. Consistent with the NCCN and EORTC guidelines, the FN rate of our DAC regimen was higher than 20%. When paclitaxel, instead of docetaxel, was used in combination with anthracycline +/− cyclophosphamide, the FN rate fell into the 10–20% range. In the NCCN guidelines, docetaxel every 21 days and CMF regimens are considered intermediate-risk regimens. However, in our population, these two regimens had a low risk of FN ($<$10%)[5], consistent with the EORTC guidelines [3]. Therefore, physicians should summarize the FN rate of each regimen in their own population to gain reliable reference information for clinical decision making. Applying any of the guidelines without prior validation is not appropriate.

### Validation of Jenkin's Model in the Population

Developing a predictive model for FN is important. In patients who receive high-risk regimens with the support of prophylactic CSF, an accurate model may enable the identification of those who may still have FN and the subsequent dose deduction. Patients could also be well informed about the possible compli-

**Table 3.** Validation of Jenkin's model and Modified Jenkin's model.

| Group* | ANC (×10^9/L) | ALC (×10^9/L) | AMC (×10^9/L) | Total No. | FN in the 1st cycle No. | FN in the 1st cycle % | P† |
|---|---|---|---|---|---|---|---|
| Jenkin's model | | | | | | | |
| Group I | >5.2 | >2.4 | n/a | 155 | 15 | 9.7 | NS |
| Group II | ≤5.2 | ≤2.4 | n/a | 93 | 9 | 9.7 | |
| Group III | ≤4.4 | ≤2.1 | n/a | 72 | 14 | 19.4 | |
| Group IV | ≤3.8 | ≤1.8 | n/a | 69 | 13 | 18.8 | |
| Group V (High-risk subgroup) | ≤3.1 | ≤1.5 | n/a | 39 | 4 | 10.3 | |
| Model-A | | | | | | | |
| Low-risk subgroup (Group I & II) | >4.4 | >2.1 | n/a | 248 | 24 | 9.7 | <0.05 |
| High-risk subgroup (Group III,IV & V) | ≤4.4 | ≤2.1 | n/a | 180 | 31 | 17.2 | |
| Model-B | | | | | | | |
| Low-risk subgroup (Group I,II & III) | >3.8 | >1.8 | n/a | 320 | 38 | 11.9 | NS |
| High-risk subgroup(Group IV & V) | ≤3.8 | ≤1.8 | n/a | 108 | 17 | 15.7 | |
| Model-C | | | | | | | |
| Low-risk subgroup | Not fulfill the criteria of high-risk group | | | 337 | 34 | 10.1 | <0.01 |
| High-risk subgroup | ≤4.4 | ≤2.1 | ≤0.28 | 91 | 21 | 23.1 | |

*In Jenkin's model, patients were classified into different groups without overlaps. For example, group IV comprises patients with ANC ≤3.8 and ALC ≤1.8 who do not fulfil the criteria for group V.
†Chi-square test was used.

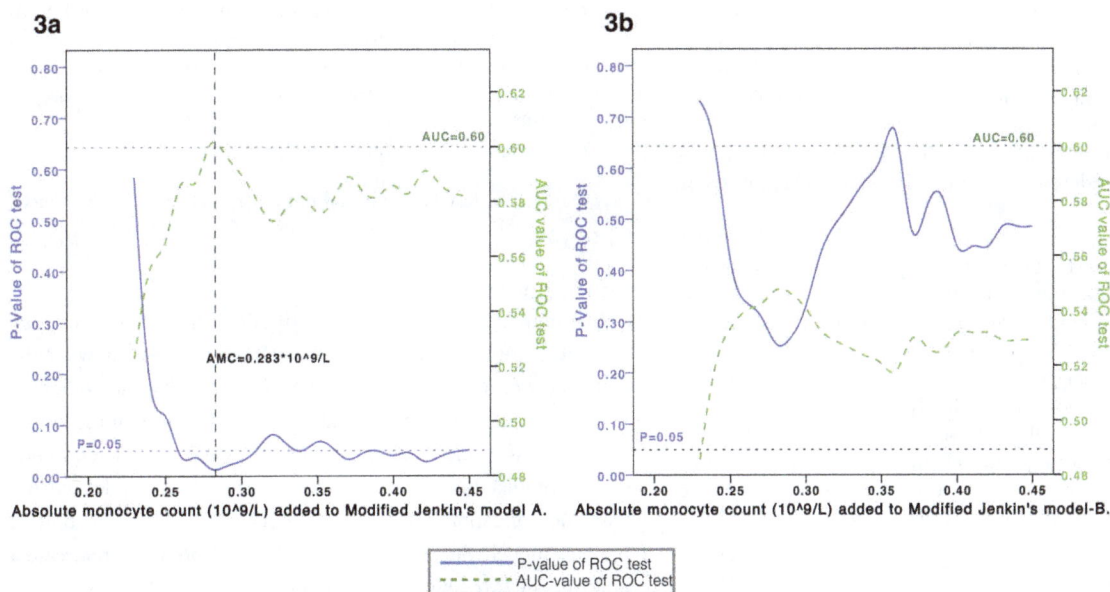

**Figure 3. Optimal threshold of AMC.** To incorporate AMC into Model-A (3a) or Model-B (3b), we calculated the AUC and P-value of the new model when different threshold of AMC was used. A new model (Model-C) could be developd from Model-A (3a) with the highest AUC value and lowest P value, when the threshold of AMC = 0.283*10^9/L. No valid model could be established when AMC was incorporated into Model-B (3b).

cations. A predictive model could also be helpful for patients with an intermediate risk of FN (10–20%) when the use of prophylactic CSF is determined by the physician. Several models have been developed and widely validated in cancer patients[9,14,16,19,22,24]. However, few models have been developed specifically for breast cancer patients. The INC-EU (Impact of Neutropenia in Chemotherapy European study group) reported a multivariate model in breast cancer patients[15], but they did not present it as an applicable formula or nomogram for external validation. In the present study, we tested whether Jenkin's model is valid in our patients. Prior to that, we screened our pretreatment hematological parameters and found that only the ANC was marginally associated with FN status. ANC, ALC or AMC alone was not associated with FN. Similar findings were also observed in one of Jenkin's studies, in which the ANC and ALC were not by themselves correlated with the frequency of FN. However, their patients, when combined into five groups based on the Jenkin's model, had significant differences in the risk of FN in any cycle or in the 1st cycle[21]. When testing the Jenkin's model in our population, we noticed that group V patients (ANC$\leq 3.1 \times 10^9$/L & ALC$\leq 1.5 \times 10^9$/L), who are defined as a high-risk subgroup in the Jenkin's model, did not have an FN rate higher than 20%. The following explanations for the failure of the Jenkin's model were considered:

1) The distribution of baseline hematological parameters differed among our population and Jenkin's. This explanation could be ruled out because we compared the mean and median values of the WBC, ANC and ALC in our populations with those in the Jenkin's studies and did not observe any significant differences (Table 2). In addition, the number of the patients distributed in the different subgroups was also similar among the populations (see Figure S1 and Table S1).

2) The FN rate among our populations (12.8%) and those in Jenkin's studies are different (8% and 6% in the 2009 and 2012 studies, respectively). In addition, Jenkin et al. used the same regimen (CEF in the 2009 study and TEC in the 2012

study) in their population, whereas different chemotherapy regimens were used in our patients. These might be the most likely reasons that cannot be ruled out. Our study did not have a sufficiently large sample size to validate Jenkin's model in patients receiving the same chemotherapy regimens.

3) In Jenkin's model, they considered patients in Group V to be the high-risk subgroup. Because Group V patients did not have a significant higher risk of FN in our populations, we tried to use different thresholds of Jenkin's model by combining the five subgroups into two and generated Model-A and -B (described in the Methods and Results sections). As shown in Table 3, Model-A and -B did not perform well either.

Taken together, our data suggested that the Jenkin's model may not be valid in our population.

## Incorporation of AMC into the Jenkin's Model

To improve the Jenkin's model, we incorporated the AMC as a predictor based on our hypothesis that the combination of ANC, ALC and AMC could comprehensively reflect the bone marrow granulocyte reservoir and, therefore, predict the chemotherapy-induced FN. Kondo et al. and Oguz et al. reported that an AMC$< 0.15 \times 10^9$/L was an independent factor for FN in solid tumors[13,24]. With the same threshold, Moreau's study also suggested that the baseline AMC could independently predict FN in hematological malignancies[26]. In our study, the quintile values of AMC were $0.23 \times 10^9$/L, $0.30 \times 10^9$/L, $0.36 \times 10^9$/L and $0.45 \times 10^9$/L. There were only 16 (3.7%) patients with a pretreatment AMC$< 0.15 \times 10^9$/L, and none of them had FN events. Therefore, an AMC$< 0.15 \times 10^9$/L may not be an optimal threshold. Our study revealed that the AMC threshold should be higher than $0.28 \times 10^9$/L to enable the AUC to reach a significant level (Figure 3). We applied $0.28 \times 10^9$/L as the AMC threshold in Model-C, which identified patients with a significantly high risk of FN (23%). This result is very surprising because AMC only constitutes a small percentage of the WBC but plays such a critical role in risk assessment. Model-C might be able to reflect the patients' internal reasons that determine their predisposition to FN. In addition, the predictive ability of Model-C was independent of the chemotherapy regimens, as shown by our multivariate analysis. Therefore, to comprehensively evaluate the risk of FN, we propose that the pretreatment ANC, ALC and AMC values should all be considered, in addition to the chemotherapy regimens.

All of the patients received surgical treatment in our study. However, it is unknown whether the sequence of chemotherapy and surgery would have any influences on the model predicting accuracy. As a confounding factor, neoadjuvant chemotherapy was associated with FN in univariate analysis, but not in multivariate analysis, suggesting that the sequence of chemotherapy and surgery was not independently associated with FN. In multivariate analysis, we also assessed but did not observe any interaction between neoadjuvant chemotherapy and Model-C, which indicated that the surgical treatment or not would have no impact on the model prediction accuracy in this study.

## Limitations of our Study

Several limitations of our study should be addressed.

1) We only focused on the FN that occurred during the $1^{st}$ cycle of chemotherapy. We are uncertain whether our model can be predictive for FN occurring for the duration of chemotherapy. However, because approximately 80% of FN occurred during the $1^{st}$ cycle of thermotherapy, our study may still be valid for testing the predictive models. To predict the risk of FN occurred in the $2^{nd}$ cycle of chemotherapy or later, more "post-chemo" hematological parameters could be incorporated to improve the model performance.

2) The sample size of our population was not sufficiently large to assess the performance of the models in each chemotherapy regimen. The dosage of chemotherapy regimen might also have influences on model prediction, which could not be assessed in this study. In addition, we had no patients who received dose-dense chemotherapy, which is presently widely used. However, the multivariate analysis in our study suggested that Model-C is an independent predictor of FN when adjusted for the chemotherapy regimens. Thus, we believe that our Model-C, with AMC as one of the predictors, could predict the patient's predisposition for FN regardless of the chemotherapy regimens.

3) Chia et al.[17] had studied the association between chronic comorbid condition and the risk of FN and showed that congestive heart failure, osteoarthritis, previous cancer and

thyroid disorder were associated with increased risk of FN. In addition, the pretreatment renal function, liver function and chemotherapy dosage, which were shown to be associated with FN, were not included in this study. Therefore, it remains unknown whether these factors may affect the performance of the models in our study.

4) We do not have an external dataset to validate our Model-C.

## Conclusions

In summary, our study suggested that 1) the FN rate of each chemotherapy regimen should be evaluated prior to following any guidelines on the prophylactic use of CSF. 2) The chemotherapy regimen is critical as an external factor when assessing the risk of FN in breast cancer patients. Hematological parameters alone cannot predict FN in our population. 3) Jenkin's model did not pass the validation test in our populations. 4) Modification of Jenkin's model with AMC incorporated as a predictor to create a new model (Model-C) was developed with excellent predictive capability.

Further investigations, including external validation of our new model, are needed. Can our model be used to predict the FN rate for the entire duration of chemotherapy or in metastatic breast cancer patients? Can additional parameters, such as indexes of the liver or renal function, be incorporated to improve our model? Can our model be used in patients receiving dose-dense chemotherapy with prophylactic CSF support? Are there any differences of the performance of our model when used in patients with different regimens of chemotherapy? Future studies are needed to help clarify these issues.

## Acknowledgments

We appreciate all the support from the staff at our breast tumor center, Sun Yat-Memorial Hospital.

## Author Contributions

Conceived and designed the experiments: XD XZ FS. Performed the experiments: XZ WJ LZ. Analyzed the data: KC WJ LZ FS. Contributed reagents/materials/analysis tools: XZ WJ FS HD. Wrote the paper: KC LZ.

## References

1. Dale DC (2002) Colony-stimulating factors for the management of neutropenia in cancer patients. Drugs 62 Suppl 1: 1–15.
2. Renner P, Milazzo S, Liu JP, Zwahlen M, Birkmann J, et al. (2012) Primary prophylactic colony-stimulating factors for the prevention of chemotherapy-induced febrile neutropenia in breast cancer patients. Cochrane Database Syst Rev 10: CD007913.
3. Aapro MS, Bohlius J, Cameron DA, Dal Lago L, Donnelly JP, et al. (2011) 2010 update of EORTC guidelines for the use of granulocyte-colony stimulating factor to reduce the incidence of chemotherapy-induced febrile neutropenia in adult patients with lymphoproliferative disorders and solid tumours. Eur J Cancer 47: 8–32.
4. Crawford J, Caserta C, Roila F (2010) Hematopoietic growth factors: ESMO Clinical Practice Guidelines for the applications. Ann Oncol 21 Suppl 5: v248–251.
5. NCCN (2013) Myeloid Growth Factors. NCCNorg Version 2.

6. Smith TJ, Khatcheressian J, Lyman GH, Ozer H, Armitage JO, et al. (2006) 2006 update of recommendations for the use of white blood cell growth factors: an evidence-based clinical practice guideline. J Clin Oncol 24: 3187–3205.
7. Kouroukis CT, Chia S, Verma S, Robson D, Desbiens C, et al. (2008) Canadian supportive care recommendations for the management of neutropenia in patients with cancer. Curr Oncol 15: 9–23.
8. Flowers CR, Seidenfeld J, Bow EJ, Karten C, Gleason C, et al. (2013) Antimicrobial prophylaxis and outpatient management of fever and neutropenia in adults treated for malignancy: American Society of Clinical Oncology clinical practice guideline. J Clin Oncol 31: 794–810.
9. Ray-Coquard I, Borg C, Bachelot T, Sebban C, Philip I, et al. (2003) Baseline and early lymphopenia predict for the risk of febrile neutropenia after chemotherapy. Br J Cancer 88: 181–186.
10. Dittrich C, Sevelda P, Salzer H, Obermair A, Speiser P, et al. (2003) Lack of impact of platinum dose intensity on the outcome of ovarian cancer patients. 10-

year results of a prospective randomised phase III study comparing carboplatin-cisplatin with cyclophosphamide-cisplatin. Eur J Cancer 39: 1129–1140.

11. Elias A, Ryan L, Sulkes A, Collins J, Aisner J, et al. (1989) Response to mesna, doxorubicin, ifosfamide, and dacarbazine in 108 patients with metastatic or unresectable sarcoma and no prior chemotherapy. J Clin Oncol 7: 1208–1216.

12. Lyman GH, Lyman CH, Agboola O (2005) Risk models for predicting chemotherapy-induced neutropenia. Oncologist 10: 427–437.

13. Oguz A, Karadeniz C, Ckitak EC, Cil V (2006) Which one is a risk factor for chemotherapy-induced febrile neutropenia in childhood solid tumors: early lymphopenia or monocytopenia? Pediatr Hematol Oncol 23: 143–151.

14. Hosmer W, Malin J, Wong M (2010) Development and validation of a prediction model for the risk of developing febrile neutropenia in the first cycle of chemotherapy among elderly patients with breast, lung, colorectal, and prostate cancer. Supportive Care in Cancer 19: 333–341.

15. Schwenkglenks M, Pettengell R, Jackisch C, Paridaens R, Constenla M, et al. (2010) Risk factors for chemotherapy-induced neutropenia occurrence in breast cancer patients: data from the INC-EU Prospective Observational European Neutropenia Study. Supportive Care in Cancer 19: 483–490.

16. Sato I (2012) Prediction of docetaxel monotherapy-induced neutropenia based on the monocyte percentage. Oncology Letters.

17. Chia VM, Page JH, Rodriguez R, Yang SJ, Huynh J, et al. (2013) Chronic comorbid conditions associated with risk of febrile neutropenia in breast cancer patients treated with chemotherapy. Breast Cancer Res Treat 138: 621–631.

18. Lyman GH, Kuderer NM, Crawford J, Wolff DA, Culakova E, et al. (2011) Predicting individual risk of neutropenic complications in patients receiving cancer chemotherapy. Cancer 117: 1917–1927.

19. Moreau M, Klastersky J, Schwarzbold A, Muanza F, Georgala A, et al. (2008) A general chemotherapy myelotoxicity score to predict febrile neutropenia in hematological malignancies. Annals of Oncology 20: 513–519.

20. Jenkins P, Freeman S (2009) Pretreatment haematological laboratory values predict for excessive myelosuppression in patients receiving adjuvant FEC chemotherapy for breast cancer. Ann Oncol 20: 34–40.

21. Jenkins P, Scaife J, Freeman S (2012) Validation of a predictive model that identifies patients at high risk of developing febrile neutropaenia following chemotherapy for breast cancer. Ann Oncol 23: 1766–1771.

22. Choi CW, Sung HJ, Park KH, Yoon SY, Kim SJ, et al. (2003) Early lymphopenia as a risk factor for chemotherapy-induced febrile neutropenia. American Journal of Hematology 73: 263–266.

23. Ray-Coquard I, Borg C, Bachelot T, Sebban C, Philip I, et al. (2003) Baseline and early lymphopenia predict for the risk of febrile neutropenia after chemotherapy. British Journal of Cancer 88: 181–186.

24. Kondo M, Oshita F, Kato Y, Yamada K, Nomura I, et al. (1999) Early monocytopenia after chemotherapy as a risk factor for neutropenia. Am J Clin Oncol 22: 103–105.

25. Jenkins P, Freeman S (2008) Pretreatment haematological laboratory values predict for excessive myelosuppression in patients receiving adjuvant FEC chemotherapy for breast cancer. Annals of Oncology 20: 34–40.

26. Moreau M, Klastersky J, Schwarzbold A, Muanza F, Georgala A, et al. (2009) A general chemotherapy myelotoxicity score to predict febrile neutropenia in hematological malignancies. Ann Oncol 20: 513–519.

# 12

# A Prospective Cohort Study of the Effects of Adjuvant Breast Cancer Chemotherapy on Taste Function, Food Liking, Appetite and Associated Nutritional Outcomes

**Anna Boltong[1]\*, Sanchia Aranda[2,3,4], Russell Keast[5], Rochelle Wynne[4], Prudence A. Francis[6], Jacqueline Chirgwin[7], Karla Gough[3]**

1 Cancer Council Victoria, Melbourne, Australia, 2 Cancer Institute NSW, Eveleigh, NSW, Australia, 3 Department of Cancer Experiences Research, Peter MacCallum Cancer Centre, East Melbourne, Victoria, Australia, 4 Melbourne School of Health Sciences, The University of Melbourne, Carlton, Victoria, Australia, 5 Centre for Physical Activity and Nutrition Research, Deakin University, Burwood, Victoria, Australia, 6 Breast Medical Oncology, Peter MacCallum Cancer Centre, East Melbourne, Victoria, Australia, 7 Breast Medical Oncology, Eastern Health, Australia

## Abstract

**Background:** 'Taste' changes are commonly reported during chemotherapy. It is unclear to what extent this relates to actual changes in taste function or to changes in appetite and food liking and how these changes affect dietary intake and nutritional status.

**Patients and methods:** This prospective, repeated measures cohort study recruited participants from three oncology clinics. Women ($n = 52$) prescribed adjuvant chemotherapy underwent standardised testing of taste perception, appetite and food liking at six time points to measure change from baseline. Associations between taste and hedonic changes and nutritional outcomes were examined.

**Results:** Taste function was significantly reduced early in chemotherapy cycles ($p < 0.05$) but showed recovery by late in the cycle. Ability to correctly identify salty, sour and umami tastants was reduced. Liking of sweet food decreased early and mid-cycle ($p < 0.01$) but not late cycle. Liking of savory food was not significantly affected. Appetite decreased early in the cycle ($p < 0.001$). Reduced taste function was associated with lowest kilojoule intake ($r = 0.31$; $p = 0.008$) as was appetite loss with reduced kilojoule ($r = 0.34$; $p = 0.002$) and protein intake ($r = 0.36$; $p = 0.001$) early in the third chemotherapy cycle. Decreased appetite early in the third and final chemotherapy cycles was associated with a decline in BMI ($p = <0.0005$) over the study period. Resolution of taste function, food liking and appetite was observed 8 weeks after chemotherapy completion. There was no association between taste change and dry mouth, oral mucositis or nausea.

**Conclusion:** The results reveal, for the first time, the cyclical yet transient effects of adjuvant chemotherapy on taste function and the link between taste and hedonic changes, dietary intake and nutritional outcomes. The results should be used to inform reliable pre-chemotherapy education.

**Editor:** Salomon M. Stemmer, Davidoff Center, Israel

**Funding:** The contribution by first author Dr. Boltong was funded by a Victorian Cancer Agency Supportive Care in Cancer PhD Scholarship (SCS08Resub_04_Boltong). The funders had no role in study design, data collection and analysis, decision to publish, or preparation of the manuscript.

**Competing Interests:** The authors have declared that no competing interests exist.

\* Email: anna.boltong@cancervic.org.au

## Introduction

Taste is one of the five senses and interacts with smell, touch and other physiological cues to affect the wider perception of *flavor*. Taste function is defined as the perception derived when chemical molecules stimulate taste receptor fields in areas of the tongue, soft palate and oropharyngeal region of the oral cavity to perceive the five basic taste qualities (sweet, sour, salty, bitter and umami) [1], measured via standardised processes [2]. Food hedonics, which also contributes to flavour perception, encompasses food liking: the immediate experience or anticipation of pleasure from the oro-sensory stimulation of eating a food [3], and

appetite: a psychobiologically based sensation related to the maintenance of eating and a desire for specific foods [4].

Chemotherapy is known to affect other senses with ototoxicity and peripheral neuropathy recognized treatment-related toxicities, which in some cases may be permanent [5,6]. 'Taste' changes are commonly reported by people receiving chemotherapy [7] even among those who do not report nausea. It is unclear to what extent this relates to altered taste function per se or to changes to the sense of smell or touch (including oral dryness) or to hedonic aspects such as food liking, or appetite, also described colloquially by patients and clinicians as 'taste' [8].

'Taste' changes in oncology populations have been linked to adverse effects on quality of life, morbidity and mortality due to an association with inadequate energy and nutrient intake, weight loss, malnutrition [11], reduced compliance with treatment regimens [9], reduced immunity [10,11], altered food relationships [12], changed food rituals [13], emotional distress and interference with daily life [14]. The extent to which true taste problems play a role in these scenarios is unknown. The ability to perceive taste sensations guides food choice, which in itself is a determinant of health [15]. Because changes in taste function, liking of food and appetite all have the potential to underpin changes in dietary intake and nutritional status, understanding the extent of the contribution of each would help inform the development of effective interventions in future.

## Study Objectives

The primary objective of this study was to measure the effect of adjuvant breast cancer chemotherapy on taste function and food hedonics across the treatment trajectory. The primary hypothesis was that taste function and food hedonics would be adversely affected by chemotherapy and that the greatest changes to taste function and food hedonics would occur early in a chemotherapy cycle. It was also hypothesised that changes in taste function and food hedonics would be associated with alterations in dietary intake and nutritional status. A secondary objective was to assess the relationship between changes in taste function and toxicities.

## Methods

### Study Design

This was a prospective, multi-centre cohort study that recruited patients planned for adjuvant chemotherapy for breast cancer at three hospital-based oncology clinics in Melbourne, Australia from April to December 2011. Potentially eligible patients were identified via medical oncology clinics and breast cancer multidisciplinary meetings.

### Ethics statement

Institutional ethics approval was granted at Eastern Health and Peter MacCallum Cancer Centre and written informed consent was obtained from each patient before enrolment.

### Participants

Patients aged 18 years or over scheduled to receive an anthracycline and/or taxane containing chemotherapy regimen for the adjuvant treatment of resected invasive breast cancer were eligible to participate. Patients were required to be able to read and converse in English. Exclusion criteria included chemotherapy already initiated, concurrent radiotherapy, previous radiotherapy to the head and neck region, or presence of cognitive impairment that might impact study outcomes.

### Variables

Outcome measures were number of tastants identified correctly, food liking score, appetite rating, daily energy (kJ) and macronutrient (protein, fat and carbohydrate) intake, weight, body mass index (BMI) and nutritional status (Figure 1). Demographic and clinical data collected were obtained for age, years of education, smoking status, BMI, concurrent medications, presence of conditions implicated in taste function (liver or renal dysfunction, sinusitis, diabetes) and treatment related toxicities (nausea, dry mouth and oral mucositis).

## Data sources and measurement

Figure 1 details study assessment time points and data collected. Time points were selected in order to avoid days in the chemotherapy cycle when patients may be taking corticosteroids. Intra-cycle time points were chosen to assess effects early, middle and late in a cycle. Stage of chemotherapy treatment was selected based on a qualitative study with chemotherapy recipients who reported symptoms being apparent by the third chemotherapy cycle and resolving by 6–8 weeks after completion of chemotherapy treatment [16].

Demographic and clinical data were obtained from the patients' medical records and via direct questioning of the participant. Clinical assessment of relevant chemotherapy toxicities was performed at each study appointment in accordance with the US Department of Health and Human Services Common Terminology Criteria for Adverse Events (CTCAE) v.4.03, 2010.

Taste identification testing was performed in accordance with the International Standards Organization (ISO), ISO 3972:2011-Sensory Analysis-Methodology-Method of Investigating Sensitivity of Taste as part of a taste identification task. Tastants and their corresponding concentrations were: sucrose 300 mM, NaCl 200 mM, citric acid 5 mM, caffeine 10 mM, MSG 200 mM. These solutions were prepared in the Deakin University sensory laboratory from food grade chemicals and deionised water in the 7 day period prior to testing. At testing, five 2 ml solutions corresponding to the five basic taste qualities (sweet, salty, sour, bitter and umami) were each tasted in a single 'sip and spit' technique to determine the total number and individual tastants identified correctly at each time point. The mouth was rinsed with room temperature purified water three times before and after sampling and expectorating each solution. Perceived taste quality was identified by selecting one of seven choices. Correct responses were *sweet* for sucrose, *salty* for NaCl, *sour* for citric acid, *bitter* for caffeine, and *savoury* for MSG. Additional choices were *none* or *metallic*. Taste identification score was assigned as 0–5 correct choices.

Food liking was assessed using a 9-point hedonic scale [17] to measure liking of a standard sweet (chocolate) and umami (soup) food item from *Like extremely* (9) to *Dislike extremely* (1). Appetite was rated on a 10-point scale from *Best appetite* (10) to *Worst appetite* (1). Before all taste tests, participants were asked to refrain from smoking, chewing gum, using toothpastes or other oral care products, or eating or drinking anything other than water for a minimum of one hour.

Dietary intake data for the preceding 24 hour period was collected by a dietitian via telephone according to the United States Department of Agriculture (USDA) automated multiple-pass approach (AMPA) [18]. Dietary data were analysed using FoodWorks 2007 (Xyris software, Queensland, Australia) and daily nutrient intake was quantified as kilojoules and grams of protein per kg of body weight and carbohydrate and fat as a proportion of daily energy intake. Investigator assisted height and self-reported weight were used to calculate BMI (kg/m$^2$). The Patient-Generated Subjective Global Assessment (PG-SGA) [19] is a validated method of assessing and classifying nutritional status in oncology populations and was used at baseline (T0) and 8 weeks after completion of chemotherapy (T6) [20].

## Sample size

Sample size requirements for this study were determined based on estimates available for the hedonic scale and a difference between baseline and final follow-up (where attrition would be highest). In this case, sample size calculations were based on a paired-samples t-test with an alpha level of 0.05, 80% power, a

| Data collected | Time point | | | | | |
| --- | --- | --- | --- | --- | --- | --- |
| | Baseline (1-27 days prior to chemotherapy commencement)<br><br>(T0) | Day 4-6 (early) of third chemotherapy cycle<br><br>(T1) | Day 8-10 (middle) of third chemotherapy cycle<br><br>(T2) | Day 12-13 or 19-20[a] (late) of third chemotherapy cycle<br><br>(T3) | Day 4-6 (early) of final chemotherapy cycle<br><br>(T4) | 8 weeks (+/- 2 weeks) post chemotherapy completion<br><br>(T5) |
| Taste identification | ✓ | ✓ | ✓ | ✓ | ✓ | ✓ |
| Food liking | ✓ | ✓ | ✓ | ✓ | ✓ | ✓ |
| Appetite | ✓ | ✓ | ✓ | ✓ | ✓ | ✓ |
| Dietary intake | | ✓ | ✓ | ✓ | ✓ | |
| Height | ✓ | | | | | |
| Weight | ✓ | ✓ | ✓ | ✓ | ✓ | ✓ |
| PG-SGA (nutritional status) | ✓ | | | | | ✓ |
| Comorbidities | ✓ | ✓ | ✓ | ✓ | ✓ | ✓ |
| Concurrent medication | ✓ | ✓ | ✓ | ✓ | ✓ | ✓ |
| Treatment toxicities | ✓ | ✓ | ✓ | ✓ | ✓ | ✓ |
| Smoker status | ✓ | ✓ | ✓ | ✓ | ✓ | ✓ |

**Figure 1. Summary of outcome data collected at each study time point.** [a]Day 12–13 of the third chemotherapy cycle if receiving 14 day chemotherapy cycles. Cycle 3, Day 19–20 if receiving 21 day chemotherapy cycles.

difference of 0.8 points in food liking and a standard deviation of 2.1 [17] (a standardised difference of 0.42). Given these specifications, a total sample of 47 patients was required at final follow-up. Assuming attrition of up to 10%, a minimum of 52 patients were needed at baseline.

## Statistical analysis

Recruitment bias was assessed by comparing the age, treatment centre and cancer stage of patients who consented to participate and those who declined participation using t-tests and chi-squared (or Fisher's exact) tests as appropriate. Analysis of food liking and appetite was carried out by fitting a linear mixed model to each outcome separately; a reference cell model was used to generate estimates of baseline means and differences between baseline and follow-up assessments with 95% confidence intervals and tests of significance. An unstructured covariance type was used to model the covariance structure among repeated measures and all models were estimated by maximum likelihood. McNemar's test was used to assess differences between proportions of participants correctly identifying all five tastants at follow-up assessments compared with baseline. Differences were also assessed for each tastant individually. An SPSS macro created by Garcia-Granero was used to perform this test. [21] Confidence intervals generated by this macro are based on methods developed by Newcombe [22]. Kendall's Tau-b was used to examine associations of change scores for number of tastants correctly identified and liking of sweet and savoury test food items with change in BMI and PG-SGA score. Frequency statistics were used to summarise treatment toxicities at each time point and Kendall's Tau-b was used to examine associations of change scores for number of tastants correctly identified with treatment toxicities at corresponding follow-up assessments. Correlation coefficients were interpreted as follows: 0.1, small association; 0.3, medium association; and 0.5, large association [23]. SPSS Windows Version 21 (Chicago, IL, USA) was used for all analyses. No adjustments were made for multiplicity.

## Results

Fifty-two participants were enrolled in the study. Figure 2 summarises numbers of participants screened, approached and recruited.

There were no differences between patients who consented to participate and those who declined participation in terms of age, treatment centre or stage of disease (all $p > 0.05$). Compliance with data collection was high at $\geq 96\%$ for clinical variables, $\geq 94\%$ for demographic variables and $\geq 92\%$ for all outcome measures. Demographic, clinical and social characteristics of the sample are shown in Table 1.

## Change in taste function

Before adjuvant chemotherapy, 33% of participants correctly identified all five tastants (Table 2). Taste function was reduced with significantly fewer participants correctly identifying all five tastants early cycle 3 (difference $-18\%$, 95% CI $-33$, $-3$; $p = 0.043$) and early final cycle (difference $-20\%$; 95% CI $-35$, $-3$; $p = 0.039$) compared with baseline. Fewer participants correctly identified all five tastants mid cycle 3 (difference $-13\%$, 95% CI $-28$, 2; $p = 0.15$) but this difference was not significant and any effect had predominantly resolved by late cycle 3 (difference $-4\%$, 95% CI $-20$, 12; $p = 0.79$). There was no difference between the proportions of participants who correctly identified all five tastants pre-chemotherapy and 2 months post-chemotherapy (difference 0%, 95% CI $-15$, 15; $p = 0.77$).

At baseline and at all subsequent time points, sucrose as sweet and caffeine as bitter were the most and least accurately identified tastants respectively (Table 2). Further, compared with baseline, there were no differences between the proportions of participants who correctly identified either of these tastants at any follow-up time point (all $p > 0.05$). Conversely, there was a significant reduction in the proportions of participants who correctly identified MSG as savoury early cycle 3 (difference $-16\%$, 95% CI $-29$, $-2$; $p = 0.046$) and NaCl as salty mid cycle 3 (difference $-20\%$, 95% CI $-35$, $-3$; $p = 0.039$) and early final cycle

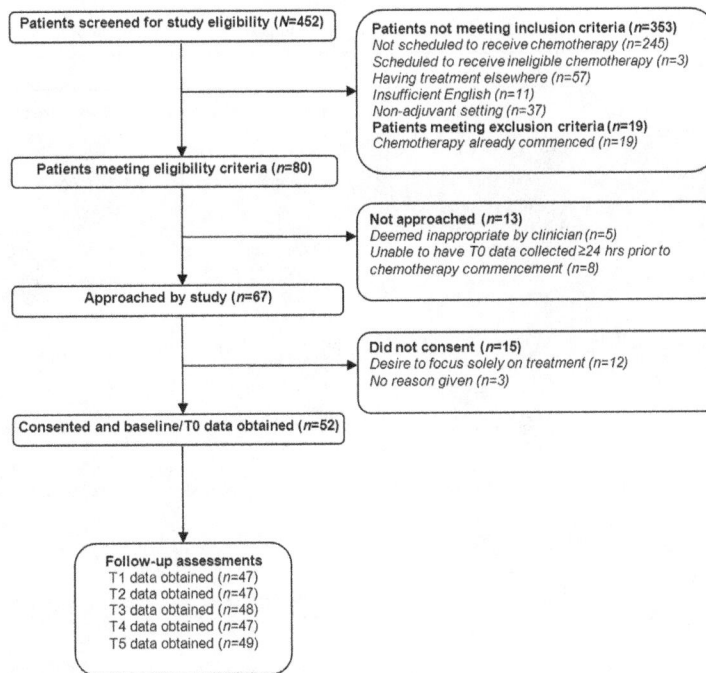

**Figure 2. CONSORT diagram reporting numbers of individuals at each stage of the study.**

(difference −23%, 95% CI −39, −6; $p = 0.022$). Compared with baseline, fewer participants correctly identified citric acid as sour at all subsequent time points (Table 2) but only the difference between early final cycle and baseline reached significance (difference −27%, 95% CI −41, −11; $p = 0.004$).

### Change in food hedonics

Food liking and appetite (Table 3) exhibited similar patterns of differences as taste function indexed by total number of tastants correctly identified. Compared with baseline, appetite was significantly lower early cycle 3 (difference 2.1, 95% CI −2.9, −1.3; $p < 0.0005$) and early final cycle (difference 2.1, 95% CI −3.0, −1.2; $p < 0.0005$). Liking of sweet food was also significantly lower early cycle 3 (difference 0.9, 95% CI −1.5, −0.4; $p = 0.002$) and early final cycle (difference 1.1, 95% CI −1.7, −0.5; $p = 0.001$), as well as mid cycle 3 (difference 0.8, 95% CI −1.4, −0.3; $p = 0.003$), compared with before chemotherapy. Compared with baseline, none of the differences in liking of savoury food at subsequent time points were significant (all $p > 0.05$).

### Association between changes in taste function and appetite and nutritional outcomes

**Changes in taste function.** There was a significant, medium-sized association between a change in taste function and kilojoule intake early cycle 3 (Tau-b = 0.31, $p = 0.008$). Participants whose ability to correctly identify all five tastants deteriorated consumed fewer kilojoules per kilogram (Table 4).

**Changes in appetite.** There were significant, medium-sized associations between reduced appetite early cycle 3 and reduced kilojoule and protein intake (Tau-b = 0.34, $p = 0.002$; and Tau-b = 0.36, $p = 0.001$, respectively) and decline in BMI early cycle 3 compared to baseline (Tau-b = 0.31, $p = 0.004$). There was also a significant, medium-sized association between changes in reduced appetite and decline in BMI early final cycle compared to baseline (Tau-b = 0.42, $p < 0.0005$) (Table 4).

### Association between changes in taste, chemotherapy type and nutrition related toxicities

The majority of participants reported no symptoms of dry mouth, oral mucositis or nausea at all time points assessed. Nonetheless, there was a notable increase in the percentages of patients reporting treatment-related toxicities early and mid cycle 3 and early final cycle. None of the associations between changes in taste function at follow-up time points from before chemotherapy and self-reported toxicities were significant (all $p > .05$, Table 5).

### Discussion

The results of this study investigating women receiving adjuvant chemotherapy support the hypothesis that taste function is adversely affected by chemotherapy and that chemotherapy-related effects are greatest early in a chemotherapy cycle. Further, changes in taste function are cyclical and transient, as are changes in food liking and appetite. The hypothesis that chemotherapy related taste and hedonic changes are associated with alterations in dietary intake and weight was also supported, although these effects are experienced variably. Associations between change in taste function and chemotherapy-related nausea, dry mouth and mucositis, were typically small or trivial in size. Thus this study contributes new knowledge in the area of chemotherapy-related changes in taste function, food hedonics and nutritional outcomes for women receiving adjuvant chemotherapy for breast cancer.

This is the first published study to have examined taste function more than once within a single chemotherapy cycle in a sample size greater than 10 participants and the first to assess perception of all five basic taste qualities in an adult chemotherapy population. Taste assessment in previous studies of chemotherapy populations was conducted on the day of chemotherapy administration (late cycle) when patients report symptoms are at their mildest. This flaw in methodology incorrectly suggested that taste function may be unaffected by chemotherapy [24]. Data from the

**Table 1.** Demographic, clinical and social characteristics of study participants and non-participants at baseline.

| Characteristic | Study sample | Non-participants | p value[a] |
|---|---|---|---|
| **Gender** | | | |
| Female n (%) | 52 (100) | 15 (100) | |
| **Age** | | | 0.35 |
| Range | 32–74 | 33–73 | |
| Mean | 50.4 | 53.3 | |
| SD | 9.7 | 11.6 | |
| **Treatment Centre** | | | 0.78 |
| Clinic A | 25 | 9 | |
| Clinic B | 9 | 1 | |
| Clinic C | 18 | 5 | |
| **Schooling years** | | | |
| Range | 7–21 | | |
| Mean | 14.2 | | |
| SD | 3.2 | | |
| **BMI** | | | |
| IQR range | 24.2–31.3 | | |
| Median | 26.9 | | |
| **Smoking status n (%)** | | | |
| Never smoked | 24 (46) | | |
| Ex-smoker | 24 (46) | | |
| Current smoker | 4 (8) | | |
| **Cancer stage n (%)** | | | 0.53 |
| I | 13 (25) | 3 (20) | |
| II | 23 (44) | 5 (33) | |
| III | 16 (31) | 7 (47) | |
| **Scheduled chemotherapy treatment n (%)** | | | |
| [b]Taxane based regimens | 24 (46) | | |
| [c]Anthracyline → Docetaxel | 17 (33) | | |
| [c]Anthracyline → Paclitaxel | 11 (21) | | |

[a]for comparison of responders and non-responders;
[b]Taxane based regimens were: TC(4): Docetaxel 75 mg/m$^2$ plus cyclophosphamide 600 mg/m$^2$ every 3 weeks ×4 cycles: n = 20 patients (38.5%); or 6 cycles: TC(6), n = 1 (1.9%); TCarbo: Docetaxel 75 mg/m$^2$ plus carboplatin AUC 6 every 3 weeks ×6 cycles: n = 3 (5.8%);
[c]Sequential anthracycline → taxane regimens were: AC(4)-T(4): Doxorubicin 60 mg/m$^2$ plus cyclophosphamide 600 mg/m$^2$ every 3 weeks ×4 cycles followed by docetaxel 100 mg/m$^2$ every 3 weeks ×4 cycles: n = 4 (7.7%); ddAC(4)-T(4): Doxorubicin 60 mg/m$^2$ plus cyclophosphamide 600 mg/m$^2$ every 2 weeks ×4 cycles followed by paclitaxel 175 mg/m$^2$ every 2 weeks ×4 cycles (with G-CSF during each of 8 cycles): n = 5 (9.6%); AC(4)-T(12): Doxorubicin 60 mg/m$^2$ plus cyclophosphamide 600 mg/m$^2$ every 3 weeks ×4 cycles followed by paclitaxel 80 mg/m$^2$ weekly ×12 cycles: n = 2 (3.8%); ddAC(4)-T(12): Doxorubicin 60 mg/m$^2$ plus cyclophosphamide 600 mg/m$^2$ every 2 weeks by 4 cycles (with G-CSF during each of 4 cycles) followed by paclitaxel 80 mg/m$^2$ weekly ×12 cycles: n = 4 (7.7%); FEC(3)-D(3): 5-fluorouracil 500 mg/m$^2$ plus epirubicin 100 mg/m$^2$ plus cyclophosphamide 500 mg/m$^2$ every 3 weeks followed by docetaxel 100 mg/m$^2$ every 3 weeks ×3 cycles: n = 13 (25.0%).
*Notes.* Cancer stage as per AJCC Cancer Staging Manual. Seventh edition. Numbers in parentheses are total chemotherapy cycles received for each type. dd = dose dense (given over a 2-week cycle).

current study supports a recommendation that future research incorporates early-mid cycle taste measurements in its design. It has been shown previously that chemotherapy related taste changes resolve some time between the end of treatment and 3 months after [25]. This study provides new evidence that for breast cancer patients, taste problems experienced in the first 4–6 days after chemotherapy administration will likely resolve over the course of a single chemotherapy cycle, repeat with each cycle and resolve completely in as little as two months after chemotherapy completion. These findings equip clinicians with accurate information to provide breast cancer patients regarding expected nature and duration of symptoms.

Given that patients undergoing chemotherapy commonly report a reversal in preference for sweet or savoury foods and aversions to items such as chocolate and coffee [26], the difference between change in liking of the prototypical sweet food and prototypical savoury food is noteworthy. It is not known whether a change in taste function per se is responsible for the changes in liking of food observed or whether this is driven more by changes in appetite or as a result of other factors such as chemotherapy induced nausea. It is postulated that the absence of a demonstrated decrease in ability to identify sweet and bitter tastants may account for this observation, suggesting these sweet and bitter taste qualities are disproportionally (and aversively) perceptible over others. It has been shown previously that hedonic scores for sucrose solutions

**Table 2.** Correct identification of standardised tastants: proportions of sample identifying all five correct at baseline and differences in proportion at subsequent time points (N = 52).

| | [a]T0: Pre-chemo (baseline) | [b]T1: Early cycle 3 Difference | p | [b]T2: Mid cycle 3 Difference | p | [b]T3: Late cycle 3 Difference | p | [b]T4: Early final cycle Difference | p | [b]T5: 2 months post-chemo Difference | p |
|---|---|---|---|---|---|---|---|---|---|---|---|
| **All tastants** | 33 | **−18 [−33, −3]** | 0.043 | −13 [−28, 2] | 0.15 | −4 [−20, 12] | 0.79 | **−20 [−35, −3]** | 0.039 | 0 [−15, 15] | 0.77 |
| **Sweet** | 98 | 0 [−8, 8] | 1.00 | −4 [−14, 4] | 0.48 | −4 [−14, 4] | 0.48 | −2 [−11, 6] | 1.00 | 0 [−7, 7] | 1.00 |
| **Salty** | 87 | −13 [−29, 3] | 0.181 | **−20 [−35, −3]** | 0.039 | −4 [−19, 10] | 0.77 | **−23 [−39, −6]** | 0.022 | −4 [−15, 6] | 0.62 |
| **Sour** | 77 | −20 [−36, −2] | 0.052 | −19 [−36, −1] | 0.067 | −23 [−42, −2] | 0.070 | **−27 [−41, −11]** | 0.004 | −18 [−34, −2] | 0.052 |
| **Bitter** | 52 | −16 [−32, 2] | 0.15 | −6 [−22, 10] | 0.61 | −2 [−16, 12] | 1.00 | −13 [−29, 5] | 0.24 | −2 [−16, 12] | 1.00 |
| **Umami** | 79 | **−16 [−29, −2]** | 0.046 | −15 [−30, 0] | 0.10 | −6 [−17, 4] | 0.37 | −9 [−23, 6] | 0.39 | 0 [−11, 11] | 0.68 |

*Notes.* [a]Pre-chemo data are percentage correct.
[b]All other data are differences in percentages correct (follow-up assessment minus baseline assessment) with 95% CI. All *p* are continuity-corrected.

**Table 3.** Food hedonics: estimates of food liking and appetite at baseline and differences at subsequent time points (N = 52).

| | [a]T0: Pre-chemo (baseline) | [b]T1: Early cycle 3 Difference | p | [b]T2: Mid cycle 3 Difference | p | [b]T3: Late cycle 3 Difference | p | [b]T4: Early final cycle Difference | p | [b]T5: 2 months post-chemo Difference | p |
|---|---|---|---|---|---|---|---|---|---|---|---|
| **Liking of sweet food** | 7.8 (0.2) | **−0.9 [−1.5, −0.4]** | 0.002 | **−0.8 [−1.4, −0.3]** | 0.003 | −0.3 [−0.7, 0.1] | 0.16 | **−1.1 [−1.7, −.5]** | 0.001 | −0.1 [−0.4, −0.2] | 0.70 |
| **Liking of savoury food** | 5.5 (0.3) | −0.5 [−1.1, 0.1] | 0.085 | −0.4 [−1.0, 0.2] | 0.19 | 0.0 [−0.6, 0.6] | 0.97 | −0.4 [1.0, 0.2] | 0.23 | −0.1 [−0.7, 0.4] | 0.65 |
| **Appetite** | 7.8 (0.3) | **−2.1 [−2.9, −1.3]** | <0.0005 | −0.7 [−1.5, 0.1] | 0.089 | 0.3 [−0.4, 0.9] | 0.45 | **−2.1 [−3.0, −1.2]** | <0.0005 | 0.2 [−0.5, 0.85] | 0.58 |

*Notes.* [a]Pre-chemo data are mean scores at baseline with the standard error of estimate in brackets.
[b]All other data are within-group changes in mean scores (follow-up assessment minus pre-chemo assessment) with 95% CI at specified time point.

**Table 4.** Associations with taste and appetite changes from baseline to assessment points early in the third and final chemotherapy cycles.

| | Taste change from baseline | | | | Appetite change from baseline | | | |
| --- | --- | --- | --- | --- | --- | --- | --- | --- |
| | T1: Early cycle 3 | | T4: Early final cycle | | T1: Early cycle 3 | | T4: Early final cycle | |
| | Tau-b | p value | Tau-b | p value | Tau-b | p value | Tau-b | p value |
| **kJ per kg consumed** | **0.31** | 0.008 | 0.10 | 0.37 | **0.34** | 0.002 | 0.14 | 0.19 |
| Protein (g) per kg consumed | 0.17 | 0.13 | 0.06 | 0.62 | **0.36** | 0.001 | 0.13 | 0.23 |
| Proportion of daily energy intake as fat | 0.07 | 0.54 | −0.08 | 0.45 | 0.15 | 0.16 | 0.03 | 0.75 |
| Proportion of daily energy intake as CHO | 0.12 | 0.31 | 0.12 | 0.28 | −0.13 | 0.22 | −0.06 | 0.55 |
| Change in PG−SGA across study period | −0.07 | 0.56 | 0.02 | 0.88 | −0.11 | 0.33 | 0.18 | 0.092 |
| **BMI change** | −0.01 | 0.91 | 0.12 | 0.28 | **0.31** | 0.004 | **0.42** | <0.0005 |

Notes. CHO = Carbohydrate. BMI change calculated for the relevant taste/appetite change period. Medium-sized associations in bold for emphasis.

decrease at high concentrations in patients with poorest appetites [27] suggesting that those with poorest appetites have greatest aversion to intensely sweet items.

This study adds to limited existing evidence for the link between taste and hedonic changes, dietary behaviour and nutritional outcomes. Although a reduction in taste function was associated with a lower kJ intake, appetite loss was more strongly related to dietary inadequacy and weight loss than was change in taste sensitivity. Reduced appetite had a medium-sized association with reduced BMI and a small-sized association with worsening nutritional status, however not all participants suffering taste or appetite deficits lost weight. The relationship between taste and food hedonics and alterations in dietary quality and nutritional outcomes was specific to early breast cancer populations in this study and should be tested in other clinical scenarios not least because of bidirectional weight change and its variable clinical implications.

Varying use of anti-nausea medications may be a confounding factor in this study as nausea has previously been associated with learned food aversions during chemotherapy treatment [28]. It is postulated that degree of nausea control is likely to influence self-rated appetite and food liking. Future studies should consider incorporating a standardised anti-emetic regimen. Previous studies of taste and food hedonics in chemotherapy populations suffered from methodological issues of heterogeneity in cancer type, stage and prescribed chemotherapy. This was not a factor in the current study. However, time lapse between assessments did vary between individuals within the sample due to differing number of chemotherapy cycles administered, chemotherapy cycle length, and treatment delays. The post-chemotherapy time point (T5) represented a period of 5–8 months from the baseline assessment. This variability has implications for nutritional outcome measures as weight gain has previously been shown to vary with duration of treatment in studies of women receiving adjuvant chemotherapy for breast cancer [29].

## Conclusions

Despite the stated limitations, this study characterised, for the first time, changes in taste perception and food hedonics over repeated chemotherapy cycles in women with early breast cancer and provided evidence that taste per se, as opposed to other elements of flavour is adversely affected at key points during chemotherapy. Findings will inform the design of future studies seeking to understand the mechanisms of changes in taste perception during chemotherapy, and ultimately, the design of interventions aimed at reducing the negative nutritional consequences of chemotherapy treatment. Understanding more about sensory risk factors for weight gain in breast cancer groups should be prioritised in future clinical research, given the link between obesity and poorer outcomes in this population.

### Implementation of findings into practice

Patients do not systematically receive specific information regarding the possible nature, timing of onset and duration of taste problems by health professionals, nor are possible consequences of changes or management strategies routinely discussed. This research has generated new evidence to guide assessment and predictors of chemotherapy induced sensory and hedonic changes. Findings of the study will shape tailored patient information provision in preparation for chemotherapy.

**Table 5.** Presence of mouth dryness, oral mucositis and nausea at each time point and association between each toxicity and change in taste function.

| | T0: Pre-chemo (baseline) | T1: Early cycle 3 | T2: Mid cycle 3 | T3: Late cycle 3 | T4: Early final cycle | T5:2 months post-chemo |
|---|---|---|---|---|---|---|
| **Mouth dryness** | | | | | | |
| Grade 0 | 92.3 | 55.6 | 63.8 | 81.3 | 63.8 | 87.8 |
| Grade 1 | 7.7 | 40.0 | 29.8 | 16.7 | 29.8 | 12.2 |
| Grade 2 | 0.0 | 4.4 | 6.4 | 2.1 | 6.4 | 0.0 |
| Correlation with change in taste function | | −0.052 | −0.019 | −0.078 | 0.059 | 0.043 |
| p value | | 0.70 | 0.88 | 0.55 | 0.65 | 0.76 |
| **Oral mucositis** | | | | | | |
| Grade 0 | 96.2 | 88.9 | 85.1 | 87.5 | 83.0 | 93.9 |
| Grade 1 | 3.8 | 6.7 | 10.6 | 10.4 | 10.6 | 6.1 |
| Grade 2 | | 4.4 | 2.1 | 2.1 | 4.3 | |
| Grade 3 | | | 2.1 | | 2.1 | |
| Correlation with change in taste function | | −0.018 | 0.072 | −0.12 | −0.063 | −0.029 |
| p value | | 0.89 | 0.59 | 0.35 | 0.63 | 0.83 |
| **Nausea** | | | | | | |
| Grade 0 | 96.2 | 57.8 | 73.9 | 89.4 | 76.6 | 91.8 |
| Grade 1 | 1.9 | 13.3 | 10.9 | 6.4 | 6.4 | 4.1 |
| Grade 2 | 1.9 | 28.9 | 15.2 | 4.3 | 17.0 | 4.1 |
| Correlation with change in taste function | | 0.003 | −0.11 | −0.091 | −0.096 | −0.10 |
| p value | | 0.98 | 0.40 | 0.49 | 0.46 | 0.46 |

Notes. Data on presence of mouth dryness, oral mucositis and nausea are percentages.

## Author Contributions

Conceived and designed the experiments: AB SA RK RW PF JC KG. Performed the experiments: AB. Analyzed the data: KG AB. Contributed reagents/materials/analysis tools: RK. Contributed to the writing of the manuscript: AB SA KG. Data acquisition: AB. Quality control of data and algorithms: AB SA. Manuscript editing and review: AB SA RW RK PF JC KG.

## References

1. Breslin PA, Spector AC (2008) Mammalian taste perception. Curr Biol 18(4): R148–55. Epub 2008/02/28.

2. International Organization for Standardization (2011) ISO 3972: 2011 - Sensory Analysis – Methodology – Method of investigating sensitivity of taste. Geneva: ISO.

3. Mela DJ (2006) Eating for pleasure or just wanting to eat? (2006) Reconsidering sensory hedonic responses as a driver of obesity. Appetite 47(1): 10–7. Epub 2006/05/02.

4. Blundell JE (1979) Hunger, appetite and satiety-constructs in search of identities. In: Turner M, editor. Nutrition and Lifestyles. London: Applied Science Publishers. pp. 21–42.

5. Gilmer-Knight KR, Kraemer DF, Neuwelt EA (2005) Ototoxicity in Children Receiving Platinum Chemotherapy: Underestimating a Commonly Occurring Toxicity That May Influence Academic and Social Development. J Clin Oncol 23(34): 8588–96.

6. Quasthoff S, Hartung HP (2002) Chemotherapy-induced peripheral neuropathy. J Neurol. 249(1): 9–17.

7. Zabernigg A, Gamper EM, Giesinger JM, Rumpold G, Kemmler G, et al. (2010) Taste alterations in cancer patients receiving chemotherapy: a neglected side effect? Oncologist 15(8): 913–20. Epub 2010/07/30.

8. Boltong A, Keast R, Aranda S (2011) Talking About Taste: How do Oncology Clinicians Discuss and Document Taste Problems? Cancer Forum 35(2): 81–7.

9. Doty RL, Shah M, Bromley SM (2008) Drug-induced taste disorders. Drug Saf 31(3): 199–215. Epub 2008/02/28.

10. Schiffman SS, Sattely-Miller EA, Taylor EL, Graham BG, Landerman LR, et al. (2007) Combination of flavor enhancement and chemosensory education improves nutritional status in older cancer patients. J Nutr Health Aging 11(5): 439–54.

11. Schiffman SS (2007) Critical illness and changes in sensory perception (2007) Proc Nutr Soc. 66(3): 331–45. Epub 2007/07/20.

12. Schiffman SS, Graham BG (2000) Taste and smell perception affect appetite and immunity in the elderly. European journal of clinical nutrition (Suppl 3): S54–S63.

13. Bernhardson B (2003) 5 themes described the experiences of patients with chemotherapy induced oral mucositis. Evid Based Nurs 6(2): 62–.

14. Bernhardson BM, Tishelman C, Rutqvist LE (2007) Chemosensory changes experienced by patients undergoing cancer chemotherapy: a qualitative interview study. J Pain Symptom Manage 34(4): 403–12.

15. McQuestion M, Fitch M, Howell D (2011) The changed meaning of food: Physical, social and emotional loss for patients having received radiation treatment for head and neck cancer. Eur J Oncol Nurs 15(2): 145–51. Epub 2010/09/25.

16. Boltong A, Keast R, Aranda S (2012) Experiences and consequences of altered taste, flavour and food hedonics during chemotherapy treatment Support Care Cancer 20(11): 2765–74.

17. Peryam DR, Pilgrim FJ (1957) Hedonic scale method of measuring food preferences. Food Technology 11, Suppl: 9–14.

18. Raper N, Perloff B, Ingwersen L, Steinfeldt L, Anand J (2004) An overview of USDA's Dietary Intake Data System. J Food Comp Anal 17(3–4): 545–55.

19. Ottery F (2000) Patient-Generated Subjective Global Assessment. In: McCallum P & Polisena C, editor (2000) The Clinical Guide to Oncology Nutrition Chicago: American Dietetic Association. pp. 11–23.

20. Bauer J, Capra S, Ferguson M (2002) Use of the scored Patient-Generated Subjective Global Assessment (PG-SGA) as a nutrition assessment tool in patients with cancer. Eur J Clin Nutr 56: 779–85.

21. Garcia-Granero M (2011) Two proportions test (related) - SPSS. Available: http://www.how2stats.net/2011/09/two-proportions-test-related-spss.html. Accessed 2014 Jul 06.

22. Newcombe R (1998) Interval estimation for the difference between independent proportions: comparison of eleven methods. Stat Med 17(8): 873–90.

23. Cohen J (1998) Set Correlation and Contingency Tables. Appl Psych Meas 12(4): 425–34.

24. Boltong A, Keast R (2012) The influence of chemotherapy on taste perception and food hedonics: A systematic review. Cancer Treat Rev 38(2): 152–63.

25. Steinbach S, Hummel T, Bohner C, Berktold S, Hundt W, et al. (2009) Qualitative and quantitative assessment of taste and smell changes in patients undergoing chemotherapy for breast cancer or gynecologic malignancies. J Clin Oncol 27(11): 1899–905.

26. Boakes RA, Tarrier N, Barnes BW, Tattersall MH (1993) Prevalence of anticipatory nausea and other side-effects in cancer patients receiving chemotherapy. Eur J Cancer. 29A(6): 866–70. Epub 1993/01/01.

27. Trant AS, Serin J, Douglass HO (1982) Is taste related to anorexia in cancer patients? Am J Clin Nutr 36(1): 45–58. Epub 1982/07/01.

28. Schwartz MD, Jacobsen PB, Bovbjerg DH (1996) Role of nausea in the development of aversions to a beverage paired with chemotherapy treatment in cancer patients. Physiol Behav 59(4–5): 659–63. Epub 1996/04/01.

29. Heasman K, Sutherland H, Campbell J, Elhakim T, Boyd N (1985) Weight gain during adjuvant chemotherapy for breast cancer. Breast Cancer Res Tr 5(2): 195–200.

# 13

# Analysis of Combination Drug Therapy to Develop Regimens with Shortened Duration of Treatment for Tuberculosis

George L. Drusano[1]*, Michael Neely[2], Michael Van Guilder[2], Alan Schumitzky[2], David Brown[1], Steven Fikes[1], Charles Peloquin[3], Arnold Louie[1]

1 Institute for Therapeutic Innovation, College of Medicine, University of Florida, Lake Nona, Florida, United States of America, 2 Laboratory of Applied Pharmacokinetics, School of Medicine, University of Southern California, Los Angeles, California, United States of America, 3 Infectious Diseases PK Laboratory, College of Pharmacy, University of Florida, Gainesville, Florida, United States of America

## Abstract

*Rationale:* Tuberculosis remains a worldwide problem, particularly with the advent of multi-drug resistance. Shortening therapy duration for *Mycobacterium tuberculosis* is a major goal, requiring generation of optimal kill rate and resistance-suppression. Combination therapy is required to attain the goal of shorter therapy.

*Objectives:* Our objective was to identify a method for identifying optimal combination chemotherapy. We developed a mathematical model for attaining this end. This is accomplished by identifying drug effect interaction (synergy, additivity, antagonism) for susceptible organisms and subpopulations resistant to each drug in the combination.

*Methods:* We studied the combination of linezolid plus rifampin in our hollow fiber infection model. We generated a fully parametric drug effect interaction mathematical model. The results were subjected to Monte Carlo simulation to extend the findings to a population of patients by accounting for between-patient variability in drug pharmacokinetics.

*Results:* All monotherapy allowed emergence of resistance over the first two weeks of the experiment. In combination, the interaction was additive for each population (susceptible and resistant). For a 600 mg/600 mg daily regimen of linezolid plus rifampin, we demonstrated that >50% of simulated subjects had eradicated the susceptible population by day 27 with the remaining organisms resistant to one or the other drug. Only 4% of patients had complete organism eradication by experiment end.

*Discussion:* These data strongly suggest that in order to achieve the goal of shortening therapy, the original regimen may need to be changed at one month to a regimen of two completely new agents with resistance mechanisms independent of the initial regimen. This hypothesis which arose from the analysis is immediately testable in a clinical trial.

**Editor:** Andres R. Floto, Cambridge University, United Kingdom

**Funding:** This work was funded by National Institute of Allergy and Infectious Diseases (R01 AI079578); Bill and Melinda Gates Foundation TB Accelerator Program; Pfizer, Inc for the Hollow Fiber System evaluation. The funders had no role in study design, data collection and analysis, decision to publish, or preparation of the manuscript.

**Competing Interests:** The authors have no competing interests with respect to Pfizer, Inc. and this applies to employment, consultancy, patents, products in development, marketed products, etc.

* Email: gdrusano@ufl.edu

## Introduction

*Mycobacterium tuberculosis* (Mtb) infects one-third of the world's population. The World Health Organization estimates that in 2011 there were 8.7 million new cases and 1.4 million deaths caused by this microbe [1]. Standard treatment for drug susceptible Mtb consists of two months of rifampin, isoniazid, pyrazinamide and ethambutol during the intensive phase of therapy followed by four months of rifampin and isoniazid during the continuation phase [2]. Treatment failure caused by initially drug-susceptible (DS) Mtb is sometimes due to emergence of antibiotic-resistant isolates. The major gap for optimal TB therapy is the absence of an effective short (circa 2 months) regimen that is

active against both DS- and Multi-Drug Resistant (MDR)-TB. The ability to obtain maximal rates of kill of Mtb while suppressing resistance emergence is our best hope of markedly shortening duration of therapy.

Recently a number of anti-TB drugs have entered clinical trials (e.g. bedaquiline, delamanid, PA-824, SQ109, sutezolid) or are approved for the treatment of other infections (clofazimine) [3,4–6]. A unifying theme shared by these drugs is that their unique mechanisms of action do not confer cross resistance to current first and second line drugs.

Combination therapy is a proven method for suppressing resistance emergence in patients with active Mtb infection [7]. Choosing the right drugs in combination is critical to achieving the goal of rapid kill with resistance suppression. Isoniazid is antagonistic with PZA and perhaps rifampin in the standard regimen in a murine evaluation [8]. Our laboratory has demonstrated in the Hollow Fiber Infection Model (HFIM) that moxifloxacin and rifampin are antagonistic for bacterial cell kill but do provide good suppression of amplification of resistant subpopulations; the antagonism has been validated in the murine aerosol challenge model [9,10].

We need to develop a methodology for rationally identifying optimal combinations for clinical trial. Our HFIM has evaluated a large number of anti-TB agents, both alone and in combination [11–16] with the results correlating with both murine data as well as clinical data.

In this evaluation we examined linezolid and rifampin, alone and in combination against Log-phase *M. tuberculosis*. Rifampin was chosen because it is one of our best agents against both Log-phase organisms as well as organisms in Non-Replicative Persister phase [9]. Linezolid has shown promising activity as a single agent in patients with XDR TB [17].

Greco and colleagues developed the Universal Response Surface Approach (URSA) in the oncology realm [18] as a mathematically rigorous approach to determining the interaction of drugs (synergy, additivity, antagonism). We have extended this approach by also considering *a priori* drug-resistant subpopulations.

Because the approach is fully parametric, the results can be submitted for Monte Carlo simulation. In so doing, we can identify drug doses that will 1) obtain maximal bacterial cell kill and 2) suppress resistant subpopulation amplification for both drugs and do so for a population of simulated patients. This will provide a rational way forward to choose optimal combinations that will lead to shortened therapy durations.

## Results

### MIC determination and mutation frequency

The H37Rv strain used for these experiments had an MIC to linezolid of 1.0 mg/L and 0.25 mg/L to rifampin. The mutational frequency to resistance for linezolid was $-6.93\pm0.44$ $\mathrm{Log_{10}}$ (CFU) at 2 mg/L (2xMIC); for rifampin, it was $-5.77\pm0.48$ $\mathrm{Log_{10}}$(CFU) at the critical concentration of 1 mg/L.

### HFIM evaluation of linezolid and rifampin alone and in combination

Non-protein-bound drug exposures (Area Under the concentration-time Curve–AUC) of rifampin consistent with doses of 200, 600 and 900 mg daily and of linezolid at exposures of 150, 300 and 600 mg daily were examined. These agents were also examined in combination in all possible two-drug regimens (9 regimens). A no-treatment-control was also included. The single agent regimens (including control) total colony counts are displayed in Figure 1 Panel A. No single agent regimen produced any substantial change in total colony counts over the 28 days of observation. In addition, samples were also quantitatively cultured on plates infused with twice the MIC of linezolid (2×1 mg/L) or with the rifampin critical concentration of 1 mg/L (4×MIC). All single agent regimens allowed emergence of resistance (Figure 1, Panel C, D). Resistant isolates were recovered after 7–10 days.

Combination therapy regimens effect on the total Mtb population is shown in Figure 1, Panel B. Surprisingly, most combination regimens also allowed resistance emergence (Figure 1, Panels E, F). These regimens, did, however result in a multi-Log decline in total bacterial population in some instances. Only regimens with 600 mg or 900 mg of rifampin daily in combination

with 600 mg daily of linezolid had no organisms recoverable on resistance plates by experiment end.

## Mathematical population model for all regimens

In this model, we examined the concentration-time curves of each agent either alone or in combination. These concentration-time profiles were analyzed by the first two differential equations (see Methods for a full model description). The third differential equation described the impact of drug exposure on the total bacterial population, which included the population fully susceptible to both agents, the subpopulation resistant to rifampin, but sensitive to linezolid and the subpopulation resistant to linezolid, but susceptible to rifampin. The fourth and fifth differential equations described the impact of combination therapy on subpopulations resistant to drug 1/sensitive to drug 2 and resistant to drug 2/sensitive to drug 1. No organisms resistant to both drugs were recovered at baseline.

The fit of the model to the data was acceptable, as seen below:

1) Observed-Predicted Regression for All Linezolid Concentrations
   $\mathbf{Observed = 0.993x\, Pr\, edicted + 0.004; r^2 = 0.983; p < 0.001}$

2) Observed-Predicted Regression for All Rifampin Concentration
   $\mathbf{Oberved = 1.000x\, Pr\, edicted - 0.0014; r^2 = 0.997; p \ll 0.001}$

3) Observed-Predicted Regression for All Total Colony Counts
   $\mathbf{Observed = 0.978x\, Pr\, edicted + 0.071; r^2 = 0.908; p < 0.001}$

4) Observed-Predicted Regression for All Colony Counts (Linezolid-Resistant)
   $\mathbf{Observed = 0.926x Predicted + 0.182; r^2 = 0.978; p < 0.001}$

5) Observed-Predicted Regression for All Colony Counts (Rifampin-Resistant)
   $\mathbf{Observed = 0.954x\, Pr\, edicted - 0.078; r^2 = 0.870; p \ll 0.001}$

These regressions represent the observed-predicted plots using the Bayesian-posterior estimates. The median parameter vector was employed to obtain the Bayesian estimates for each system output. The point estimates of all the mean and median parameter values and standard deviations are displayed in Table 1.

The value of the interaction parameter "$\alpha$" for each of the populations determines the drug interaction (synergy, additivity, antagonism) for the combination regimens. The value of these parameters and attendant 95% confidence interval is displayed in Table 2.

As can be seen, all $\alpha$ values are negative. However, for each, the 95% confidence interval overlaps zero, meaning the combination tends toward antagonism (the negative $\alpha$-value), but is not significant and would be accorded a definition of additivity.

Of equal or greater importance, we can obtain Bayesian estimates of the interaction parameters for each of the 9 combination therapy regimens. These values of $\alpha$ are displayed by regimen in Figure 2 panels A–C. It is apparent by inspection that some values of $\alpha$ are positive (tending to synergy), but that these positive values are distributed in different parts of the space for each population/subpopulation, meaning that identifying a regimen optimal for each of these populations/subpopulations is not straightforward.

## Monte Carlo simulation

The greatest decrement of total bacterial population while maintaining suppression of amplification of resistant subpopulations is only attained by combination regimens of linezolid 600 mg daily in combination with either 600 or 900 mg of rifampin daily (Figure 1). The exposure targets for these simulated regimens are

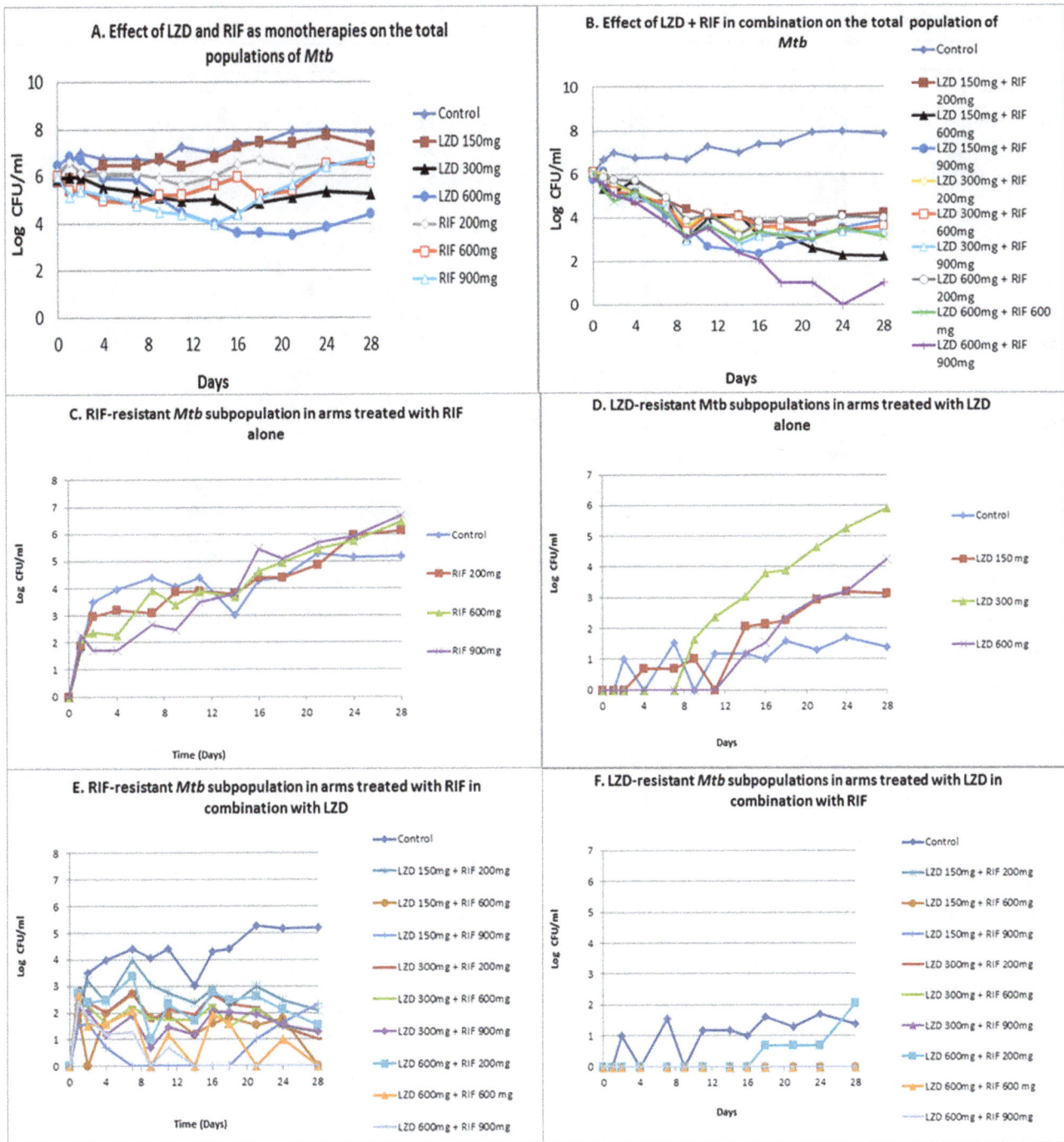

Figure 1. Effect of Linezolid (LZD) or Rifampin (RIF) alone and in combination on the total colony counts of *Mycobacterium tuberculosis* (Mtb) (Panels A and B) and on the less susceptible subpopulations (Panels C–F) as determined in a Hollow Fiber Infection Model.

AUC/MIC ratios of 98.9 of linezolid plus 84.6 of rifampin for the first regimen and 98.9 of linezolid and 123.2 for rifampin for the second regimen.

We generated a 1000-subject Monte Carlo simulation for Area Under the concentration-time Curve (AUC) for the combination of 600 mg/600 mg of linezolid/rifampin. We employed previous determinations of rifampin and linezolid penetration into the Epithelial Lining Fluid (ELF) [19–21]. The values employed were for total ELF values, as we are unaware of any information regarding free fraction in ELF. The percent penetration (AUC$_{ELF}$/AUC$_{Plasma}$ Ratio) was employed to calculate the distributions of AUC$_{ELF}$ for linezolid. To obtain this distribution, we were kindly provided with the data from the publication of McGee et al [22]. The subset of the patients (infected with *M. tuberculosis*) who received linezolid 600 mg daily were subjected to population pharmacokinetic modeling with NPAG. The first distribution calculated was for 1,000 simulated patients for AUC$_{Plasma}$. This distribution was then multiplied by percent

**Table 1.** Parameter Values From a Combination Chemotherapy Mathematical Model.

| Parameter | Units | Mean | Median | S.D. |
|---|---|---|---|---|
| $V_1$ | L | 83.5 | 81.9 | 22.4 |
| $CL_1$ | L/h | 6.20 | 6.19 | 0.748 |
| $V_2$ | L | 139 | 141 | 10.9 |
| $CL_2$ | L/h | 30.8 | 31.5 | 1.77 |
| POPMAX | CFU/ml | $7.85 \times 10^9$ | $7.24 \times 10^8$ | $1.75 \times 10^{10}$ |
| $K_{gs}$ | $h^{-1}$ | 0.100 | 0.107 | 0.0464 |
| $K_{ks}$ | $h^{-1}$ | 0.235 | 0.170 | 0.130 |
| $E_{501s}$ | mg/L | 0.527 | 0.358 | 0.389 |
| $E_{502s}$ | mg/L | 2.72 | 2.33 | 2.38 |
| $\alpha_s$ | ----- | −0.954 | −0.232 | 4.73 |
| $K_{gr1}$ | $h^{-1}$ | 0.0232 | 0.0198 | 0.0116 |
| $K_{kr1}$ | $h^{-1}$ | 0.274 | 0.318 | 0.113 |
| $E_{50\_1r1}$ | mg/L | 13.5 | 13.8 | 2.49 |
| $\alpha_{r1}$ | ----- | −4.55 | −6.11 | 3.39 |
| $K_{gr2}$ | $h^{-1}$ | 0.127 | 0.133 | 0.0757 |
| $K_{kr2}$ | $h^{-1}$ | 0.251 | 0.190 | 0.112 |
| $E_{50\_2r2}$ | mg/L | 5.92 | 6.01 | 0.829 |
| $\alpha_{r2}$ | ----- | −0.431 | −0.950 | 2.48 |
| $H_{1s}$ | ----- | 4.60 | 4.64 | 1.85 |
| $H_{2s}$ | ----- | 2.26 | 2.35 | 1.07 |
| $H_{1r1}$ | ----- | 18.4 | 20.3 | 6.73 |
| $H_{2r2}$ | ----- | 15.3 | 15.8 | 3.23 |
| $INIT_4$ | CFU/ml | 1.88 | 2.72 | 1.87 |
| $INIT_5$ | CFU/ml | 1.50 | 1.98 | 1.14 |

**S.D. = Standard Deviation.**

penetration into ELF. We employed the average penetration of the calculated penetration of the studies of Honeybourne et al [19] and Boselli et al [20]. For rifampin, the analysis of Goutelle et al [21] provided an explicit parameter vector that allowed direct calculation of the $AUC_{ELF}$ for a 600 mg dose.

We then determined the frequency with which these regimens would achieve the AUC/MIC targets for linezolid/rifampin of 98.9/123.2 as measured in the HFIM. To ultimately obtain an expectation for target attainment we employed the MIC distribution for linezolid from the paper of Ahmed et al [23] and for rifampin from the paper of van Klingeren et al [24]. For a regimen of linezolid 600 mg plus rifampin 600 mg, the exposure which suppressed resistance amplification, but which did not achieve the maximal cell kill the AUC/MIC was attained (expectation over the MIC distribution) 96% of the time for

linezolid and 60% of the time for rifampin. Assuming orthogonality of probabilities, both exposures would be attained 57.6% of the time.

For the linezolid 600 mg daily plus rifampin 900 mg daily regimen, we employed the data from a pharmacokinetic evaluation of higher rifampin doses in TB-infected patients by Boeree et al [25]. The abstract did not provide measures of variability, but did provide point estimates of the mean AUC for doses of 10, 20, 25 and 30 mg/kg per day, as determined on day 7 of dosing. We used the ratio of AUC's of 10 mg/kg/day to 20, 25 and 30 mg/kg/day, which were 4.28, 5.11 and 7.20, respectively. These increases in $AUC_{Plasma}$ were employed as multipliers for the $AUC_{ELF}$ as determined above from the data of Goutelle et al [21].

For the 20 mg/kg/day dose, the rifampin expected target attainment was 88.0% and the combined regimen expected target

**Table 2.** Interaction parameters ($\alpha$) for fully susceptible (S), resistant to linezolid (L), and resistant to rifampin (R) organism populations and 95% confidence intervals.

| | $\alpha$ Susceptible | $\alpha$ L-resistant | $\alpha$ R-resistant |
|---|---|---|---|
| Mean | −0.709 | −4.347 | −0.436 |
| Median | −0.232 | −5.725 | −0.917 |
| 95% CI | −8.701–7.295 | −11.309–2.615 | −4.85–4.422 |

**A.**

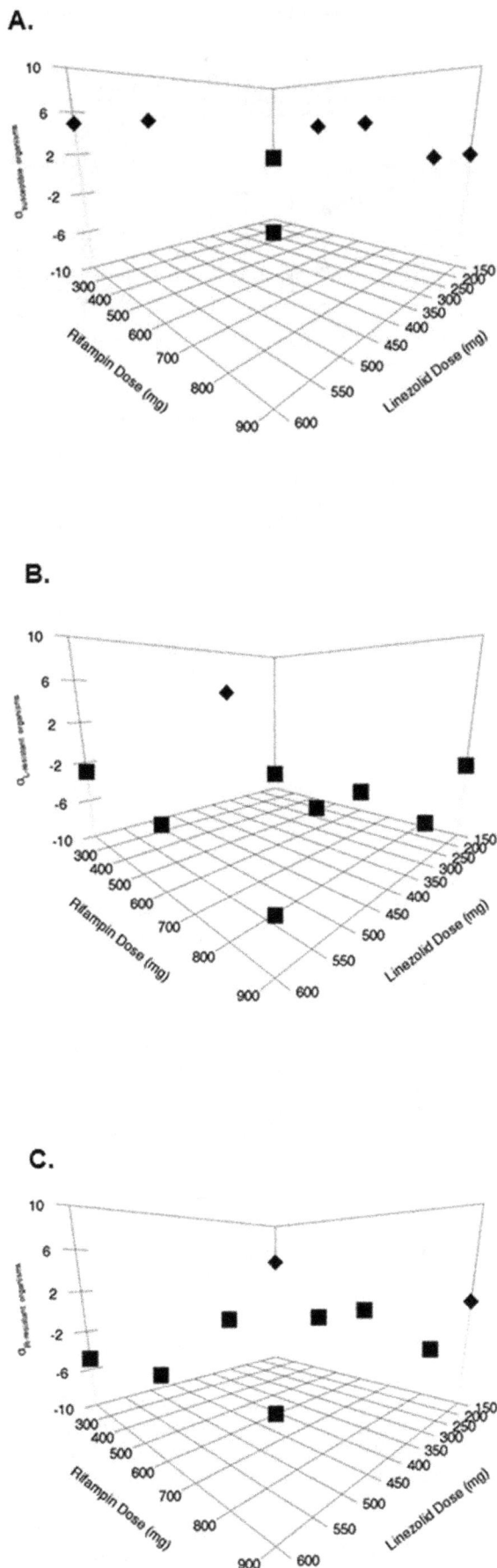

**Figure 2. Plots of the α-values (an index of drug interaction for effect) for different combination regimens of linezolid plus rifampin for A. Fully-Susceptible Organisms; B. Linezolid-Resistant Organisms; C. Rifampin-Resistant Organisms.** Diamonds indicate positive α-values; Squares indicates negative α-values.

attainment was 84.5%. For the 25 mg/kg/day dose, these values were 91.4% for rifampin and 87.7% for the combination. For the 30 mg/kg/day rifampin dose, these results were 96.9% for rifampin and 93.0% for the combination.

We also wished to show the utility of the fully parametric modeling approach and performed a 1,000 subject simulation from the full model. In Figure 3, we show the median ± standard deviation colony counts from the simulation for a regimen of linezolid 600 mg daily plus rifampin 600 mg daily. The regimen impact upon the total bacterial population, as well as the subpopulations fully susceptible to both drugs and those resistant to either linezolid or rifampin are shown. With time, all standard deviations show an increase, because any fixed-dose regimen will generate a broad range of exposures for each drug and, consequently, for both drugs in the combination. Some will be large exposures and suppress resistance, while others will be in the range optimal to amplify resistant subpopulations for one or the other drug or both.

In the total population, the regimen produces a decline just below 2 $Log_{10}(CFU/ml)$, which then regrows slightly because of resistant subpopulation amplification. Both resistant populations decline (at the median), but amplify back up with time (minimum counts for linezolid and rifampin of 0.892 and 1.585 $Log_{10}(CFU/ml)$, with hour 648 counts of 1.321 and 1.650 $Log_{10}(CFU/ml)$, respectively.

Examination of the impact of the combination chemotherapy on the fully susceptible population is most important (Figure 3B). Here, we see first order decline. By the end of the experiment slightly greater than 50% of simulated subjects had extinguished this population. Given the responses of the resistant subpopulations, we are, in essence, trading fully susceptible organisms for their resistant subpopulations which some sub-optimal exposures are amplifying.

Among the 1000 iterates, 40/1000 (4.0%) had total population eradication by day 27 (Hour 648), while 316/1000 and 318/1000 had eradication of linezolid-resistant or rifampin-resistant populations, respectively.

**B.**

## Discussion

Currently, no rational way of identifying optimal combinations of agents is available. In this work we have set forth a mathematical model to allow evaluation of combination regimens both for cell kill and suppression of resistance. Because the model is fully parametric, Monte Carlo simulation can be performed to inform us about the behavior of the regimen for a population of patients. This allows explicit translation of the mathematical results to the clinic, demonstrating the impact of true between-patient variability in pharmacokinetics of both agents on the ability of the regimen to kill organisms and suppress emergence of resistance.

There are two major issues with regard to shortening therapy duration. The first is to identify a regimen that will kill organisms at as high a rate as possible. Such a regimen will then have the shortest time to an extinction event. It is also important that a regimen be robust for resistance suppression. Having multiple agents does not guarantee resistance suppression. Examination of

**C.**

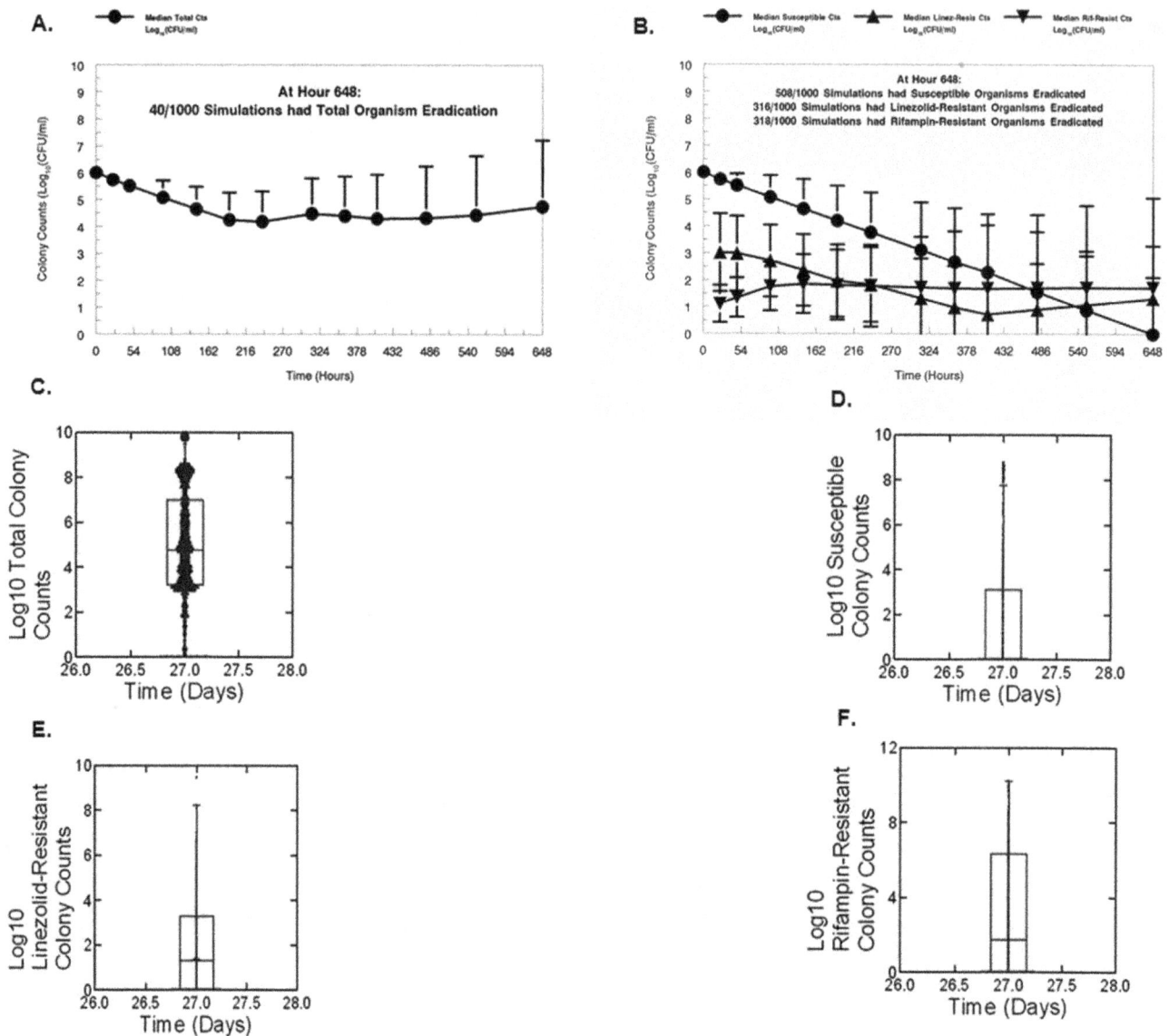

**Figure 3. System simulation (1,000 iterate Monte Carlo simulation) for total colony counts (A), susceptible counts and subpopulations less-susceptible to the study drugs (LZD and RIF) from the Bayesian posterior parameter vectors (B).** In Panels A and B, the median values and the standard deviations are displayed. In Panels C–F, the box and whisker plots (median-line; 25th and 75th percentiles at the bottom and top of the box; 95th percentile is displayed at the top of the figure) show the distribution of colony counts for the total population (Panel C), the susceptible population (Panel D) and the less-susceptible populations for LZD (Panel E) and RIF (Panel F) simulated at the last day of the experiment.

Figure 1 shows that several combination regimens demonstrated excellent early rates of kill only to have resistance emergence ultimately occur. In order to reach the goal of shortening regimen duration, both aims need to be attained.

In this set of studies, we used our hollow fiber infection model to examine the impact of rifampin and linezolid, alone and in combination against Log-phase Mtb. For the single agent evaluations, there were exposure-responses demonstrated early on. However, in all single agent evaluations, this early exposure-response was lost due to the amplification of a less-susceptible population of organisms (Figure 1, Panels C, D).

There were nine combination therapy regimens (all possible combinations of three exposures for each agent). Surprisingly, only two of these combination regimens provided optimal resistance

suppression. Only one fulfilled the task of reaching a very low total bacterial burden in addition to suppressing resistance.

Linezolid and rifampin interact in an additive way with a non-significant tendency to antagonism for kill of the WT population. The "α" value for interaction for the WT population was 4.935 for the 600 mg/600 mg regimen and was −0.265 for the 600 mg/ 900 mg regimen. For the resistant subpopulations, all "α" values were substantially more negative and ranged from −2.45 to − 6.245. As can be seen in Figure 1, a resistant subpopulation amplified for linezolid in only 1 of 9 combination regimens (linezolid 600 mg daily/rifampin 200 mg daily). The 600 mg linezolid dose provides substantial selective pressure and the rifampin dose of 200 mg daily is not high on the exposure-response curve, allowing linezolid resistant isolates to amplify. The "α" value of −2.995 tends to antagonism for the linezolid-resistant isolates, providing another reason for the amplification of a linezolid-resistant population. Even though the rifampin dose was low at 200 mg daily, it produced sufficient selective pressure to allow resistant subpopulation amplification for this agent; the "α" value for the regimen for rifampin-resistant isolates was negative at −4.85.

We employed Monte Carlo simulation for the regimen of 600 mg daily of linezolid plus 600 mg daily of rifampin. We undertook two different approaches. In the first, we simply took the optimal cell kill and resistance suppression exposures and calculated how often a regimen of linezolid/rifampin of 600 mg/ 600 mg of the combination achieved those exposures. The results were clear cut. The optimal exposures for both were only achieved circa 58% of the time. Higher rifampin doses (20–30 mg/kg/day [25] increased the target attainment to 84–93%). Peloquin had first suggested earlier [26] that we were not administering optimal exposures to rifampin and these data are concordant with that suggestion.

We also employed the full mathematical model to perform a 1,000 subject simulation to calculate the total population burden, the fully susceptible population, as well as the burden of linezolid- and rifampin-resistant organisms over time. We again chose the 600 mg/600 mg (both daily) regimen for this evaluation. The results are displayed in Figure 3. The median ± SD of the different populations is displayed in Panels A and B. The first important issue is that when a specific drug regimen is administered to a population of patients, the results will vary significantly because of inter-patient variability in the handling of both agents in the combination. Figure 3A shows the range of impact of a 600 mg linezolid plus 600 mg of rifampin regimen administered daily on the total bacterial population.

Panel B displays delineation of the disparate effects on the different subpopulations. The combination regimen of 600 mg/ 600 mg of linezolid/rifampin drives first order decline in the fully-susceptible subpopulation. By experiment end, over 50% of simulated subjects have eradicated this subpopulation. For those with lower exposures of one drug, the other or both, there is some amplification of subpopulations resistant to linezolid or rifampin. In the last portion of the experiment, we are, for many simulated subjects, simply trading off fully susceptible organisms for resistant isolates.

Figure 3, panels C–F show the range of the impact on the total, fully susceptible and drug-resistant populations at experiment end. An eradication event (all populations) was achieved in 40/1000 iterates (4%). It should be noted that this outcome assumes the MIC is that of the isolate studied in these experiments. Resistant subpopulations were eradicated in slightly greater than 30% of instances for each drug in the combination.

The analysis demonstrates that additive combinations have an easier time having a major impact on the fully susceptible population relative to the resistant subpopulations. This is because the second drug is required to be high on the exposure-response curve in order to be able to suppress or kill the bacterial population less-susceptible to the other agent. The other factor to have an impact is the size of the change in MIC between the susceptible and resistant organisms. In this combination, rifampin has a major change in MIC (>32-fold increase). This means that the second drug (linezolid) is, in essence, acting alone on these organisms and suboptimal exposures straightforwardly lead to amplification of the population.

This may be modified if the two agents are highly synergistic instead of additive or antagonistic. Nonetheless, if we cannot find a synergistic pair, it becomes important to recognize that after a time the first combination regimen will have produced its maximal effect. It may then be wise to switch to a completely new regimen to help achieve an eradication event in a very high proportion of patients. The fully susceptible population will be eradicated in many subjects and much of the remaining organism burden will be resistant to one drug or another. A new regimen taking over at approximately one month will solve this problem if the new agents are independent of the resistance mechanisms affecting the first pair. In addition, because many patients will have a reduced bacterial burden because of the initial regimen, the probability of resistant subpopulation amplification will be reduced for the follow-on regimen.

It is important to emphasize that these findings are for Log-phase organisms. It is felt that there are other metabolic states of Mtb, such as slower growing organisms in acid environments as well as non-replicative persister phenotype organisms. Organisms also persist intracellularly. These other populations make the problem more complex. Nonetheless, as we learn more about the impact of combination therapy on these separate populations over time, the necessity to switch regimens during therapy becomes more important if we are to achieve the goal of markedly reducing the duration of therapy, while suppressing resistance.

We must emphasize that in order to kill optimally and suppress resistance amplification, it is not sufficient just to have a combination regimen. Preferably, the regimen should be synergistic or at least additive in all instances. Further, the doses chosen for each drug in the combination should be sufficient to suppress the amplification of the pre-existent, less-susceptible populations for each drug. The intensity of exposure that is optimal for each drug will be a function of the size of the change in MIC value between the wild-type isolate and the resistant mutant. As an example here, the MIC-value change for rifampin is so large that rifampin-resistant clones are being suppressed only by the second drug (linezolid in this instance).

It is critical to properly use the new drugs that are entering our therapeutic armamentarium. We have the opportunity to choose wisely so that we can achieve the dual goal of rapid bacterial kill and resistance amplification suppression. The mathematical model set forth here along with the Hollow Fiber Infection Model allows rational choice of combination regimens. Monte Carlo simulation allows between-patient variability in drug exposures to be accounted for and identify the rates of attainment of target exposures which will achieve the stated goals. Wise choices will prolong the therapeutic utility of new agents as well as allowing the greatest probability of identifying a regimen that will allow a shorter therapeutic duration.

## Materials and Methods

### Bacterium

*Mycobacterium tuberculosis* (*Mtb*) strain H37Rv was used. Stocks of the bacterium were stored at −80°C. For each experiment, an aliquot of the bacterial stock was inoculated into filter-capped T-flasks containing 7H9 Middlebrook broth that was supplemented with 0.05% Tween 80 and 10% oleic acid, albumen, dextrose and catalase (OADC). The culture was incubated at 37°C, 5% $CO_2$ on a rocker platform for 4 to 5 days to achieve log phase growth.

Log-phase bacteria: Log phase growth bacteria were generated as described above. The bacteria were washed with fresh Middlebrook broth and were then transferred to pre-warmed 7H9 broth supplemented with 10% ADC (ADC-broth). The bacteria were adjusted to the desired concentration with pre-warmed ADC-broth and were inoculated into the hollow fiber cartridges. Log phase growth was maintained by continuously replacing the medium within the hollow fiber systems with fresh ADC-broth. Quantitative cultures of the starting inocula were conducted to confirm that the desired bacterial concentrations were placed into the hollow fiber systems. By serial dilution plating, quantitative estimations of the control bacterial cultures were conducted to confirm that bacteria were in log-phase throughout the course of the experiment.

## Drugs

Pharmaceutical grade linezolid was purchased as a solution for injection from CuraScript (St. Mary, FL). Rifampin powder was purchased from Sigma-Aldrich (St. Louis, MO). The drugs were stored according to the manufacturers' instructions.

Rifampin powder was dissolved in DMSO and then added to medium to the desired concentration. The working solutions of rifampin were stored at $-80°C$. Aliquots of the working solutions were thawed on the day of use and were used immediately. Linezolid solution for injection was dissolved with sterile water to the desired concentrations. The ADC-broth used in all arms of the hollow fiber experiments was supplemented with DMSO (final concentration: 0.3% DMSO). The growth of the *Mtb* in log phase was not affected by concentrations of DMSO as high as 1% (data not shown).

## Agar susceptibility testing

Susceptibility studies for linezolid and rifampin were conducted with log phase growth *Mtb* using the agar proportional method described by the CLSI (Susceptibility testing for Mycobacteria, Nocardiae, and Other Aerobic Actinomycetes; Approved Standard, Document A24-A, Wayne, PA) and the absolute serial dilution method on 7H10 agar +10% OADC and 0.3% DMSO. The MICs were read after 4 weeks of incubation at 37°C, 5% $CO_2$. For the agar proportional method, the lowest concentration of a drug that provided a 99% reduction in the bacterial density relative to the no-drug control was read as the MIC. For the absolute serial dilution method, the MIC was read as the lowest concentration of drug for which there was no growth on the agar plate.

## Mutation frequency studies

Mutation frequencies were determined for 2.5x the MIC of linezolid and for the critical concentration of 1 µg/mL of rifampin. MICs to the test drug were determined for a subset of the mutants that were derived from the mutation frequency studies to define the change in MIC values in the drugs between the parent and mutant strains.

## Overview of the *In vitro* hollow fiber system

The methods for the HFIM for *Mycobacterium tuberculosis* study have been described elsewhere [9]. An *in vitro* hollow fiber system allows the investigator to expose a microbe to any concentration-time profile of antibiotics and can simulate the pharmacokinetic profile for any drug and any half-life within the system.

Syringe pumps infuse the drug(s) into the hollow fiber system at a rate to simulate an intravenous or oral route of administration of the compound(s) and the drug-containing medium is replaced with drug-free medium to simulate the desired half-life of the drug(s). Medium samples are taken from the central compartment for measurement of drug content by liquid chromatography dual mass spectrometry (LC/MS/MS) to confirm achievement of the targeted PK profile. The peripheral compartment is sampled for quantitative culture of the bacterium over the course of an experiment. Bacterial samples are plated on drug-free agar and

agar supplemented with the antibiotic(s) infused into that hollow fiber system to characterize the effect of the treatment regimen on the total and less-susceptible bacterial populations.

Dose-range combination study for bolus dosed linezolid and rifampin against log phase growth *Mtb*. Different half-lives were developed in the system simultaneously employing the approach of Blaser [27]. Three dosages of linezolid and rifampin were administered alone and together as 2 h infusions on a once-daily schedule of administration. The simulated half-life for linezolid was 8.5 hours. The simulated half-life for rifampin was 3 hours.

## Population Combination Therapy Model

Population mixture modeling was performed employing the Non-Parametric Adaptive Grid (NPAG) program of Leary et al [28] and with an approach previously published by our laboratory [29]. Monte Carlo simulation was performed with the ADAPT V package of D'Argenio et al [30] and with PMetrics [31]. This approach allows us to apply classical properties of drug interaction for effect (Synergy, Additivity, Antagonism) to multiple populations simultaneously because of the mixture model approach. The original Greco model did not allow this and ignored the possibility of a resistant subpopulation. The first two differential equations are those required to describe the concentration-time profiles for each of the drugs in the combination. This requires 4 parameters, as the drug administration pumps will be set to describe a mono-exponential decline profile. The parameters are Volume (V in Liters) for $Drug_1$ ($V_1$) and $Drug_2$ ($V_2$) and Clearance for the 2 drugs, $CL_1$ and $CL_2$. These differential equations are displayed below:

(1) $dX_1/dT = R_1 - (CL_1/V_1) \times X_1$; where $R_1$ is the piecewise input function for $Drug_1$ and $X_1$ is the $Drug_1$ amount in the central compartment.

(2) $dX_2/dT = R_2 - (CL_2/V_2) \times X_2$; where $R_2$ is the piecewise input function for $Drug_2$ and $X_2$ is the $Drug_2$ amount in the central compartment.

The next two differential equations describe the growth and death of the drug-susceptible populations for Drug1 and Drug2. Differently from previous modeling we have done, the kill function will be the equation of the Universal Response Surface Approach (URSA) of Greco. This approach has been employed by our lab in the past for cell kill analysis. It is appropriate to employ this combination approach here, as the differential equation describes the growth (front part of the equation) and kill (back part of the equation) of the susceptible population.

(3) $dN_S/dT = K_{gmax-S} \times N_S \times G - K_{kmax-S} \times M_S \times N_S$; where $N_S$ is the number of organisms susceptible to $Drug_1$ and $Drug_2$, $K_{gmax-S}$ is the maximal growth rate constant for the population sensitive to both $Drug_1$ and $Drug_2$, G is a logistic carrying function, which allows the population to achieve stationary phase, $K_{kmax-S}$ is the maximal kill rate constant for $Drug_1$ and $Drug_2$ in combination for the susceptible population and $M_S$ incorporates the URSA equation of Greco [18] for the $Drug_1$ and $Drug_2$-Susceptible population. Because the Greco equation is not in closed form, the parameters must be estimated via a bi-directional root finder. This has been implemented in the NPAG program, along with code to allow simultaneous handling of two agents by Van Guilder, Neely, Schumitzky and Jelliffe.

(4) $dN_{R1}/dT = K_{gmax-R1} \times N_{R1} \times G - K_{kmax-R1} \times M_{R1} \times N_{R1}$; where $N_{R1}$ is the number of organisms resistant to $Drug_1$ and sensitive to $Drug_2$, $K_{gmax-R1}$ is the maximal growth rate constant for the $Drug_1$-resistant organisms, G is a logistic carrying function, which allows the population to achieve stationary phase, $K_{kmax-R1}$ is the maximal kill rate constant for $Drug_1$ and $Drug_2$ in combination for the $Drug_1$-resistant population and $M_{R1}$

incorporates the URSA equation of Greco for the $Drug_1$-resistant, $Drug_2$-sensitive population.

(5)  $dNR_2/dT = K_{gmax\text{-}R2} \times NR_2 \times G - K_{kmax\text{-}R2} \times M_{R2} \times N_{R2}$; where $N_{R2}$ is the number of organisms resistant to $Drug_2$ and sensitive to $Drug_1$, $K_{gmax\text{-}R2}$ is the maximal growth rate constant for the $Drug_2$-resistant organisms, G is a logistic carrying function, which allows the population to achieve stationary phase, $K_{kmax\text{-}R2}$ is the maximal kill rate constant for $Drug_1$ and $Drug_2$ in combination for the $Drug_2$-resistant population and $M_{R2}$ incorporates the URSA equation of Greco for the $Drug_2$-resistant, $Drug_1$-sensitive population.

Normally, there would be a requirement for a sixth differential equation, describing the population resistant to both $Drug_1$ and $Drug_2$. However, we have not found such strains at baseline experimentally in our experiments.

$$G = (1 - (N_S + N_{R1} + N_{R2})/POPMAX)$$

$$M = (1 - \text{Fractional Effect})$$

as derived from Greco URSA model; in this circumstance, $E_{con}$ is set to 1.0.

For the Greco URSA model:

$$1 = \frac{drug1}{IC_{50D1} x (E/E_{con} - E)^{1/HD1}} + \frac{[drug2]}{IC_{50D2} x (E_{con} - E)^{1/HD2}}$$
$$+ \frac{\alpha x [drug1 x drug2]}{IC_{50D1} x IC_{50D2} x (E_{con} - E)^{(1/2HD1 + 1/2HD2)}}$$

where [drug 1] is the concentration of $Drug_1$; [drug 2] is the concentration of $Drug_2$; $IC_{50D1}$ is the concentration for which the effect is half maximal for Drug 1; $IC_{50D2}$ is the concentration for which the effect is half maximal for $Drug_2$; $HD_1$ and $HD_2$ are Hill's constants for $Drug_1$ and $Drug_2$, respectively; $E_{con}$ is the effect for the control; $\alpha$ is the interaction parameter; and $E$ is the fractional effect.

If $\alpha$ and its attendant 95% confidence bound cross zero, the effect is additive. If $\alpha$ and its attendant 95% confidence bound do not cross zero and are positive, the effect is synergistic. If $\alpha$ and its attendant 95% confidence bound do not cross zero and are negative, the effect is antagonistic.

The use of a mixture model allows independent identification of interaction parameters ($\alpha_1$ through $\alpha_3$) that identify the interaction of the drugs for the fully susceptible population ($\alpha_1$), as well as subpopulations resistant to $Drug_1$ or $Drug_2$ ($\alpha_2$ and $\alpha_3$). This will allow identification of regimens optimal for overall bacterial cell kill as well as resistance suppression for both agents.

System Outputs: System outputs 1 & 2, associated with differential equations 1 and 2 are the measured $Drug_1$ and $Drug_2$ concentrations in the central compartment

$Output_1 = X_1/V_1$; $Output_2 = X_2/V_2$.

System Output 3 is the Total Organism Number which is the Population sensitive to $Drug_1$ and $Drug_2$ plus population resistant to $Drug_1$, sensitive to $Drug_2$ plus population resistant to $Drug_2$ and sensitive to $Drug_1$ (as above, a population resistant to both $Drug_1$ and $Drug_2$ has not yet been observed). This output is measured by plating on antibiotic-free plates.

System Output 4 is the Population resistant to $Drug_1$ and sensitive to $Drug_2$. This output is measured by plating on agar into which $Drug_1$ has been incorporated. The actual concentration employed will differ, depending upon the step size of the resistance mechanism that we are attempting to capture in any experiment with different drugs.

System Output 5 is the Population resistant to $Drug_2$ and sensitive to $Drug_1$. This output is measured by plating on agar into which $Drug_2$ has been incorporated. The actual concentration employed will differ, depending upon the step size of the resistance mechanism that we are attempting to capture in any experiment with different drugs.

System Output 6 is the Population resistant to $Drug_1$ and to $Drug_2$. This output is measured by plating on agar into which $Drug_1$ and $Drug_2$ have been incorporated. The actual concentrations employed will differ, depending upon the step size of the resistance mechanism that we are attempting to capture. As above, we have not yet observed the need for this system output.

This approach to modeling combination chemotherapy with a mixture model and the URSA equation will allow the "inverted U" mountain type of response to be modeled as was demonstrated in our previous publication [32]. Because of the fully parametric nature of this approach, it allows Monte Carlo simulation to be conducted and allows powerful bridging to man. This approach allows us to explore combination chemotherapy for cell kill as well as resistance suppression for *Mycobacterium tuberculosis*, and also for any other circumstance requiring combination chemotherapy.

## Acknowledgments

We thank K Fennelly, M Lauzardo, N Jumbe, R Hafner, S Schmidt for critical discussions and reading of the manuscript.

## Author Contributions

Conceived and designed the experiments: GLD AL. Performed the experiments: DB SF AL. Analyzed the data: MN MVG AS CP. Contributed reagents/materials/analysis tools: MN MVG AS. Wrote the paper: GLD AL.

## References

1. World Health Organization (2012) Global Tuberculosis Report. Geneva, Switzerland: WHO.

2. World Health Organization (2009) Treatment of tuberculosis guidelines. 4th edition. Geneva Switzerland: WHO.

3. FDA Package insert for bedaquiline. Available: http://www.accessdata.fda.gov/Scripts/cder/drugsatfda/index.cfm. Accessed: 2014 Jun 17.

4. Lienhardt C, Raviglione M, Spigelman M, Hafner R, Jaramillo E, et al. (2012) New Drugs for the treatment of tuberculosis: needs, challenges, promise, and prospects for the future. J. Infect. Dis. 205: S241–S249.

5. Grosset J, Tyagi S, Almeida DV, Converse PJ, Li SY, et al. (2013) Assessment of clofazimine activity in a second-line regimen for tuberculosis in mice. Am J Respir Crit Care Med. 188:608–612.

6. Zhang M, Sala C, Hartkoorn RC, Dhar N, Mendoza-Losana A, et al. (2012) Streptomycin-starved *Mycobacterium tuberculosis* 18b, a drug discovery tool for latent tuberculosis. Antimicrob. Agents Chemother. 56: 5782–5789.

7. Selkon JB, Devadatta S, Kullarna KG, Mitchison DA, Narayana AS, et al. (1964) The emergence of isoniazid-resistant cultures in patients with pulmonary tuberculosis during treatment with isoniazid alone or isoniazid plus PAS. Bull World Health Organ. 31:273–94.

8. Almeida D, Nuermberger E, Tasneen R, Rosenthal I, Tyagi S, et al. (2009) Paradoxical effect of isoniazid on the activity of rifampin-pyrazinamide combination in a mouse model of tuberculosis. Antimicrob Agents Chemother. . 53:4178–4184.

9. Drusano GL, Sgambati N, Eichas A, Brown DL, Kulawy R, et al. (2010) The Combination of Rifampin plus Moxifloxacin is Synergistic for Resistance Suppression, but is Antagonistic for Cell Kill for *Mycobacterium tuberculosis* as Determined in a Hollow Fiber Infection Model. mBio 1:3 e00139–10.

10. Balasubramanian V, Solapure S, Gaonkar S, Mahesh Kumar KN, Shandil RK, et al. (2012) Effect of Co-administration of Moxifloxacin and Rifampin on

*Mycobacterium tuberculosis* in a Murine Aerosol Infection Model. Antimicrob Agents Chemother 56:3054–3057.

11. Gumbo T, Louie A, Deziel MR, Parsons LM, Salfinger M, et al. (2004) Selection of a Moxifloxacin Dose that Suppresses *Mycobacterium tuberculosis* Resistance Using an In Vitro Pharmacodynamic Infection Model and Mathematical Modeling. J Infect Dis 190:1642–1651.

12. Gumbo T, Louie A, Deziel MR, Drusano GL (2005) Pharmacodynamic evidence that ciprofloxacin failure against tuberculosis is not due to poor microbial kill, but to rapid emergence of resistance. Antimicrob Agents Chemother 49:3178–3181.

13. Gumbo T, Louie A, Liu W, Ambrose PG, Bhavnani SM, et al. (2007) Isoniazid's bactericidal activity ceases because of the emergence of resistance, not depletion of Mycobacterium tuberculosis in the log phase of growth. J Infect Dis 195:194–201.

14. Gumbo T, Louie A, Brown D, Ambrose PG, Bhavnani SM, et al. (2007) Isoniazid bactericidal activity and resistance emergence: integrating pharmacodynamics and pharmacogenomics to predict efficacy in different ethnic populations. Antimicrob Agents Chemother. 51: 2329–2336.

15. Gumbo T, Louie A, Deziel MR, Liu W, Parsons LM, et al. (2007) Concentration-dependent *Mycobacterium tuberculosis* killing and prevention of resistance by rifampin. Antimicrob Agents Chemother 51:3781–3788.

16. Drusano GL, Sgambati N, Eichas A, Brown DL, Kulawy R, et al. (2011) Effect of administering moxifloxacin plus rifampin against *Mycobacterium tuberculosis* 7 of 7 Days versus 5 of 7 Days in an *in Vitro* pharmacodynamic system. mBio. 2:e00108–11.

17. Lee M, Lee J, Carroll MW, Choi H, Min S, et al. (2012) Linezolid for treatment of chronic extensively drug-resistant tuberculosis. N Engl J Med. 367:1508–1518.

18. Greco WR, Bravo G, Parsons JC (1995). The search for synergy: a critical review from a response surface perspective. Pharmacol. Rev. 47:331–385.

19. Honeybourne D, Tobin C, Jevons G, Andrews J, Wise R (2003) Intrapulmonary penetration of linezolid. J Antimicrob Chemother. 51:1431–1434.

20. Boselli E, Breilh D, Rimmelé T, Djabarouti S, Toutain J, et al. (2005) Pharmacokinetics and intrapulmonary concentrations of linezolid administered to critically ill patients with ventilator-associated pneumonia. Crit Care Med 33:1529–1533.

21. Goutelle S, Bourguignon L, Maire PH, Van Guilder M, Conte JE Jr, et al. (2009) Population modeling and Monte Carlo simulation study of the pharmacokinetics and antituberculosis pharmacodynamics of rifampin in lungs. Antimicrob Agents Chemother. 53;2974–2981.

22. McGee B, Dietze R, Hadad DJ, Molino LP, Maciel EL, et al. (2009) Population pharmacokinetics of linezolid in adults with pulmonary tuberculosis. Antimicrob Agents Chemother. 53:3981–3984.

23. Ahmed I, Jabeen K, Inayat R, Hasan R. (2013) Susceptibility testing of extensively drug-resistant and pre-extensively drug-resistant Mycobacterium tuberculosis against levofloxacin, linezolid and amoxicillin-clavulanate. Antimicrob Agents Chemother. 57:2511–2525.

24. Van Klingern B, Dessens-Kroon M, van der Laan T, Kremer K, van Soolingen D. (2007) Drug susceptibility testing of *Mycobacterium tuberculosis* complex by use of a high-throughput, reproducible, absolute concentration method. J Clin Microbiol. 45: 2662–2668.

25. Boeree M, Diacon A, Dawson R. et al. (2013) What is the "right" dose of rifampin? Paper #148LB. 20th Conference on Retroviruses and Opportunistic Infections. March 3–6. Atlanta, GA.

26. Peloquin C (2003) What is the "right" dose of rifampin? Int J Tuberc Lung Dis. 7:3–5.

27. Blaser J (1985) In-vitro model for simultaneous simulation of the serum kinetics of two drugs with different half-lives. J Antimicrob Chemother. 15 Suppl A:125–130.

28. Leary RH, Jelliffe R, Schumitzky A, Van Guilder M (2001) An adaptive grid non-parametric approach to population pharmacokinetic/dynamic (PK/PD) population models. Proceedings, 14th IEEE symposium on Computer Based Medical Systems 1:389–394.

29. Jumbe N, Louie A, Leary R, Liu W, Deziel MR, et al. (2003) Application of a mathematical model to prevent *in-vivo* amplification of antibiotic-resistant bacterial populations during therapy. J Clin Invest 112:275–285.

30. D'Argenio DZ, Schumitzky A, Wang X (2009) ADAPT 5 User's Guide: Pharmacokinetic/Pharmacodynamic Systems Analysis Software. Biomedical Simulations Resource, Los Angeles.

31. Neely MN, van Guilder MG, Yamada WM, Schumitzky A, Jelliffe RW (2012) Accurate Detection of Outliers and Subpopulations with Pmetrics, a Nonparametric and Parametric Pharmacometric Modeling and Simulation Package for R. Therapeutic Drug Monitoring. 34:467–476.

32. Drusano GL, Liu W, Fregeau C, Kulawy R, Louie A (2009) Differing effect of combination chemotherapy with meropenem and tobramycin on cell kill and suppression of resistance on wild-type Pseudomonas aeruginosa PA01 and its isogenic MexAB efflux pump over-expressed mutant. Antimicrob Agents Chemother. 53:2266–2273.

# 14

# Prognostic Significance of CD26 in Patients with Colorectal Cancer

**Colin Siu-Chi Lam**[1,3], **Alvin Ho-Kwan Cheung**[1], **Sunny Kit-Man Wong**[1,3], **Timothy Ming-Hun Wan**[1,3], **Lui Ng**[1,3], **Ariel Ka-Man Chow**[1,3], **Nathan Shiu-Man Cheng**[1,3], **Ryan Chung-Hei Pak**[1], **Hung-Sing Li**[1,3], **Johnny Hon-Wai Man**[1,3], **Thomas Chung-Cheung Yau**[2], **Oswens Siu-Hung Lo**[1], **Jensen Tung-Chung Poon**[1], **Roberta Wen-Chi Pang**[1,3]*, **Wai Lun Law**[1]

**1** Department of Surgery, Li Ka Shing Faculty of Medicine, The University of Hong Kong, Hong Kong SAR, China, **2** Department of Clinical Oncology, Li Ka Shing Faculty of Medicine, The University of Hong Kong, Hong Kong SAR, China, **3** Centre for Cancer Research, Li Ka Shing Faculty of Medicine, The University of Hong Kong, Hong Kong SAR, China

## Abstract

*Background:* CD26, dipeptidyl peptidase IV, was discovered firstly as a membrane-associated peptidase on the surface of leukocyte. We previously demonstrated that a subpopulation of CD26+ cells were associated with the development of distant metastasis, enhanced invasiveness and chemoresistance in colorectal cancer (CRC). In order to understand the clinical impact of CD26, the expression was investigated in CRC patient's specimens. This study investigated the prognostic significance of tumour CD26 expression in patients with CRC. Examination of CD26+ cells has significant clinical impact for the prediction of distant metastasis development in colorectal cancer, and could be used as a selection criterion for further therapy.

*Methods:* Tumour CD26 expression levels were studied by immunohistochemistry using Formalin-fixed paraffin embedded (FFPE) tissues in 143 patients with CRC. Tumour CD26 expression levels were correlated with clinicopathological features of the CRC patients. The prognostic significance of tumour tissue CD26 expression levels was assessed by univariate and multivariate analyses.

*Result:* CD26 expression levels in CRC patients with distant metastasis were significantly higher than those in non-metastatic. High expression levels of CD26 were significantly associated with advanced tumour staging. Patients with a high CD26 expression level had significantly worse overall survival than those with a lower level (p<0.001).

*Conclusions:* The expression of CD26 was positively associated with clinicopathological correlation such as TNM staging, degree of differentiation and development of metastasis. A high CD26 expression level is a predictor of poor outcome after resection of CRC. CD26 may be a useful prognostic marker in patients with CRC.

**Editor:** Hiromu Suzuki, Sapporo Medical University, Japan

**Funding:** The authors have no support or funding to report.

**Competing Interests:** The authors have declared that no competing interests exist.

* E-mail: robertap@hku.hk

## Introduction

Colorectal cancer (CRC) is the third most common malignancy and leading cause of cancer death in the world [1]. Approximately 50% of patients with CRC develop liver metastases, cancer patients with metastasis have higher mortality than just primary tumour alone [2,3]. Liver is the most common site of distant metastasis in CRC patients with poor prognosis. Therefore, understanding the biological mechanism of metastasis is important for prognosis of metastasis in CRC.

CD26 – also known as dipeptidyl peptidase IV, is a 110-kDa cell surface glycoprotein protein with multiple functions, and is widely expressed in most cell types including T lymphocytes, endothelial and epithelial cells. It is a type II membrane-bound protein and member of prolyl peptidase family with carboxy terminus facing extracellular space. It is also composed of a transmembrane region

and a short cytoplasmic domain. CD26 acts as other prolyl peptidase family: its carboxy terminal extracellular domain regulates the activities of a number of cytokines and chemokines through removal of the N-terminal dipeptide from polypeptides with proline or alanine in the penultimate position [4,5]. CD26 can hydrolyse amino acid on matrix metalloproteinase [6]. CD26 was demonstrated as a binding partner with fibronectin and collagen in a variety of experimental conditions [7,8,9]. CD26 interacts with type I and III collagens and fibronectin, which proteolysis the ECM and result in facilitating the tumour cells migration, invasion and metastasis [10,11,12,13]. Based on its ability to regulate biological molecules through its enzymatic activity, CD26 can act as a tumour suppressor or activator.

Our lab previously demonstrated that a subpopulation of CD26+ cells were associated with the development of distant

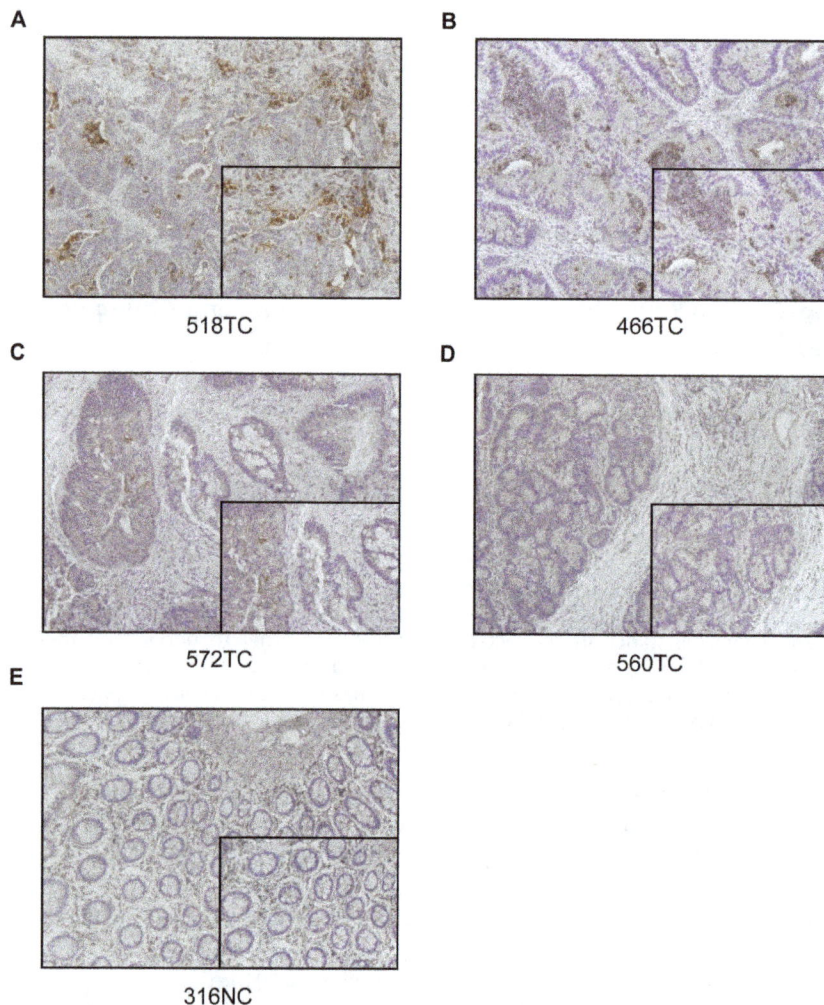

**Figure 1. Immunostaining for CD26 on normal colon and CRC patient's specimen.** (A-D) Colorectal cancer patient specimen with strong, moderate, weak and negative CD26 staining, respectively. (E) Normal colon. Magnification with 200x and 400x.

metastasis in colorectal cancer through binding to extracellular matrix components such as fibronectin and collagen, and regulating the expression of EMT markers [13]. Besides its expression on tumour cell surface, the truncated form (sCD26/DPPIV) is also present in body fluids such as serum, and its levels are correlated with tumour status and behaviour for certain cancers. Serum CD26 levels were suggested as an early diagnosis and predictive marker of colorectal cancer [14]. Higher levels of circulating CD26 have been identified in CRC patients with metastatic disease [15]. All of these studies suggested that CD26 is a potential biomarker for CRC diagnosis and prognosis. The patient's specimens are another way to be used for detecting CD26 expression level by immunohistochemistry. Therefore, the aim of the present study was to clarify the prognostic significance of CD26 expression in patients with colorectal cancer.

## Patients and Methods

One hundred and forty three patients (81 men and 62 women; median age 73, range 29–92 years) who underwent resection of CRC at Queen Mary Hospital, The University of Hong Kong, between August 2008 and November 2011 were studied. No patient had received any preoperative treatment. The specimens were fixed with formalin and embedded with paraffin wax. The

study was approved by Institutional Review Board of the University of Hong Kong/Hospital Authority Hong Kong West Cluster (HKU/HA HKW IRB), and the written informed consent was obtained from the patients for participation.

To evaluate the prognostic significance of CD26 expression in CRC patients, the association between CD26 expression and survival was studied. Five micrometres tissue sections were cut and antigen retrieval was achieved by boiling the sections in citric buffer, pH 8.0, in an oven for 10 mins. Adjacent normal colorectal tissues were used as controls, and negative controls were performed by replacing the CD26 antibody (Novus Biologicals, LLC) with phosphate buffered saline. Positive signals were evaluated by two independent assessors who were unaware of clinical outcomes, in five fields under light microscopy at a magnification of 400X. Staining intensity was scored as follows: 0-negative staining; 1-weak staining; 2-moderate staining and 3-strong staining.

All clinicopathological data and follow-up results were collected prospectively in a computerized database. Tumours were staged according to the pathological tumour node metastasis (TNM) classification. All patients were monitored every 3 months for detection of any recurrence or distant metastasis. The last patient in the cohort had been followed for 21 months.

**Table 1.** CD26 expression categorized by clinicopathological data of CRC patients.

| Variable | | No. of cases[a] | CD26 Expression[a] | | P* |
|---|---|---|---|---|---|
| | | | Low(n = 98) | High(n = 45) | |
| Age (years old): | >65 | 42 | 24 | 18 | 0.075 |
| | ≤65 | 101 | 74 | 27 | |
| Gender: | Male | 81 | 56 | 25 | 0.858 |
| | Female | 62 | 42 | 20 | |
| Tumour size (cm³): | >5 | 51 | 35 | 16 | 1.000 |
| | ≤5 | 92 | 63 | 29 | |
| Degree of Differentiation: | Well and moderate | 132 | 94 | 38 | **0.029** |
| | Poor | 7 | 2 | 5 | |
| TNM stage: | Stage I/II | 66 | 57 | 9 | **<0.001** |
| | Stage III/IV | 76 | 40 | 36 | |
| Metastasis status[b]: | No metastasis | 116 | 92 | 24 | **<0.001** |
| | Metastasis | 27 | 6 | 21 | |
| Liver Metastasis: | No | 123 | 92 | 31 | **<0.001** |
| | Yes | 20 | 6 | 14 | |

TNM, tumour node metastasis.
[a]The total number of cases may be less than 143 because of missing information.
[b]Patients with distant metastasis were classified as "Metastasis".
*$\chi^2$ test (or Fisher exact test in 2-sided)

## Statistical analysis

The $\chi^2$ test (or Fisher exact test where appropriate) was used for nominal variables. Survival rates were calculated by the Kaplan Meier method and compared between groups by the log rank test. Multivariate analysis of prognostic factors was performed by the Cox proportional hazard model. All statistical analyses were performed by SPSS 16 for Windows statistical software (SPSS, Chicago, IL). P value <0.05 was considered statistically significant.

## Results

CD26 was expressed in CRC tumour specimens with different expression levels which were classified into four groups according to their staining intensity (strong, moderate, weak and negative staining) (Fig. 1). The CD26 expression level was further classified into high (staining intensity 2, 3) and low (staining intensity 0, 1) expression. The possible association between CD26 expression level and clinicopathological data was also examined (Table 1). There was no significant relationship observed between CD26 expression level and age, gender or tumour size. However, significantly higher CD26 expression was correlated with poorly differentiated tumour, late TNM stage, and presence of metastasis (especially liver metastasis). Moreover, CD26 expression was significantly associated with TNM stage III and stage IV (Table 2).

The median follow-up duration of the 143 patients with CRC was 32 months (range 0–60). The 1-, 3- and 5-year overall survival rates were 91, 66 and 66 per cent respectively in patients with high CD26 expression, and 96, 94 and 78 per cent respectively in those with low CD26 levels (P<0.001) (Fig. 2A). The survival curve of CRC patients included in this study is plotted in Figure 2B. The median disease-free survival time was 33 months (range 0–60) and the percentages of tumour recurrence were 25.2% and 5.1% for patients with high and low CD26 expression in five years, respectively. It means that the disease-free survival of patients with

**Table 2.** CD26 expression categorized by TNM stage of CRC patients.

| Variable | No. of cases[a] | Percentage | CD26 Expression[a] | | P* |
|---|---|---|---|---|---|
| | | | Low | High | |
| TNM stage (I, II and III, n = 115): | | | | | |
| Stage I/II | 66 | 57% | 57 | 9 | 0.037 |
| Stage III | 49 | 43% | 34 | 15 | |
| TNM stage (I, II and IV, n = 93): | | | | | |
| Stage I/II | 66 | 71% | 57 | 9 | <0.001 |
| Stage IV | 27 | 29% | 6 | 21 | |

TNM, tumour node metastasis.
[a]The total number of cases may be less than 143 because of missing information.
*$\chi^2$ test (or Fisher exact test in 2-sided)

**A**

**B**

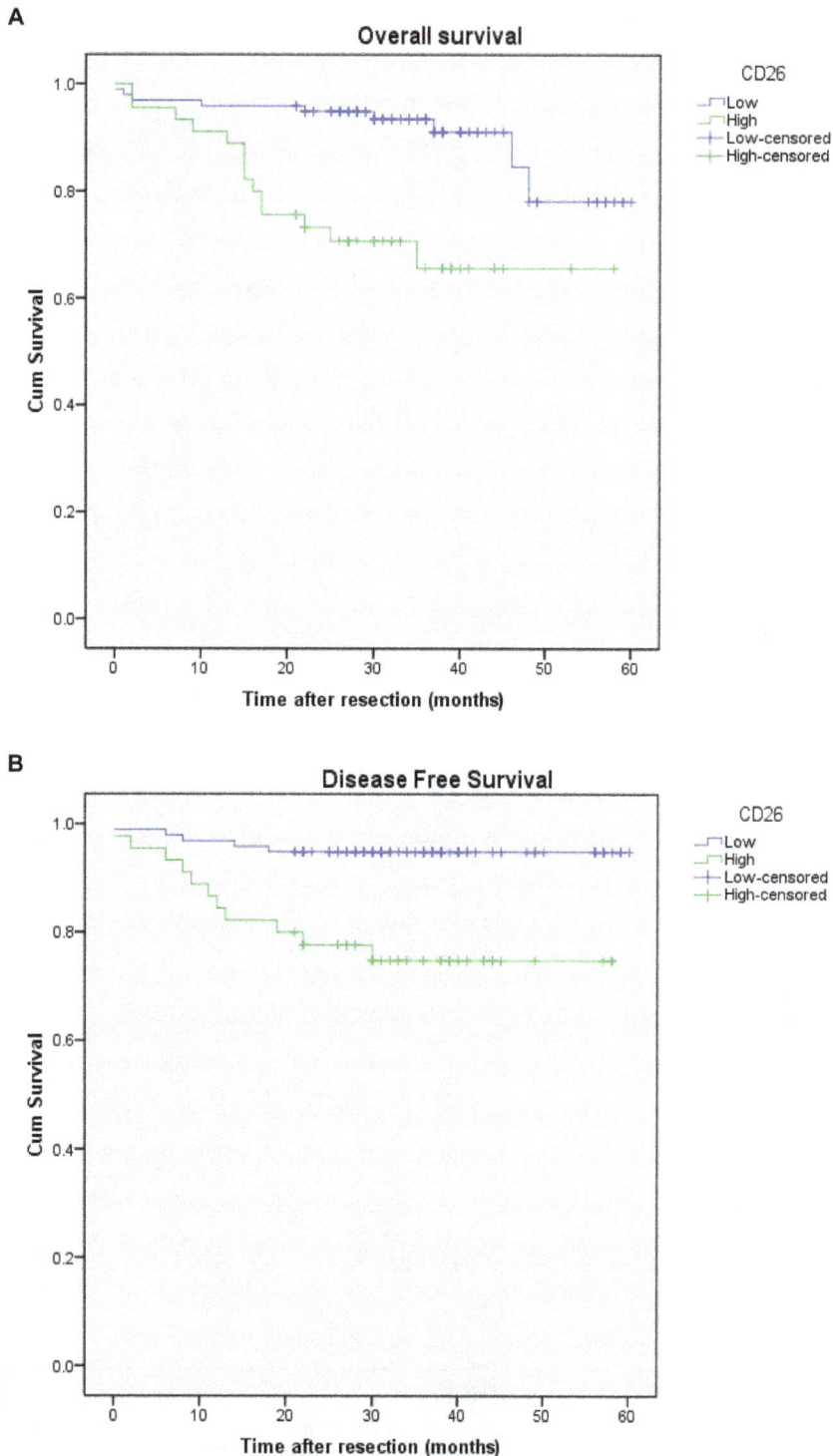

**Figure 2. High CD26 expression associated with worse overall and disease free survival of colorectal cancer patients.** A) Kaplan-Meier cumulative overall survival curves of CRC patients with high (expression level 3 and 2) and low CD26 expression. P<0.001 (log rank test). B) Kaplan-Meier disease free survival for CRC patients stratified by high and low CD26 expression. P = 0.001 (log rank test).

high CD26 expression was significantly worse than that of patients with low CD26 level (P= 0.001). Results shown in Figure 3 suggest that there was significant differences between patients with metastasis and those without metastasis in either overall survival (P<0.001) or disease-free survival (P<0.001). The percentages of

tumour recurrence were 44.4% and 3.4% for patients with distant metastasis and without distant metastasis in five years, respectively.

Besides CD26 expression, table 3 shows the results of a univariate analysis of patient's clinicopathological features which might affect prognosis. From these parameters, only TNM stage,

**A**

**B**

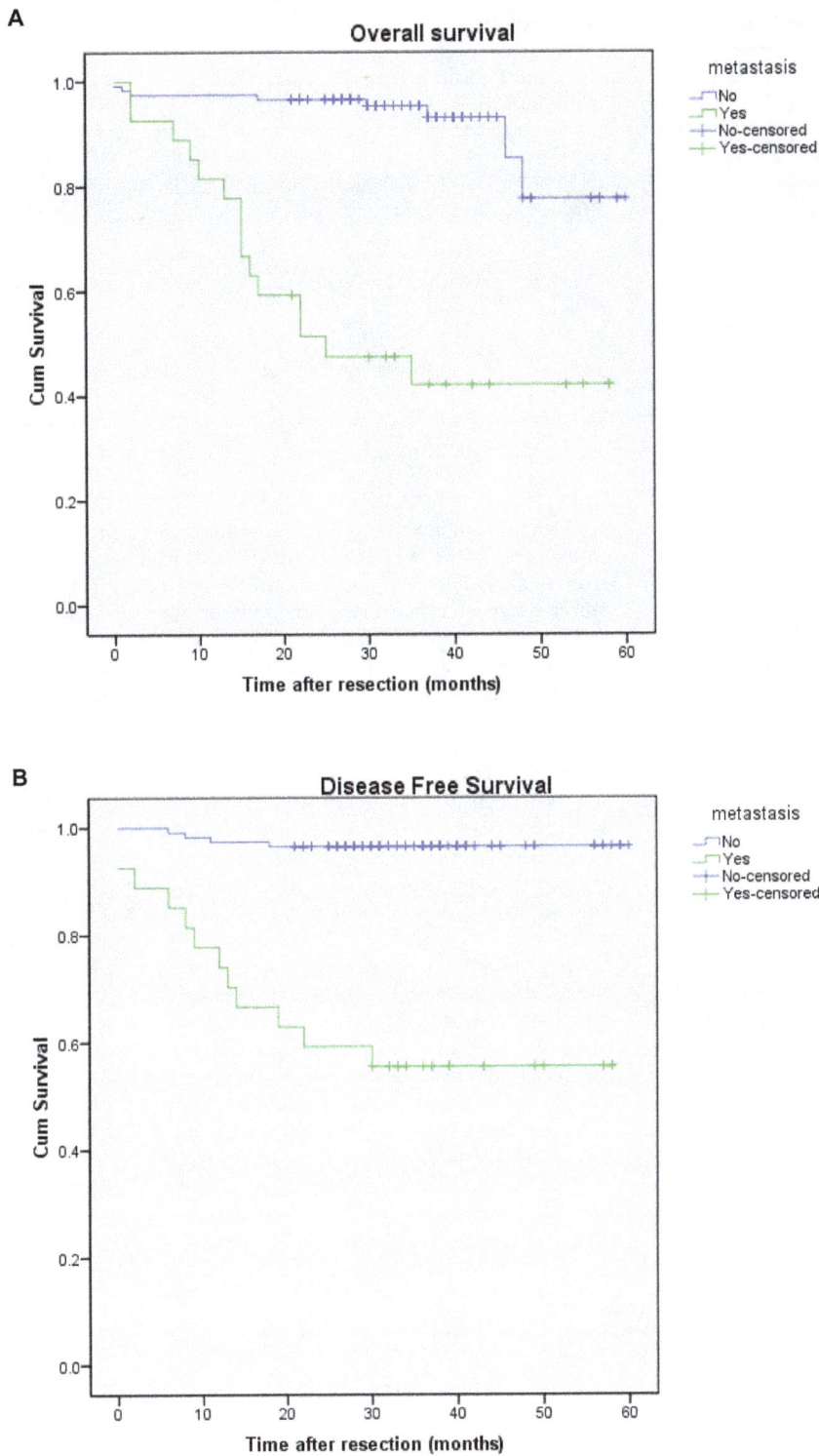

**Figure 3. Metastasis associated with worse overall and disease free survival of colorectal cancer patients.** A) Kaplan-Meier cumulative overall survival curves of CRC patients with metastasis and no metastasis. P<0.001 (log rank test). B) Kaplan-Meier disease free survival for CRC patients stratified by metastasis and no metastasis. P<0.001 (log rank test).

metastatic status and liver metastasis had significant long-term outcome in this study.

When CD26 expression (high versus low levels) was entered into a Cox regression analysis together with these three factors, only metastatic status was identified as independent prognostic factors of overall survival (Table 4A). However, CD26 expression level was an independent prognostic factor of overall survival when CD26 expression was entered into a Cox regression analysis together without metastatic status (Table 4B).

**Table 3.** Significant prognostic factors of overall survival by univariate analysis.

| Variable | No. of cases | 5-year survival (%) | P* |
|---|---|---|---|
| TNM stage: | | | |
| Stage I/II | 64 | 92.4 | 0.021 |
| Stage III/IV | 78 | 77.6 | |
| Metastasis status: | | | |
| No metastasis | 116 | 93.1 | <0.001 |
| Metastasis | 27 | 44.4 | |
| Liver metastasis: | | | |
| No | 123 | 90.2 | <0.001 |
| Yes | 30 | 45 | |

*Log rank test

To study the response of chemotherapy, CRC patients with different CD26 expression were analysed with or without chemotherapy (5-Fu or oxaliplatin) (Fig. 4). The result showed that high CD26 expression was associated with worse overall survival whether with or without chemotherapy (P = 0.013 and 0.012 respectively). On the other hand, there was no significant effect of chemotherapy on CRC patients with high or low CD26 expression (Fig. 5). Figure 5A suggest that CRC patients with high CD26 expression seems have better survival for the first year with chemotherapy, but the survival became worse afterwards.

## Discussion

Colorectal cancer (CRC) is one of the most leading cause of cancer deaths in the world due to asymptomatic early stage and mostly diagnosis in advanced stages [1]. The 5 year survival rate of CRC patients with metastatic disease is less than 10% [16]. Colonoscopy and faecal occult blood test (FOBT) in stool are the two most common screening tool for CRC [17,18,19]. However, they have different disadvantages and limitations such as high cost for the population with low risk, discomfort of patients or low sensitivity [20]. Besides an asymptomatic early stage, metastasis is the major cause of high mortality in CRC. In order to predict the outcome of colorectal cancer accurately, there has been great interest to develop factors which can help for diagnosis or prognosis because survival can be dramatically improved at early detection and treatment of CRC [21].

CD26 is a multifunctional cell surface glycoprotein protein with intrinsic dipeptidyl peptidase IV (DPPIV) activity which widely expressed in most cell types. Cell surface proteases participate in cancer progression and malignant transformation by facilitating tumour cell invasion and metastasis [22]. Yamada K et al. recently demonstrated that anti-CD26 monoclonal antibody induced nuclear localization of CD26 from cell surface which can inhibit tumour cell growth [23]. Several studies have indicated that serum CD26 can be an early diagnostic marker for colorectal cancer [15,24,25]. However, they did not clarify whether CD26 expression had any independent prognostic significance. Moreover, the reports were conflicted in the concentration of soluble CD26 in CRC patients: one study found out that soluble CD26 was significantly higher in healthy donors, but another report showed higher level of soluble CD26 was detected in CRC patients. It varies among different papers, which may due to different detection methods in the study (one used ELISA assay and another one used an assay for enzyme activity).

Our previous study has clearly demonstrated that a subpopulation of cancer cells with CD26 expression were associated with the metastatic progression and chemoresistance of colorectal cancer [13]. Based on our previous findings, we further investigated the potential prognostic properties of CD26 expression on CRC patient's specimens.

In this study, our results showed that the high CD26 expression level was a significant predictor of both reduced overall survival (P<0.001, log rank test) and disease free survival (P = 0.001) in

**Table 4.** Prognostic factors of overall survival by Cox regression analysis.

| A: Variable | Hazard ratio | P* |
|---|---|---|
| TNM stage (I/II versus III/IV) | 0.466 (0.089, 2.44) | 0.366 |
| CD26 expression (Low versus High) | 1.953 (0.674, 5.656) | 0.218 |
| Metastasis status (No Metastasis versus Metastasis) | 10.556 (1.731, 64.367) | 0.011 |
| Liver Metastasis (No versus Yes) | 1.279 (0.392, 4.176) | 0.683 |
| B: Variable | Hazard ratio | P* |
| TNM stage (I/II versus III/IV) | 1.029 (0.301, 3.514) | 0.964 |
| CD26 expression (Low versus High) | 2.967 (1.122, 7.83) | 0.028 |
| Liver Metastasis (No versus Yes) | 4.897 (1.772, 13.536) | 0.002 |

Values in parentheses are 95% confidence intervals.
*Log rank test

**A**

**B**

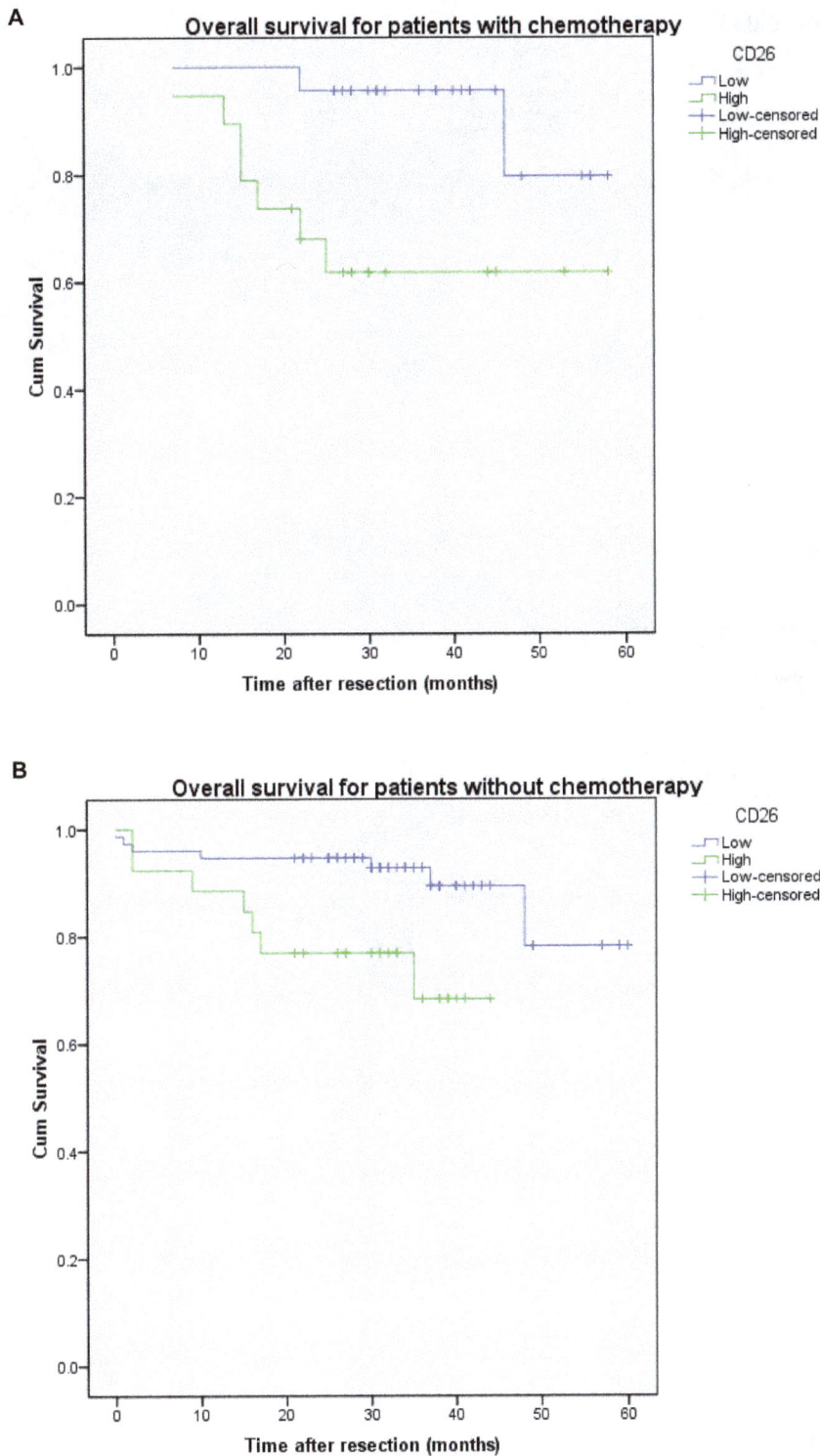

**Figure 4. High CD26 expression associated with worse overall survival of colorectal cancer patients with or without chemotherapy.** Kaplan-Meier cumulative overall survival curves of CRC patients with (A) and without (B) chemotherapy. P = 0.013 and 0.012 respectively (log rank test).

patients with CRC under univariate analysis, which means that higher CD26 expression has worse survival rate and higher rate of recurrence. Even though there is no correlation between CD26 expression and age, gender or tumour size, a significant difference in degree of differentiation ($P = 0.029$, chi-square test), TNM stage ($P<0.001$) or metastatic status ($P<0.001$) show that CD26 expression was positively associated with tumour differentiation, invasion and metastasis. It indicated that higher CD26 expression had poorer differentiation and higher potential for developing distant metastasis. Moreover, CD26 also has significant higher

**A**

**B**

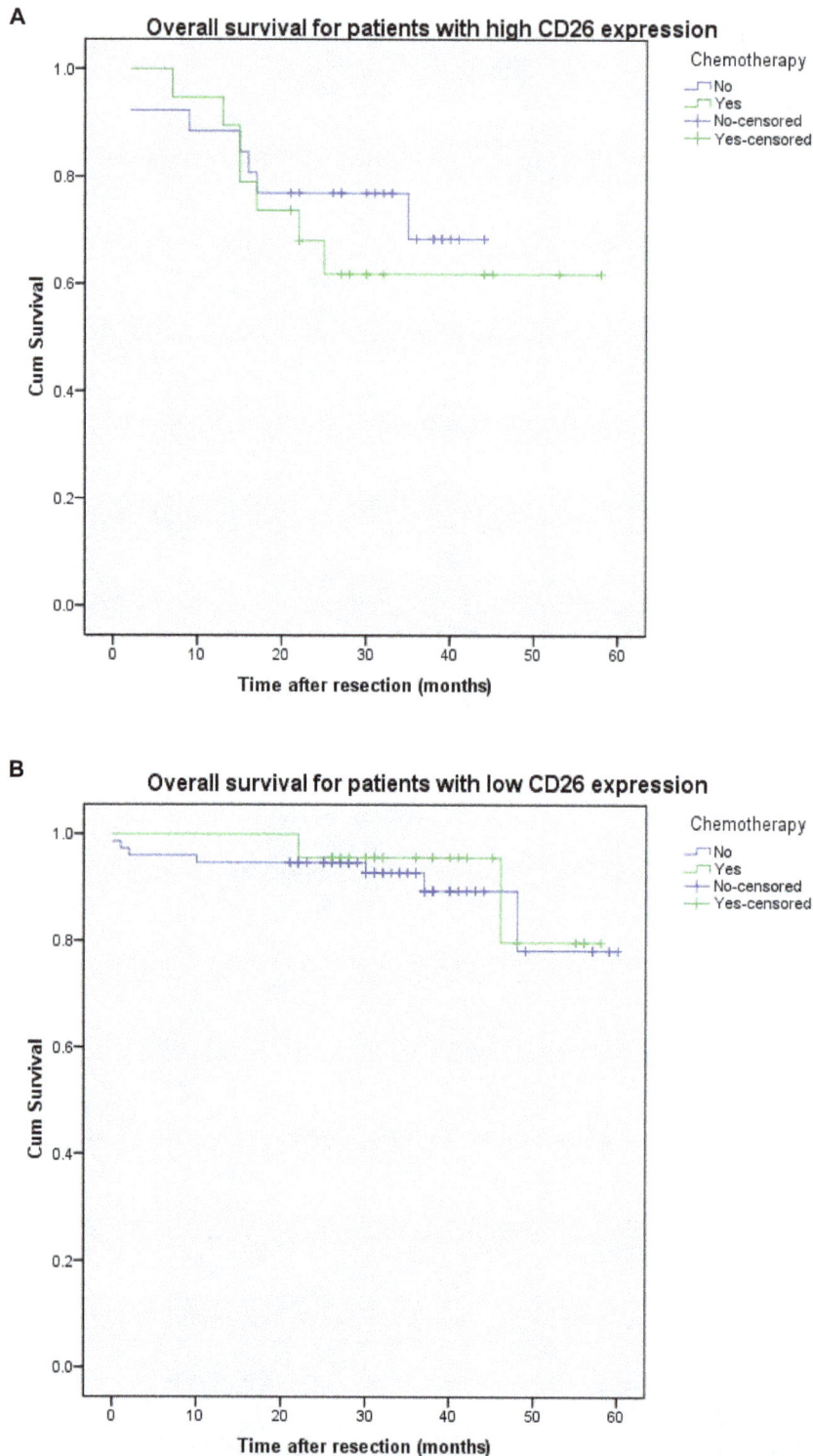

**Figure 5. Chemotherapy has no effect on overall survival of colorectal cancer patients with high or low CD26 expression.** Kaplan-Meier cumulative overall survival curves of CRC patients with high (A) or low (B) CD26 expression. P = 0.514 and 0.661 respectively (log rank test).

expression on TNM stage III ($P = 0.037$) or stage IV ($P < 0.001$), which demonstrated that high expression of CD26 was associated with late TNM stage. In multivariate analysis, CD26 expression is a long-term survival independent pathological variable which have clinical implications when comparing with tumour stage ($P = 0.028$). It indicated that CD26 expression was a more significant prognostic marker than TNM stage. However, in the multivariate analysis including metastatic status, CD26 expression was not an independent predictor of overall survival which may due to dominant effect of metastatic status on patient survival.

CD26 has a function of binding to extracellular matrix proteins which may have a role in tumour migration and metastasis.

Recent studies have demonstrated that CD26 binds to fibronectin and type 1 collagen, which are major components of the extracellular matrix, to facilitate the metastatic progression and invasive phenotype in CRC through down-regulation of E-cadherin [26,27,28]. Additionally, CD26+ cells were shown to possess greater cancer stem cell properties and chemoresistance when compared with CD26- cells [13]. Our previous findings also suggest that the CD26 protein in CD26+ cells does not only provide them with adhesion to both fibronectin and type I collagen but also give them EMT-like attributes, which contributes to the invasive phenotype and metastatic capacity of the CD26+ cells. It is consistent with our findings that CD26 expression is significantly associated with metastatic status ($P<0.001$). Taken together, it provides a potential explanation as to why higher CD26 expression is associated with poorer survival in CRC patients.

The new metastases is still frequently developed even the tumour response has been improved for systemic chemotherapy on CRC. There are more than 80% in situ tumour recurrences for CRC patients even after apparently complete radiological response to chemotherapy for liver metastasis [29]. As demonstrated in our previous in vitro and in vivo studies, CD26+ cancer stem cell subpopulation had enhanced chemoresistance [13]. Therefore, CRC patients with high CD26 expression may fail to eradicate the CD26+ cells under chemotherapeutic treatments which led to enrichment of CD26+ cells and ultimately cause further metastasis and worse survival after first year of treatment. Chemotherapy (5-Fu and oxaliplatin) didn't show improvement on

CRC patients survival after surgical resection, it is crucial for development new therapeutic strategies targeting such CD26+ cancer stem cell.

Carcinoembrynoic antigen (CEA) is a tumour-associated antigen which was identified in CRC tissue in 1965 [30]. Patient's sera CEA level, who have tumours of digestive tract, was used as a most common diagnostic and prognostic marker for CRC [31,32,33,34]. However, the postoperative CEA values were stabilized after 12th post-operative week and the mean time of detectable rise in CEA for CRC patients is more than 3 months [35], which may lose the most suitable time for adjuvant therapy. On the contrary, the CD26 expression level can be detected after operation and the result can be used for prognosis.

In conclusion, our findings suggest that the specimen CD26 expression level is an independent prognostic marker which predicts survival significantly before development of metastasis, and it can provide additional prognostic information and allow selection of CRC patients at high risk of tumour recurrence or development metastasis for adjuvant or neoadjuvant therapy. CD26 expression may be a useful prognostic marker in patients with CRC after surgical resection.

## Author Contributions

Conceived and designed the experiments: CSL WLL RWP. Performed the experiments: CSL AHC SKW. Analyzed the data: CSL RCP. Contributed reagents/materials/analysis tools: CSL TMW AKC LN NSC HSL JHM AHC TCY OSL JTP. Wrote the paper: CSL WLL RWP.

## References

1. Jemal A, Siegel R, Ward E, Hao Y, Xu J, et al. (2009) Cancer statistics, 2009. CA: a cancer journal for clinicians 59: 225–249.
2. Hunter KW, Crawford NP, Alsarraj J (2008) Mechanisms of metastasis. Breast Cancer Res 10 Suppl 1: S2.
3. Boyle P, Ferlay J (2005) Cancer incidence and mortality in Europe, 2004. Annals of oncology: official journal of the European Society for Medical Oncology/ESMO 16: 481–488.
4. Mentlein R (1999) Dipeptidyl-peptidase IV (CD26)—role in the inactivation of regulatory peptides. Regulatory peptides 85: 9–24.
5. Tanaka T, Camerini D, Seed B, Torimoto Y, Dang NH, et al. (1992) Cloning and functional expression of the T cell activation antigen CD26. Journal of immunology 149: 481–486.
6. Wolf M, Albrecht S, Marki C (2008) Proteolytic processing of chemokines: implications in physiological and pathological conditions. Int J Biochem Cell Biol 40: 1185–1198.
7. Bauvois B (1988) A collagen-binding glycoprotein on the surface of mouse fibroblasts is identified as dipeptidyl peptidase IV. The Biochemical journal 252: 723–731.
8. Piazza GA, Callanan HM, Mowery J, Hixson DC (1989) Evidence for a role of dipeptidyl peptidase IV in fibronectin-mediated interactions of hepatocytes with extracellular matrix. Biochem J 262: 327–334.
9. Loster K, Zeilinger K, Schuppan D, Reutter W (1995) The cysteine-rich region of dipeptidyl peptidase IV (CD 26) is the collagen-binding site. Biochemical and biophysical research communications 217: 341–348.
10. Gonzalez-Gronow M, Kaczowka S, Gawdi G, Pizzo SV (2008) Dipeptidyl peptidase IV (DPP IV/CD26) is a cell-surface plasminogen receptor. Front Biosci 13: 1610–1618.
11. Havre PA, Abe M, Urasaki Y, Ohnuma K, Morimoto C, et al. (2008) The role of CD26/dipeptidyl peptidase IV in cancer. Front Biosci 13: 1634–1645.
12. Sedo A, Stremenova J, Busek P, Duke-Cohan JS (2008) Dipeptidyl peptidase-IV and related molecules: markers of malignancy? Expert Opin Med Diagn 2: 677–689.
13. Pang R, Law WL, Chu AC, Poon JT, Lam CS, et al. (2010) A subpopulation of CD26+ cancer stem cells with metastatic capacity in human colorectal cancer. Cell stem cell 6: 603–615.
14. Ayude D, Paez de la Cadena M, Cordero OJ, Nogueira M, Ayude J, et al. (2003) Clinical interest of the combined use of serum CD26 and alpha-L-fucosidase in the early diagnosis of colorectal cancer. Disease markers 19: 267–272.
15. de la Haba-Rodriguez J, Macho A, Calzado MA, Blazquez MV, Gomez MA, et al. (2002) Soluble dipeptidyl peptidase IV (CD-26) in serum of patients with colorectal carcinoma. Neoplasma 49: 307–311.
16. Boyle P, Ferlay J (2005) Cancer incidence and mortality in Europe, 2004. Ann Oncol 16: 481–488.
17. Mandel JS, Bond JH, Church TR, Snover DC, Bradley GM, et al. (1993) Reducing mortality from colorectal cancer by screening for fecal occult blood. Minnesota Colon Cancer Control Study. The New England journal of medicine 328: 1365–1371.
18. Kronborg O, Fenger C, Olsen J, Jorgensen OD, Sondergaard O (1996) Randomised study of screening for colorectal cancer with faecal-occult-blood test. Lancet 348: 1467–1471.
19. Smith RA, Cokkinides V, von Eschenbach AC, Levin B, Cohen C, et al. (2002) American Cancer Society guidelines for the early detection of cancer. CA Cancer J Clin 52: 8–22.
20. Vijan S, Hwang EW, Hofer TP, Hayward RA (2001) Which colon cancer screening test? A comparison of costs, effectiveness, and compliance. Am J Med 111: 593–601.
21. Winawer SJ (2005) Screening of colorectal cancer. Surgical oncology clinics of North America 14: 699–722.
22. Hakomori S (1989) Aberrant glycosylation in tumors and tumor-associated carbohydrate antigens. Adv Cancer Res 52: 257–331.
23. Yamada K, Hayashi M, Madokoro H, Nishida H, Du W, et al. (2013) Nuclear localization of CD26 induced by a humanized monoclonal antibody inhibits tumor cell growth by modulating of POLR2A transcription. PloS one 8: e62304.
24. Hundt S, Haug U, Brenner H (2007) Blood markers for early detection of colorectal cancer: a systematic review. Cancer epidemiology, biomarkers & prevention: a publication of the American Association for Cancer Research, cosponsored by the American Society of Preventive Oncology 16: 1935–1953.
25. Cordero OJ, Ayude D, Nogueira M, Rodriguez-Berrocal FJ, de la Cadena MP (2000) Preoperative serum CD26 levels: diagnostic efficiency and predictive value for colorectal cancer. British journal of cancer 83: 1139–1146.
26. Kirkland SC (2009) Type I collagen inhibits differentiation and promotes a stem cell-like phenotype in human colorectal carcinoma cells. Br J Cancer 101: 320–326.
27. Inamoto T, Yamochi T, Ohnuma K, Iwata S, Kina S, et al. (2006) Anti-CD26 monoclonal antibody-mediated G1-S arrest of human renal clear cell carcinoma Caki-2 is associated with retinoblastoma substrate dephosphorylation, cyclin-dependent kinase 2 reduction, p27(kip1) enhancement, and disruption of binding to the extracellular matrix. Clin Cancer Res 12: 3470–3477.
28. Sato T, Yamochi T, Aytac U, Ohnuma K, McKee KS, et al. (2005) CD26 regulates p38 mitogen-activated protein kinase-dependent phosphorylation of integrin beta1, adhesion to extracellular matrix, and tumorigenicity of T-anaplastic large cell lymphoma Karpas 299. Cancer research 65: 6950–6956.
29. Benoist S, Brouquet A, Penna C, Julie C, El Hajjam M, et al. (2006) Complete response of colorectal liver metastases after chemotherapy: does it mean cure? J Clin Oncol 24: 3939–3945.

30. Gold P, Freedman SO (1965) Demonstration of Tumor-Specific Antigens in Human Colonic Carcinomata by Immunological Tolerance and Absorption Techniques. J Exp Med 121: 439–462.
31. National Cancer Institute of Canada-American Cancer Society (1972) A collaborative study of a test for carcinoembryonic antigen (CEA) in the sera of patients with carcinoma of the colon and rectum. A joint National Cancer Institute of Canada-American Cancer Society investigation. Can Med Assoc J 107: 25–33.
32. Dhar P, Moore T, Zamcheck N, Kupchik HZ (1972) Carcinoembryonic antigen (CEA) in colonic cancer. Use in preoperative and postoperative diagnosis and prognosis. JAMA 221: 31–35.
33. Lo Gerfo P, Lo Gerfo F, Herter F, Barker HG, Hansen HJ (1972) Tumor-associated antigen in patients with carcinoma of the colon. Am J Surg 123: 127–131.
34. Zamcheck N, Moore TL, Dhar P, Kupchik H (1972) Immunologic diagnosis and prognosis of human digestive-tract cancer: carcinoembryonic antigens. N Engl J Med 286: 83–86.
35. Herrera MA, Chu TM, Holyoke ED (1976) Carcinoembryonic antigen (CEA) as a prognostic and monitoring test in clinically complete resection of colorectal carcinoma. Ann Surg 183: 5–9.

# 15

# Serum YKL-40 Level is Associated with the Chemotherapy Response and Prognosis of Patients with Small Cell Lung Cancer

Chun-Hua Xu[1,2], Li -Ke Yu[1,2]*, Ke-Ke Hao[1,2]

**1** First Department of Respiratory Medicine and Nanjing Chest Hospital, Nanjing, Jiangsu, China, **2** Clinical Center of Nanjing Respiratory Diseases, Nanjing, Jiangsu, China

## Abstract

This study was to explore the association between the serum YKL-40 level and the clinical characteristics, the response to chemotherapy and prognosis in small cell lung cancer (SCLC). Serum YKL-40 levels were detected and compared in 120 patients with SCLC pre- and post-chemotherapy, and in 40 healthy controls. Receiver operating characteristics (ROC) curves were adopted for diagnosis and calculation of area under ROC curve in SCLC. The Kaplan–Meier method, univariate and multivariate Cox regression analysis were used to analyze the correlation between pre-chemotherapy serum YKL-40 levels and progression-free survival (PFS) and overall survival (OS). The pre-chemotherapy serum YKL-40 levels were significantly higher than those of the controls ($p<0.001$). The post-chemotherapy serum YKL-40 levels in the SCLC cases were lower than pre-chemotherapy serum YKL-40 levels in these cases ($p = 0.026$). The patients with high serum YKL-40 showed a poorer response to chemotherapy than those patients with low serumYKL-40 ($p = 0.031$). Univariate analysis revealed that SCLC patients with high serum YKL-40 had a shorter PFS and OS than those with low serum YKL-40 (HR of 1.74, $p = 0.033$; HR of 1.33, $p = 0.001$). Cox multivariate analysis indicated that YKL-40 was an independent prognostic indicator of PFS and OS (HR of 1.12, $p = 0.029$; HR of 1.84, $p = 0.025$). Kaplan–Meier survival curves further confirmed that patients with low serum YKL-40 have longer PFS and OS ($p = 0.016$ and $p = 0.041$, respectively). These results suggest that YKL-40 is a potential prognostic marker of chemotherapy response in SCLC.

**Editor:** Christina Lynn Addison, Ottawa Hospital Research Institute, Canada

**Funding:** This work was supported in part by a grant from "Twelve-Five Plan" the Major Program of Nanjing Medical Science and Technique Development Foundation (Molecular Mechanism Study on Metastasis and Clinical Efficacy Prediction of Non-small Cell Lung Cancer) (LK-Yu). No additional funding was received for this study. The funders had no role in study design, data collection and analysis, decision to publish, or preparation of the manuscript.

**Competing Interests:** The authors have declared that no competing interests exist.

\* E-mail: yulike_doctor@163.com

## Introduction

Lung cancer is the leading cause of cancer-related death worldwide, with more than 1.2 million deaths each year [1]. Small cell lung cancer (SCLC) accounts for up to 15% of total lung malignancies [2]. Despite the often dramatic response to chemotherapy and radiotherapy in patients with SCLC, most die from recurrent disease [3]. With rapid tumor doubling rate and early metastasis, over half of SCLC patients present with extensive disease [4]. As a result, five years survival rate in SCLC is only 10%–26% [5].

Tumor markers play a key role in patient management for many malignancies. The potential uses of serum tumor markers include aiding early diagnosis, determining prognosis, predicting response or resistance to specific therapies, and monitoring therapy in patients with advanced disease. Tumor markers that are currently available for lung cancer, such as progastrin-releasing peptide (ProGRP), carcinoembryonic antigen (CEA), and neuron-specific enolase (NSE), are not satisfactory for diagnosis at an early stage or for monitoring the disease because of their relatively low sensitivity and specificity in detecting the presence of cancer cells [6–8]. Therefore, more studies are required to discover novel biomarkers in order to predict the chemotherapy response and improve the prognosis of patients with SCLC.

YKL-40 is produced by cancer cells and may play a role in cancer cell proliferation and angiogenesis [9]. Recent studies have shown that elevations of serum YKL-40 were reported in various malignant tissues, including breast cancer, gastric cancer, and ovarian cancer [10–13]. The association between increased YKL-40 and a poor prognosis has been well documented [11–17], including lung cancer [18–20]. However, the association between serum YKL-40 level and the clinical characteristics, especially the response to chemotherapy and prognosis in SCLC remain largely unknown.

The purpose of this study was to investigate the clinical role of serum YKL-40 in SCLC patients. Our aim is to evaluate the possibility of serum YKL-40 as a biomarker in SCLC.

## Materials and Methods

### Patients

The study included 120 SCLC patients, who were diagnosed at the Nanjing Chest Hospital between January 2007 and December 2011. Mean age of the patients was $64.5\pm5.6$ years, 95 male and 25 female. All the patients underwent clinical examination, CT scans of the chest and brain, CT and ultrasonography of the upper

**Table 1.** Clinical characteristics of SCLC patients and controls.

| Characteristics | SCLC (N = 120) | Control (N = 40) | p-value |
|---|---|---|---|
| Age, yr | | | |
| Range | 46 78 | 45 74 | |
| Mean | 64.5±5.6 | 57.6±10.8 | 0.247 |
| Gender | | | |
| Male | 95 (79.17%) | 31 (75.50%) | |
| Female | 25 (20.83%) | 9 (22.50%) | 0.176 |
| Smoking condition | | | |
| Smoker | 80 (66.67%) | 29 (72.50%) | |
| Nonsmoker | 40 (33.33%) | 11 (27.50%) | 0.138 |

p values were calculated using chi-square test.

abdomen, fibreoptic bronchoscopy, bone scanning, and positron emission tomography. Staging was carried out according to the veterans administration lung cancer group (VALG) staging system [21]: Limited disease (LD) was defined as disease confined to one hemithorax including the mediastinal lymph nodes and/or the supraclavicular lymph nodes; extensive disease (ED) was defined as having limited disease or malignant pleural effusion. Smoking history was obtained from the health interview questionnaire. Current and former smokers were classified as "smoker" and never smokers as "nonsmoker". The control subjects consisted of 40 healthy volunteers (31 males and 9 females with a mean age of 57.6±10.8 years), as documented by a general health examination in the same period. They were not on any medication, and had no clinical signs or symptoms of cancer, liver, kidney or hormonal disease. The demographic features and clinical characteristics of the studied groups are illustrated in Table 1.

All SCLC patients received chemotherapies for a maximum of six cycles. Chemotherapy regimens are presented in Table 2. Computed tomography (CT) scans were performed after 2 cycles of chemotherapy. All patients had measurable disease. Response categories were defined according to the Response Evaluation Criteria in Solid Tumors (RECIST) as complete response (CR), partial response (PR), stable disease (SD) and progressive disease (PD) [22]. For data analysis, CR and PR were combined as response that was sensitive to chemotherapy, while SD and PD were grouped as non-response. Follow-up information was obtained by phone investigations. The median follow-up of surviving patients at the time of analysis was 14 months (range, 5–36 months). The date of the last follow-up was March 21, 2013.

**Table 2.** The clinicopathological characteristics of SCLC and the association with serum YKL-40 levels.

| Group | n | YKL-40 (ng/mL) | p-value |
|---|---|---|---|
| Age, yr | | | |
| <60 | 52 | 68.47±26.95 | 0.209 |
| ≥60 | 68 | 74.81±27.76 | |
| Gender | | | |
| Male | 95 | 72.85±26.94 | 0.541 |
| Female | 25 | 69.06±29.81 | |
| Smoking status | | | |
| Nonsmoker | 40 | 66.51±27.26 | 0.118 |
| Smoker | 80 | 74.84±27.33 | |
| Performance status | | | |
| 0, 1 | 86 | 73.92±26.52 | 0.265 |
| 2, 3 | 34 | 67.36±29.65 | |
| Disease stage | | | |
| Limited | 70 | 67.31±25.98 | 0.024* |
| Extended | 50 | 78.71±28.39 | |
| Chemotherapy regimen | | | |
| EP | 102 | 70.67±25.62 | 0.376 |
| IP | 18 | 73.16±27.38 | |

EP, cisplatin with etoposide; IP, cisplatin with irinotecan.
*Significant difference.

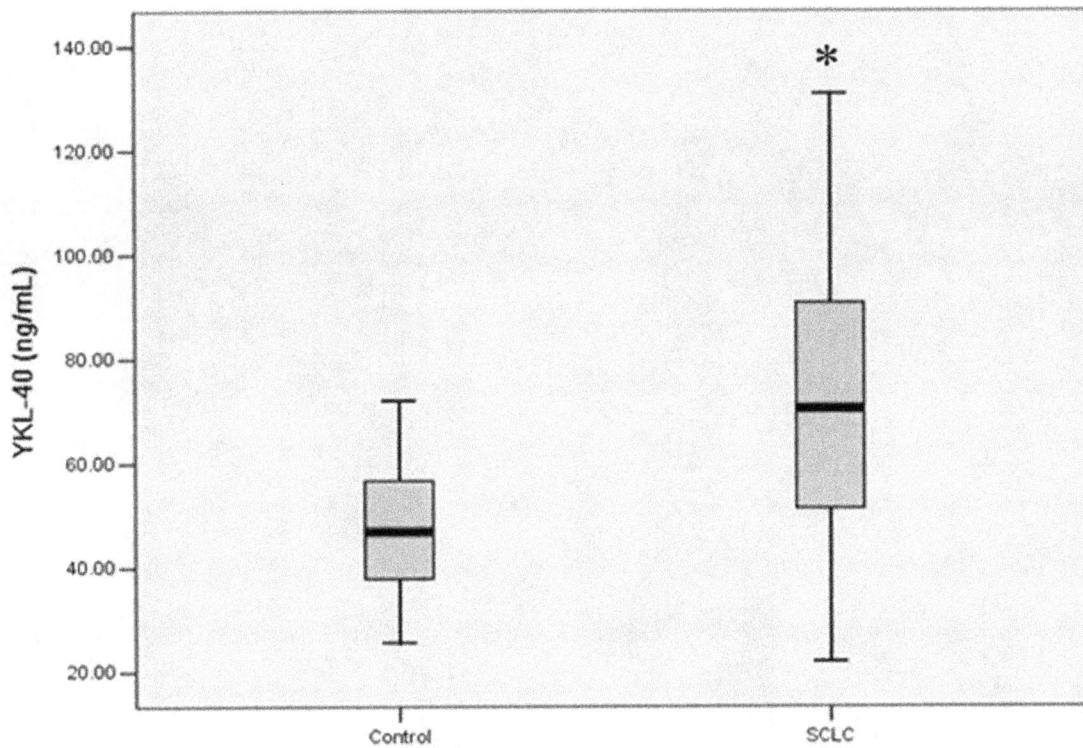

**Figure 1. Pre-chemotherapy serum YKL-40 levels in SCLC patients and healthy controls.** Among 120 SCLC patients, the serum levels of YKL-40 were (72.06±27.48) ng/mL, which were significantly higher than (48.41±13.63) ng/mL in healthy controls ($p<0.001$, $t$-test).

Progression-free survival (PFS) was defined as the time interval between the date of diagnosis and the date of disease progression or last follow-up. Overall survival (OS) was defined as the time interval between the date of diagnosis and the date of death or the last follow-up.

The protocol was approved by the Ethics Committee of the Nanjing Chest Hospital, and written informed consent was obtained from all patients and healthy controls before the study. Doctors recorded the obtainment of the written consent in patients' clinical files. After the treat agreement was signed but prior to the chemotherapy, the patients also noted in the treat

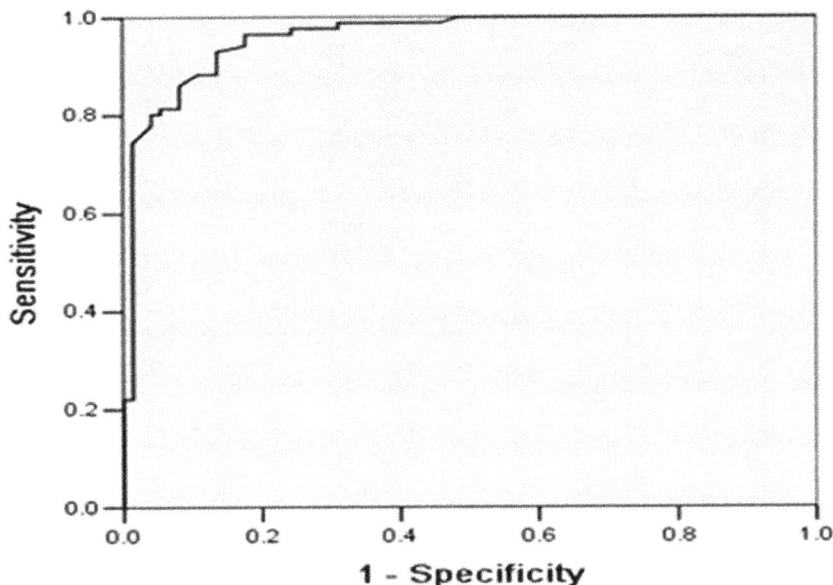

**Figure 2. ROC curve of the serum YKL-40 levels of 120 SCLC patients and 40 controls.** Serum levels of YKL-40 among 120 SCLC patients and 40 healthy controls were determined. The diagnostic potentials of YKL-40 were assessed by ROC curves. The AUC value was 0.96.

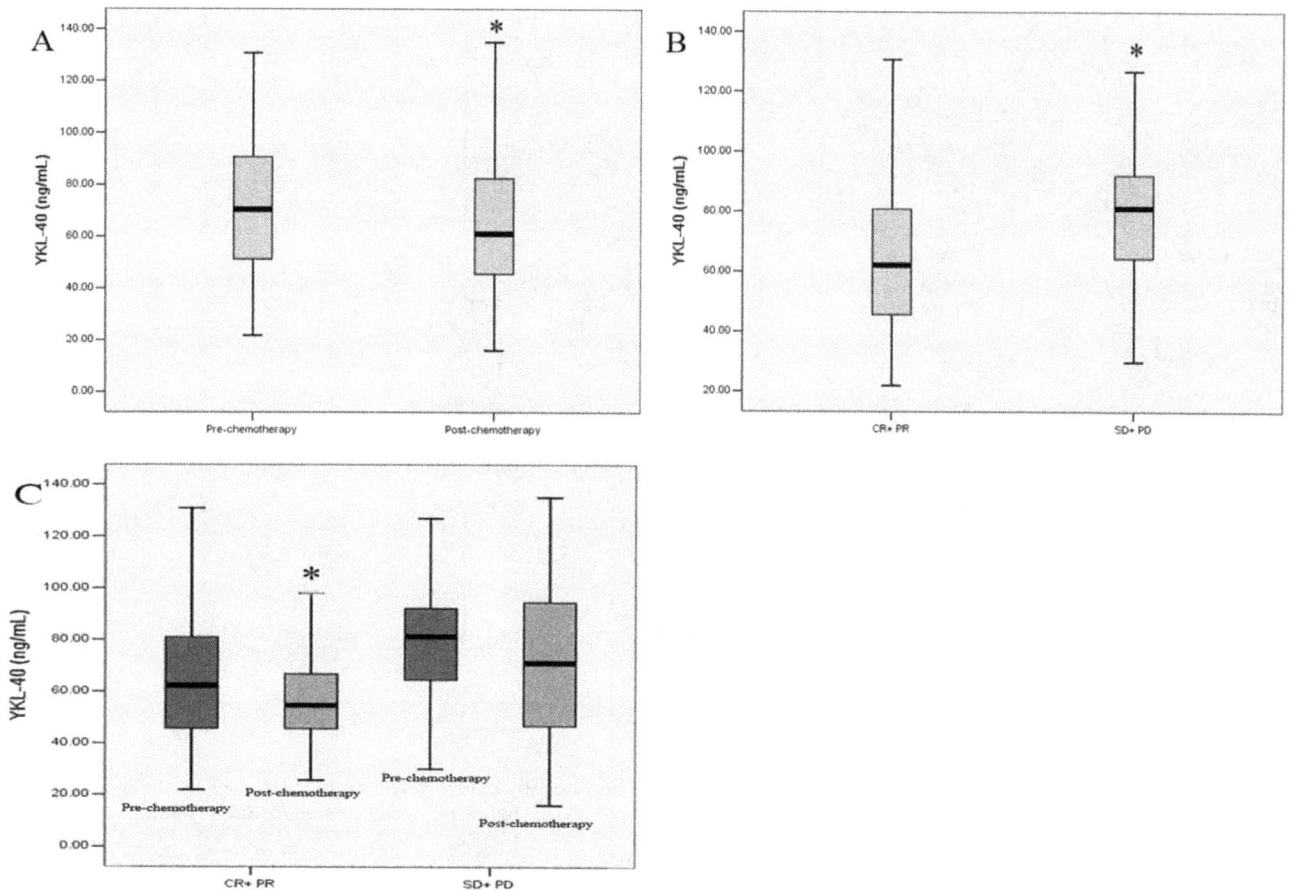

**Figure 3. Distribution of serum YKL-40 levels.** Serum YL-40 levels in the SCLC patients significantly decreased after chemotherapy ($p = 0.026$) (A). The pre-chemotherapy serum YKL-40 levels were lower in the sensitive to chemotherapy group than in the resistant to chemotherapy group ($p = 0.004$) (B). Serum YKL-40 of responders after chemotherapy were significantly decreased ($p = 0.029$), while YKL-40 of non-responders did not change significantly ($p = 0.256$) (C).

agreement that she/he was informed about and agreed to participate in this study. The Ethics Committee approved this written consent procedure and had unscheduled inspection of documents and records to assure the study was compliant.

### Serum Collection

Peripheral blood samples were obtained from the healthy controls and from the patients after diagnosis but prior to any treatments. For the 120 SCLC patients treated with chemother-

apy, serum samples were obtained 3 weeks after completion of the second chemotherapy cycle. The whole blood samples were promptly centrifuged at 3000 rpm for 15 minutes and the supernatant stored at $-80°C$ until use.

### Detection of Serum YKL-40 Levels

The serum levels of YKL-40 were measured using an YKL-40 ELISA kit ((Quidel, San Diego, CA, USA). A volume of 50 μl of 2-fold diluted samples was added to a 96-well plate

**Table 3.** Response to chemotherapy and serum YKL-40 levels.

| Clinical response | All patients | YKL-40 (high) (%) | YKL-40 (low) (%) | p-value |
|---|---|---|---|---|
| CR | 32 | 14 (43.8) | 18 (56.2) | |
| PR | 33 | 24 (72.7) | 9 (27.3) | |
| SD | 35 | 28 (80.0) | 7 (20.0) | |
| PD | 20 | 15 (75.0) | 5 (25.0) | |
| Response (CR+PR) | 65 | 38 (58.5) | 27 (41.5) | 0.031* |
| Non-response (SD+PD) | 55 | 43 (78.2) | 12 (21.8) | |

CR, complete response; PR, partial response; SD, stable disease; PD, progressive disease.
*Significant difference.

**Table 4.** Characteristics and serum YKL-40 distribution of SCLC patients with pre-and post- chemotherapy.

| Therapeutic efficacy | N | pre-chemotherapy | post-chemotherapy | p-value |
|---|---|---|---|---|
| Response (CR+PR) | 65 | 65.56±27.20 | 56.54±18.12 | 0.029* |
| Non-response (SD+PD) | 55 | 79.75±25.99 | 73.71±29.41 | 0.256 |
| Total | 120 | 72.06±27.48 | 64.41±25.47 | 0.026* |

CR, complete response; PR, partial response; SD, stable disease; PD, progressive disease.
*Significant difference.

covered with YKL-40 monoclonal antibody and incubated for 2 h at room temperature. After aspirating and washing each well four times, 50 μl of YKL-40 conjugate was added and the wells incubated for 2 h at room temperature. Each well was washed an additional four times to remove residual liquid and 200 μl of substrate solution was added to each well and the wells incubated for 30 min in darkness. After addition of stop solution, absorbance was measured at 450 nm on a Biotek-elx800 microplate reader (Roche, USA), and the YKL-40 concentration determined. The sensitivity of the ELISA was 20 ng/mL. All samples were measured in duplicate in two separate plates. For duplicate samples, intra-assay coefficient of variation of <5% and the inter-assay coefficient of variation of <6% were accepted.

## Statistical Analysis

Statistical analysis was carried out using SPSS 17.0 software. Data were expressed as mean ± standard deviation (SD). Continuous variables were compared using $t$ test. Survival curves were plotted by the Kaplan-Meier method and compared using the log-rank test. Survival data were evaluated using univariate and multivariate Cox regression analysis. Receiver operating characteristics curves (ROC) were adopted to determine the diagnostic value of YKL-40 in cancer. For each ROC, an optimal cut-off point was determined as the value of the parameter that maximized the sum of specificity and sensitivity. A value of $p < 0.05$ was considered significant.

## Results

### Pre-chemotherapy Serum YKL-40 Levels in the SCLC Patients and the Controls

As shown in Figure 1, the mean level of YKL-40 in the pre-chemotherapy serum from SCLC patients (n = 120) was (72.06±27.48 ng/mL), which was significantly higher than the controls (n = 40, 48.41±13.63 ng/mL, $p < 0.001$).

### Relationship between Pre-Chemotherapy Serum YKL-40 Levels and Clinicopathological Characteristics

Table 2 showed the pre-chemotherapy serum YKL-40 levels in SCLC with different clinicopathological characteristics. The serum YKL-40 levels were significantly correlated with disease stage ($p = 0.024$), while there were no difference with age ($p = 0.209$), gender ($p = 0.541$), smoking status ($p = 0.118$), performance status ($p = 0.265$), and chemotherapy regimen ($p = 0.376$).

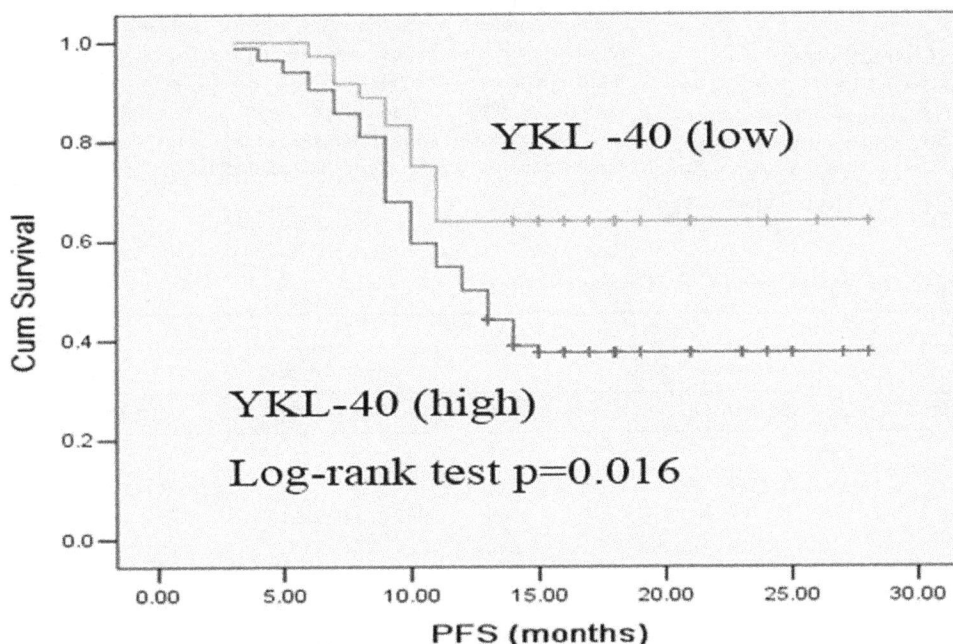

**Figure 4. Kaplan-Meier curve comparing PFS of SCLC patients with high serum YKL-40 versus those with low serum YKL-40.** Log-rank test determined that the PFS in low serum YKL-40 group was significantly longer than those of the high serum YKL-40 group ($p = 0.016$).

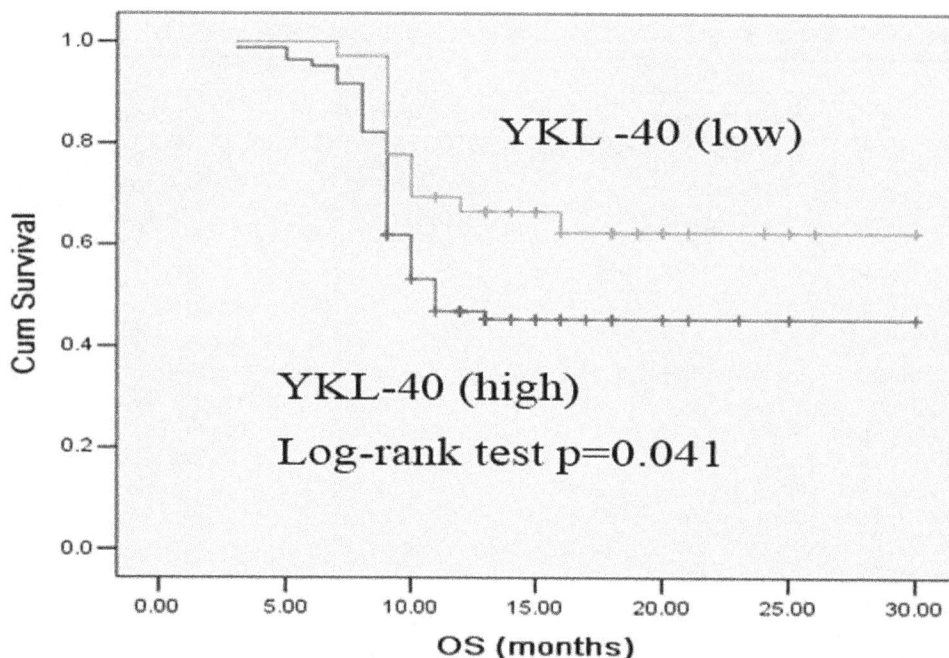

**Figure 5. Kaplan-Meier curve comparing OS of SCLC patients with high serum YKL-40 versus those with low serum YKL-40.** The Log-rank test showed that the survival times were significantly longer in patients with low serum YKL-40 than those of high serum YKL-40 ($p = 0.041$).

## Diagnostic Value of Serum YKL-40 in SCLC

ROC curves were calculated based on the serum YKL-40 levels of the 120 SCLC patients and 40 controls (Figure 2). The estimated area under the ROC curve was 0.96 (95% CI (confidence interval), 0.93–0.99). The optimal cut-off value of serum YKL-40 level was 65.7 ng/mL (low vs. high) based on the maximization of the sum of specificity and sensitivity, resulting in 67.5% sensitivity, 95.0% specificity, and 74.4% accuracy for the diagnosis of SCLC.

## Serum YKL-40 and Response to Chemotherapy

To determine the correlation between serum YKL-40 levels and chemotherapy response, the YKL-40 levels between pre- and post-chemotherapy were analyzed in SCLC patients who received 2 cycles of chemotherapy. Generally, serum YL-40 levels significantly decreased after chemotherapy ($p = 0.026$) (Figure 3A).

Among 120 patients, 32 (26.67%) patients achieved CR, 33 (27.5%) patients achieved PR, 35 (29.17%) patients achieved SD, and 20 (16.67%) patients achieved PD. Of the 81 patients with high serum YKL-40, 38 (46.91%) responded to chemotherapy with either complete response, or partial remission. Of 39 low serumYKL-40 patients, 27 (69.23%) exhibited a response to chemotherapy. The difference in response to chemotherapy between high and low serum YKL-40 patients was statistically significant (p = 0.031) (Table 3).

Pre-chemotherapy serum YKL-40 of patients who were sensitive to chemotherapy were significantly lower than that of non-responders ($p = 0.004$) (Figure 3B). Serum YKL-40 of responders after chemotherapy were significantly decreased ($p = 0.029$), while YKL-40 of non-responders did not change significantly ($p = 0.256$) (Figure 3C) (Table 4).

**Table 5.** Univariate and multivariate Cox regression analysis of variables with PFS.

| Variables | Univariate | | Multivariate | |
|---|---|---|---|---|
| | HR (95% CI) | *p*-value | HR (95% CI) | *p*-value |
| Age (<60 *vs.* ≥60) | 1.21 (0.72–2.02) | 0.475 | | |
| Gender (female *vs.* male) | 0.48 (0.22–1.04) | 0.064 | | |
| Disease stage (limited *vs.* extended) | 3.21 (1.15–8.93) | 0.025* | 2.34 (1.02–5.36) | 0.046* |
| Smoking status (smoker *vs.* nonsmoker) | 0.99 (0.96–1.02) | 0.474 | | |
| Performance status (0, 1 *vs.* 2, 3) | 1.70 (0.93–3.11) | 0.082 | | |
| Chemotherapy regimen (EP *vs.* IP) | 1.92 (0.69–1.983) | 0.673 | | |
| YKL-40 (high *vs.* low) | 1.74 (1.05–2.88) | 0.033* | 1.12 (1.01–1.23) | 0.029* |

HR, hazard ratio; CI, confidence interval; EP, cisplatin with etoposide; IP, cisplatin with irinotecan.
*Significant difference.

**Table 6.** Univariate and multivariate Cox regression analysis of variables with OS.

| Variables | Univariate | | Multivariate | |
|---|---|---|---|---|
| | HR (95% CI) | p-value | HR (95% CI) | p-value |
| Age (<60 vs. ≥60) | 0.98 (0.43–2.23) | 0.957 | | |
| Gender(female vs. male) | 0.72 (0.51–1.02) | 0.065 | | |
| Disease stage (Limited vs. Extended) | 3.16 (1.36–7.40) | 0.007* | 2.13 (1.32–3.44) | 0.002* |
| Smoking status (smoker vs. nonsmoker) | 0.99 (0.97–1.01) | 0.141 | | |
| Performance status (0, 1 vs. 2, 3) | 1.09 (0.97–1.22) | 0.089 | | |
| Chemotherapy regimen (EP vs. IP) | 1.37 (0.65–2.86) | 0.408 | | |
| YKL-40 (high vs. low) | 1.33 (0.65–2.21) | 0.001* | 1.84 (1.08–3.15) | 0.025* |

HR, hazard ratio; CI, confidence interval; EP, cisplatin with etoposide; IP, cisplatin with irinotecan.
*Significant difference.

## Association of Serum YKL-40 Levels with Survival

Low serum YKL-40 patients had significantly longer PFS and OS than high serum YKL-40 patients (Figure 4 and 5). The median PFS and OS were 6 and 10 months for high serum YKL-40 patients compared with 9 and 18 months for low serum YKL-40 patients, respectively. The 1-year survival rate was 40.7% in the 81 cases with high serumYKL-40, and 51.3% in the 39 cases with low serum YKL-40, a statistically significant difference ($p = 0.041$).

In univariate Cox analysis, the pre-chemotherapy serum YKL-40 level (dichotomized as >65.7 ng/mL vs ≤65.7 ng/mL) was associated with PFS (HR = 1.74, $p = 0.033$) and OS (HR = 1.33, $p = 0.001$) (Table 5 and Table 6). Univariate analysis of prognostic significance also showed that disease stage was significantly associated with poor survival. However, no association with the patient's prognosis was noted for age, gender, smoking, performance status and chemotherapy regimen.

In multivariate Cox analysis, the pre-chemotherapy serum level of YKL-40 was independent prognostic factor for OS and PFS in the patients with SCLC (Table 5 and Table 6).

## Discussion

YKL-40 is a chitinase-like protein. The biologic functions of YKL-40 in cancer cells are unknown, and very few studies have evaluated the functional role of YKL-40 expression in cancer cells. It has been suggested that YKL-40 plays a role in the proliferation and differentiation of malignant cells, protects the cells from undergoing apoptosis, stimulates angiogenesis, has an effect on extracellular tissue remodeling, and stimulates fibroblast activity or proliferation surrounding the cancer cells [23,24].

The objective of the current investigation was to study the association between the pre-chemotherapy serum YKL-40 level and chemotherapy response and clinical outcomes of patients with SCLC. In the present study, serum YKL-40 levels were higher in SCLC patients in line with the levels reported in most other types of cancer [25–27]. Furthermore, with a cut-off value of 65.7 ng/mL, YKL-40 had a sensitivity of 67.5% and a specificity of 95.0% for the prediction of SCLC, making it a potential adjunctive tool for diagnosis of SCLC. Importantly, the serum levels of YKL-40 were significantly correlated with disease stage, while there were no difference with age, gender, smoking status and performance status.

Reports regarding the association of YKL-40 expression with response to chemotherapy are few and varied. Gronlund et al

reported that high serum levels of YKL-40 were associated with increased risk of second-line chemoresistance in patients with ovarian cancer [28]. However, Thöm et al found that the pretreatment serum YKL-40 level had no impact on response to chemotherapy in non-small cell lung cancer (NSCLC) [20]. Our study clearly showed that high serum YKL-40 patients response to chemotherapy were poorer than those of low serum YKL-40 patients. These results probably reflect different mechanisms of carcinogenesis between SCLC and NSCLC. Additionally, we observed that the pre-chemotherapy serum YKL-40 levels of the responder groups which were sensitive to chemotherapy were significantly lower than those of the non-responder groups which were resistant to chemotherapy. Moreover, serum YKL-40 levels were significantly decreased after chemotherapy, especially in the positive response group. To date, the mechanism of YKL-40 involved in resistance to chemotherapy is currently unclear.

Many studies have shown that serum YKL-40 was an important factor to predict the prognosis of several types of cancer [11–17]. Recently, Choi et al reported that high pretreatment serum YKL-40 level in patients with NSCLC was an independent prognostic variable of poor prognosis [18]. In SCLC patients, a high serum YKL-40 at the time of diagnosis and before chemotherapy was independent of prognostic variables for survival within the first 6 months and independent of age, performance status, and serum lactate dehydrogenase [19]. In our study, we have demonstrated that serum YKL-40 level in patients with SCLC was related to their very poor prognosis, as illustrated by the short PFS and OS in SCLC patients that had the highest serum YKL-40 levels. It is noteworthy that a high serum YKL-40 level was an independent prognostic biomarker of poor survival in this patient population. The mechanism involved in the association between YKL-40 and a poor prognosis is poorly understood. Previous studies suggested that poor survival in cancer patients with elevated YKL-40 might be attributed to the promotion of angiogenesis [17,29].

In conclusion, the serum level of YKL-40 in SCLC patients was significantly higher than healthy controls. Serum YKL-40 in the positive chemotherapeutic response group was significantly lower after chemotherapy. The results not only further support that serum YKL-40 is related to chemotherapy response, but also provide clues that YKL-40 possess the potential to be a serum diagnostic and prognostic marker for SCLC. Moreover, further work is underway to both replicate these findings in a study with a larger cohort in lung cancer.

## Author Contributions

Conceived and designed the experiments: LKY. Performed the experiments: CHX. Analyzed the data: KKH. Contributed reagents/materials/analysis tools: CHX LKY KKH. Wrote the paper: CHX.

## References

1. Chen Z, Wang T, Cai L, Su C, Zhong B, et al. (2012) Clinicopathological significance of non-small cell lung cancer with high prevalence of Oct-4 tumor cells. J Exp Clin Cancer Res 31: 10.

2. Maddison P, Thorpe A, Silcocks P, Robertson JF, Chapman CJ (2010) Autoimmunity to SOX2, clinical phenotype and survival in patients with small-cell lung cancer. Lung Cancer 70: 335–339.

3. J Barata F, Costa AF (2007) Small cell lung cancer-state of the art and future perspectives. Rev Port Pneumol 13: 587–604.

4. Govindan R, Page N, Morgensztern D, Read W, Tierney R, et al. (2006) Changing epidemiology of small-cell lung cancer in the United States over the last 30 years: analysis of the surveillance, epidemiologic, and end results database. J Clin Oncol 24: 4539–4544.

5. Free CM, Ellis M, Beggs L, Beggs D, Morgan SA, et al. (2007) Lung cancer outcomes at a UK cancer unit between 1998-2001. Lung Cancer 57: 222–228.

6. Okamura K, Takayama K, Izumi M, Harada T, Furuyama K, et al. (2013) Diagnostic value of CEA and CYFRA 21-1 tumor markers in primary lung cancer. Lung Cancer 80: 45–49.

7. Tufman A, Huber RM (2010) Biological markers in lung cancer: A clinician's perspective. Cancer Biomark 6: 123–135.

8. Grunnet M, Sorensen JB (2012) Carcinoembryonic antigen (CEA) as tumor marker in lung cancer. Lung Cancer 76: 138–143.

9. Johansen JS, Jensen BV, Roslind A, Nielsen D, Price PA (2006) Serum YKL-40, a new prognostic biomarker in cancer patients? Cancer Epidemiol Biomarkers Prev 15: 194–202.

10. Bi J, Lau SH, Lv ZL, Xie D, Li W, et al. (2009) Overexpression of YKL-40 is an independent prognostic marker in gastric cancer. Hum Pathol 40: 1790–1797.

11. Schmidt H, Johansen JS, Sjoegren P, Christensen IJ, Sorensen BS, et al. (2006) Serum YKL-40 predicts relapse-free and overall survival in patients with American Joint Committee on Cancer stage I and II melanoma. J Clin Oncol 24: 798–804.

12. Yamac D, Ozturk B, Coskun U, Tekin E, Sancak B, et al. (2008) Serum YKL-40 levels as a prognostic factor in patients with locally advanced breast cancer. Adv Ther 25: 801–809.

13. Høgdall EV, Ringsholt M, Høgdall CK, Christensen IJ, Johansen JS, et al. (2009) YKL-40 tissue expression and plasma levels in patients with ovarian cancer. BMC Cancer 9: 8.

14. Dupont J, Tanwar MK, Thaler HT, Fleisher M, Kauff N, et al. (2004) Early detection and prognosis of ovarian cancer using serum YKL-40. J Clin Oncol 22: 3330–3339.

15. Jensen BV, Johansen JS, Price PA (2003) High levels of serum HER-2/neu and YKL-40 independently reflect aggressiveness of metastatic breast cancer. Clin Cancer Res 9: 4423–4434.

16. Wang D, Zhai B, Hu F, Liu C, Zhao J, et al. (2012) High YKL-40 serum concentration is correlated with prognosis of Chinese patients with breast cancer. PLoS One 7: e51127.

17. Saidi A, Javerzat S, Bellahcène A, De Vos J, Bello L, et al. (2008) Experimental anti-angiogenesis causes upregulation of genes associated with poor survival in glioblastoma. Int J Cancer 122: 2187–2198.

18. Choi IK, Kim YH, Kim JS, Seo JH (2010) High serum YKL-40 is a poor prognostic marker in patients with advanced non-small cell lung cancer. Acta Oncol 49: 861–864.

19. Johansen JS, Drivsholm L, Price PA, Christensen IJ (2004) High serum YKL-40 level in patients with small cell lung cancer is related to early death. Lung Cancer 46: 333–340.

20. Thöm I, Andritzky B, Schuch G, Burkholder I, Edler L, et al. (2010) Elevated pretreatment serum concentration of YKL-40-An independent prognostic biomarker for poor survival in patients with metastatic nonsmall cell lung cancer. Cancer 116: 4114–4121.

21. van Meerbeeck JP, Fennell DA, De Ruysscher DK (2011) Small-cell lung cancer. Lancet 378: 1741–1755.

22. Therasse P, Arbuck SG, Eisenhauer EA, Wanders J, Kaplan RS, et al. (2000) New guidelines to evaluate the response to treatment in solid tumors. European Organization for Research and Treatment of Cancer, National Cancer Institute of the United States, National Cancer Institute of Canada. J Natl Cancer Inst 92: 205–216.

23. Lee CG, Hartl D, Lee GR, Koller B, Matsuura H, et al. (2009) Role of breast regression protein 39 (BRP-39)/chitinase 3-like-1 in Th2 and IL-13- induced tissue responses and apoptosis. J Exp Med 206: 1149–1166.

24. Shao R, Hamel K, Petersen L, Cao QJ, Arenas RB, et al. (2009) YKL-40, a secreted glycoprotein, promotes tumor angiogenesis. Oncogene 28: 4456–4468.

25. Zou L, He X, Zhang JW (2010) The efficacy of YKL-40 and CA125 as biomarkers for epithelial ovarian cancer. Braz J Med Biol Res 43: 1232–1238.

26. Mitsuhashi A, Matsui H, Usui H, Nagai Y, Tate S, et al. (2009) Serum YKL-40 as a marker for cervical adenocarcinoma. Ann Oncol 20: 71–77.

27. Schultz NA, Christensen IJ, Werner J, Giese N, Jensen BV, et al. (2013) Diagnostic and prognostic impact of circulating YKL-40, IL-6, and CA 19.9 in patients with pancreatic cancer. PLoS One 8: e67059.

28. Gronlund B, Høgdall EV, Christensen IJ, Johansen JS, Nørgaard-Pedersen B, et al. (2006) Pre-treatment prediction of chemoresistance in second-line chemotherapy of ovarian carcinoma: value of serological tumor marker determination (tetranectin, YKL-40, CASA, CA 125). Int J Biol Markers 21: 141–148.

29. Mylin AK, Andersen NF, Johansen JS, Abildgaard N, Heickendorff L, et al. (2009) Serum YKL-40 and bone marrow angiogenesis in multiple myeloma. Int J Cancer 124: 1492–1494.

# 16

# Optical Imaging for Monitoring Tumor Oxygenation Response after Initiation of Single-Agent Bevacizumab followed by Cytotoxic Chemotherapy in Breast Cancer Patients

**Shigeto Ueda**[1]*, **Ichiei Kuji**[2], **Takashi Shigekawa**[1], **Hideki Takeuchi**[1], **Hiroshi Sano**[1], **Eiko Hirokawa**[1], **Hiroko Shimada**[1], **Hiroaki Suzuki**[3], **Motoki Oda**[3], **Akihiko Osaki**[1], **Toshiaki Saeki**[1]

**1** Department of Breast Oncology, International Medical Center, Saitama Medical University, Hidaka, Saitama, Japan, **2** Department of Nuclear Medicine, International Medical Center, Saitama Medical University, Hidaka, Saitama, Japan, **3** Central Research Laboratory, Hamamatsu Photonics K.K., Hamakita-ku, Hamamatsu, Japan

## Abstract

*Purpose:* Optical imaging techniques for measuring tissue hemoglobin concentration have been recently accepted as a way to assess tumor vascularity and oxygenation. We investigated the correlation between early optical response to single-agent bevacizumab and treatment outcome.

*Methods:* Seven patients with advanced or metastatic breast cancer were treated with single-agent bevacizumab followed by addition of weekly paclitaxel. Optical imaging of patient's breasts was performed to measure tumor total hemoglobin concentration (tHb) and oxygen saturation ($stO_2$) at baseline and on days 1, 3, 6, 8, and 13 after the first infusion of bevacizumab. To assess early metabolic response, 2-deoxy-2-($^{18}$F)-fluoro-D-glucose (FDG) positron emission tomography/computed tomography (PET/CT), $^{18}$F-fluoromisonidazole (FMISO)-PET/CT, and magnetic resonance imaging were performed at baseline and after two cycles of the regimen.

*Results:* Seven patients were grouped as responders (n = 4) and nonresponders (n = 3) on the basis of metabolic response measured by FDG-PET/CT. The responders showed remarkable tumor shrinkage and low accumulations of FMISO tracer relative to those of the nonresponders at the completion of two cycles of chemotherapy. Tumors of both groups showed remarkable attenuation of mean tHb as early as day 1 after therapy initiation. The nonresponders had lower baseline $stO_2$ levels compared with adjacent breast tissue $stO_2$ levels along with a pattern of steadily low $stO_2$ levels during the observation window. On the other hand, the responders appeared to sustain high $stO_2$ levels with temporal fluctuation.

*Conclusions:* Low tumor $stO_2$ level after single-agent bevacizumab treatment was characteristic of the nonresponders. Tumor $stO_2$ level could be a predictor of an additional benefit of bevacizumab over that provided by paclitaxel.

**Editor:** Elad Katz, AMS Biotechnology, United Kingdom

**Funding:** This work was supported by JSPS KAKENHI Grant Number 25830105 and Hidaka Research Grant. The funders had no role in study design, data collection and analysis, decision to publish, or preparation of the manuscript.

**Competing Interests:** Hiroaki Suzuki and Motoki Oda are employed by Hamamatsu Photonics K.K. Hamamatsu Photonics K.K. has patents related to development of TRS20 (Patent number, US5836883A, patent name, Measuring the characteristics of a scattering medium; US6104946A, Measuring method and apparatus of absorption information of scattering medium; US6567165B1, Concentration measuring method and apparatus for absorption component in scattering medium; US6704110B2, Method and apparatus for measuring internal information of scattering medium; US0100449A1, Method and device for measuring scattering-absorption body). There are no further patents, products in development or marketed products to declare.

* E-mail: syueda@saitama-med.ac.jp

## Introduction

Bevacizumab, a monoclonal antibody against vascular endothelial growth factor (VEGF) A, has demonstrated clinical efficacy in combination with chemotherapy in patients with HER2 negative breast cancer [1],[2]. To date, although it is believed that a particular subset of patients could greatly benefit from early adoption of bevacizumab in addition to chemotherapy, no specific biomarkers for assessing bevacizumab response have been consistently validated [3].

Diffuse optical spectroscopic imaging (DOSI) is a noninvasive imaging technology using near-infrared light that can measure tissue hemoglobin concentration obtained from spectroscopic oxy-hemoglobin ($O_2Hb$) and deoxy-hemoglobin (HHb) data as well as directly visualize vascularity and tissue oxygenation indicated from tHb ($O_2Hb$+HHb) and $stO_2$ ($O_2Hb$/tHb), respectively [4],[5]. DOSI has been currently integrated into several clinical neoadjuvant studies that have explored hemodynamic biomarkers for predicting early treatment response [6],[7],[8].

Zhu et al. reported that remarkable reduction in tumor tHb of primary breast cancer after early treatment cycles of neoadjuvant chemotherapy could predict favorable pathological outcome [7]. In a separate study, Roblyer et al. reported that transient increase in $O_2$Hb on day 1 after chemotherapy initiation was characteristic of responders but not nonresponders [8]. These results suggested the clinical importance of tumor oxygenation response to chemotherapy sensitivity. Jain first proposed a therapeutic concept with bevacizumab involving a "normalization window" of tumor vasculature in which more accurate remodeling of the disorganized structure and abnormal functioning of tumor vessels would improve perfusion and enhance tissue oxygenation, which would result in more efficient delivery of cytotoxic drugs [9]. We hypothesized that if vascular normalization occurs after successful vascular remodeling, tumor tHb level should decrease and $stO_2$ level should simultaneously improve.

In this clinical study, we used DOSI to monitor tumor mean tHb and $stO_2$ levels after the initiation of single-agent bevacizumab followed by cytotoxic chemotherapy in patients with advanced or metastatic breast cancer and determined if early changes in tHb and $stO_2$ over a period of single-agent bevacizumab administration could be a predictor of treatment response.

## Materials and Methods

From October 2012 through December 2013, we enrolled patients with locally advanced or metastatic HER2-negative breast cancer (TNM stage III or IV) to receive a combination chemotherapy regimen with paclitaxel and bevacizumab. Patients who have received prior chemotherapy or hormonal therapy before participating in this study were also included. Patient history, including histopathological and radiological imaging results and Ki67 proliferative index, was obtained from medical records. The treatment regimen reported in the study was standard care.

This study was approved by the institutional review board of the International Medical Center, Saitama Medical University, and written informed consent was obtained from each participant prior to inclusion (12-084).

### Chemotherapy regimen

All patients received bevacizumab (5 mg/kg body weight) intravenously on days 1 and 15 in combination with paclitaxel (80 mg/m$^2$ body surface area) on days 1, 8, and 15, repeated every 4 weeks (Figure 1) [10]. Paclitaxel infusion was omitted on the first day of the first cycle. Dexamethasone (6.6 mg) and an $H_2$ antagonist were used for supportive treatment during the course of chemotherapy; however, use of these drugs in the first infusion of bevacizumab was omitted. Breast surgery was performed for patients deemed resectable after 5–6 weeks of completion of the initial chemotherapy. Treatment continued for six cycles unless there was disease progression, unacceptable toxicity, or withdrawal of consent. If study treatment was discontinued, further local and/or systemic treatment was permitted at the investigator's discretion.

### TRS breast imaging system

To extract quantitative hemoglobin concentrations from breast tissue, we developed a system that used a time-correlated single-photon counting (TCSPC) method for measuring temporal response profiles of tissue against optical pulse inputs and enabled quantitative analysis of light absorption and scattering in tissue according to the photon diffusion theory [4],[11]. This approach

could quantify $O_2$Hb and HHb tissue levels. Details of the TRS breast imaging system have been previously published [12].

An ultrasound-assisted optical probe was used to visualize the largest tumor lesions, which were located in the center of a 10-mm square grid map that was constructed for the lesion and surrounding normal tissue. The grid map of a tumor-bearing breast basically comprised 7×7 points with a 10-mm interval between two points in the x–y dimension. For spline interpolation, custom software (DataBreastViewer, version 109; SincereTechnology Corp., Kanagawa, Japan) was used to perform 2D image processing and analysis.

### Hemodynamic biomarkers

The distribution of tHb levels of a tumor-bearing breast shows the functional vascular tumor volume, which is contrasted by that of the surrounding normal tissue. The distribution of $stO_2$ levels maps the magnitude of tissue oxygenation of breast tissue. A lesional region of interest (ROI) 2 cm in radius from the center of the tumor was constructed, and the mean levels of tHb and $stO_2$ were calculated. To demonstrate the capacity of DOSI to reveal the tumor response of bevacizumab, we monitored changes in the mean levels of tHb and $stO_2$ of a tumor-bearing breast and a normal contralateral breast at baseline (day -1) and on days 1, 3, 6, 8, and 13 after the first infusion of bevacizumab.

### Serial examination of positron emission tomography (PET)/computed tomography (CT) using 2-deoxy-2-($^{18}$F)-fluoro-D-glucose (FDG) and $^{18}$F-fluoromisonidazole (FMISO)

Biograph 6 (Siemens, Medical Systems, Inc.:Suite, Washinton, D.C., United States) was used to perform PET/CT. Details of the FDG PET/CT procedure have been described previously [13] [14]. All patients were required to fast for at least 6 h to confirm normal glucose blood levels. One hour after the administration of FDG tracer (3.7 MBq/kg), the patients were positioned prone on the whole-body PET/CT scanner couch. CT was initially performed followed by a PET emission scan that covered the identical transverse field of view. The Biograph allows simultaneous collection of 16 slices over a span of 15.8 mm with a slice thickness of 2.5 mm and a transaxial resolution of 6.3 mm. The acquisition time was 2 min per table positron. PET scans were processed, reconstructed with an ordered subset expectation maximization, and measured attenuation correction. Ordered subset expectation maximization image reconstruction was used for all data. Acquisition of PET data was operated in three-dimensional and high resolution mode.

According to protocol, FMISO-PET/CT scan was basically performed 1 day after the FDG-PET/CT scan. All patients were intravenously injected with 7.4 MBq/kg of FMISO. At 2 h after injection, FMISO-PET/CT was performed immediately after the CT scan. ROIs with 1.0-cm maximum diameters were drawn on the areas of abnormal FDG or FMISO accumulation corresponding to the baseline tumor lesions. In a series of PET/CT scans, care was taken to draw the ROI in the same lesion as shown on the baseline lesion. For deciding each ROI, CT combined with PET provided anatomical landmarks for detecting the lesion, and the maximal standardized uptake value (SUVmax) was recorded from the target. The PET/CT images were analyzed by at least two radiologists in a blinded manner. SUV was calculated according to the following formula:

SUV = activity concentration in ROI (MBq/ml)/injection dose (MBq/kg body weight). The serial FDG and FMISO PET/CT scans were scheduled before treatment initiation and after two

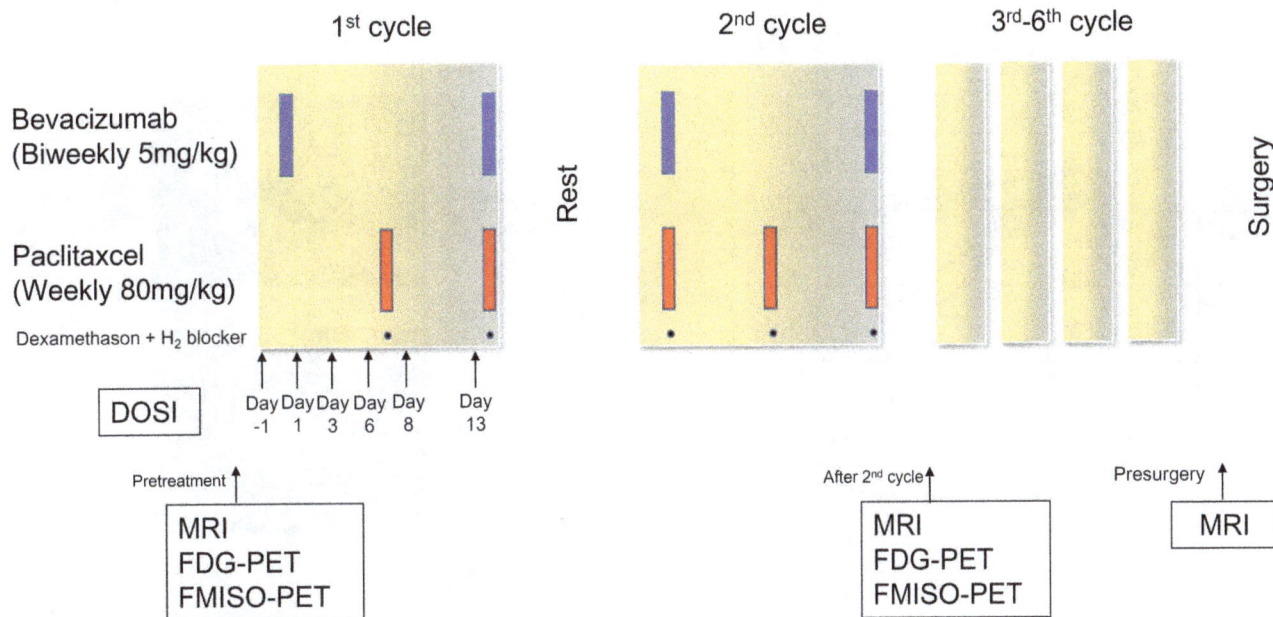

**Figure 1. The schedule of treatment and imaging tests.** Schematic of combination treatment for patients with advanced or metastatic breast cancer. All patients received bevacizumab (5 mg/kg body weight) intravenously on days 1 and 15 in combination with paclitaxel (80 mg/m$^2$ body surface area) on days 1, 8, and 15 and repeated every 4 weeks. Subsequently, the patients underwent 5 additional cycles of bevacizumab and paclitaxel. Both before treatment and after the 2$^{nd}$ cycle of chemotherapy, the patients underwent MRI, FDG-PET/CT, and FMISO-PET/CT. Imaging using diffuse optical spectroscopy was also performed on day 1 before the first infusion of bevacizumab and on days 1, 3, 6, 8, and 13 after the infusion.

cycles of chemotherapy. PET/CT scans were performed at least 2 weeks after performing a diagnostic core biopsy and after infusion of drug.

## Serial examination using breast magnetic resonance imaging (MRI)

Details of the breast MRI have been described previously [15]. The device used was a 1.5-T instrument (Avanto; Siemens, Erlangen, Germany) that used a body coil for transmission and a two-channel breast array coil for reception. For measuring maximum diameters of lesions, post-contrast coronal, axial, and sagittal images obtained by contrast-enhanced dynamic imaging were used. The percentage changes in tumor maximal size at baseline and after two cycles for lesions were assessed radiographically.

## Study end points

The schedule of imaging studies using DOSI, MRI, FDG-PET/CT, and FMISO-PET/CT is shown in Figure 1. Early tumor metabolic response assessed by serial FDG-PET/CT has been widely accepted as predictive of clinicopathological outcome for advanced breast cancer in a neoadjuvant setting [16],[17]. An optimal cutoff value between 40% and 65% of the baseline SUV has been suggested for potential early identification of nonresponders. In this study, we employed a reduction rate of 40% as a cutoff value for FDG-SUV to separate responders from nonresponders (Figure 2A).

## Criteria for morphological response

Patients underwent MRI tests to compare size reduction between baseline and the completion of treatment according to the RECIST guideline [18]. The protocol stipulated that the initial treatment should be discontinued in patients who showed progressive disease (PD) (20% or more increase in size) or appearance of new metastatic lesions and that such patients should be excluded from further participation in the study.

## Assessment of pathological response

Pathological tumor response was determined on the basis of the General Rules of Criteria and Pathological Recording of Breast Cancer 2007 by at least two pathologists [19]. Surgical specimens were cut in 0.5-cm-thick slices and evaluated for the presence of microscopic tumor cells in the invasive area as well as areas with marked fibrosis or scarring, and the presence of ductal component and lymph nodal metastasis was not evaluated. No residual invasive cancer cells in all areas of the surgical specimens was defined as pathological complete response or pCR (grade 3). The disappearance or marked degeneration of two-thirds or more of the tumor cells was defined as substantially effective (grade 2). The disappearance or marked degeneration of one-third to less than two-thirds was defined as moderately effective (grade 1b). The disappearance or marked degeneration of less than one-third of the tumor cells or mild tumor cell degeneration, regardless of the percentage, was defined as mildly effective (grade 1a). Almost no change in cancer cells after treatment was defined as not effective (grade 0).

## Statistics

MedCalc software (Mariakerke, Belgium) was used to perform statistical evaluations. Continuous variables were presented as means, median, and standard deviations (SD). A paired Student's $t$-test was used to analyze changes in variables. Differences at a p value of less than 5% were considered to be statistically significant.

(A)

(B)

(C)

(D)

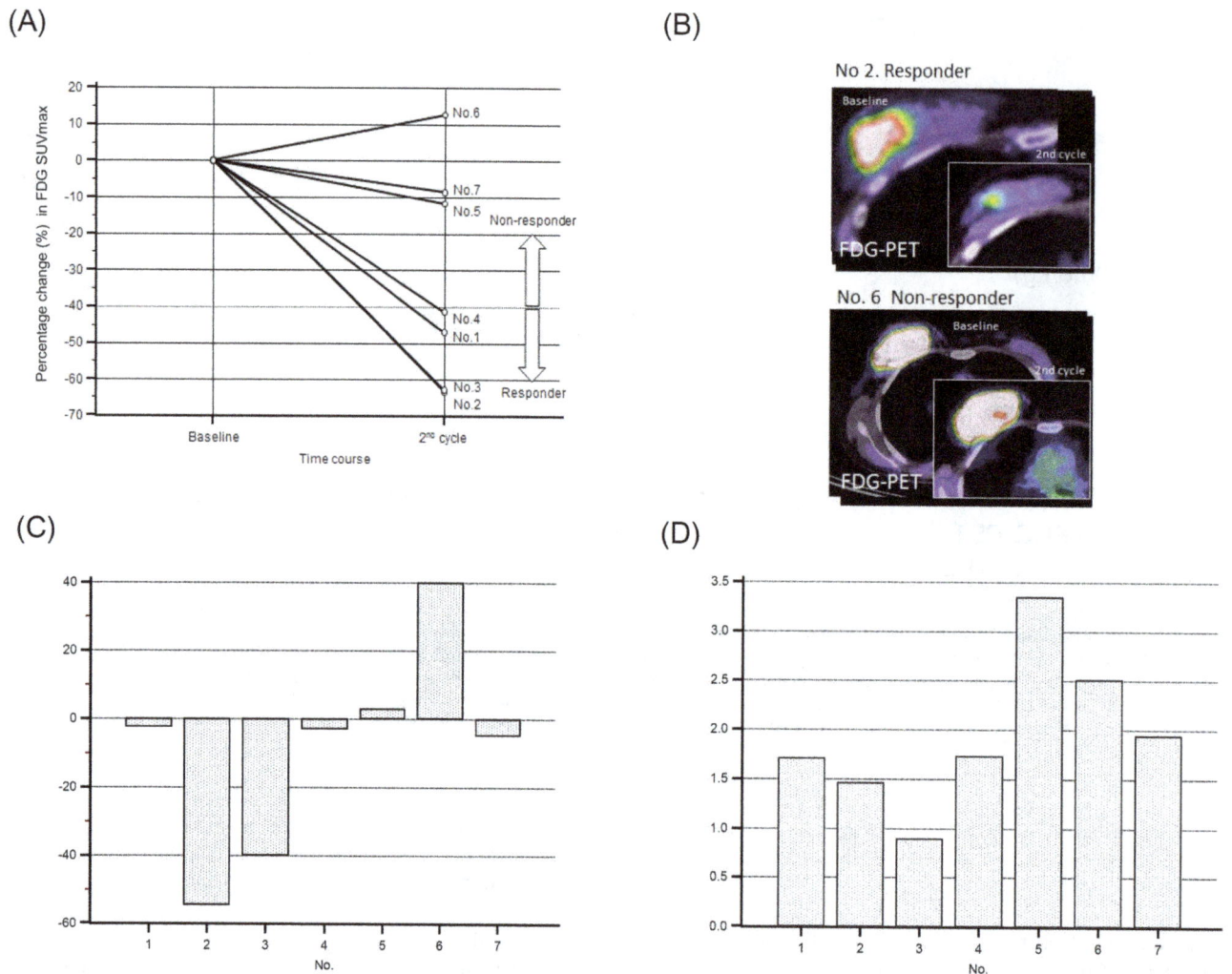

**Figure 2. Results of tumor shrinkage and hypoxia after 2nd cycle of chemotherapy.** A. Percentage change in 18F-fluorodeoxyglucose uptake expressed as standardized uptake value (%SUV) from baseline after 2nd cycle of chemotherapy regimen. Patients with %SUV >-40% were considered as responders and others were as nonresponders. B. Representative examples of transversal fused PET/CT scans at baseline and after 2nd cycle of chemotherapy with responders (No. 2) and nonresponders (No. 6) are shown. C. Percentage change in maximal size as measured by breast MRI at baseline and after 2nd cycle of chemotherapy. Patient Nos. 1, 2, 3, and 4 were responders and Nos. 5, 6 and 7 were nonresponders. There were no significant difference between responders (mean $-24.9\% \pm 26.4$ SD) and nonresponders ($12.7 \pm 23.9$ SD, p=0.1). D. Lesion maximal SUV (SUVmax) as measured by FMISO-PET/CT at the completion of the 2nd cycle of chemotherapy. The intensity of SUVmax indicates hypoxic activity of the tumor. Nonresponders (mean $2.6 \pm 0.7$ SD) had significantly higher FMISO-SUVmax than responders (mean $1.4 \pm 0.4$ SD, p=0.03)

## Results

### Baseline characteristics

We enrolled seven women in this study. All patients received at least two cycles of the regimen. One patient (No. 3) declined further treatment after the completion of two cycles and was therefore withdrawn from the study. Another patient (No. 6) discontinued the study treatment because of a paclitaxel-induced infusion reaction and then received further chemotherapy using nab-particle paclitaxel on a triweekly basis. All patients underwent DOSI, MRI, FDG-PET/CT, and FMISO-PET/CT imaging tests on treatment.

The baseline characteristics of the seven patients are shown in Table 1. The median age of the patients was 52.6 years (range, 36–63 years), and the median tumor size was 51.7 mm (range, 30–67 mm) assessed by breast MRI. Based on breast MRI and FDG-PET/CT examination, five patients were determined to have TNM stage III and two patient had stage IV with lung and

multiple bone metastases. One patient (No. 1) had previously received hormonal therapy, and the other six patients had not previously received systemic therapy. Five patients had histologically invasive ductal carcinoma (IDC) with luminal subtype, and two patients had IDC with triple-negative subtype.

### Assessment of therapeutic response

Employing a reduction rate of 40% as a cutoff value for FDG-PET/CT metabolic response, tumors with reductions ≥40% were defined as responders (n = 4), and tumors with <40% reductions were defined as nonresponders (n = 3) (Figure 2A and B). Figure 2C showed that the responders achieved remarkable tumor shrinkage (mean, $-24.9\% \pm 26.4$ SD) and Figure 2D showed low levels of FMISO-SUV (mean, 1.4, $\pm 0.4$ SD) at the completion of the 2nd cycle of chemotherapy. On the other hand, the nonresponders showed no evidence of tumor shrinkage (mean, $12.7\% \pm 23.9$ SD) but still sustained high levels of FMISO-SUV (mean, $2.6 \pm 0.7$ SD)

**Table 1.** Patient demographics.

| No. | Age (year) | Rt/Lt | Histology | Size (mm) | TNM stage | ER (%) | PgR (%) | HER2 | Ki67 (%) |
|---|---|---|---|---|---|---|---|---|---|
| 1 | 58 | Lt | IDC | 43 | T4N1M1 | 50 | 0 | 0 | 30 |
| 2 | 51 | Rt | IDC | 44 | T4N1M0 | 90 | 50 | 1 | 35 |
| 3 | 45 | Lt | IDC | 30 | T4N1M0 | 90 | 10 | 1 | 20 |
| 4 | 56 | rt | IDC | 67 | T3N1M0 | 0 | 0 | 1 | 15 |
| 5 | 61 | Rt | IDC | 67 | T3N1M0 | 90 | 90 | 1 | 20 |
| 6 | 36 | Rt | IDC | 50 | T4N3M0 | 50 | 50 | 1 | 70 |
| 7 | 63 | Lt | IDC | 61 | T4N1M1 | 0 | 0 | 0 | 65 |

Lt, left; Rt, right; IDC, invasive ductal carcinoma; ER, estrogen receptor; PgR, progesteron receptor; HER2; c-erb-B 2.

at the same time point. There was significant difference of FMISO-SUV level between responders and nonresponders (p = 0.03).

All nonresponding patients included PD on the basis of RECIST criteria and/or histopathologically no response (grade 0) following surgery. On the other hands, all responding patients included partial response (PR) and/or histopathologically marked or moderate response (grade 2 or grade 1b) (Table 2).

## Assessment of hemodynamic biomarkers

Figure 3A and B showed three dimensional reconstruction mapping of tHb and $stO_2$ levels of tumor-bearing breast and contralateral normal breast. All patients had a hotspot corresponding to tumor lesion and significantly higher tHb of tumor-bearing breast (mean, 60.5 $\mu$M$\pm$38.5 SD) compared with that of contralateral normal breast (mean, 15.2 $\mu$M$\pm$5.1 SD, p = 0.009). Responding tumors (mean, 37.2%$\pm$9.5 SD) had significantly lower level of tHb compared to nonresponding tumors (mean, 91.6%$\pm$42.1 SD, p = 0.04). In contrast, for $stO_2$ maps, there was no difference between tumor (mean, 67.3%$\pm$9.3 SD) and normal tissue (mean, 67.3%$\pm$5.1 SD, p = 0.9). Responding tumors appeared an elevation of $stO_2$ level corresponding to tumor lesion and surrounding normal tissue, while nonresponding tumors showed a dip of $stO_2$ level compared to surrounding normal tissue.

Figures 4 present serial maps of the distribution of tHb (A) and $stO_2$ (B) levels in tumor-bearing breasts of all the patients over the observed time window during treatment.

Figure 5A shows the change in the mean tumor tHb levels from baseline during treatment. The mean tumor tHb level at baseline (mean, 60.5 $\mu$M$\pm$38.5 SD) was compared with those at day 1 (mean, 49.6 $\mu$M$\pm$26.3 SD, p = 0.5), day 3 (mean, 47.5 $\mu$M$\pm$32.3 SD, p = 0.5), day 6 (mean, 54.6 $\mu$M$\pm$41.9 SD, p = 0.7), day 8 (mean, 50.5 $\mu$M$\pm$30.9 SD, p = 0.6), and day 13 (mean, 58.8 $\mu$M$\pm$40.7 SD, p = 0.9). There were no significant difference of tumor tHb level between responders and nonresponders on each time point.

Figure 5B shows the observed mean tumor $stO_2$ percentage at baseline and during the treatment. The mean $stO_2$ percentage at baseline did not differ between responders (mean, 70.9%$\pm$10.5 SD) and nonresponders (mean, 62.4%$\pm$5.4 SD, p = 0.1), but the mean $stO_2$ percentage was significantly higher in responding tumors at day 1 (mean, 71.1%$\pm$4.2 SD), day 3 (mean, 69.9%$\pm$9.6 SD), day 6 (mean, 71.6%$\pm$3.7SD) compared to nonresponding tumors at day 1 (mean, 58.7%$\pm$5.4 SD, p = 0.02), day 3 (mean, 55.3%$\pm$6.0 SD, p = 0.04), day 6 (mean, 58.7%$\pm$7.5 SD, p = 0.03). There were no significant difference at day 8 and 13 between two groups.

## Discussion

In this study, the breast cancer patients showed considerable variation in the early responses to single-agent bevacizumab. Our initial experience illustrates at least two patterns of tumor hemodynamics. When the patients were grouped into responders and nonresponders on the basis of the serial FDG-PET/CT results, both groups showed remarkably elevated tHb in lesions relative to the adjacent breast tissue tHb levels. Figure 5A shows that a transient decrease from the baseline tumor tHb level occurred in the responders and nonresponders during the first 1 weeks. This finding indicates that a decrease in tumor vascularity could not be a biomarker of substantially therapeutic response to bevacizumab but may be an indicator of other pharmacological effects of bevacizumab; for example, blockage of VEGF, which induces vasoconstriction [20]. Van der Veldt et al. reported that

**Table 2.** Therapeutic outcome of patients after administration of the initial chemotherapy.

| No. | Completed cycles of initial chemotherapy | % change in tumor size after initial chemotherapy | RECIST criteria | Intervention after initial chemotherapy | Post-surgical pathological assessment | Baseline FDG-SUV$_{max}$ | % change in SUV$_{max}$ at 2nd cycle | Metabolic response at 2nd cycle | Comments |
|---|---|---|---|---|---|---|---|---|---|
| 1 | 6 | −25.6 | PR | Surgery | Grade 2 | 9.8 | −47.1 | Response | The patient received endocrine therapy and showed no progression of disease for 6 months after surgery |
| 2 | 6 | −54.5 | PR | Surgery | Grade 2 | 8.5 | −63.3 | Response | The patient received adjuvant endocrine therapy and no evidence of relapse was found by routine imaging for 8 months after surgery |
| 3 | 2 | −40 | PR | - | - | 10.3 | −63 | Response | The patient declined further treatment after the completion of 2 cycles and was therefore withdrawn from the study |
| 4 | 6 | −25.4 | PR | Surgery | Grade 1b | 4.4 | −41.4 | Response | The patient received adjuvant endocrine therapy and no evidence of relapse was found by routine imaging for 7 months after surgery |
| 5 | 5 | −13.4 | SD | Surgery | Grade 0 | 6.8 | −11.8 | Nonresponse | The patient received adjuvant endocrine therapy and locoregional radiotherapy and no evidence of relapse was found by routine imaging for 7 months after surgery |
| 6 | 2 | 40 | PD | Surgery | Grade 0 | 23.2 | 12.7 | Nonresponse | The patient underwent adjuvant chemotherapy and locoregional radiotherapy, but relapse in the lung and bones was detected by CT scans 6 months after surgery. |
| 7 | 2 | −4.9 | PD | 2nd line chemotherapy | - | 17.8 | −8.5 | Nonresponse | Disease progression of primary and metastatic lesions of the lung and bones was detected by FDG-PET/CT scan after administration of 2 cycles of the initial chemotherapy |

PR,partial response; SD,stable disease; PD,progressive disease; Grade 2, disappearance or marked degeneration of two-thirds or more of tumor cells; Grade 1b, disappearance or marked degeneration of one-third to less than two-thirds of tumor cells; Grade 0, no change in tumor cells.

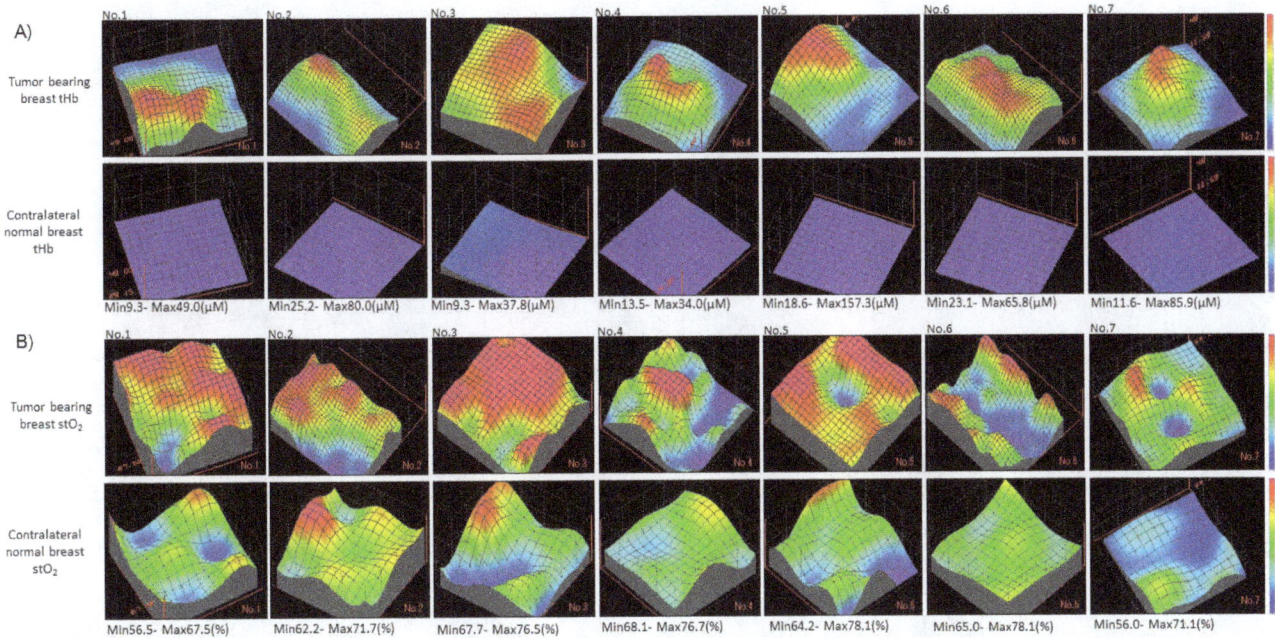

**Figure 3. Baseline maps of breast tHb and stO₂.** Three dimensional reconstruction mapping of baseline tHb (A) and stO₂ (B) of tumor-bearing breast and contralateral normal breast. Tumor-bearing breast map shows a 6×6-cm measurement area that included the tumor located at the center and surrounding normal tissues at the margins. Contralateral normal breast map includes a 4×4-cm measurement area corresponding a mirror image location.

patients who received single-agent bevacizumab had a significant decrease in plasma levels of circulating VEGF at 3 h after bevacizumab administration and the majority of patients had a substantial recovery in VEGF level after 4 days [21]. This trend of circulating VEGF level is consistent with our results of early tHb response to bevacizumab.

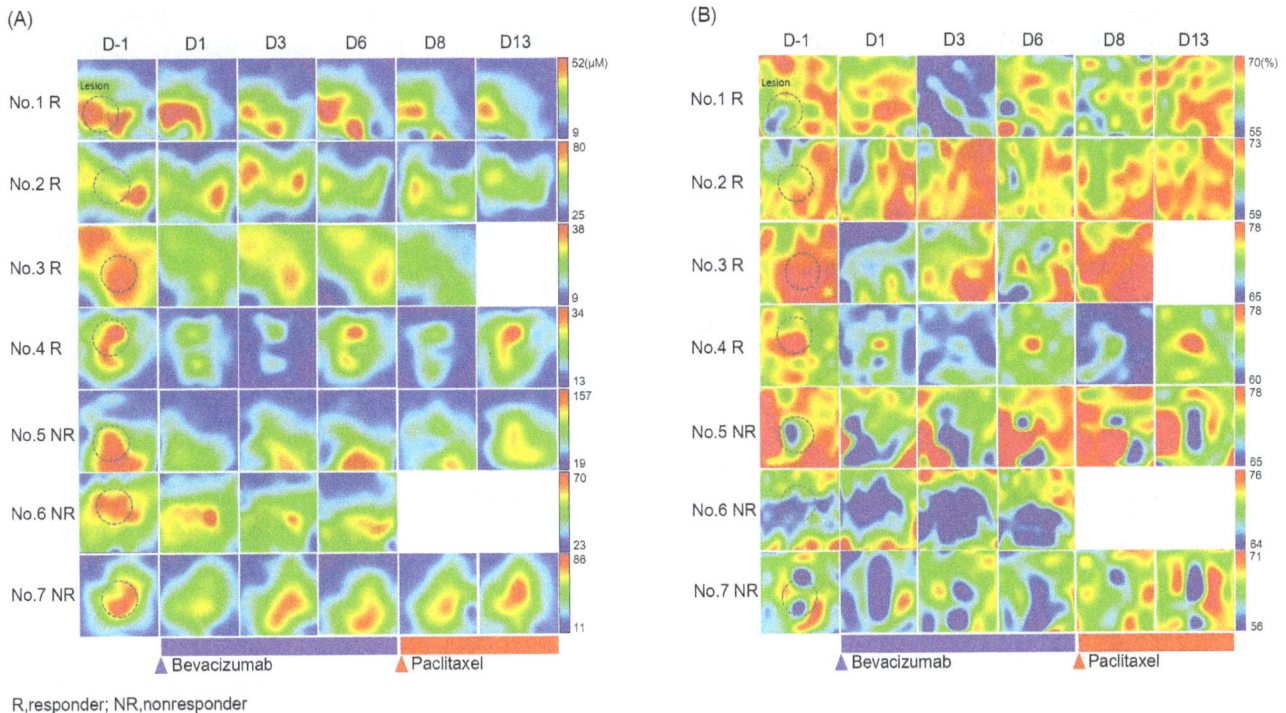

R, responder; NR, nonresponder

**Figure 4. Serial maps of tumor-bearing breast tHb and stO₂ on treatment.** Serial maps of tumor-bearing breast tHb (A) and stO₂ (B) during bevacizumab treatment at baseline (day −1) and on days 1, 3, 6, 8, and 13 after the initiation of bevacizumab. The measurement points of stO₂ were exactly identical to those of tHb during treatment.

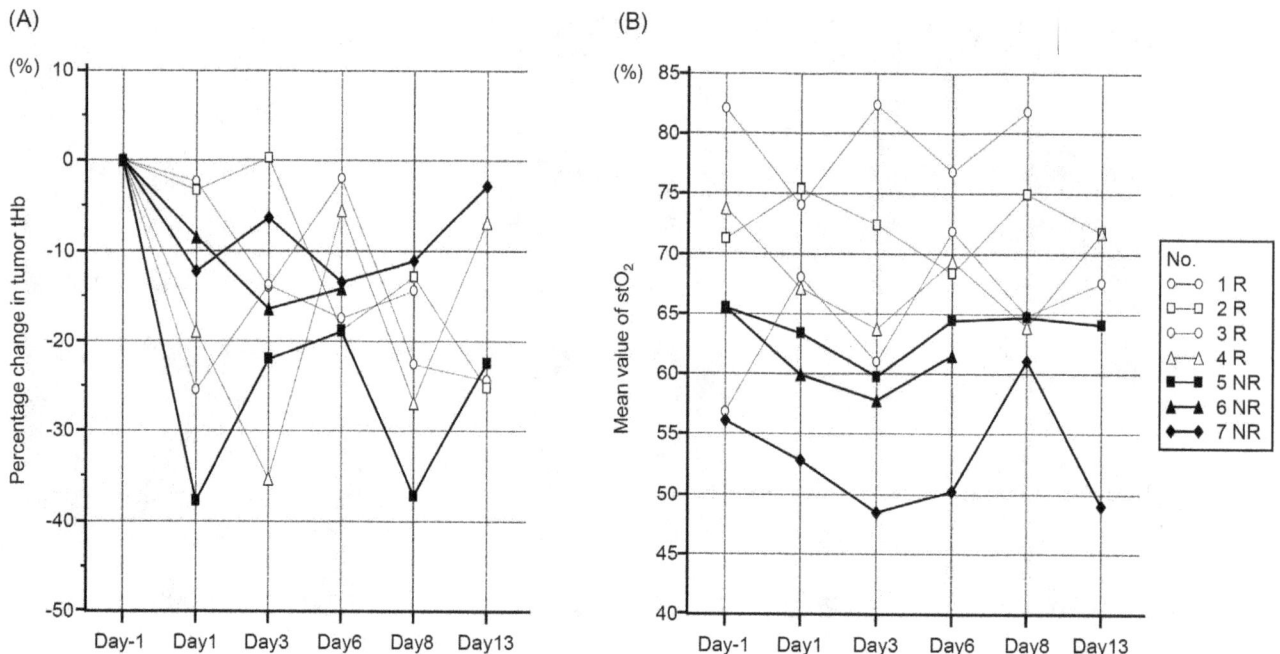

R,responder; NR,nonresponder

**Figure 5. Results of serial monitoring of tumor tHb and stO$_2$ during bevacizumab treatment.** A. Percentage change in tumor tHb on days 1, 3, 6, 8, and 13 after the initiation of bevacizumab relative to the baseline level. There were no significant difference of the value between responders and non-responders during the time points. B. The mean value of stO$_2$ at baseline (Day −1) and on days 1, 3, 6, 8, and 13 after the initiation of bevacizumab. The value of nonresponders was significantly lower than that of responders on day 1, day 3, and day 6 (p<0.05).

Figure 3B shows that the baseline stO$_2$ values of nonresponding tumors (Nos. 5, 6 and 7) were lower than those of the surrounding normal breast tissues, and sequential maps of figure 4B showed that relatively low levels of tumor stO$_2$ were sustained over the observation time window. In fact, these two patients had unfavorable pathological outcomes based on surgical findings and the other patient had progression of both primary and distant metastatic lesions after treatment. This result may indicate that severe chronic hypoxia was present at baseline with insufficient vascular remodeling and failure to normalize even after infusion of bevacizumab. On the other hand, the observed mean stO$_2$ levels of figure 5B at different time points in responding tumors fluctuated depending on the patient, but they apparently trended higher than those of the adjacent normal tissues during the observation time window. For example, the No. 2 patient had a responding tumor that showed a gradual increase in stO$_2$ on days 1 and 3 despite attenuation of tHb. This result may explain the effect of bevacizumab, which contributes to normalization of the tumor vasculature and enhances oxygenation. In fact, the No. 2 patient had a better pathological outcome with minimally invasive components at surgery. In the other patients defined as responders, the tumor stO$_2$ levels also varied greatly in response to bevacizumab but remained high during the observation time window. However, these tumors substantially improved stO$_2$ after paclitaxel and then achieved favorable pathological results. Thus, the concomitant change in tumor stO$_2$ may indicate how efficiently tumor oxygenation has recovered following vascular remodeling due to VEGF blockage.

In a retrospective study that examined 41 breast cancer patients who underwent neoadjuvant chemotherapy, Ueda et al. reported

that elevated baseline levels of tumor stO$_2$ significantly correlated with pCR [22]. In addition, the investigators claimed that tumor reoxygenation exhibited by elevation of tumor O$_2$Hb as early as day 1 after the initiation of cytotoxic chemotherapy, which is called O$_2$Hb flare, was adequate to discriminate nonresponding tumors from both partial and complete responders [8]. These findings were consistent with the current result that showed the significance of tumor oxygenation to improve chemotherapy response.

In essence, vascular normalization is considered to occur only in regions of the tumor where the abnormal and immature vasculature of the tumor microenvironment has been corrected by proper dosing and timing of bevacizumab, which would result in sufficient oxygen delivery [23]. In other words, our experience suggests that if vascular remodeling fails, bevacizumab-induced vessel regression may cause more severe hypoxia in the tumor microenvironment. However, a limitation of this preliminary study is that the number of patients was too limited to confirm this speculation. A larger number of patients is needed to verify our findings and provide sufficient evidence to support our speculation concerning the possible effect of bevacizumab in patients with failure of vascular remodeling.

In conclusion, this noninvasive optical imaging technique for visualizing vascularity and oxygenation could be useful for tracking the vascular normalization window. Although our findings are not definitive, the initial results suggest that a further study to identify a particular subset of patients who would benefit from bevacizumab may be beneficial.

## Acknowledgments

The authors thank Noriko Wakui for her excellent technical assistance and Yukio Ueda, PhD and Yutaka Yamashita, Central Research Laboratory, Hamamatsu Photonics K.K. for their sincere cooperation of this research.

## Author Contributions

Conceived and designed the experiments: SU T. Saeki IK. Performed the experiments: SU T. Shigekawa H. Shimada H. Sano EH AO HT. Analyzed the data: SU MO IK. Contributed reagents/materials/analysis tools: H. Suzuki MO. Wrote the paper: SU T. Saeki IK.

## References

1. Miller K, Wang M, Gralow J, Dickler M, Cobleigh M, et al. (2007) Paclitaxel plus bevacizumab versus paclitaxel alone for metastatic breast cancer. N Engl J Med 357: 2666–2676.

2. Bear HD, Tang G, Rastogi P, Geyer CE Jr, Robidoux A, et al. (2012) Bevacizumab added to neoadjuvant chemotherapy for breast cancer. N Engl J Med 366: 310–320.

3. Jain RK, Duda DG, Willett CG, Sahani DV, Zhu AX, et al. (2009) Biomarkers of response and resistance to antiangiogenic therapy. Nat Rev Clin Oncol 6: 327–338.

4. Patterson MS, Chance B, Wilson BC (1989) Time resolved reflectance and transmittance for the non-invasive measurement of tissue optical properties. Appl Opt 28: 2331–2336.

5. Cerussi A, Shah N, Hsiang D, Durkin A, Butler J, et al. (2006) In vivo absorption, scattering, and physiologic properties of 58 malignant breast tumors determined by broadband diffuse optical spectroscopy. J Biomed Opt 11: 044005.

6. Tromberg BJ, Cerussi A, Shah N, Compton M, Durkin A, et al. (2005) Imaging in breast cancer: diffuse optics in breast cancer: detecting tumors in premenopausal women and monitoring neoadjuvant chemotherapy. Breast Cancer Res 7: 279–285.

7. Zhu Q, DeFusco PA, Ricci A Jr, Cronin EB, Hegde PU, et al. (2013) Breast cancer: assessing response to neoadjuvant chemotherapy by using US-guided near-infrared tomography. Radiology 266: 433–442.

8. Roblyer D, Ueda S, Cerussi A, Tanamai W, Durkin A, et al. (2011) Optical imaging of breast cancer oxyhemoglobin flare correlates with neoadjuvant chemotherapy response one day after starting treatment. Proc Natl Acad Sci U S A 108: 14626–14631.

9. Jain RK (2005) Normalization of tumor vasculature: an emerging concept in antiangiogenic therapy. Science 307: 58–62.

10. Aogi K, Masuda N, Ohno S, Oda T, Iwata H, et al. (2011) First-line bevacizumab in combination with weekly paclitaxel for metastatic breast cancer: efficacy and safety results from a large, open-label, single-arm Japanese study. Breast Cancer Res Treat 129: 829–838.

11. Ueda Y, Yoshimoto K, Ohmae E, Suzuki T, Yamanaka T, et al. (2011) Time-resolved optical mammography and its preliminary clinical results. Technol Cancer Res Treat 10: 393–401.

12. Ueda S, Nakamiya N, Matsuura K, Shigekawa T, Sano H, et al. (2013) Optical imaging of tumor vascularity associated with proliferation and glucose metabolism in early breast cancer: clinical application of total hemoglobin measurements in the breast. BMC Cancer 13: 514.

13. Ueda S, Saeki T, Shigekawa T, Omata J, Moriya T, et al. (2012) 18F-fluorodeoxyglucose positron emission tomography optimizes neoadjuvant chemotherapy for primary breast cancer to achieve pathological complete response. Int J Clin Oncol 17: 276–282.

14. Imabayashi E, Matsuda H, Yoshimaru K, Kuji I, Seto A, et al. (2011) Pilot data on telmisartan short-term effects on glucose metabolism in the olfactory tract in Alzheimer's disease. Brain Behav 1: 63–69.

15. Mizukoshi W, Kozawa E, Inoue K, Saito N, Nishi N, et al. (2013) (1)H MR spectroscopy with external reference solution at 1.5 T for differentiating malignant and benign breast lesions: comparison using qualitative and quantitative approaches. Eur Radiol 23: 75–83.

16. Wang Y, Zhang C, Liu J, Huang G (2012) Is 18F-FDG PET accurate to predict neoadjuvant therapy response in breast cancer? A meta-analysis. Breast Cancer Res Treat 131: 357–369.

17. Mghanga FP, Lan X, Bakari KH, Li C, Zhang Y (2013) Fluorine-18 fluorodeoxyglucose positron emission tomography-computed tomography in monitoring the response of breast cancer to neoadjuvant chemotherapy: a meta-analysis. Clin Breast Cancer 13: 271–279.

18. Eisenhauer EA, Therasse P, Bogaerts J, Schwartz LH, Sargent D, et al. (2009) New response evaluation criteria in solid tumours: revised RECIST guideline (version 1.1). Eur J Cancer 45: 228–247.

19. Kurosumi M, Akashi-Tanaka S, Akiyama F, Komoike Y, Mukai H, et al. (2008) Histopathological criteria for assessment of therapeutic response in breast cancer (2007 version). Breast Cancer 15: 5–7.

20. Robinson ES, Khankin EV, Choueiri TK, Dhawan MS, Rogers MJ, et al. (2010) Suppression of the nitric oxide pathway in metastatic renal cell carcinoma patients receiving vascular endothelial growth factor-signaling inhibitors. Hypertension 56: 1131–1136.

21. Van der Veldt AA, Lubberink M, Bahce I, Walraven M, de Boer MP, et al. (2012) Rapid decrease in delivery of chemotherapy to tumors after anti-VEGF therapy: implications for scheduling of anti-angiogenic drugs. Cancer Cell 21: 82–91.

22. Ueda S, Roblyer D, Cerussi A, Durkin A, Leproux A, et al. (2012) Baseline tumor oxygen saturation correlates with a pathologic complete response in breast cancer patients undergoing neoadjuvant chemotherapy. Cancer Res 72: 4318–4328.

23. Goel S, Duda DG, Xu L, Munn LL, Boucher Y, et al. (2011) Normalization of the vasculature for treatment of cancer and other diseases. Physiol Rev 91: 1071–1121.

# 17

# ATO/ATRA/Anthracycline-Chemotherapy Sequential Consolidation Achieves Long-Term Efficacy in Primary Acute Promyelocytic Leukemia

Zi-Jie Long[1,9], Yuan Hu[1,9], Xu-Dong Li[1], Yi He[1], Ruo-Zhi Xiao[1], Zhi-Gang Fang[1], Dong-Ning Wang[1], Jia-Jun Liu[1], Jin-Song Yan[3], Ren-Wei Huang[1]*, Dong-Jun Lin[1]*, Quentin Liu[1,2]*

1 Department of Hematology, Third Affiliated Hospital, Sun Yat-sen University, Sun Yat-sen Institute of Hematology, Sun Yat-sen University, Guangzhou, China, 2 Institute of Cancer Stem Cell, Dalian Medical University, Dalian, China, 3 Department of Hematology, Second Affiliated Hospital, Dalian Medical University, Dalian, China

## Abstract

The combination of all-trans retinoic acid (ATRA) and arsenic trioxide ($As_2O_3$, ATO) has been effective in obtaining high clinical complete remission (CR) rates in acute promyelocytic leukemia (APL), but the long-term efficacy and safety among newly diagnosed APL patients are unclear. In this retrospective study, total 45 newly diagnosed APL patients received ATRA/chemotherapy combination regimen to induce remission. Among them, 43 patients (95.6%) achieved complete remission (CR) after induction therapy, followed by ATO/ATRA/anthracycline-based chemotherapy sequential consolidation treatment with a median follow-up of 55 months. In these patients, the estimated overall survival (OS) and the relapse-free survival (RFS) were 94.4%±3.9% and 94.6±3.7%, respectively. The toxicity profile was mild and reversible. No secondary carcinoma was observed. These results demonstrated the high efficacy and minimal toxicity of ATO/ATRA/anthracycline-based chemotherapy sequential consolidation treatment for newly diagnosed APL in long-term follow-up, suggesting a potential frontline therapy for APL.

**Editor:** Francesco Bertolini, European Institute of Oncology, Italy

**Funding:** The authors have no support or funding to report.

**Competing Interests:** The authors have declared that no competing interests exist.

* Email: liuq9@mail.sysu.edu.cn (QL); lindj@mail.sysu.edu.cn (DJL); huangrw56@163.com (RWH)

9 These authors contributed equally to this work.

## Introduction

Acute promyelocytic leukemia (APL), characterized by the t (15, 17) chromosomal translocation and leukemogenic PML-RARα fusion protein, is accumulated of abnormal promyelocytes in the bone marrow and causes severe bleeding tendency [1]. The treatment of APL with chemotherapy achieved complete remission (CR) in two-thirds of newly diagnosed patients, however, the 5-year disease-free survival (DFS) was still very poor [1–3]. The induction of all-trans retinoic acid (ATRA) in the treatment and optimization of the anthracycline-based regimens resulted in terminal differentiation of APL cells with a 90–95% CR and the 5-year DFS up to 74% [1,4,5], although approximately 5–30% of patients developed disease recurrence [6].

As one of the most potential drugs in APL, arsenic trioxide ($As_2O_3$, ATO) targets PML/RARα and exerts dose-dependent dual effects on APL cells, with low concentrations inducing differentiation and high concentrations triggering apoptosis [7]. Since 1990s, the use of ATO has improved the clinical benefit of refractory or relapsed as well as newly diagnosed APL [8–11]. ATO injection for APL patients who developed disease recurrence or failed to respond to standard treatment was later approved by the US FDA. Moreover, molecular remission is obtainable in patients from 72% to 91% after CR by ATO alone [12,13]. Strong synergistic anti-leukemic effects of ATO in combination with ATRA were found in both APL cell lines and APL animal

models, with induction catabolism of the PML-RARα fusion protein [14–17]. Importantly, previous clinical trials showed that the combination of ATO and ATRA yielded a longer survival rate compared to either ATRA or ATO monotherapy [18–23]. Moreover, ATO consolidation therapy spared anthracycline exposure [24], and improved both event-free survival (EFS) and overall survival (OS) in newly diagnosed APL [25]. Yet, a standard ATO/ATRA consolidation regimen for newly diagnosed APL remains to be further validated.

In this retrospective study, ATRA/chemotherapy combination regimen was applied to induce remission for newly diagnosed APL patients. A regimen consisting of ATO, ATRA and anthracycline-based chemotherapy was used sequentially as consolidation therapy for the patients who obtained CR. The long-term efficacy and safety of ATO/ATRA/anthracycline-based chemotherapy consolidation regimen were evaluated.

## Methods

### Patients

This retrospective study consisted of 45 patients with newly diagnosed APL in the Third Affiliated Hospital, Sun Yat-sen University, from March 1, 2000 to August 31, 2012. The median age was 29 years (10–62 years). Pertinent patient clinical reports of this study were obtained with patients' written consent and the approval of the Ethical Board of The Third Affiliated Hospital,

Sun Yat-sen University ([2013]2-69). Parental written consent was obtained for underage participants.

APL diagnosis was established according to clinical presentations, morphological criteria of the French-American-British classification, cytogenetic assay for t (15; 17) (q22; q21) and RT-PCR analysis for PML-RARα transcripts. The exclusion criteria for this retrospective study included: dysfunction of liver or kidney; any heart diseases or cardiac functional insufficiency; patients who died before initiation of the therapy. Standard induction therapy was administered for the 45 newly diagnosed APL patients (Figure 1). Two patients died during induction treatment. The remaining 43 patients received consolidation therapy. The clinical features of patients were described in Table 1.

### Remission Induction Therapy

Induction therapy for these newly diagnosed patients with APL was a combination of ATRA and daunorubicin plus cytarabine. Once the diagnosis was suspected on the basis of clinical features and the peripheral blood smear, ATRA was administered orally at $40 \text{ mg/m}^2$/day (divided into two equal doses) until CR was achieved. Patients with WBC counts $\geq 10 \times 10^9$/L additionally received hydroxycarbamide orally until the WBC count was down to less than $10 \times 10^9$/L. ATRA was continued for 3 to 15 days to ameliorate the coagulopathy before initiating chemotherapy (daunorubicin $40 \text{ mg/m}^2$/day for 3 days, cytarabine 100 mg/q12 h for 7 days).

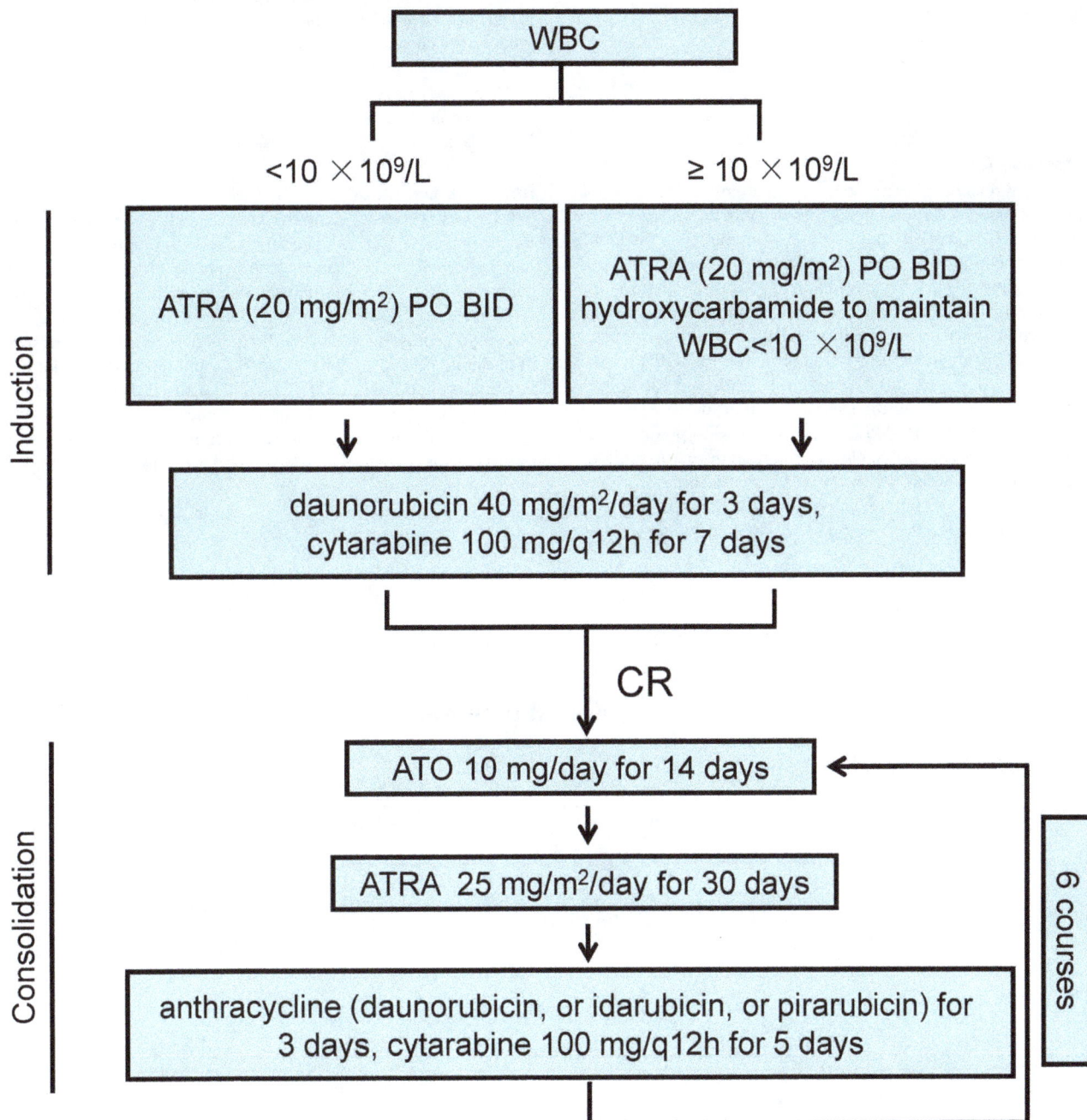

**Figure 1. A chart review of patients treated with standard of induction and consolidation therapy.**

**Table 1. Clinical data of the patients.**

|  | N = 45 |
|---|---|
| Gender, male/female | 20/25 |
| Median age, years | 29 (10–62) |
| WBC, ×109/L |  |
| Median | 2.3 (0.2–47.5) |
| <10 | 1.9 (0.2–7.8, 84.4%) |
| ≥10 | 37.9 (13.2–47.5, 15.6%) |
| Median Hb, g/L | 81.0 (38.0–120.0) |
| Median platelet, ×109/L | 23.0 (5.0–120.0) |
| Clinical CR | 95.6% |
| Median days to clinical CR | 30 (20–60) |
| Median months to molecular CR | 6 (2–12) |

## Supportive Care

During induction of remission, examinations including whole peripheral blood cell counts, renal and hepatic function tests were performed. Coagulation and fibrinolysis parameters including fibrinogen, D-dimmers, fibrin degradation product (FDP), pro-thrombin time (PT), and activated partial thromboplastin time (APTT) were monitored to identify the requirement of platelet, fresh plasma, or cryoprecipitate transfusions. Supportive treatment was based on maintaining platelet counts $>30 \times 10^9$/L until coagulopathy disappearance. Electrocardiogram and sonography were used for monitoring the cardiac function for patients. APL differentiation syndrome (APLDS) was treated with prednisone or dexamethasone until clear resolution of symptoms. Drug toxicities were documented using the National Cancer Institute-Common Toxicity Criteria, version 3.0. Symptomatic therapy was performed for the side effects of ATO, ATRA and anthracycline.

Patients with chronic hepatitis B were treated with lamivudine or telbivudine for prevention of virus activation.

## Consolidation Therapy

Patients were monitored to confirm that the bone marrow morphology and recovery of peripheral blood cell counts. Consolidation therapy included 6 courses was initiated once CR was achieved, and each course included three consecutive regimens: (1) ATO, 10 mg/day for 14 days intravenously; (2) ATRA, 25 mg/m$^2$/day for 30 days orally; (3) anthracycline-based regimens: daunorubicin (40 mg/m$^2$/day), or idarubicin (8 mg/m$^2$/day), or pirarubicin (25 mg/m$^2$/day) for 3 days plus cytarabine 100 mg/q12 h for 5 days. The three regimens of consolidation therapy were administered sequentially every month in the first year after achieving CR. In the second year, each regimen of consolidation therapy was administered sequentially every two months. Six courses were given totally.

All patients received intrathecal therapy (methotrexate 15 mg, cytarabine 50 mg, dexamethasone 8 mg) when CR was achieved. Prophylaxis was performed 4–6 times altogether.

## Response Definition

CR was defined according to clinical presentations and morphological criteria, including cellular bone marrow blasts and abnormal promyelocytes≤5% with an absolute neutrophil count $\geq 1.0 \times 10^9$/L and platelet count $\geq 100 \times 10^9$/L. Clinical recurrence was defined as the presence of $\geq 5\%$ blasts, or abnormal promyelocytes in the bone marrow, or the appearance of leukemic cells in peripheral blood, or abnormal promyelocytes in cerebrospinal fluid (CSF). RT-PCR for the PML-RARα fusion transcript was performed on the bone marrow follow-up every 2 months for monitoring molecular remission. After molecular remission, the examination was still performed every 3 months for monitoring relapse.

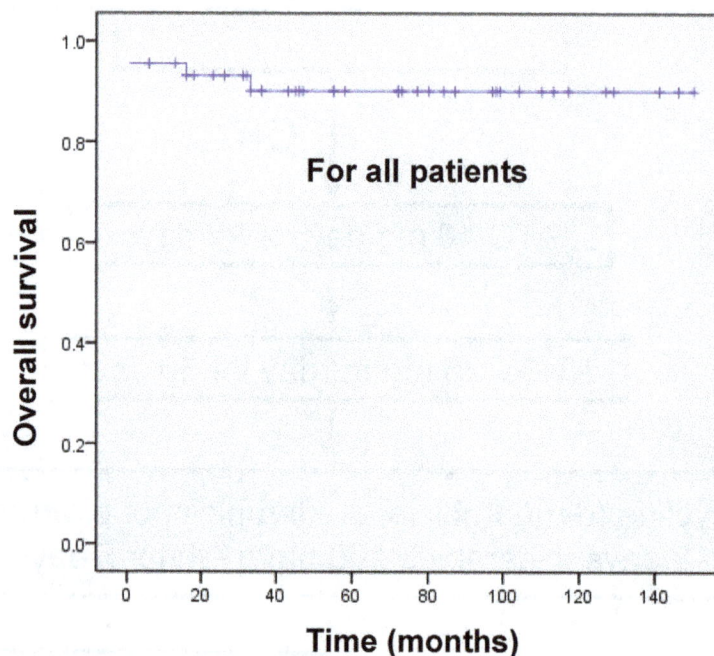

**Figure 2. Survival analysis.** The OS for all 45 patients.

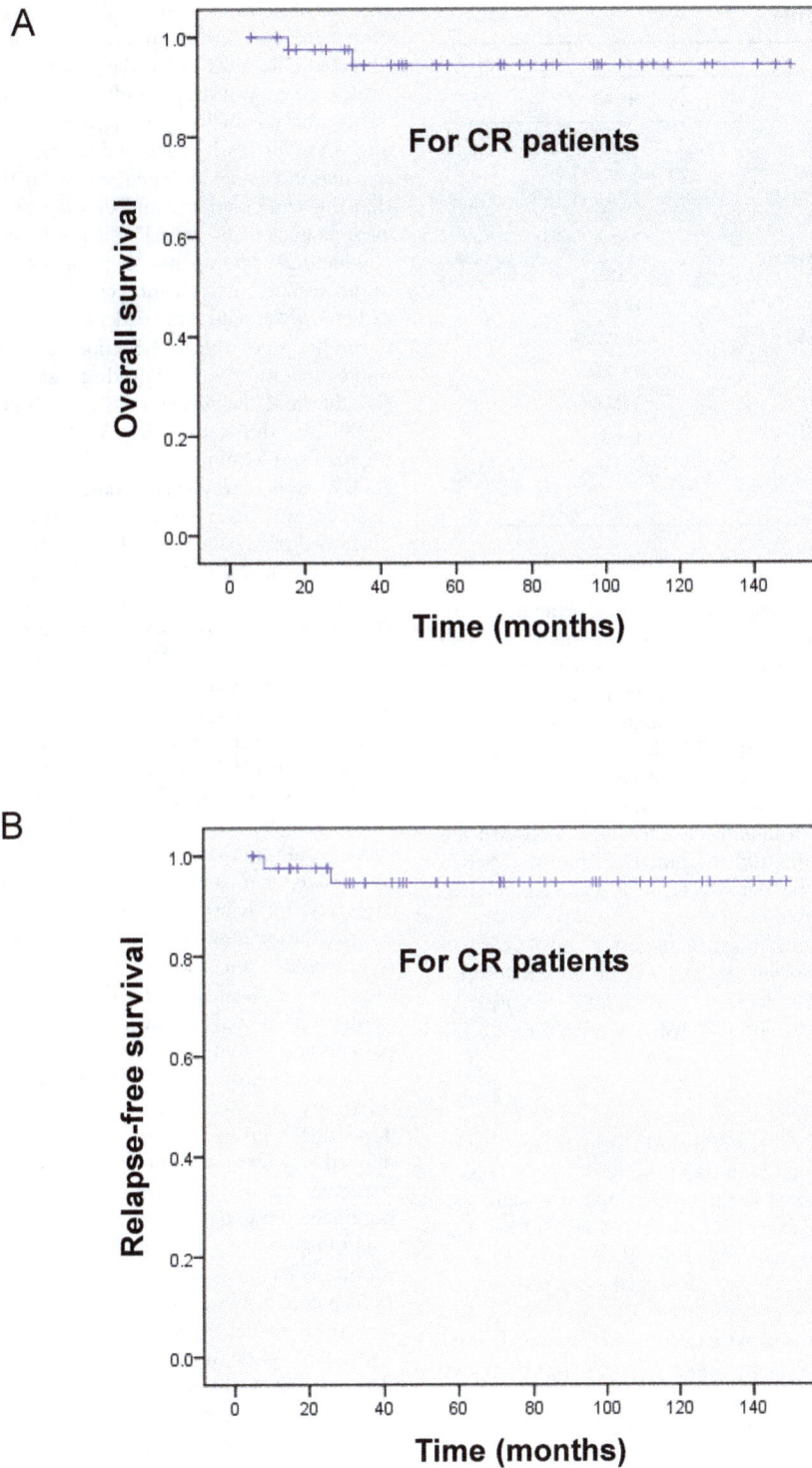

**Figure 3. Survival analysis.** The OS (A) and RFS (B) for the 43 patients who obtained CR.

## Statistical Analysis

OS was defined as the time from the initiation of induction therapy to death. RFS was defined as the time from CR to relapse. Survival analysis was performed using Kaplan-Meier estimate methods. Statistical analysis was performed using SPSS16.0 for windows software.

## Results

### Outcomes

As seen in Table 1, among total 45 patients, 43 (95.6%) achieved CR in remission introduction therapy. The median time to achieve CR was 30 days (range: 20–60 days). Two patients suffered from early death within 15 days during the induction

**Table 2. Toxicity profile.**

|  | N = 43 |
|---|---|
| Hepatotoxicity | 7 (16.3%) |
| Grade I | 6 (14.0%) |
| Grade II | 1 (2.3%) |
| Grade III | 0 (0%) |
| Grade IV | 0 (0%) |
| Skin reaction | 19 (44.2%) |
| Headache | 13 (30.2%) |
| Neutropenia | 8 (18.6%) |
| Gastrointestinal reaction | 6 (14.0%) |
| Cardiac arrhythmia | 1 (2.3%) |
| APLDS | 2 (4.7%) |
| Fever | 4 (9.3%) |

therapy due to intracranial hemorrhage (1 case), or acute tumor lysis syndrome (1 case). For the 43 patients who entered CR, all received ATO/ATRA/anthracycline-based chemotherapy for consolidation therapy. The median follow-up was 55 months (range: 6–150 months), and the median months to molecular CR was 6 months (range: 2–12 months). Till the end of this study, 41 patients remained in good clinical and molecular remission. Two patients relapsed: one presented with central nervous system (CNS) leukemia in the 27th month and the other developed full bone marrow relapse in the 10th month. Both patients died 6 months after relapse. No patient developed a secondary myelodysplastic syndrome or carcinoma.

As shown in Figure 2 and Figure 3, the estimated 3-year OS rates for all 45 patients and for those who achieved CR (n = 43) were 90.2% ± 4.7% (Figure 2) and 94.4% ± 3.9% (Figure 3A), respectively. The RFS rates for CR patients were 94.6 ± 3.7% (Figure 3B).

## Toxicity Profile

The main side effect of ATRA is the APLDS whereas that of ATO is liver dysfunction. Both ATRA- and ATO- based treatments were tolerated well in the present study. As shown in Table 2, APLDS was diagnosed in 2 patients (4.7%). Other side effects of ATRA, such as skin reactions (19 patients, 44.2%), headache (13 patients, 30.2%), gastrointestinal tract reactions (6 patients, 14.0%) and fever (4 patients, 9.3%), were mild and overcame by administration of symptomatic medication. During consolidation, 6 of 41 patients developed tolerable and reversible grade I liver dysfunction and 1 patients developed grade II liver dysfunction, whereas no grade III–IV liver toxicity was observed. Hepatic function returned to normal in all of these patients after supportive therapy. No one needed termination of ATO therapy because of severe liver damage. Therapy-related neutropenia were observed in 8 patients (18.6%). One 62-year-old patient presented with chronic cardiac insufficiency in the 18th month after CR, which might be due to the accumulation of anthracycline for the elderly. In addition, all the 8 hepatitis B patients did not show any virus reactivation during consolidation.

## Discussion

ATRA in combination with anthracycline-based chemotherapy is considered as the standard for the induction and consolidation

therapy of newly diagnosed APL. However, cumulative incidence of relapse still occurs in one third of the patients who have obtained CR. ATO induced catabolism of the PML-RARα fusion protein, demonstrating an effective targeted therapy in APL. In 1990s, the possibility of using a triad of chemotherapy, ATRA, and ATO for newly diagnosed patients in APL was discussed at a meeting in Shanghai. Then studies in the mouse model showed that this combination could dramatically prolong the survival or even eradicate disease. These results encouraged physicians to conduct new therapeutic approaches based on ATO/ATRA/anthracycline-based chemotherapy combination for the treatment of newly diagnosed APL patients.

Indeed, since the introduction of ATRA/ATO-based combination treatment for newly diagnosed APL and recurrence, the CR rate and the 5-year DFS have been greatly improved [18–23,26]. In this study, the ATRA/chemotherapy combination regimen was administered to induce remission, and the ATO plus ATRA and anthracycline-based chemotherapy consolidation regimen was used to maintain long-term efficacy for newly diagnosed APL patients. In 45 de novo patients, CR was achieved in 43 patients (95.6%), whereas the median time to achieved CR was 30 days. The estimated 3-year OS rate for all patients was 90.2% ± 4.7%. For patients who achieved CR (n = 43), the OS and RFS rates were 94.4% ± 3.9% and 94.6% ± 3.7%, respectively. Our data were consistent with recent studies [23], which reported a long-term outcome in the ATRA/ATO-based regimen.

The therapeutic benefit of ATO as a single agent for the treatment of APL has been reported previously [27,28], thus using ATO as the post-remission therapy for the APL patients in CR was reasonable. Importantly, ATO consolidation produced a good survival rate no matter which method was used in CR induction and eliminated the need for maintenance therapy [29–31]. However, the relatively high incidence of ATO-induced hepatotoxicity during remission induction remains unclear and worthy of note, though the side effects of ATO were considered to be moderate. Reversible grade III–IV hepatotoxicity was seen in a small proportion of patients [27]. Overtreatment in the majority of patients was potentially associated with a risk of treatment-related death during early disease remission as well as longer-term risks of secondary carcinoma or anthracycline-related cardiomyopathy. Thus in the present study, ATRA-based induction regimen was applied and ATO was not added to the remission regimen. Either the daily or the total dosage of ATO for consolidation was minimal (10 mg/day for 14 days each course), which APL patients could benefit from ATO by consolidation without overtreatment during each course. In fact, during the consolidation, no grade III–IV hepatotoxicity was documented in our patients. Only 7 patients developed tolerable and reversible grade I–II liver dysfunction, and their hepatic function returned to normal after consolidation therapy. Other side effects were minimal during post-remission treatment. Another major concern associated with long-term exposure to ATO is secondary tumors, and we found no cases in the present study developed secondary tumors. Besides, our analysis showed that incorporation of ATRA drastically achieved long-term efficacy. Importantly, patients in our study showed a very low incidence of APLDS (4.7%). While the dosage of ATO was relatively small, APL patients could benefit from the consolidation with ATO and ATRA, thus usage of ATO/ATRA combination as the post-remission therapy for the APL patients in CR contributed to high efficacy and low side effects.

The therapeutic benefit of ATRA/ATO use in relapsed APL has been described previously [32–35]. However, in a randomized study of 10 cases, the ATRA/ATO combination regimen failed to induce synergistic effect [36]. In our study, the beneficial effects

**Table 3. Review of clinical studies of APL in different groups.**

| Clinical Studies | No. of patients | Age (median) | Sanz Risk (low/int/high) | Induction Therapy | CR | Consolidation Therapy | Maintenance Therapy | Survival Outcome |
|---|---|---|---|---|---|---|---|---|
| Long ZJ, et al. present study | 45 (20/25) | 29 (10-62) | low/int 38; high 7 | ATRA+DNR+Ara-C | 95.6% | ATO+ATRA+IDA+Ara-C, 6 courses | | 3-year OS 90.2%, RFS 94.6% |
| Zhang YM, et al. 2013 [37] | 33 (18/15) | 65 (60-79) | 6/22/5 | ATO | 87.9% | ATO, 4 years | | 10-year OS 69.3%, DFS 64.8%, CSS 84.8% |
| Lo-Coco F, et al. 2013 [38] | A: 77 (40/37); B: 79 (36/43) | A: 44.6 (19.1-70.2); B: 46.6 (18.7-70.2) | A: low/int 33/44; B: low/int 27/52 | A: ATRA+ATO; B: ATRA+IDA | A: 100%; B: 95% | A: ATO+ATRA, 28 weeks; B: ATRA+IDA/MTZ, 3 cycles | B: MTX, 6-MP, ATRA, 2 years | A: 2-year OS 99%, DFS 97%; B: 2-year OS 91%, DFS 90% |
| Iland HJ, et al. 2012 (APML4) [39] | 124 (62/62) | 44 (3-78) | 32/67/24 | ATRA+IDA+ATO | 95% | ATO+ATRA, 2 cycles | ATRA, MTX, 6-MP, 8 cycles | 2-year RFS 97.5%, FFS 88.1%, OS 93.2% |
| Avvisati G, et al. 2011 (AIDA 0493) [40] | 828 (438/390) | 37.2 (1.4-74.7) | 157/432/231 | ATRA+IDA | 94.3% | IDA+Ara-C, MTZ+VP-16, IDA+Ara-C+6-TG, 3 courses | 6-MP, MTX, ATRA, 2 years | 12-year EFS 68.9%, OS 76.5%, DFS 70.8% |
| Sanz MA, et al. 2010 (LPA2005) [41] | 402 (209/193) | 42 (3-83) | 84/200/118 | ATRA+IDA | 99%/95%/83% | IDA, ATRA, MTZ, Ara-C, 3 courses | 6-MP, MTX, ATRA, 2 years | 4-year DFS 90% (93%/92%/82%), OS 88% (96%/91%/79%) |
| Powell BL, et al. 2010 (C9710) [25] | A: 244 (123/121); B: 237 (124/113) | 15-60 year 207/197; >60 year 37/40 | A: 69/120/55; B: 67/112/58 | A: ATRA+Ara-C+DNR; B: ATRA+Ara-C+DNR | A: 90%; B: 90% | A: ATO, 2 cycles+(ATRA+DNR), 2 cycles; B: (ATRA+DNR), 2 cycles | ATRA±6-MP/MTX, 1 year | 3-year EFS 80%/63%, OS 86%/81%, DFS 90%/70% |
| Hu J, et al. 2009 [23] | 85 (47/38) | >55 year 14; ≤55 year 71 | low/int 66; high 19 | ATRA+ATO | 94.1% | DNR+Ara-C, Ara-C pulse, HHT+Ara-C, 3 cycles | ATRA, ATO, MTX/6-MP, 5 cycles | 5-year OS 91.7%, RFS 94.8% |
| Lengfelder E, et al. 2009 (AMLCG) [42] | 142 (59/83) | 40 (16-60) | 33/72/37 | ATRA+TAD (6-TG, Ara-C, DNR)+HAM (Ara-C, MTZ) | low/int 95.2%; high 83.8% | TAD, 1 cycle | Ara-C, DNR, 6-TG, CTX, 3 years | 6-year EFS 78.3%/67.3%, OS 84.4%/73.0%, RFS 82.1%/80.0% |
| Asou N et al. 2007 (APL97) [31] | 283 (158/125) | 48 (15-70) | low/int 232; high 51 | ATRA±IDA/Ara-C | 94% | MTZ+Ara-C, DNR+VP-16+Ara-C, IDA+Ara-C, 3 courses | BHAC, DNR, 6-MP, MTZ, VP-16, VDS, ACR, 6 courses | 6-year DFS 68.5%, OS 83.9% |

Abbreviations: low/int/high: low/intermediate/high; OS: overall survival; DFS: disease-free survival; CSS: cause-specific survival; FFS: failure-free survival; Ara-C: cytarabine; BHAC: behenoyl Ara-C; DNR: daunorubicin; IDA: idarubicin; MTX: methotrexate; 6-MP: mercaptopurine; MTZ: mitoxantrone; VP-16: etoposide; VDS: vindesin; ACR: aclarubicin; 6-TG: 6-thioguanine; HHT: homoharringtonine; CTX: cyclophosphamide.

were observed in the newly diagnosed APL, in contrast to that report. The reason might be that majority of the relapsed patients lost sensitivity to ATRA due to previous exposure, making it difficult to expect a full efficacy of the synergism between ATRA and ATO in those patients. In addition, parts of recent studies about different risks of patients were summarized in Table 3 [23,25,31,37–42] to make a comparison and we found that there was no strong evidence about the recommended strategy for different risk groups. However, the addition of ATO was proved to improve the long-term survival of patients with different risks, which gave support to our present study.

Mechanically, ATRA and ATO targets PML/RARα and exerts dose-dependent differentiation and apoptosis. Microarray, proteomics, and bioinformatics revealed that synergistic effect in combination therapy was due to transcriptional remodeling induced by ATRA-induced differentiation and ATO-related proteome level change. Importantly, enhanced degradation of PML-RARα might be considered for the efficacy of combination therapy in patients: ATO targeted PML, while ATRA aimed to RARα. Besides RA signaling and ubiquitin-proteasome pathway,

some self-renewal and differentiation related molecules were newly revealed to be involved in the ATO/ATRA synergistic effect, such as c-myc, Bmi-1 [14,43]. Thus, further studies should attempt to identify the network by which ATO/ATRA regulates in APL cells.

In summary, we reported that the ATO/ATRA-based regimen incorporating chemotherapy for consolidation therapy for newly diagnosed APL yielded an encouraging long-term survival rate with alleviated side effects, thus reinforcing its potential use as frontline therapy for APL.

## Acknowledgments

We thank members of Department of Hematology, Third Affiliated Hospital, Sun Yat-sen University for their critical comments.

## Author Contributions

Conceived and designed the experiments: QL RWH DJL. Performed the experiments: XDL YH RZX ZGF DNW JJL. Analyzed the data: ZJL YH XDL. Contributed reagents/materials/analysis tools: QL DJL RWH. Wrote the paper: ZJL YH JSY.

## References

1. Wang ZY, Chen Z (2008) Acute promyelocytic leukemia: From highly fatal to highly curable. Blood 111: 2505–2515.
2. Cunningham I, Gee TS, Reich LM, Kempin SJ, Naval AN, et al. (1989) Acute promyelocytic leukemia: treatment results during a decade at Memorial Hospital. Blood 73: 1116–1122.
3. Sanz MA, Jarque I, Martín G, Lorenzo I, Martínez J, et al. (1988) Acute promyelocytic leukemia: therapy results and prognostic factors. Cancer 61: 7–13.
4. Huang ME, Ye YC, Chen SR, Chai JR, Lu JX, et al. (1988) Use of all-trans retinoic acid in the treatment of acute promyelocytic leukemia. Blood 72: 567–572.
5. Tallman MS, Andersen JW, Schiffer CA, Appelbaum FR, Feusner JH, et al. (2002) All-trans retinoic acid in acute promyelocytic leukemia: Longterm outcome and prognostic factor analysis from the North American Intergroup protocol. Blood 100: 4298–4302.
6. Tallman MS (2007) Treatment of relapsed or refractory acute promyelocytic leukemia. Best Pract Res Clin Haematol 20: 57–65.
7. Chen GQ, Shi XG, Tang W, Xiong SM, Zhu J, et al. (1997) Use of arsenic trioxide (As₂O₃) in the treatment of acute promyelocytic leukemia (APL): As2O3 exerts dosedependent dual effects on APL cells. Blood 89: 3345–3353.
8. Shen ZX, Chen GQ, Ni JH, Li XS, Xiong SM, et al. (1997) Use of arsenic trioxide (As₂O₃) in the treatment of acute promyelocytic leukemia (APL): II. Clinical efficacy and pharmacokinetics in relapsed patients. Blood 89: 3354–3360.
9. Sun HD, Ma L, Hu XC, Zhang TD (1992) Ai-Lin I treated 32 cases of acute promyelocytic leukemia. Chin J Integrat Chin West Med 12: 170–171.
10. Zhang P, Wang SY, Hu LH (1996) Arsenic trioxide treated 72 cases of acute promyelocytic leukemia. Chin J Hematol 17: 58–62.
11. Niu C, Yan H, Yu T, Sun HP, Liu JX, et al. (1999) Studies on treatment of acute promyelocytic leukemia with arsenic trioxide: remission induction, follow-up, and molecular monitoring in 11 newly diagnosed and 47 relapsed acute promyelocytic leukemia patients. Blood 94: 3315–3324.
12. Shigeno K, Naito K, Sahara N, Kobayashi M, Nakamura S, et al. (2005) Arsenic trioxide therapy in relapsed or refractory Japanese patients with acute promyelocytic leukemia: updated outcomes of the phase II study and postremission therapies. Int J Hematol 82: 224–229.
13. Soignet SL, Frankel SR, Douer D, Tallman MS, Kantarjian H, et al. (2001) United States multicenter study of arsenic trioxide in relapsed acute promyelocytic leukemia. J Clin Oncol 19: 3852–3860.
14. Zheng PZ, Wang KK, Zhang QY, Huang QH, Du YZ, et al. (2005) Systems analysis of transcriptome and proteome in retinoic acid/arsenic trioxide-induced cell differentiation/apoptosis of promyelocytic leukemia. Proc Natl Acad Sci USA 102: 7653–7658.
15. Gianni M, Koken MH, Chelbi-Alix MK, Benoit G, Lanotte M, et al. (1998) Combined arsenic and retinoic acid treatment enhances differentiation and apoptosis in arsenic-resistant NB4 cells. Blood 91: 4300–4310.
16. Jing Y, Wang L, Xia L, Chen GQ, Chen Z, et al. (2001) Combined effect of all-trans retinoic acid and arsenic trioxide in acute promyelocytic leukemia cells in vitro and in vivo. Blood 97: 264–269.
17. Lallemand-Breitenbach V, Guillemin MC, Janin A, Daniel MT, Degos L, et al. (1999) Retinoic acid and arsenic synergize to eradicate leukemic cells in a mouse model of acute promyelocytic leukemia. J Exp Med 189: 1043–1052.
18. Shen ZX, Shi ZZ, Fang J, Gu BW, Li JM, et al. (2004) All-trans retinoic acid/ As₂O₃ combination yields a high quality remission and survival in newly diagnosed acute promyelocytic leukemia. Proc Natl Acad Sci USA 101: 5328–5335.
19. Aribi A, Kantarjian HM, Estey EH, Koller CA, Thomas DA, et al. (2007) Combination therapy with arsenic trioxide, all-trans retinoic acid, and gemtuzumab ozogamicin in recurrent acute promyelocytic leukemia. Cancer 109: 1355–1359.
20. Estey E, Garcia-Manero G, Ferrajoli A, Faderl S, Verstovsek S, et al. (2006) Use of all-trans retinoic acid plus arsenic trioxide as an alternative to chemotherapy in untreated acute promyelocytic leukemia. Blood 107: 3469–3473.
21. Wang G, Li W, Cui J, Gao S, Yao C, et al. (2004) An efficient therapeutic approach to patients with acute promyelocytic leukemia using a combination of arsenic trioxide with low-dose all-trans retinoic acid. Hematol Oncol 22: 63–71.
22. Li X, Sun WJ, Li ZJ, Zhao YZ, Li YT, et al. (2007) A survival study and prognostic factors analysis on acute promyelocytic leukemia at a single center. Leuk Res 31: 765–771.
23. Hu J, Liu YF, Wu CF, Xu F, Shen ZX, et al. (2009) Long-term efficacy and safety of all-trans retinoic acid/arsenic trioxide-based therapy in newly diagnosed acute promyelocytic leukemia. Proc Natl Acad Sci U S A 106 (9): 3342–3347.
24. Gore SD, Gojo I, Sekeres MA, Morris L, Devetten M, et al. (2010) Single cycle of arsenic trioxide-based consolidation chemotherapy spares anthracycline exposure in the primary management of acute promyelocytic leukemia. J Clin Oncol 28(6): 1047–1053.
25. Powell BL, Moser B, Stock W, Gallagher RE, Willman CL, et al. (2010) Arsenic trioxide improves event-free and overall survival for adults with acute promyelocytic leukemia: North American Leukemia Intergroup Study C9710. Blood 116(19): 3751–3757.
26. Quezada G, Kopp L, Estey E, Wells RJ (2008) All-trans-retinoic acid and arsenic trioxide as initial therapy for acute promyelocytic leukemia. Pediatr Blood Cancer 51: 133–135.
27. Mathews V, George B, Lakshmi KM, Viswabandya A, Bajel A, et al. (2006) Single-agent arsenic trioxide in the treatment of newly diagnosed acute promyelocytic leukemia: Durable remissions with minimal toxicity. Blood 107: 2627–2632.
28. Ghavamzadeh A, Alimoghaddam K, Ghaffari SH, Rostami S, Jahani M, et al. (2006) Treatment of acute promyelocytic leukemia with arsenic trioxide without ATRA and/or chemotherapy. Ann Oncol 17: 131–134.
29. Dai CW, Zhang GS, Shen JK, Zheng WL, Pei MF, et al. (2009) Use of all-trans retinoic acid in combination with arsenic trioxide for remission induction in patients with newly diagnosed acute promyelocytic leukemia and for consolidation/maintenance in CR patients. Acta Haematol 121 (1): 1–8.
30. Coutre SE, Othus M, Powell B, Willman CL, Stock W, et al. (2014) Arsenic trioxide during consolidation for patients with previously untreated low/ intermediate risk acute promyelocytic leukaemia may eliminate the need for maintenance therapy. Br J Haematol doi: 10.1111/bjh.12775.
31. Asou N, Kishimoto Y, Kiyoi H, Okada M, Kawai Y, et al. (2007) A randomized study with or without intensified maintenance chemotherapy in patients with acute promyelocytic leukemia who have become negative for PML-RARalpha transcript after consolidation therapy: the Japan Adult Leukemia Study Group (JALSG) APL97 study. Blood 110(1):59–66.
32. Au WY, Chim CS, Lie AK, Liang R, Kwong YL (2002) Combined arsenic trioxide and all-trans retinoic acid treatment for acute promyelocytic leukemia recurring from previous relapses successfully treated using arsenic trioxide. Br J Haematol 117: 130–132.

33. Grigg A, Kimber R, Szer J (2003) Prolonged molecular remission after arsenic trioxide and all-trans retinoic acid for acute promyelocytic leukemia relapsed after allogeneic stem cell transplantation. Leukemia 17: 1916–1917.

34. Galimberti S, Papineschi F, Carmignani A, Testi R, Fazzi R, et al. (1999) Arsenic and all-trans retinoic acid as induction therapy before autograft in a case of relapsed resistant secondary acute promyelocytic leukemia. Bone Marrow Transplant 24: 345–348.

35. Rock N, Mattiello V, Judas C, Huezo-Diaz P, Bourquin JP, et al. (2014) Treatment of an acute promyelocytic leukemia relapse using arsenic trioxide and all-trans-retinoic in a 6-year-old child. Pediatr Hematol Oncol 31(2):143–148.

36. Raffoux E, Rousselot P, Poupon J, Daniel MT, Cassinat B, et al. (2003) Combined treatment with arsenic trioxide and all-trans-retinoic acid in patients with relapsed acute promyelocytic leukemia. J Clin Oncol 21: 2326–2334.

37. Zhang Y, Zhang Z, Li J, Li L, Han X, et al. (2013) Long-term efficacy and safety of arsenic trioxide for first-line treatment of elderly patients with newly diagnosed acute promyelocytic leukemia. Cancer 119(1):115–125.

38. Lo-Coco F, Avvisati G, Vignetti M, Thiede C, Orlando SM, et al. (2013) Retinoic acid and arsenic trioxide for acute promyelocytic leukemia. N Engl J Med 369(2):111–121.

39. Iland HJ, Bradstock K, Supple SG, Catalano A, Collins M, et al. (2012) All - trans-retinoic acid, idarubicin, and IV arsenic trioxide as initial therapy in acute promyelocytic leukemia (APML4). Blood 120(8):1570–1580.

40. Avvisati G, Lo-Coco F, Paoloni FP, Petti MC, Diverio D, et al. (2011) AIDA 0493 protocol for newly diagnosed acute promyelocytic leukemia: very long-term results and role of maintenance. Blood 117(18):4716–4725.

41. Sanz MA, Montesinos P, Rayón C, Holowiecka A, de la Serna J, et al. (2010) Risk-adapted treatment of acute promyelocytic leukemia based on all-trans retinoic acid and anthracycline with addition of cytarabine in consolidation therapy for high-risk patients: futher improvements in treatment outcome. Blood 115(25): 5137–5146.

42. Lengfelder E, Haferlach C, Saussele S, Haferlach T, Schultheis B, et al. (2009) High dose ara-C in the treatment of newly diagnosed acute promyelocytic leukemia: long-term results of the German AMLCG. Leukemia 23(12):2248–2258.

43. Dos Santos GA, Kats L, Pandolfi PP (2013) Synergy against PML-RARa: targeting transcription, proteolysis, differentiation, and self-renewal in acute promyelocytic leukemia. J Exp Med 210(13):2793–2802.

# 18

# Diabetes, Prediabetes and the Survival of Nasopharyngeal Carcinoma

Pu-Yun OuYang[1], Zhen Su[1], Jie Tang[1], Xiao-Wen Lan[1], Yan-Ping Mao[1], Wuguo Deng[2☺¶], Fang-Yun Xie[1*☺¶]

1 Department of Radiation Oncology, Sun Yat-sen University Cancer Center, State Key Laboratory of Oncology in South China, Collaborative Innovation Center for Cancer Medicine, Guangzhou, Guangdong, China, 2 Department of Experimental Research, Sun Yat-sen University Cancer Center, State Key Laboratory of Oncology in South China, Collaborative Innovation Center for Cancer Medicine, Guangzhou, Guangdong, China

## Abstract

*Background:* The incidence of diabetes is increasing. But the impact of diabetes and prediabetes on survival of patients with nasopharyngeal carcinoma (NPC) has received little evaluation.

*Methods:* In a cohort of 5,860 patients, we compared the disease specific survival (DSS), locoregional relapse-free survival (LRFS) and distant metastasis-free survival (DMFS) of patients with diabetes, prediabetes and normoglycemia defined by pretreatment fasting plasma glucose (FPG) using Kaplan–Meier method, log-rank test and Cox proportional hazards model.

*Results:* Comparing to normoglycemic patients, the diabetic and the prediabetic were generally older, fatter, had hypertension, heart diseases and hyperlipaemia and usually received radiotherapy alone. But both the diabetic and the prediabetic had similar DSS, LRFS and DMFS to normoglycemic patients, even adjusting for such important factors as age, gender, smoking, drinking, hypertension, heart diseases, body mass index, hyperlipaemia, titer of VCA-IgA and EA-IgA, pathology, T-stage, N-stage, chemotherapy and radiotherapy ($P>0.05$ for all). Additionally, the findings remained unchanged in sensitivity analysis by excluding patients with known diabetes history and in subgroups of the various factors.

*Conclusions:* The diabetic and prediabetic NPC patients had similar survival to normoglycemic NPC patients. These data, in the largest reported cohort, are the first to evaluate the association between diabetes, prediabetes and the survival in NPC. The findings are relevant to patient management and provided evidence of the effect on this disease exerted by comorbidities.

Editor: Chang-Qing Gao, Central South University, China

Funding: The authors have no support or funding to report.

Competing Interests: The authors have declared that no competing interests exist.

* Email: xiefy@sysucc.org.cn

☺ These authors contributed equally to this work.

¶ These authors are senior authors on this work.

## Introduction

The incidence of diabetes is increasing worldwide. Epidemiologic evidence suggests that people with diabetes are at an increased risk of cancers of liver, biliary tract, pancreatic, colorectal, as well as leukemia and melanoma [1–3]. Importantly, clinical studies observed a significantly poorer survival in several kinds of cancer patients with elevated blood glucose levels than those with normoglycemia, including extranodal natural killer (NK)/T-cell lymphoma (nasal type) [4], lung cancer [5], pancreatic cancer [6], breast cancer [7–9], acute lymphocytic leukemia [10] or colorectal cancer [11,12].

However, no studies found significant association between diabetes and a higher risk of head and neck cancer [13,14]. And Stott-Miller even observed weak inverse associations between type 2 diabetes and head and neck squamous cell cancer (HNSCC) [13], which was quite similar to the relation of diabetes with a lower risk of larynx cancer in the study by Atchison et al [3]. Additionally, nasopharyngeal carcinoma (NPC) is a non-lymphomatous, squamous-cell carcinoma that occurs in the epithelial lining of the nasopharynx. Of particular importance, it has distinct epidemiology, etiology [15], pathologic characteristics, clinical manifestation and treatment modes [16] compared to other cancers, including other types of head and neck cancer. Therefore, the finding that other types of cancer patients with diabetes had a lower survival than those without diabetes cannot be directly applied to the patients with NPC. To our best knowledge, only one study had reported the association between diabetes and the survival of NPC patients [17]. Unfortunately, only 37 patients with diabetes at diagnosis of NPC were enrolled into that study, and the influence of obesity, smoking, hypertension, heart diseases and hyperlipaemia were not taken into account.

In this largest study, with adjustment for various important covariates, we would provide convincing evidence of the association between diabetes, prediabetes defined by fasting plasma glucose (FPG) and the survival of NPC patients.

## Materials and Methods

### Patients

The study was reviewed and approved by the Human Ethics Approval Committee at Sun Yat-sen University Cancer Center. As a retrospective analysis of routine data, we therefore requested and were granted a waiver of individual informed consent from the ethics committee. Between January 2005 and December 2010, 6034 newly diagnosed, biopsy-proven, non-metastatic and hospitalized NPC patients who were at the age of 20 or >20 years were potentially eligible for this study. After excluding cases with missing data, we eventually enrolled 5860 patients who had complete pretreatment evaluation including history and physical examination, haematology and biochemistry profiles, fiberoptic nasopharyngoscopy with biopsy, magnetic resonance imaging (MRI) of the nasopharynx and neck, chest radiography, abdominal sonography and Technetium-99m-methylene diphosphonate (Tc-99-MDP) whole-body bone scan. The following pretreatment data were anonymously extracted and analyzed, including age, gender, smoking status, drinking status, hypertension history, heart diseases history, diabetes history, FPG, body mass index (BMI), total cholesterol (CHO), triglycerides (TG), high density lipoprotein cholesterol (HDL-C), low density lipoprotein cholesterol (LDL-C), titer of immunoglobulin A against viral capsid antigen (VCA-IgA) and early antigen (EA-IgA) and histological type.

All the included patients were restaged according to the seventh edition of the UICC/AJCC Staging System for NPC [18]. And all were treated by definitive intensity-modulated radiotherapy (IMRT) or conventional radiotherapy (CRT) with or without chemotherapy; further details of the radiation techniques had been described previously [19]. Institutional guidelines recommended no chemotherapy for patients in early stage, and induction, concurrent and adjuvant chemotherapy or combined treatment for those in locoregionally advanced stage. Induction or adjuvant chemotherapy consisted of cisplatin with 5-fluorouracil, cisplatin with taxane or triplet of cisplatin and 5-fluorouracil plus taxane every 3 weeks for two to three cycles. Concurrent chemotherapy consisted of cisplatin given on weeks 1, 4 and 7 of radiotherapy or cisplatin given weekly. Deviation from the institutional guidelines was result from organ dysfunction, treatment intolerance and/or patient refusal.

Patients were examined every 3–6 months during the first 3 years, with follow-up examinations every 6–12 months thereafter or until death. The assessment included history and physical examination and a series of conventional examination equipment at each follow-up visit, to detect the possible relapse or distant metastasis. Local relapses were confirmed by biopsy, MRI scan, or both. Regional relapses were diagnosed by clinical examination and an MRI scan of the neck and, in doubtful cases, by fine needle aspiration of the lymph nodes. Distant metastases were diagnosed by clinical symptoms, physical examinations, and imaging methods including chest radiography, bones scan, MRI, and abdominal sonography. Patients with relapse, distant metastasis or in persistent disease were delivered with salvage treatment including reirradiation, chemotherapy and surgery. Those patients without recent examination tests in the medical records were followed up by telephone call.

### Diabetes and prediabetes assessment

According to the 2014 diagnosis and classification of diabetes mellitus by American Diabetes Association (ADA) [20], patients were classified into the normoglycemic (FPG <5.6 mmol/L), the prediabetic (FPG 5.6–6.9 mmol/L) and the diabetic (FPG ≥ 7.0 mmol/L) group based on FPG only. Patients with known diabetes at diagnosis were classified into the diabetic group and were excluded in sensitivity analysis.

### End points

The primary end point was disease specific survival (DSS), defined as the time from treatment to death resulting from NPC or treatment complications [21]. Secondary end points were locoregional relapse-free survival (LRFS) and distant metastasis-free survival (DMFS), defined as the time from treatment to the first locoregional relapse and distant metastasis, respectively.

### Statistical analysis

Statistical analyses were performed using IBM SPSS Statistics version 20.0. Clinical parameters, including CHO, TG, HDL-C and LDL-C, were stratified into normal and abnormal group. Age and titer of VCA-IgA and EA-IgA were classified according to the criteria adopted in the previous studies [22,23]. Comparisons of categorical characteristics were performed using $\chi^2$ statistic. Univariate stratified survival analyses were performed using Kaplan–Meier methods and log-rank test [24]. Multivariate analyses for hazard ratios (HRs) and 95% confidence intervals (CIs) were performed using the Cox proportional hazards model [25] with forward selection method for important covariates such as gender, smoking and BMI, and enter method for FPG. Two-sided $P$-values <0.05 were considered to be significant.

## Results

### Patients

The median follow-up duration (from the first day of therapy) was 55.6 months (range, 3.1–119.2 months), with 612 (10.4%) cases of lost-to-follow up. There were 569 (9.7%) cases of locoregional relapse, 762 (13.0%) cases of distant metastasis and 889 (15.2%) cases of disease-cause death, respectively. The 5-year survival rates were as follows: DSS 84.9%, LRFS 89.2% and DMFS 86.0%.

The clinicopathologic characteristics of the 5860 patients were shown in Table 1. Of the 121 patients who had known diabetes at diagnosis, 17 patients had a FPG level <5.6 mmol/L and 44 patients <7.0 mmol/L. Drinking, HDL-C level, titer of VCA-IgA and EA-IgA, histological type, T-stage, N-stage, clinical stage and radiotherapy did not significantly differ for group of the diabetic versus the normoglycemic or the prediabetic versus the normoglycemic. Comparing to normoglycemic patients, the diabetic and the prediabetic were generally older, fatter, had hypertension, heart diseases and higher levels of CHO, TG and LDL-C and usually received radiotherapy alone. In the diabetic group, we observed a significantly higher proportion of smoker.

### Diabetes, prediabetes and survival

In contrast with normoglycemic patients, Kaplan-Meier curves displayed the non-significant differences of DSS, LRFS and DMFS rates for patients with diabetes or prediabetes. (Figure 1)

Since diabetes or prediabetes was usually accompanied with age, obesity, smoking, hypertension, heart diseases and hyperlipaemia, the actual survival differences between diabetic, prediabetic and normoglycemic NPC patients cannot be disclosed exactly without excluding the influence of these covariates. However, after

**Table 1.** Clinicopathologic characteristics of 5860 patients with nasopharyngeal carcinoma.

| Characteristics | Normoglycemia | Diabetes | Prediabetes | P1 | P2 |
|---|---|---|---|---|---|
| | No. (%) | No. (%) | No. (%) | | |
| **Total** | 3949 | 345 | 1566 | | |
| **Age** | | | | <0.001 | <0.001 |
| 20–30 | 254 (6.4) | 3 (0.9) | 26 (1.7) | | |
| 30–40 | 1138 (28.8) | 26 (7.5) | 290 (18.5) | | |
| 40–50 | 1286 (32.6) | 104 (30.1) | 553 (35.3) | | |
| 50–60 | 875 (22.2) | 104 (30.1) | 445 (28.4) | | |
| ≥60 | 396 (10.0) | 108 (31.3) | 252 (16.1) | | |
| **Gender** | | | | 0.072 | 0.133 |
| Male | 2916 (73.8) | 270 (78.3) | 1187 (75.8) | | |
| Female | 1033 (26.2) | 75 (21.7) | 379 (24.2) | | |
| **Smoking** | | | | 0.004 | 0.862 |
| Yes | 1677 (42.5) | 174 (50.4) | 661 (42.2) | | |
| No | 2272 (57.5) | 171 (49.6) | 905 (57.8) | | |
| **Drinking** | | | | 0.495 | 0.107 |
| Yes | 477 (12.1) | 46 (13.3) | 165 (10.5) | | |
| No | 3472 (87.9) | 299 (86.7) | 1401 (89.5) | | |
| **Hypertension** | | | | <0.001 | 0.012 |
| Yes | 169 (4.3) | 67 (19.4) | 92 (5.9) | | |
| No | 3780 (95.7) | 278 (80.6) | 1474 (94.1) | | |
| **Heart disease** | | | | <0.001 | <0.001 |
| Yes | 25 (0.6) | 46 (13.3) | 28 (1.8) | | |
| No | 3924 (99.4) | 299 (86.7) | 1538 (98.2) | | |
| **BMI (kg/m$^2$) §** | | | | <0.001 | <0.001 |
| <18.5 | 346 (8.8) | 11 (3.2) | 85 (5.4) | | |
| 18.5–22.9 | 1819 (46.1) | 85 (24.6) | 562 (35.9) | | |
| 22.9–27.5 | 1505 (38.1) | 194 (56.2) | 744 (47.5) | | |
| ≥ 27.5 | 279 (7.1) | 55 (15.9) | 175 (11.2) | | |
| **CHO (mmol/L) ¶** | | | | <0.001 | <0.001 |
| ≤6.47 | 3629 (91.9) | 296 (85.8) | 1367 (87.3) | | |
| >6.47 | 320 (8.1) | 49 (14.2) | 199 (12.7) | | |
| **TG (mmol/L) ¶** | | | | <0.001 | 0.003 |
| ≤1.7 | 2826 (71.6) | 190 (55.1) | 1058 (67.6) | | |
| >1.7 | 1123 (28.4) | 155 (44.9) | 508 (32.4) | | |
| **HDL-C (mmol/L) ¶** | | | | 0.954 | 0.402 |
| ≥0.78 | 3848 (97.4) | 336 (97.4) | 1532 (97.8) | | |
| <0.78 | 101 (2.6) | 9 (2.6) | 34 (2.2) | | |
| **LDL-C (mmol/L) ¶** | | | | 0.001 | <0.001 |
| ≤3.4 | 2416 (61.2) | 179 (51.9) | 839 (53.6) | | |
| >3.4 | 1533 (38.8) | 166 (48.1) | 727 (46.4) | | |
| **VCA-IgA #** | | | | 0.085 | 0.334 |
| ≤80 | 988 (25.0) | 73 (21.2) | 418 (26.7) | | |
| 80–320 | 2024 (51.3) | 198 (57.4) | 771 (49.2) | | |
| >320 | 937 (23.7) | 74 (21.4) | 377 (24.1) | | |
| **EA-IgA #** | | | | 0.076 | 0.293 |
| ≤10 | 1755 (44.4) | 136 (39.4) | 673 (43.0) | | |
| 10–40 | 1260 (31.9) | 130 (37.7) | 534 (34.1) | | |
| >40 | 934 (23.7) | 79 (22.9) | 359 (22.9) | | |
| **Histological type *** | | | | 0.598 | 0.097 |

**Table 1.** Cont.

| Characteristics | Normoglycemia No. (%) | Diabetes No. (%) | Prediabetes No. (%) | P1 | P2 |
|---|---|---|---|---|---|
| WHO I+II | 279 (7.1) | 27 (7.8) | 131 (8.4) | | |
| WHO III | 3670 (92.9) | 318 (92.2) | 1435 (91.6) | | |
| **T-stage** | | | | **0.804** | **0.070** |
| T1+T2 | 1450 | 129 | 616 | | |
| T3+T4 | 2499 | 216 | 950 | | |
| **N-stage** | | | | **0.246** | **0.124** |
| N0+N1 | 3017 | 254 | 1205 | | |
| N2+N3 | 932 | 91 | 333 | | |
| **Clinical stage** | | | | **0.139** | **0.221** |
| I | 223 (5.6) | 12 (3.5) | 102 (6.5) | | |
| II | 918 (23.2) | 81 (23.5) | 395 (25.2) | | |
| III | 1569 (39.7) | 146 (42.3) | 618 (39.5) | | |
| IVa | 1047 (26.5) | 82 (23.8) | 382 (24.4) | | |
| IVb | 192 (4.9) | 24 (7.0) | 69 (4.4) | | |
| **Chemotherapy** | | | | **0.003** | **0.005** |
| No | 725 (18.4) | 86 (24.9) | 339 (21.6) | | |
| Yes | 3224 (81.6) | 259 (75.1) | 1227 (78.4) | | |
| **Radiotherapy** | | | | **0.632** | **0.084** |
| IMRT | 1161 (29.4) | 109 (31.6) | 456 (29.1) | | |
| 3DCRT | 59 (1.5) | 4 (1.2) | 37 (2.4) | | |
| 2DCRT | 2729 (69.1) | 232 (67.2) | 1073 (68.5) | | |

Note: BMI = body mass index, CHO = total cholesterol, TG = triglycerides, HDL-C = high density lipoprotein cholesterol, LDL-C = low density lipoprotein cholesterol, VCA = viral capsid antigen, EA = early antigen, IgA = immunoglobulin A, IMRT = intensity-modulated radiotherapy, 3DCRT = three-dimensional conformal radiotherapy, 2DCRT = two-dimensional conventional radiotherapy.

P1 – diabetes vs normoglycemia; P2 – prediabetes vs normoglycemia.

§According to the World Health Organization classifications for Asian populations.

¶Stratified into normal and abnormal group.

#In accordance with the criteria adopted in the previous study.

*Based on the criteria of WHO histological type (1991): I - Squamous-cell carcinomas, II - Differentiated non-keratinising carcinoma, III - Undifferentiated non-keratinising carcinoma.

adjusting for age, gender, smoking, drinking, hypertension, heart diseases, BMI, levels of CHO, TG, HDL-C and LDL-C, titer of VCA-IgA and EA-IgA, histological type, T-stage, N-stage, chemotherapy and radiotherapy, we still found no significant differences of DSS, LRFS and DMFS when comparing patients with diabetes to those with normoglycemia ($P = 0.894$ for DSS, $P = 0.351$ for LRFS and $P = 0.530$ for DMFS) and comparing patients with prediabetes to those with normoglycemia ($P = 0.335$ for DSS, $P = 0.613$ for LRFS and $P = 0.671$ for DMFS). (Table 2)

To fully eliminate the effect of the discrepancies as a result of the normal or prediabetic FPG level for the 121 patients with known diabetes history, we did sensitivity analysis by excluding them. Consequently, the above results remained unchanged, as shown in Table S1.

In addition, we performed second analyses stratified by several important subgroups. (Table 3) Resultantly, multivariate analyses indicated that neither diabetes nor prediabetes was significantly associated with DSS in subgroups of age ($\leq$45 and>45 y), gender, smoking, drinking, hypertension, heart diseases, BMI ($<$25 and $\geq$ 25 kg/m$^2$), CHO, TG, HDL-C, LDL-C, T-stage (T1+T2 and T3+T4), N-stage (N0+N1 and N2+N3), clinical stage (I+II and III+IV), chemotherapy and radiotherapy (2DCRT and IMRT + 3DCRT).

## Discussion

Based on 5860 patients and thoroughly adjusting for the influence of age, obesity, smoking, drinking, hypertension, heart diseases, hyperlipaemia, tumor stage and treatment modality, our study concluded that the diabetic and prediabetic NPC patients had similar survival to the normoglycemic NPC patients.

In contrast to our present study, Liu et al [17] detected a lower disease-free survival in patients with diabetes (n = 37) than those without diabetes (n = 897); nevertheless, this study did not account for all the various potential confounders, such as obesity, smoking, hypertension, heart diseases and hyperlipaemia. Similar studies also found the significant association between hyperglycemia and the survival of patients with extranodal natural killer (NK)/T-cell lymphoma (nasal type) [4] or acute lymphocytic leukemia [10], and between DM and the survival of patients with lung cancer [5], pancreatic cancer [6], breast cancer [7,8] or colorectal cancer [11,12]. But this is hardly convincing as the small sample size of these studies [4–6,10] is very likely to cause the skewed results.

Actually, Zhou et al [26] recruited 26,460 men and 18,195 women aged 25–90 years from 17 European population-based or occupational cohorts and found that diabetes was not significantly associated with the mortality of male patients with cancers of

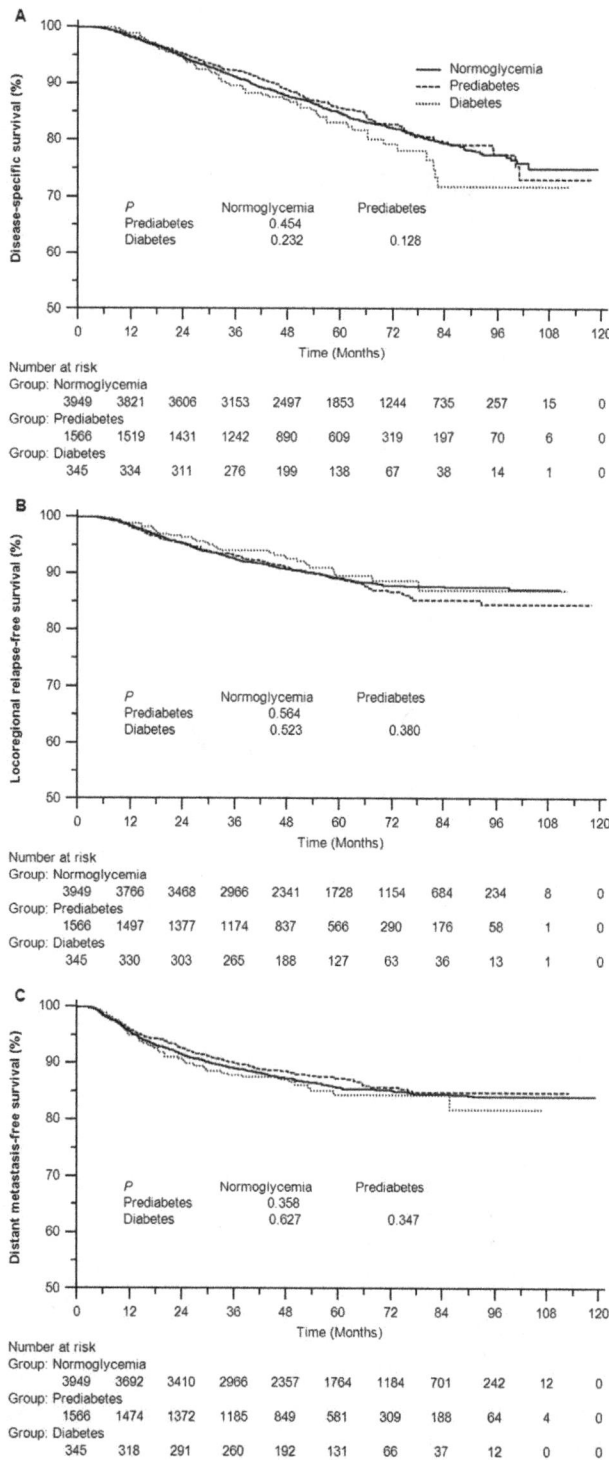

Figure 1. Kaplan-Meier curves of disease specific survival (A), locoregional relapse-free survival (B) and distant metastasis-free survival (C) for patients with normoglycemia, prediabetes and diabetes mellitus defined by fasting plasma glucose.

**Table 2.** Multivariate analysis for disease specific survival (DSS), locoregional relapse-free survival (LRFS) and distant metastasis-free survival (DMFS) *.

| Factor | DSS | | | LRFS | | | DMFS | | |
|---|---|---|---|---|---|---|---|---|---|
| | HR | 95% CI | P | HR | 95% CI | P | HR | 95% CI | P |
| Normoglycemia | 1.00 | | | 1.00 | | | 1.00 | | |
| Diabetes | 0.98 | 0.75–1.29 | 0.894 | 0.83 | 0.57–1.22 | 0.351 | 1.10 | 0.81–1.49 | 0.530 |
| Prediabetes | 0.93 | 0.79–1.08 | 0.335 | 1.05 | 0.87–1.27 | 0.613 | 0.96 | 0.82–1.14 | 0.671 |
| Gender | 0.64 | 0.54–0.76 | <0.001 | 0.65 | 0.53–0.80 | <0.001 | 0.64 | 0.54–0.77 | <0.001 |
| Age | 1.47 | 1.38–1.57 | <0.001 | 1.09 | 1.01–1.18 | 0.030 | 1.09 | 1.02–1.16 | 0.017 |
| T-stage | 1.53 | 1.42–1.64 | <0.001 | 1.28 | 1.18–1.39 | <0.001 | 1.45 | 1.35–1.57 | <0.001 |
| N-stage | 1.61 | 1.51–1.72 | <0.001 | 1.27 | 1.16–1.39 | <0.001 | 1.72 | 1.61–1.85 | <0.001 |
| BMI | 0.81 | 0.74–0.88 | <0.001 | NS | | | 0.84 | 0.76–0.92 | <0.001 |

NOTE: HR = hazard ratio, CI = confidence interval, BMI = body mass index.
*Adjusting for age, gender, smoking, drinking, hypertension, heart diseases, BMI, levels of total cholesterol, triglycerides, high density lipoprotein cholesterol and low density lipoprotein cholesterol, titer of VCA-IgA and EA-IgA, histological type, T-stage, N-stage, chemotherapy and radiotherapy with forward selection method.

pancreas, bronchus/lung, prostate and kidney/bladder, or the mortality of female patients with cancers of stomach or colon – rectum, bronchus/lung, breast and kidney/bladder. Also, Höfner et al [27] enrolled 1140 patients with localized renal cell carcinoma and revealed that type 2 diabetes at the time of

**Table 3.** Subgroup analysis of disease specific survival by patients' characteristics*.

| Factor | Diabetes | | | Prediabetes | | |
|---|---|---|---|---|---|---|
| | HR | 95% CI | P | HR | 95% CI | P |
| **Age (year)** § | | | | | | |
| ≤45 | 1.51 | 0.86–2.64 | 0.155 | 1.06 | 0.80–1.40 | 0.691 |
| >45 | 0.98 | 0.72–1.33 | 0.877 | 0.88 | 0.73–1.06 | 0.184 |
| **Gender** | | | | | | |
| Male | 1.13 | 0.85–1.51 | 0.388 | 0.90 | 0.75–1.07 | 0.215 |
| Female | 0.83 | 0.57–1.22 | 0.351 | 1.07 | 0.75–1.54 | 0.701 |
| **Smoking** | | | | | | |
| Yes | 0.98 | 0.69–1.39 | 0.893 | 0.93 | 0.75–1.16 | 0.535 |
| No | 0.96 | −.62–1.48 | 0.835 | 0.90 | 0.71–1.13 | 0.364 |
| **Drinking** | | | | | | |
| Yes | 0.97 | 0.49–1.94 | 0.934 | 1.19 | 0.81–1.76 | 0.377 |
| No | 1.00 | 0.74–1.34 | 0.986 | 0.89 | 0.75–1.06 | 0.180 |
| **Hypertension** | | | | | | |
| Yes | 0.73 | 0.34–1.58 | 0.428 | 0.93 | 0.48–1.80 | 0.824 |
| No | 1.02 | 0.76–1.38 | 0.872 | 0.94 | 0.79–1.10 | 0.415 |
| **Heart diseases** | | | | | | |
| Yes | 0.49 | 0.20–1.20 | 0.118 | 0.41 | 0.14–1.22 | 0.109 |
| No | 0.99 | 0.74–1.33 | 0.937 | 0.94 | 0.80–1.10 | 0.422 |
| **BMI (kg/m$^2$)** § | | | | | | |
| <25 | 0.91 | 0.64–1.29 | 0.600 | 0.87 | 0.72–1.05 | 0.152 |
| ≥25 | 1.03 | 0.66–1.62 | 0.884 | 0.98 | 0.74–1.32 | 0.914 |
| **CHO (mmol/L)** | | | | | | |
| ≤6.47 | 0.97 | 0.72–1.30 | 0.833 | 0.93 | .79–1.10 | 0.394 |
| >6.47 | 0.92 | 0.43–2.00 | 0.837 | 0.78 | 0.48–1.26 | 0.309 |
| **TG (mmol/L)** | | | | | | |
| ≤1.7 | 1.23 | 0.88–1.72 | 0.230 | 0.96 | 0.79–1.16 | 0.669 |
| >1.7 | 0.66 | 0.41–1.06 | 0.084 | 0.87 | 0.65–1.15 | 0.324 |
| **HDL-C mmol/L)** | | | | | | |
| ≥0.78 | 0.93 | 0.70–1.23 | 0.595 | 0.91 | 0.78–1.07 | 0.912 |
| <0.78 | 1.39 | 0.44–4.36 | 0.577 | 1.30 | 0.59–2.83 | 0.518 |
| **LDL-C (mmol/L)** | | | | | | |
| ≤3.4 | 0.92 | 0.62–1.36 | 0.666 | 1.03 | 0.84–1.28 | 0.759 |
| >3.4 | 1.03 | 0.71–1.51 | 0.873 | 0.83 | 0.65–1.05 | 0.114 |
| **T-stage** | | | | | | |
| T1+T2 | 1.10 | 0.65–1.84 | 0.730 | 0.80 | 0.58–1.13 | 0.203 |
| T3+T4 | 0.89 | 0.64–1.22 | 0.464 | 0.95 | 0.79–1.13 | 0.534 |
| **N-stage** | | | | | | |
| N0+N1 | 0.72 | 0.49–1.06 | 0.093 | 0.89 | 0.73–1.09 | 0.269 |
| N2+N3 | 1.08 | 0.72–1.63 | 0.699 | 0.91 | 0.70–1.17 | 0.465 |
| **Clinical stage** | | | | | | |
| I+II | 1.07 | 0.55–2.09 | 0.846 | 0.70 | 0.46–1.08 | 0.106 |
| III+ IV | 0.89 | 0.66–1.20 | 0.440 | 0.95 | 0.80–1.12 | 0.512 |
| **Chemotherapy** | | | | | | |
| Yes | 1.04 | 0.77–1.42 | 0.784 | 0.98 | 0.83–1.16 | 0.811 |
| No | 0.63 | 0.34–1.14 | 0.124 | 0.68 | 0.45–1.02 | 0.060 |
| **Radiotherapy** | | | | | | |
| 2DCRT | 1.11 | 0.82–1.51 | 0.498 | 0.90 | 0.75–1.08 | 0.256 |
| IMRT + 3DCRT | 0.68 | 0.37–1.28 | 0.231 | 1.03 | 0.76–1.40 | 0.860 |

NOTE: HR = hazard ratio, CI = confidence interval, BMI = body mass index, CHO = total cholesterol, TG = triglycerides, HDL-C = high density lipoprotein cholesterol, LDL-C = low density lipoprotein cholesterol, VCA = viral capsid antigen, EA = early antigen, IgA = immunoglobulin A, 2DCRT = two-dimensional conventional radiotherapy, IMRT = intensity-modulated radiotherapy, 3DCRT = three-dimensional conformal radiotherapy.
*Adjusting for age, gender, smoking, drinking, hypertension, heart diseases, BMI, levels of total cholesterol, triglycerides, high density lipoprotein cholesterol and low density lipoprotein cholesterol, titer of VCA-IgA and EA-IgA, histological type, T-stage, N-stage, chemotherapy and radiotherapy.
§According to the stratification criteria for the risk factor of age and BMI mentioned in the 2014 diagnosis and classification of diabetes mellitus by American Diabetes Association (ADA).

surgery had no significant impact on cancer-specific and recurrence-free survival. In the study by Kiderlen et al [8], relapse-free period was better in elderly breast cancer patients with diabetes compared with patients without diabetes if taking competing mortality into account; patients with diabetes without other comorbidity had a similar overall survival as patients without any comorbidity. Additionally, the ORIGIN trial found no evidence for increased cancer incidence or mortality in patients with impaired glucose metabolism or early type 2 diabetes [28]. Overall, despite of absence of straight evidence regarding the impact of FPG on survival of other types of head and neck cancer, our findings of neutral impact in NPC patients were not unreasonable. Finally, the non-significant association between diabetes and risk of head and neck cancer from the prior pooled analysis [13] and meta-analysis [14], along with the inverse relationship between diabetes and development of larynx cancer in another cohort study [3], at least indirectly suggested no impact of FPG on the survival of NPC.

Previous research showed that cancer patients with diabetes may have increased tumor cell proliferation and metastatic capacity as a consequence of the high insulin or increased free insulin-like growth factor (IGF-1) levels in hyperinsulinemic states [29]. But this was denied by a recent study [30], in which incident insulin users, exposure to insulin and glargine insulin in particular was not associated with any deleterious effect on overall and site specific cancer mortality of lung, colorectal, female genital, liver and urinary tract cancer. What is more, Margel et al [31] discovered that increased cumulative duration of metformin exposure after prostate cancer diagnosis was associated with decreases in both all-cause and cancer-specific mortality among diabetic men. But this similar protective effect from metformin exposure was not supported in NPC patients with diabetes in our study.

Certainly, the pooled analysis by Stott-Miller et al [13] showed a modest association between diabetes and the incidence of head and neck cancer among never smokers. And Atchison et al [3] assumed that smoking and BMI were two important factors potentially contributed to the inverse relationship between diabetes and development of larynx cancer. As observed in our study, a higher percentage of diabetic patients were indeed smokers and overweight or obese. Additionally, according to recent studies, NPC patients with smoking history had poorer survival [32] whereas those with higher BMI had favorable survival [33]. Therefore, the contradictory effect of smoking and BMI maybe just right principally confounded the impact of FPG

on survival of NPC. However, in the stratum of patients who had normal BMI and never smoked (n = 1461), multivariate analysis showed that both diabetic and prediabetic patients had similar DSS, LRFS and DMFS rates to euglycemic patients ($P = 0.298$, $P = 0.613$ and $P = 0.433$ for DSS; $P = 0.554$, $P = 0.315$ and $P = 0.693$ for LRFS; $P = 0.434$, $P = 0.747$ and $P = 0.458$ for DMFS, respectively).

Considering the influence of mortality from such hyperglycemia-related complications as hypertension, heart diseases and various hyperlipaemia, we set DSS as the primary endpoint, adjusted for these covariates and conducted subgroup analyses; finally, diabetes or prediabetes still had null influence to NPC survival. Moreover, there were no significant differences with respect to the distribution of tumor stage and radiotherapy, and diabetes or prediabetes remained to be irrelevant to the survival in these subgroups. Particularly, patients with diabetes or prediabetes usually received radiotherapy alone with a higher percentage than that of patients with normoglycemia. But this rarely affected the DSS of the diabetic or prediabetic subgroups.

To our knowledge, this is the largest and most detailed study to evaluate the relation between diabetes, prediabetes before treatment and the survival of NPC patients. Clinicopathologic and survival data were verified by review of individual patient records. Our findings were derived from complete adjustment and particular stratification of various important covariates. The conclusions are relevant to patient management and provided evidence of the effect on the disease of NPC exerted by comorbidities. Indeed, albeit that FPG is the primary routine test in clinic, further study with data on standard 2-hour oral glucose tolerance test (OGTT) and hemoglobin A1c (HbA1c) is warranted. Apart from that, the effect of glycemic control during radiotherapy and chemotherapy on the survival is essential to be studied.

## Author Contributions

Conceived and designed the experiments: PYOY FYX WD. Performed the experiments: PYOY. Analyzed the data: PYOY. Contributed reagents/materials/analysis tools: PYOY ZS JT XWL YPM. Wrote the paper: PYOY.

## References

1. Giovannucci E, Harlan DM, Archer MC, Bergenstal RM, Gapstur SM, et al. (2010) Diabetes and cancer: a consensus report. Diabetes Care 33: 1674–1685.
2. Bosetti C, Rosato V, Polesel J, Levi F, Talamini R, et al. (2012) Diabetes mellitus and cancer risk in a network of case-control studies. Nutr Cancer 64: 643–651.
3. Atchison EA, Gridley G, Carreon JD, Leitzmann MF, McGlynn KA (2011) Risk of cancer in a large cohort of U.S. veterans with diabetes. Int J Cancer 128: 635–643.
4. Cai Q, Luo X, Liang Y, Rao H, Fang X, et al. (2013) Fasting blood glucose is a novel prognostic indicator for extranodal natural killer/T-cell lymphoma, nasal type. Br J Cancer 108: 380–386.

5. Luo J, Chen YJ, Chang LJ (2012) Fasting blood glucose level and prognosis in non-small cell lung cancer (NSCLC) patients. Lung Cancer 76: 242–247.
6. Chu CK, Mazo AE, Goodman M, Egnatashvili V, Sarmiento JM, et al. (2010) Preoperative diabetes mellitus and long-term survival after resection of pancreatic adenocarcinoma. Ann Surg Oncol 17: 502–513.
7. Erickson K, Patterson RE, Flatt SW, Natarajan L, Parker BA, et al. (2011) Clinically defined type 2 diabetes mellitus and prognosis in early-stage breast cancer. J Clin Oncol 29: 54–60.
8. Kiderlen M, de Glas NA, Bastiaannet E, Engels CC, van de Water W, et al. (2013) Diabetes in relation to breast cancer relapse and all-cause mortality in

elderly breast cancer patients: a FOCUS study analysis. Ann Oncol 24: 3011–3016.

9.  Minicozzi P, Berrino F, Sebastiani F, Falcini F, Vattiato R, et al. (2013) High fasting blood glucose and obesity significantly and independently increase risk of breast cancer death in hormone receptor-positive disease. Eur J Cancer 49: 3881–3888.

10. Sonabend RY, McKay SV, Okcu MF, Yan J, Haymond MW, et al. (2009) Hyperglycemia during induction therapy is associated with poorer survival in children with acute lymphocytic leukemia. J Pediatr 155: 73–78.

11. Luo J, Lin HC, He K, Hendryx M (2014) Diabetes and prognosis in older persons with colorectal cancer. Br J Cancer 110: 1847–1854.

12. Meyerhardt JA, Catalano PJ, Haller DG, Mayer RJ, Macdonald JS, et al. (2003) Impact of diabetes mellitus on outcomes in patients with colon cancer. J Clin Oncol 21: 433–440.

13. Stott-Miller M, Chen C, Chuang SC, Lee YC, Boccia S, et al. (2012) History of diabetes and risk of head and neck cancer: a pooled analysis from the international head and neck cancer epidemiology consortium. Cancer Epidemiol Biomarkers Prev 21: 294–304.

14. Schmid D, Behrens G, Jochem C, Keimling M, Leitzmann M (2013) Physical activity, diabetes, and risk of thyroid cancer: a systematic review and meta-analysis. Eur J Epidemiol 28: 945–958.

15. Chang ET, Adami HO (2006) The enigmatic epidemiology of nasopharyngeal carcinoma. Cancer Epidemiol Biomarkers Prev 15: 1765–1777.

16. Wei WI, Sham JS (2005) Nasopharyngeal carcinoma. Lancet 365: 2041–2054.

17. Liu H, Xia Y, Cui N (2006) Impact of diabetes mellitus on treatment outcomes in patients with nasopharyngeal cancer. Med Oncol 23: 341–346.

18. Edge SB, Byrd DR, Compton CC, Fritz AG, Greene FL, et al. (2010) AJCC cancer staging handbook from the AJCC cancer staging manual; Edge SB, Byrd DR, Compton CC, Fritz AG, Greene FL et al., editors. New York: Springer.

19. Lai SZ, Li WF, Chen L, Luo W, Chen YY, et al. (2011) How does intensity-modulated radiotherapy versus conventional two-dimensional radiotherapy influence the treatment results in nasopharyngeal carcinoma patients? Int J Radiat Oncol Biol Phys 80: 661–668.

20. (2014) American Diabetes Association. Diagnosis and classification of diabetes mellitus. Diabetes Care 37 Suppl 1: S81–90.

21. Sun X, Su S, Chen C, Han F, Zhao C, et al. (2014) Long-term outcomes of intensity-modulated radiotherapy for 868 patients with nasopharyngeal carcinoma: An analysis of survival and treatment toxicities. Radiother Oncol 110: 398–403.

22. Liu N, Chen NY, Cui RX, Li WF, Li Y, et al. (2012) Prognostic value of a microRNA signature in nasopharyngeal carcinoma: a microRNA expression analysis. Lancet Oncol 13: 633–641.

23. Ouyang PY, Su Z, Mao YP, Liang XX, Liu Q, et al. (2013) Prognostic impact of family history in southern Chinese patients with undifferentiated nasopharyngeal carcinoma. Br J Cancer 109: 788–794.

24. Kaplan EL, Meier P (1958) Nonparametric estimation from incomplete observation. J Am Stat Assoc 53: 457–481.

25. Cox DR (1972) Regression models and life tables. J R Stat Soc B 34: 187–220.

26. Zhou XH, Qiao Q, Zethelius B, Pyorala K, Soderberg S, et al. (2010) Diabetes, prediabetes and cancer mortality. Diabetologia 53: 1867–1876.

27. Hofner T, Zeier M, Hatiboglu G, Eisen C, Schonberg G, et al. (2013) The impact of type 2 diabetes on the outcome of localized renal cell carcinoma. World J Urol.

28. Gerstein HC, Bosch J, Dagenais GR, Diaz R, Jung H, et al. (2012) Basal insulin and cardiovascular and other outcomes in dysglycemia. N Engl J Med 367: 319–328.

29. Richardson LC, Pollack LA (2005) Therapy insight: Influence of type 2 diabetes on the development, treatment and outcomes of cancer. Nat Clin Pract Oncol 2: 48–53.

30. Ioacara S, Guja C, Ionescu-Tirgoviste C, Fica S, Roden M (2014) Cancer specific mortality in insulin-treated type 2 diabetes patients. PLoS One 9: e93132.

31. Margel D, Urbach DR, Lipscombe LL, Bell CM, Kulkarni G, et al. (2013) Metformin use and all-cause and prostate cancer-specific mortality among men with diabetes. J Clin Oncol 31: 3069–3075.

32. Ouyang PY, Su Z, Mao YP, Liang XX, Liu Q, et al. (2013) Prognostic impact of cigarette smoking on the survival of patients with established nasopharyngeal carcinoma. Cancer Epidemiol Biomarkers Prev 22: 2285–2294.

33. Huang PY, Wang CT, Cao KJ, Guo X, Guo L, et al. (2013) Pretreatment body mass index as an independent prognostic factor in patients with locoregionally advanced nasopharyngeal carcinoma treated with chemoradiotherapy: findings from a randomised trial. Eur J Cancer 49: 1923–1931.

# 19

# Aberrant Promoter Methylation of Caveolin-1 is Associated with Favorable Response to Taxane-Platinum Combination Chemotherapy in Advanced NSCLC

**Seth A. Brodie**[1,2,6]**, Courtney Lombardo**[2,6]**, Ge Li**[2,6]**, Jeanne Kowalski**[6,7]**, Khanjan Gandhi**[4,6,7]**, Shaojin You**[1,5]**, Fadlo R. Khuri**[2,6]**, Adam Marcus**[2,6]**, Paula M. Vertino**[3,6]**, Johann C. Brandes**[1,2,6]*

1 Atlanta VA Medical Center, Atlanta, Georgia, United States of America, 2 Departments of Hematology and Medical Oncology, School of Medicine, Emory University, Atlanta, Georgia, United States of America, 3 Department of Radiation Oncology, School of Medicine, Emory University, Atlanta, Georgia, United States of America, 4 Department of Human Genetics, School of Medicine, Emory University, Atlanta, Georgia, United States of America, 5 Department of Pathology, School of Medicine, Emory University, Atlanta, Georgia, United States of America, 6 Winship Cancer Institute, Emory University, Atlanta, Georgia, United States of America, 7 Department of Biostatistics and Bioinformatics, Rollins School of Public Health, Atlanta, Georgia, United States of America

## Abstract

*Purpose:* Aberrant promoter DNA methylation can serve as a predictive biomarker for improved clinical responses to certain chemotherapeutics. One of the major advantages of methylation biomarkers is the ease of detection and clinical application. In order to identify methylation biomarkers predictive of a response to a taxane-platinum based chemotherapy regimen in advanced NSCLC we performed an unbiased methylation analysis of 1,536 CpG dinucleotides in cancer-associated gene loci and correlated results with clinical outcomes.

*Methods:* We studied a cohort of 49 patients (median age 62 years) with advanced NSCLC treated at the Atlanta VAMC between 1999 and 2010. Methylation analysis was done on the Illumina GoldenGate Cancer panel 1 methylation microarray platform. Methylation data were correlated with clinical response and adjusted for false discovery rates.

*Results:* Cav1 methylation emerged as a powerful predictor for achieving disease stabilization following platinum taxane based chemotherapy (p = 1.21E-05, FDR significance = 0.018176). In Cox regression analysis after multivariate adjustment for age, performance status, gender, histology and the use of bevacizumab, CAV1 methylation was significantly associated with improved overall survival (HR 0.18 (95%CI: 0.03–0.94)). Silencing of CAV1 expression in lung cancer cell lines(A549, EKVX)by shRNA led to alterations in taxane retention.

*Conclusions:* CAV1 methylation is a predictor of disease stabilization and improved overall survival following chemotherapy with a taxane-platinum combination regimen in advanced NSCLC. CAV1 methylation may predict improved outcomes for other chemotherapeutic agents which are subject to cellular clearance mediated by caveolae.

**Editor:** Sumitra Deb, Virginia Commonwealth University, United States of America

**Funding:** Support was provided by the Veterans' Health Administration Career Development Award 7-IK2BX001283-03 to JCB; NCI- 5 P50 CA128613-02 Career Development Project to JCB; NCI-P30CA138292 pilot grant to JCB; CHEST Foundation/Lungevity Foundation Clinical Lung Cancer Research Award to JCB; Uniting against Lung Cancer / Lungevity Foundation Research Award to JCB; SunTrust Scholar Award to JCB; Cohen Family Scholar Award to JCB; and Elsa U Pardee Foundation Research Award to JCB. This research project was supported in part by the Emory University Integrated Cellular Imaging Microscopy Core and the Biostatistics and Bioinformatics Shared Resource of the Winship Cancer Institute of Emory University under award number P30CA138292. The content is solely the responsibility of the authors and does not necessarily represent the official views of the National Institutes of Health or the Department of Veterans Affairs. The funders had no role in study design, data collection and analysis, decision to publish, or preparation of the manuscript.

**Competing Interests:** The authors' have read the journal's policy and the authors of this manuscript have the following competing interests: the Suntrust Scholar Award was an unconditional philanthropic gift of Suntrust Bank to the Winship Cancer Institute of Emory University to support pilot projects. The authors never had a direct connection with this commercial source. Rather, the authors' project was chosen by the Director of the Winship Cancer institute for funding based on the results of a peer review.

* Email: johann.brandes@emory.edu

## Introduction

With the exception of patients whose tumors harbor a targetable driver mutation, response rates following first-line chemotherapy in patients with advanced non-small lung cancer (NSCLC) remain poor[1] [2]. Predictive biomarkers hold the promise to better select patients for specific cytotoxic chemotherapy agents, enabling the physician to choose the most appropriate treatment regimen, thus improving overall response rates and preventing unnecessary toxicity. In modern combination regimens, taxanes are the class of drugs most commonly combined with a platinum backbone. Alternatives include pemetrexed, vinorelbine or gemcitabine. The availability of these active alternatives justifies an effort to identify biomarkers that are predictive of improved response and survival following taxane- or pemetrexed based chemotherapy in NSCLC. Expression of thymidylate synthase has been shown to be a predictor of pemetrexed sensitivity [3].

We have recently identified reduced protein expression of the mitotic checkpoint gene CHFR as powerful predictor of taxane sensitivity in NSCLC [4]. Patients with reduced CHFR expression had a significantly higher likelihood of achieving a clinical benefit and had significantly improved overall survival. Challenges in standardizing and quantifying immunohistochemistry for CHFR, however, are potential limitations of this biomarker.

The detection of aberrant promoter methylation and subsequent epigenetic silencing of genes involved in the cellular response to chemotherapy has been proposed as a qualitative biomarker for chemotherapy response [5]. The major advantage of this approach is that the detection of aberrant methylation by PCR based assays is easier than the detection of a reduction in protein expression and less susceptible to variations in experimental conditions compared with IHC [6]. Well established examples for the role of promoter methylation in the prediction of chemosensitivity are a) MGMT methylation for the prediction of response to alkylating agents such as temozolomide in glioblastoma multiforme [6,7], b) FANCF methylation as predictor for platinum sensitivity in ovarian cancer [8] and c) CHFR methylation as predictor for taxane sensitivity in gastric [9], cervical [10] and possibly also colon cancer [11].

To identify novel predictive methylation markers for improved outcomes after taxane-based chemotherapy in NSCLC, we performed an unbiased methylation analysis of 1,536 CpG dinucleotides on the Illumina GoldenGate methylation array and correlated results with clinical outcome data amongst NSCLC patients who had received platinum/taxane chemotherapy.

## Materials and Methods

### Study design

The study was approved by the Institutional Review Board of Emory University and the Research and Development Committee of the Atlanta VAMC. Waivers for informed consent requirements were granted due to the retrospective and blinded nature of the clinical data to protected health information (PHI). Patients with stage IV NSCLC who received first-line treatment with a platinum-taxane combination between the years 1999–2010 were initially identified from the local cancer registry at the Atlanta VAMC. We had previously correlated CHFR expression with clinical outcomes in this cohort [4]. Given the different requirements for tissue sections, tumor content and amount of available genomic DNA, not all patients with available tissue blocks qualified for both studies. The registry data were then validated by review of the individual medical records. The following variables were recorded: Age, Sex, Race, chemotherapy regimen, number and type of subsequent therapies, clinical response at first restaging exam, ECOG performance status, tumor histology, date of first diagnosis and overall survival. Patients were further categorized based on the ECOG performance status into good (0 and 1) vs. poor (2 and 3) status. Imaging studies were reviewed individually and response assessment was done by "Response Evaluation Criteria In Solid Tumors (RECIST 1.1)" criteria. Patients who had received at least 2 cycles of therapy and had available paraffin-embedded blocks with sufficient tumor tissue to cut at least 4 sections at 5 uM thickness were eligible.

### Histopathology

Paraffin blocks were cut in sections of 5 uM thickness. One slide was stained with hematoxylin and eosin (H&E) and analyzed by microscopy for tumor type and tumor cell percentage. Only samples with at least 40% viable tumor cell content were used for subsequent analysis. At least 2 additional unstained sections were obtained for DNA extraction.

### DNA extraction and RNA extraction

DNA was extracted from slides 2 and 3 using the E.Z.N.A$^{TM}$ FFPE DNA extraction kit from Omega Biotek (Norcross, GA). RNA was extracted from slides 4 and 5 using the E.Z.N.A$^{TM}$ FFPE RNA extraction kit from Omega Biotek (Norcross, GA). Nucleic acid content was quantified using an Eppendorf Biophotometer Plus (Eppendorf, Hauppauge, NJ) with Hellma Tray Cell (Hellma, Mullheim, Germany).

### Quantitative polymerase chain reaction

mRNA was reversed transcribed using a mix of random hexamer and oligo-dT primers using the Super Script III First strand synthesis kit (LifeTechnologies). qRT-PCR was carried out at a Tm of 55C on a Step One Plus thermocycler (Life Technologies). Primer sequences are available upon request.

### Methylation microarray

High-throughput methylation profiling was done using the Illumina GoldenGate Methylation Cancer Panel I microarray platform. DNA quality control by picogreen, bisulfite-conversion by the EZ DNA methylation kit (Zymo, Irvine, CA) and array hybridization, according to manufacturer's specifications, were performed by Emory Integrated Genomics Core facility.

### Statistical analysis

Data preprocessing and normalization of intensities used the methylumi bioconductor package [12]. In specific, samples were removed that did not pass quality control criteria in terms of an average methylation intensity detection p-value of at least 0.15 or had a low tumor content (below 50%), resulting in 33 patient samples (15 progressive disease (PD), 9 partial response (PR) and 9 stable disease (SD)) for analysis of beta values. A three-way analysis comparing mean beta values among PR versus PD versus SD using an F-statistic based on an ANOVA, applying an FDR corrected p-value of less than 0.05, resulted in the selection of two genes, CAV1 and TEK. Partek Genomics Suite Software (Partek, Inc.) was used for generating heat-maps and clustering of results.

The multivariate survival analysis was conducted by entering sex, race, ECOG performance status, age, race, histology, and Avastin use into a Cox proportional hazard model.

### Cell culture

A549, HOP-62 and EKVX NSCLC cell lines were grown in RPMI media, supplemented with 10% fetal calf serum (Invitrogen). All cell lines were a gift from Dr. Paula Vertino who originally obtained the lines from American Type Culture Collection (ATCC), Manassas, VA. Cell lines were authenticated by STR analysis by Biosynthesis Inc. (Lewisville, TX).

### Constructs and transfection

Small hairpin RNA (shRNA) against Caveolin-1 and non-effective scrambled shRNA in pRFP-C-RS vector were obtained from Origene (Rockville,MD). 1.5 μg of vector were transfected into A549, Hop-62 and EKVX cell lines using Lipofectamine-2000 (Invitrogen). Stably transfected clones were selected and expanded after incubation in Puromycin containing selection media (2.4 µg/mL final). Successful transfection of the clones was determined by fluorescent microscopy and visualization of red fluorescence as well as by subsequent immunoblot for caveolin-1.

## Immunoblotting

Cells were lysed in 1x cell lysis buffer (Cell Signaling), containing Complete protease inhibitor and Phostop (Roche) and 1 mM PMSF. Cells were sonicated briefly and lysates clarified by centrifugation. Following SDS-PAGE and semi-dry transfer the following antibodies were used: Caveolin-1 (1:1000, Cell Signaling), beta-actin (1:10000 Sigma), E-cadherin (1:1000 BD), MDR1 (1:1000 Cell Signaling), Focal-adhesion kinase (FAK) (1:1000, Cell Signaling), phospho-Y397-FAK (1:1000, Cell Signaling).

## Colony Forming Assay

Cell lines indicated were seeded at 1000 cells per well in a 6 well cluster plate. 24 hours post seeding, the cells were treated with docetaxel at 50 nM for 1 hour. The media was exchanged and colonies were allowed to develop for up to three weeks. The cells were fixed with 4% formaldehyde/PBS and stained with crystal violet for imaging and analysis. Image J software was used to quantify the results by measuring the area fraction of each well containing colonies after applying a threshold to the images to eliminate background. Data are reported as fold change over mock treated control.

## Wound healing assay

A549 cells lines bearing either shCAV1 or scrambled control were seeded to 75% confluence in 6 well dishes. 16 hours post seeding, the cell monolayers were scratched with a 20–200 ul pipette tip and imaged under 5X power at the indicated time points. The denuded area was measured using Image J software. Technical triplicates were averaged and values reported as area recovered compared to the zero-hour time point.

## Live Cell Imaging

A549 stable cell lines bearing RFP-expressing shCAV1 or scramble controls were enriched to near 100% purity using a BD-FACS Aria cell sorter and subsequently seeded into Cellview 35 mm glass bottom dishes (Greiner Bio-One). The cells were allowed to attach to the plate overnight. The dish was set on a PE Ultraview spinning disc confocal live cell imaging system. Cells were treated with 2 µM Flutax-1(Santa Cruz Biotechnology) and imaged at 20X in both red and green channels at maximum speed. Three fields of each condition were imaged. After 50 cycles, the media containing Flutax was removed and replaced with Flutax-free media. The samples were imaged for an additional 35–50 cycles. The resulting image sets were analyzed using Cell Profiler software. Analysis of Flutax uptake and turnover, termed Flutax flux, was accomplished by selecting all red positive cells as regions of interest and measuring the change of intensity in the green channel in said regions. This intensity change was measured over 50 cycles (approximately 1.2 cycles per min, 45 minutes total). Reported values are intensities averaged over three fields. Areas under the curves were calculated by trapezoid rule [13].

## Correlation of CAV1 expression and overall survival in independent cohorts

We utilized datasets of 1,715 tumors which had previously been profiled by Affymetrix microarray analysis (www.kmplot.com) [14]. 144 of these tumors also had information on overall survival, clinical stage and on the administration of chemotherapy. CAV1 expression (probe ID: 203065_S_at) was divided by the median into high vs. low expression. Survival analysis by Kaplan-Meier and Cox Proportional Hazard analysis with stage and CAV1 expression as multivariable were performed.

## Results

### Methylation microarray analysis identifies CAV1 methylation as predictor of achieving stable disease after platinum-taxane based combination chemotherapy

Between the years of 1999 to 2010, a total of 178 patients received platinum plus taxane-based chemotherapy for stage IV NSCLC at the Atlanta VAMC. Of these, 106 had a biopsy confirmation of disease and had received at least 2 cycles of chemotherapy. Paraffin embedded tissue was available for sixty-one of these patients of which forty-six met the inclusion criteria. Thirteen of the samples did not fulfill the quality control criteria for successful hybridization to the array. A total of thirty-three samples were available for final analysis (Table 1). Differential methylation (a comparison of individual probe mean beta values) was then correlated with clinical outcomes (partial response (PR), stable disease (SD) and progressive disease (PD)). Of the 807 genes included on the methylation array, 141 genes correlated to a specific outcome with a p-value <0.05. However after adjustments for false discoveries, only methylation for caveolin-1 (CAV1) (position: −169) and loss of methylation for the TEK receptor tyrosine kinase (position: −526) were statistically significantly correlated with stable disease response (Fig. 1A and 1B). Since loss of methylation is challenging to translate into the development of a clinically useful biomarker, we focused on Cav-1 methylation for subsequent experiments.

In order to correlate CAV1 methylation with overall survival in this cohort, we performed univariate and multivariate Cox-regression analyses. In the multivariate analysis and after adjusting for age, performance status, race, histology and the use of bevacizumab, Cav1 methylation was significantly correlated with improved overall survival (hazard ratio (HR) for death: 0.18 (95%CI: 0.03–0.94), p = 0.04) (Table 2), highlighting the potential relevance of Cav1 methylation as clinical biomarker.

### Cav1- mRNA expression is reduced in NSCLC with stable disease response, but correlation is weaker than between response and methylation

Promoter methylation generally results in epigenetic silencing of gene transcription [5]. Due to frequent admixtures of stromal or inflammatory cells, methylation analysis frequently correlates better with outcomes following chemotherapy than analysis of mRNA or protein expression [6]. In order to evaluate the correlation between Cav1 methylation and mRNA expression and between mRNA expression and response, we determined Cav1 mRNA levels by qRT-PCR (Fig. 1C). A trend towards reduced Cav1 mRNA levels was observed in patients with stable disease, as would have been expected in specimens with a higher rate of CAV1 promoter methylation, suggesting that CAV methylation may be a more powerful predictive biomarker than CAV1 expression.

### Loss of Cav1 expression induced epithelial mesemchymal transition (EMT)

In order to determine the biologic relevance of a loss of Cav1 expression, we stably transfected A549, HOP-62 and EKVX NSCLC cell lines with a shRNA against CAV1 or non-silencing scrambled controls. In A549 cells, loss of CAV1 was associated

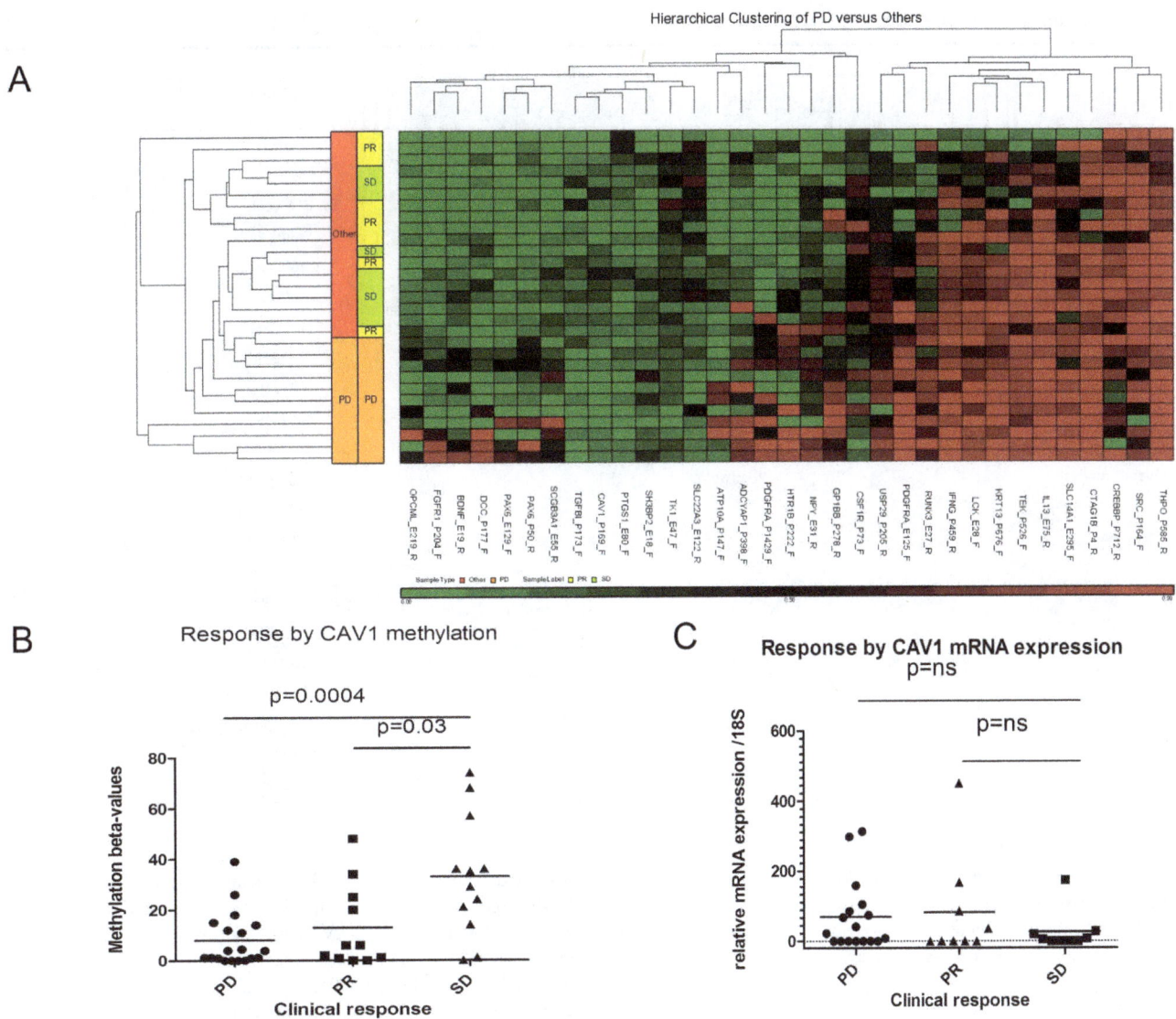

**Figure 1. A three way analysis between Progressive Disease (PD), stable disease (SD) and Partial Response (PR) was performed based on an F-statistic based ANOVA with a FDR corrected p-value <0.05.** A) Hierarchical clustering of the most prominent changes in relationship at clinical response. B) CAV1 methylation is (by methylation beta-value) is statistically significantly associated with stable disease. C) differences in CAV1 m-RNA expression by qRT-PCR between the three groups of clinical outcomes show a statistically non-significant trend towards decreased expression in patients with SD.

with a distinct morphologic change towards spindle cell shape, consistent with EMT (Fig. 2A). At the molecular level, we observed a loss of E-cadherin and an increase of Slugprotein expression consistent with EMT (Fig. 2B). EKVX and HOP-62 are cell lines that display features of EMT at baseline and their phenotype was not altered by CAV1 knockdown. Consistent with the acquisition of an EMT phenotype, shCAV1 transfected A549 cells display increased migration in wound healing assays (Fig. 2C, D). The increased migratory capabilities of CAV1 deficient A549 cells were associated with increased phosphorylation of the focal adhesion kinase (FAK), a well known migration marker [15].

## Loss of CAV1 expression sensitizes lung cancer cell lines to the effects of docetaxel by altering cellular efflux

EMT has long been considered to be an important mediator of chemo-resistance in cancer [16,17,18], which is in contradiction to

the clinical results observed in this study. In order to directly test the role of CAV1 silencing on chemo-sensitivity following exposure to cisplatin and docetaxel, we conducted colony formation experiments on the previously mentioned CAV1 or scrambled shRNA transfected NSCLC lines (A549, HOP62). Interestingly, we observed that CAV1 deficient cell lines were more sensitive to docetaxel than their non-silenced counterparts (Fig. 3A). This is in contrast to treatment with cisplatin which produced comparable cytotoxicity regardless of CAV1 expression (Fig. 3B).

In order to determine if loss of CAV1 expression alters intracellular kinetics of taxane in- and efflux, we performed life-cell imaging after addition of the fluorescently labeled taxol-derivative Flutax-1 (Santa Cruz Biotechnologies). We detected a statistically higher area under the curve (AUC) for Flutax1 in CAV1 deficient cells, suggesting that either increased taxane influx or decreased efflux are likely responsible for the observed

**Table 1.** Clinical characteristics.

| | | |
|---|---|---|
| Sex | Male | 49 (100%) |
| | Female | 0(0%) |
| Age | Median | 62 years |
| | SD | 7.6 years |
| Race | Caucasian | 33(67%) |
| | AA | 16(33%) |
| Histology | SCC | 11(22%) |
| | NOS | 15(31%) |
| | LCC | 8 (16%) |
| | AC | 15 (31%) |
| Chemotherapy | CDDP/TAX | 41 (84%) |
| | CDDP/TAX/Bev | 8 (16%) |
| Overall survival | Median | 0.59 years |
| | SD | 0.51 years |
| Response | PR | 11 (32%) |
| | SD | 15 (24%) |
| | PD | 21 (44%) |
| PS | 0 | 13(28%) |
| | 1 | 20(44%) |
| | 2 | 7 (15%) |
| | 3 | 6 (13%) |
| CAV1 M | >= 15% | 17 (35%) |
| | <15% | 32 (65%) |

increased cytotoxicity in the colony formation assays (Fig. 3C). Multidrug resistance protein MDR1 (also known p-glycoprotein) is an ATPase pump which serves as one of the major cellular detoxifiers. Given its association with caveolae and its known involvement in taxane resistance, expression levels were analyzed and were found to be reduced after CAV1 knockdown in HOP-62 cells (Fig. 3D). However, CAV1 knockdown induced sensitization to taxanes in A549 cells was observed despite a lack of MDR-1 expression, suggesting a mechanism that is at least partially independent from MDR-1 expression.

## Reduced CAV-1 expression predicts improved survival only in NSCLC patients treated with chemotherapy

In order to test the hypothesis that CAV1 specifically plays a role in mediating chemoresistance rather than being associated

with poor prognosis independently from treatment, we analyzed existing genomically and clinically characterized datasets. After adjusting for stage high CAV1 expression correlated with inferior overall survival in patients who received chemotherapy (HR 2.86; 95% CI 1.28–6.36, p<0.01), but did not predict survival in patients who did not receive chemotherapy (HR 1.23 95%CI 0.57–2.65, p = 0.6) (Fig. 4). These findings support the hypothesis that CAV1 expression is predictive of chemosensitivity and not merely prognostic marker.

## Discussion

This is the first report to show a correlation between promoter methylation of CAV1 with favorable outcomes following combination chemotherapy with paclitaxel and carboplatin in NSCLC. These findings are important because they may help establish

**Table 2.** Multivariate analysis.

| | HR (95%CI) | p |
|---|---|---|
| CAV1 P-169-F | 0.18(0.03–0.94) | 0.04 |
| PS good vs poor | 0.42(0.16–1.13) | 0.09 |
| age >=65 vs <65 | 0.77 (0.31–1.85) | 0.56 |
| Avastin use | 0.88(0.33–2.1) | 0.78 |
| Race C vs AA | 1.88 (0.77–4.95) | 0.17 |
| Histo SCC vs non-SCC | 1.11(0.40–2.83) | 0.83 |

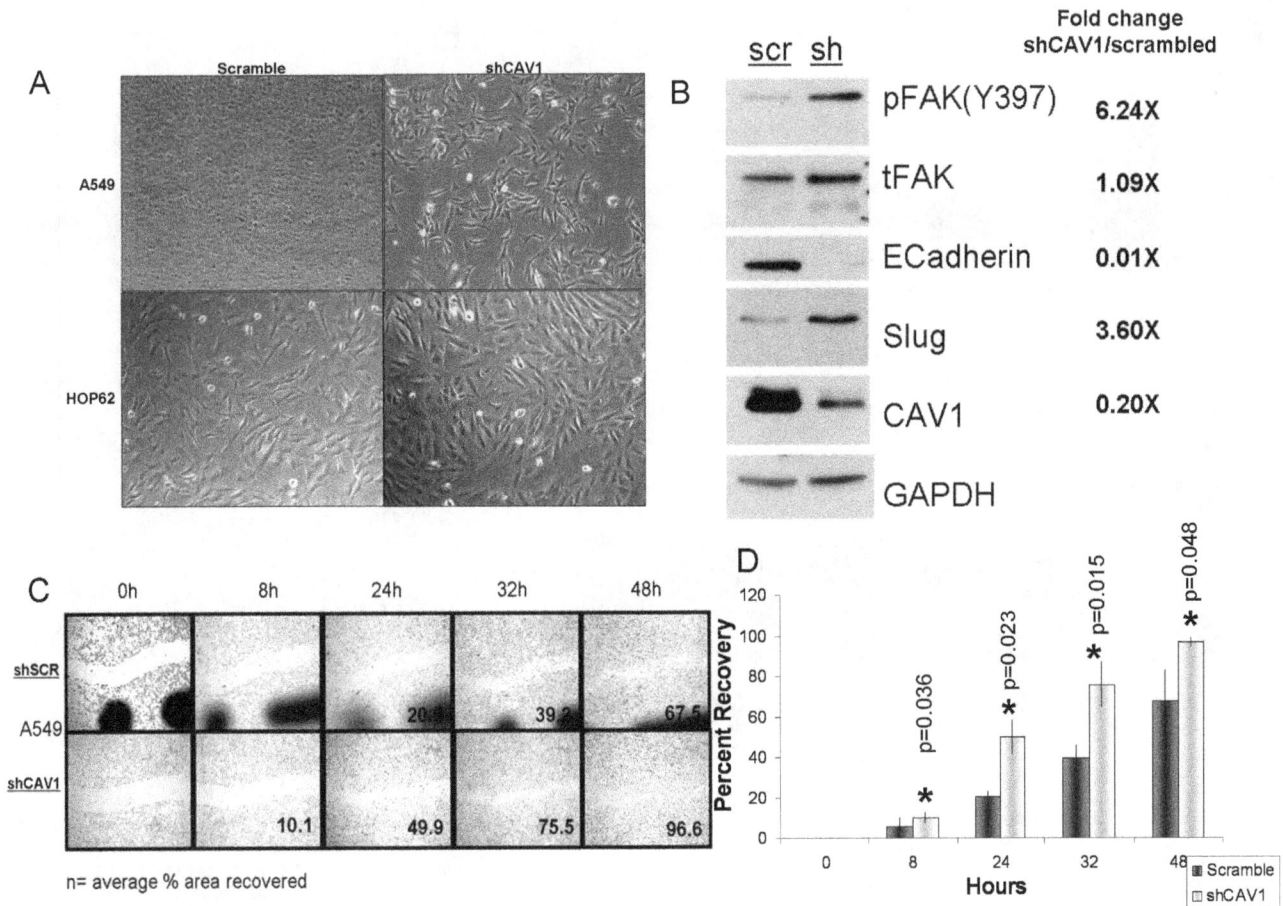

Figure 2. Stable shRNA knockdown induced an epithelial mesenchymal transformation phenotype in A549 cells. A) morphologic changes toward spindle shaped cells after CAV1 shRNA knockdown are observed in A549 cells compared to scrambled shRNA. No such changes are observed in HOP-62 cells which have undergone EMT already. B) CAV1 silencing is associated with reduced expression of E-cadherin and an increase in SLUG expression, both consistent with EMT. Increased FAK-phosphorylation (Y397) signaling serves as a marker for a pro-migratory phenotype C) CAV1 silencing increases cell migration in a wound healing assay D) Quantification of wound healing assays p values (two tailed Student's t) 8 hr p=0.036, 24 hr p=0.023, 32 hr p=0.015, 48 hr p=0.045.

CAV1 methylation as clinically relevant biomarker, which could aid in the selection of treatments that lead to a higher likelihood of survival. Our results suggest that CAV1 methylation is a better discriminator for clinical outcomes than mRNA expression. Similar findings have been previously observed for MGMT methylation vs. expression as predictor for response to alkylating agents in glioblastoma [6].

Before CAV1 methylation can be firmly established as predictive marker for taxane sensitivity in lung cancer, three important questions need to be discussed. Is it mechanistically plausible that CAV1 mediates taxane resistance? Is CAV1 silencing specifically associated only with taxane sensitivity or do intracellular pharmacokinetics of other chemotherapeutics converge on the same mechanism? Finally, could CAV1 methylation or expression be a prognostic marker that is associated with favorable prognosis independent of treatment.

CAV1 serves as integral part of caveolae, special lipid rafts which play major functions in cell signaling and endocytosis [19]. In lung cancer both tumor suppressive as well as tumor promoting roles have been described [20]. In small cell lung cancer (SCLC), loss of CAV1expression has been found to promote anchorage independent colony formation. In NSCLC reports about tumor promoting vs. tumor suppressive roles of CAV1 are conflicting and

vary among different cell lines used. For example, in H1299 cells CAV1 shRNA knockdown led to a decrease in proliferation [20], while in H460 cells increased metastatic potential and proliferation were observed [21]. In multidrug resistant cell lines, MDR1 co-localized to the low density detergent-insoluble membrane fractions which are characteristic of caveolae, suggesting a possible association between caveolae and multidrug resistance. Our data however prove a direct effect of CAV1 silencing on taxane sensitivity and intracellular uptake or retention in an MDR1 independent fashion, possibly by affecting other multidrug transporters. Support for these findings comes from several reports in the literature of taxane resistant A549 cell lines where CAV1 and MDR1 expression were either discordant or localized to different compartments of the cell membrane [22,23].

Even though our data show that CAV1 silencing increases taxane- but not platinum sensitivity the possibility exists that intracellular pharmacokinetics of other drugs used in lung cancer therapy such as gemcitabine or etoposide may be dependent on CAV1 mediated mechanisms as well. This is due to the fact that no cellular in-or efflux mechanisms have so far been described that are exclusively specific for taxanes which could at least in part explain the observations that lung cancer patients with high CAV1

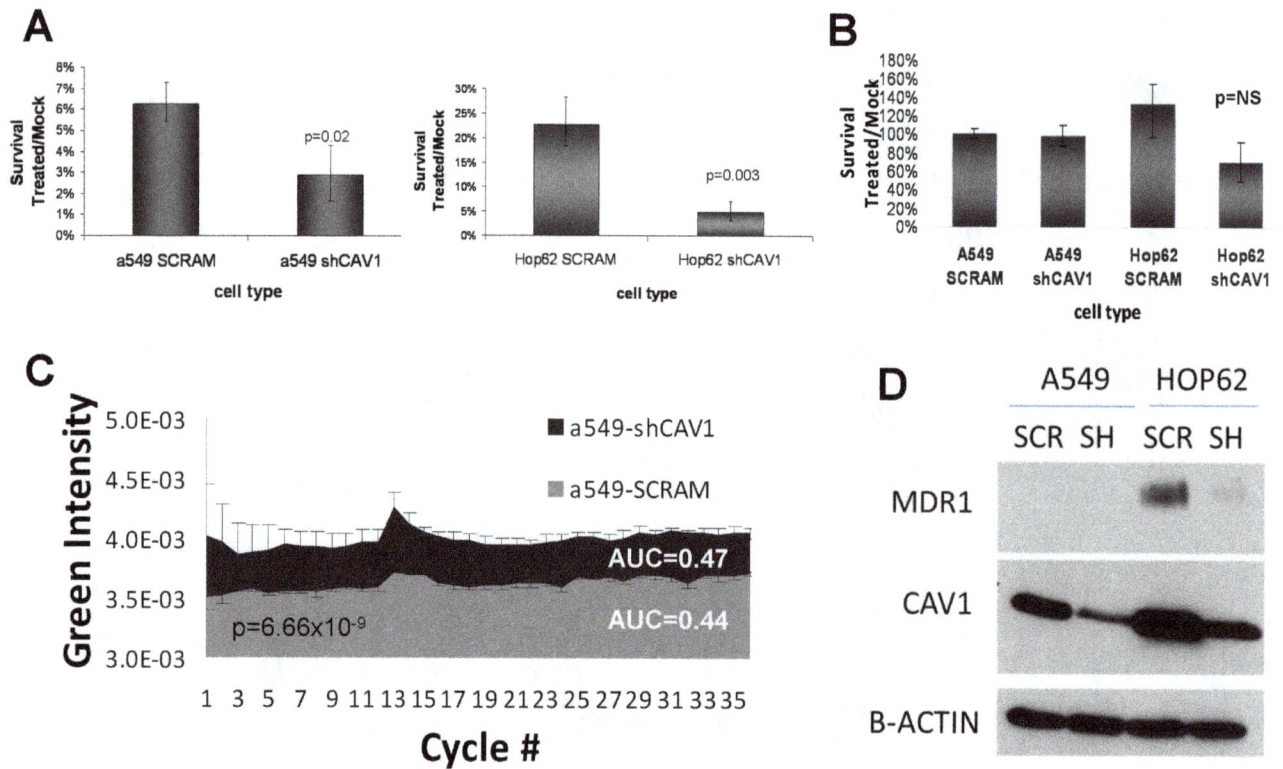

**Figure 3. Loss of CAV1 increases taxane sensitivity, by decreasing taxane turnover independent of loss of MDR1.** A: CAV1 silencing increases taxane sensitivity in colony formation assays in a549 and HOP62 NSCLC cell lines. Error bars represent standard deviations, p-value <0.05. B: No impact of CAV1 silencing is observed in relationship to cisplatin sensitivity. C: CAV1 silencing leads to increased intracellular taxol concentrations. Live cell microscopy assays were performed in the presence of fluorescently labeled taxol (Flutax). Red- and green fluorescent images were obtained at a frequency of 1.2 images/min. Green fluorescence was analyzed in red-fluorescent cells and plotted over 50 cycles. Statistical analysis was by trapezoid rule (p-value $p = 6.66 \times 10^{-9}$). D: CAV1 silencing is associated with reduced protein expression of MDR-1 in Hop-62 cells but not in A549 cells.

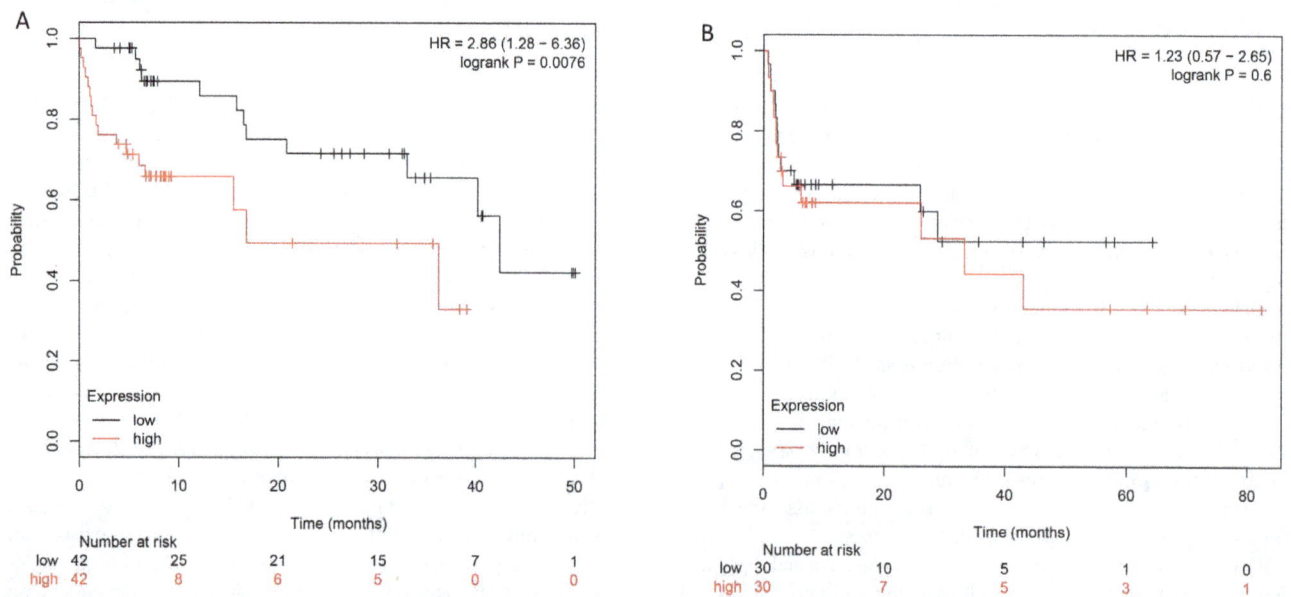

**Figure 4. Overall survival was analyzed by CAV1 expression status as determined by Affymetrix gene-expression array in patients who received chemotherapy and those who did not.** Out of 1,715 datasets, 144 had clinical information on both stage and overall survival. After adjusting for stage in a multivariate analysis reduced CAV1 expression was associated with improved survival only in patients who received chemotherapy (A) but not in patient who did not (B).

expression levels had inferior survival compared to those with low expression when gemcitabine based chemotherapy was given [24].

While we have established CAV1 methylation is a predictive biomarker for taxane based chemotherapy response in lung cancer, a possible prognostic value independent from treatment needs to be considered as well. In NSCLC, CAV1 overexpression has been associated with higher disease stage and inferior survival in patients with adenocarcinoma, but a robust correction of the survival data for stage and treatment was not done in these studies [24,25,26]. Our findings and other reports in the literature that CAV1 loss induces EMT and increases proliferation, migration and metastatic potential argue against an inherently better prognosis of CAV1 methylated tumors [21]. Further support comes from our findings that overall survival in untreated patients with lung cancer does not differ by CAV1 expression status.

In summary, we have shown that CAV1 methylation is associated with high rates of stable disease and improved overall survival in patients with advanced NSCLC following chemotherapy with platinum-taxane based regimens. CAV1 methylation could serve as biomarker for taxane sensitivity and could help identify subsets of patients who are more likely to benefit from this cytotoxic chemotherapy.

## Author Contributions

Conceived and designed the experiments: SAB CL GL JCB AIM PMV FRK. Performed the experiments: SAB CL GL JCB. Analyzed the data: SAB CL GL JK KG JCB PMV AIM. Contributed reagents/materials/analysis tools: SY. Contributed to the writing of the manuscript: SAB JCB PMV FRK.

## References

1. Schiller JH, Harrington D, Belani CP, Langer C, Sandler A, et al. (2002) Comparison of four chemotherapy regimens for advanced non-small-cell lung cancer. N Engl J Med 346: 92–98.
2. Rigas JR (2004) Taxane-platinum combinations in advanced non-small cell lung cancer: a review. Oncologist 9 Suppl 2: 16–23.
3. Takezawa K, Okamoto I, Okamoto W, Takeda M, Sakai K, et al. (2011) Thymidylate synthase as a determinant of pemetrexed sensitivity in non-small cell lung cancer. Br J Cancer 104: 1594–1601.
4. Pillai RN, Brodie SA, Sica G, You S, Varma V, et al. (2013) CHFR protein expression predicts outcomes to taxane-based first line therapy in metastatic NSCLC. Clin Cancer Res.
5. Herman JG, Baylin SB (2003) Gene silencing in cancer in association with promoter hypermethylation. N Engl J Med 349: 2042–2054.
6. Esteller M, Garcia-Foncillas J, Andion E, Goodman SN, Hidalgo OF, et al. (2000) Inactivation of the DNA-repair gene MGMT and the clinical response of gliomas to alkylating agents. The New England journal of medicine 343: 1350–1354.
7. Hegi ME, Diserens AC, Gorlia T, Hamou MF, de Tribolet N, et al. (2005) MGMT gene silencing and benefit from temozolomide in glioblastoma. The New England journal of medicine 352: 997–1003.
8. Taniguchi T, Tischkowitz M, Ameziane N, Hodgson SV, Mathew CG, et al. (2003) Disruption of the Fanconi anemia-BRCA pathway in cisplatin-sensitive ovarian tumors. Nat Med 9: 568–574.
9. Satoh A, Toyota M, Itoh F, Sasaki Y, Suzuki H, et al. (2003) Epigenetic inactivation of CHFR and sensitivity to microtubule inhibitors in gastric cancer. Cancer research 63: 8606–8613.
10. Banno K, Yanokura M, Kawaguchi M, Kuwabara Y, Akiyoshi J, et al. (2007) Epigenetic inactivation of the CHFR gene in cervical cancer contributes to sensitivity to taxanes. International journal of oncology 31: 713–720.
11. Pelosof L, Yerram SR, Ahuja N, Delmas A, Danilova L, et al. (2014) CHFR silencing or microsatellite instability is associated with increased antitumor activity of docetaxel or gemcitabine in colorectal cancer. Int J Cancer 134: 596–605.
12. Davis S, Du P, Bilke S, Triche T, Bootwalla M (2012) methylumi: Handle Illumina methylation data. R package version 2.4.0.
13. Marcus AI, O'Brate AM, Buey RM, Zhou J, Thomas S, et al. (2006) Farnesyltransferase inhibitors reverse taxane resistance. Cancer Res 66: 8838–8846.
14. Gyorffy B, Surowiak P, Budczies J, Lanczky A (2013) Online survival analysis software to assess the prognostic value of biomarkers using transcriptomic data in non-small-cell lung cancer. PLoS One 8: e82241.
15. Sieg DJ, Hauck CR, Ilic D, Klingbeil CK, Schaefer E, et al. (2000) FAK integrates growth-factor and integrin signals to promote cell migration. Nat Cell Biol 2: 249–256.
16. Wang H, Zhang G, Zhang H, Zhang F, Zhou B, et al. (2014) Acquisition of epithelial-mesenchymal transition phenotype and cancer stem cell-like properties in cisplatin-resistant lung cancer cells through AKT/beta-catenin/Snail signaling pathway. Eur J Pharmacol 723: 156–166.
17. Canadas I, Rojo F, Taus A, Arpi O, Arumi-Uria M, et al. (2014) Targeting epithelial-to-mesenchymal transition with Met inhibitors reverts chemoresistance in small cell lung cancer. Clin Cancer Res 20: 938–950.
18. Ren J, Chen Y, Song H, Chen L, Wang R (2013) Inhibition of ZEB1 reverses EMT and chemoresistance in docetaxel-resistant human lung adenocarcinoma cell line. J Cell Biochem 114: 1395–1403.
19. Doherty GJ, McMahon HT (2009) Mechanisms of endocytosis. Annu Rev Biochem 78: 857–902.
20. Sunaga N, Miyajima K, Suzuki M, Sato M, White MA, et al. (2004) Different roles for caveolin-1 in the development of non-small cell lung cancer versus small cell lung cancer. Cancer Res 64: 4277–4285.
21. Song Y, Xue L, Du S, Sun M, Hu J, et al. (2012) Caveolin-1 knockdown is associated with the metastasis and proliferation of human lung cancer cell line NCI-H460. Biomed Pharmacother 66: 439–447.
22. Belanger MM, Gaudreau M, Roussel E, Couet J (2004) Role of caveolin-1 in etoposide resistance development in A549 lung cancer cells. Cancer Biol Ther 3: 954–959.
23. Yang CP, Galbiati F, Volonte D, Horwitz SB, Lisanti MP (1998) Upregulation of caveolin-1 and caveolae organelles in Taxol-resistant A549 cells. FEBS Lett 439: 368–372.
24. Ho CC, Kuo SH, Huang PH, Huang HY, Yang CH, et al. (2008) Caveolin-1 expression is significantly associated with drug resistance and poor prognosis in advanced non-small cell lung cancer patients treated with gemcitabine-based chemotherapy. Lung Cancer 59: 105–110.
25. Yoo SH, Park YS, Kim HR, Sung SW, Kim JH, et al. (2003) Expression of caveolin-1 is associated with poor prognosis of patients with squamous cell carcinoma of the lung. Lung Cancer 42: 195–202.
26. Zhan P, Shen XK, Qian Q, Wang Q, Zhu JP, et al. (2012) Expression of caveolin-1 is correlated with disease stage and survival in lung adenocarcinomas. Oncol Rep 27: 1072–1078.

# 20

# Early Treatment Response in Non-Small Cell Lung Cancer Patients using Diffusion-Weighted Imaging and Functional Diffusion Maps

**Carolin Reischauer**[1,2,3]*, **Johannes Malte Froehlich**[1], **Miklos Pless**[4], **Christoph Andreas Binkert**[3], **Dow-Mu Koh**[5,6], **Andreas Gutzeit**[1,3]

**1** Institute of Radiology and Nuclear Medicine, Clinical Research Unit, Hirslanden Hospital St. Anna, Lucerne, Switzerland, **2** Department of Radiology, Cantonal Hospital Winterthur, Winterthur, Switzerland, **3** Department of Radiology, Paracelsus Medical University Salzburg, Salzburg, Austria, **4** Department of Oncology, Cantonal Hospital Winterthur, Winterthur, Switzerland, **5** Academic Department of Radiology, Royal Marsden NHS Foundation Trust, Sutton, Surrey, United Kingdom, **6** CR-UK and EPSRC Cancer Imaging Centre, Institute of Cancer Research, Sutton, Surrey, United Kingdom

## Abstract

*Objective:* The aim of this study was to prospectively evaluate the feasibility of monitoring treatment response to chemotherapy in patients with non-small cell lung carcinoma using functional diffusion maps (fDMs).

*Materials and Methods:* This study was approved by the Cantonal Research Ethics Committee and informed written consent was obtained from all patients. Nine patients (mean age = 66 years; range = 53–76 years, 5 females, 4 males) with overall 13 lesions were included. Imaging was performed within two weeks before initiation of chemotherapy and at one, two, and six weeks after initiation of chemotherapy. Imaging included a respiratory-triggered diffusion-weighted sequence including three b-factors (100, 600, and 800 s/mm$^2$). Treatment response was defined by change in tumor diameter on computed tomography (CT) after two cycles of chemotherapy. Changes in the apparent diffusion coefficient (ADC) on a per-lesion basis and the percentages of voxel with significantly increased or decreased ADCs on fDMs were analyzed using repeated measures analysis of variance (ANOVA). Changes in tumor size were used as covariate to examine the ability of ADCs and fDM parameters to predict treatment response.

*Results:* Repeated measures ANOVA revealed that the percentage of voxels with increased ADCs on fDMs (p = 0.002) as well as the mean ADC increase (p = 0.011) were significantly higher in good responders with a large reduction in tumor size on CT.

*Conclusion:* Our results indicate that the percentage of voxels with significantly increased ADCs on fDMs seems to be a promising biomarker for early prediction of treatment response in patients with non-small cell lung carcinoma. Contrary to averaged values, this approach allows the spatial heterogeneity of treatment response to be resolved.

**Editor:** Andreas-Claudius Hoffmann, West German Cancer Center, Germany

**Funding:** The authors have no support or funding to report.

**Competing Interests:** The authors have declared that no competing interests exist.

* Email: carolin.reischauer@hirslanden.ch

## Introduction

Response to anticancer drugs of non-small cell lung cancer is usually evaluated as tumor shrinkage on computed tomography (CT) after two cycles of chemotherapy in agreement with the response evaluation criteria in solid tumors (RECIST) [1]. Novel chemotherapies as well as new targeted therapies are being progressively introduced, therefore new biomarkers that permit early treatment monitoring and the prediction of treatment response are warranted so that treatment can be more rapidly adapted, avoiding unnecessary adverse effects from ineffective treatment and rendering anticancer therapies more cost efficient.

Diffusion-weighted imaging (DWI) is a promising tool for evaluating treatment response to anticancer therapy at an earlier stage than tumor size measurement, since cellular death and vascular changes precede changes in lesion size [2]. Using DWI, the apparent diffusion coefficient (ADC) can be calculated which has been shown to be a useful quantitative response biomarker to anticancer drugs in brain tumors [3], breast cancer [4–6], head and neck tumors [7,8], cervical cancer [9], liver cancer [10], rectal cancer [11], soft-tissue sarcomas [12], bone metastases [13,14], and non-small cell lung carcinoma [15].

More recently, the functional diffusion map (DM) has been investigated as a method of voxelwise ADC analysis that is potentially more sensitive in detecting treatment response than

ADCs averaged over entire lesions [16,17]. The fDM characterizes and quantifies heterogeneity of treatment response by segmenting the tumor on a voxelwise basis into three distinct regions with significantly increased (red voxels), significantly decreased (blue voxels) and unchanged ADCs (green voxels) under therapy. Using this method, studies have up until now focused largely on the investigation of brain tumors [16–19]. The translation to body regions prone to motion is challenging due to the requirement of precise coregistration of the pre- and post-treatment ADC maps as a mandatory preprocessing step for calculating fDMs. Hence, fDM analysis of lesions in the lung is particularly challenging due to respiratory motion and susceptibility-related artifacts caused by tissue-air interfaces.

Thus, the aim of the present pilot study was to prospectively evaluate the feasibility of monitoring and predicting treatment response in patients with non-small cell lung cancer using fDMs compared with reduction in tumor size on CT after two cycles of therapy as the reference standard.

## Materials and Methods

### Study Population

This study was approved by the Cantonal Research Ethics Committee and informed written consent was obtained from all patients in our prospective clinical study conducted between August 2010 and August 2012. Nine patients (mean age = 66 years; range = 53–76 years, 5 females, 4 males) with overall 13 lung tumors who fulfilled all inclusion and exclusion criteria were included. The inclusion criteria were: histological proven non-small-cell lung cancer (adenocarcinoma, stage IV) without any previous oncologic treatment in a palliative, non-surgical setting with planned systemic therapy. The exclusion criteria were: unwillingness to participate in the study, contraindications to magnetic resonance imaging (MRI) or inability to tolerate MRI because of high grade dyspnea or reduced general health conditions.

### Diagnosis and Treatment of Lung Cancer

In all patients, the diagnosis of lung cancer was histologically proven with transbronchial biopsy by a board-examined pulmologist. Within 14 days of diagnosis, all included patients were examined using a standardized contrast-enhanced CT and a baseline MRI examination. Therapeutic response was categorized by a radiologist (AG) with 13 years of experience in thoracic imaging using RECIST 1.1 criteria [1] by evaluating changes in the maximum tumor axial diameter on CT after two cycles of chemotherapy. Specific therapy, length of progression-free interval, and lesion size on CT before and after treatment are listed for each patient in Table 1. Note that patient 2 deceased after the second course of chemotherapy due to causes unrelated to lung cancer. At the time of death there was no tumor progression. Data for this patient was included until termination of the second course of chemotherapy.

### MRI Examination

MRI was performed at a maximum of 14 days before onset of treatment and repeated at one, two, and six weeks after initiation of the first course of chemotherapy. Imaging of the thorax was performed on a 1.5 T MRI scanner (Achieva, Philips Healthcare, Best, the Netherlands, Release 3.2.2.0) with the patient in the supine position using a 16-element sensitivity-encoding torso receive-only coil array (Philips Healthcare, Best, the Netherlands) covering the chest.

Axial Imaging of the thorax was performed using $T_1$-weighted fast spin-echo as well as dual-echo fast gradient-echo imaging, together with axial DWI, using three b-values of 100, 600 and 800 s/mm$^2$. The lower b-value was chosen to diminish perfusion effects [2]. The imaging parameters are summarized in Table 2. To minimize the effects of respiratory motion, imaging was performed using a respiratory-triggering technique with a navigator placed on the right dome of the diaphragm.

During the baseline scan prior to therapy, the DWI scan was acquired twice to allow for the calculation of the thresholds for the fDMs (see further details below). Therefore, the first scan session was longer than the follow-up scans. The scan times for baseline was about 20 minutes and for follow-up examinations approximately 14 minutes. Due to the respiratory-triggered DWI acquisition, the individual scan times varied between subjects.

### Diffusion Data Analysis

Data analysis was performed using in-house software written in Matlab (The Mathworks, Natick, MA, USA, Release 2010a). First, eddy current-induced image warping was corrected in the in-vivo data sets using a correlation-based affine registration algorithm [20]. Second, ADC maps were calculated using a mono-exponential fit of all b-factor images at each measurement time point. This resulted in altogether five ADC maps per patient, two pretreatment as well as three posttreatment ADC maps. Third, the second pretreatment ADC map and all posttreatment ADC maps were coregistered to the corresponding first pretreatment ADC map for each patient individually. Coregistration was performed using a robust multiresolution alignment algorithm [21] that was implemented in Matlab. The algorithm was extended to allow for affine transformations. As a quality indicator of coregistration, Pearson's correlation coefficients of the two pretreatment ADC maps of each patient were calculated before and after coregistration. Thereby, the correlation coefficient was computed over the entire data sets.

**Region of Interest Analysis.** The lesion borders were defined manually on the ADC maps taking into account the diagnostic information of CT and the corresponding conventional anatomical MRI. The regions of interest (ROIs) were drawn over each tumor bearing slice on the ADC maps across the entire metastases by a single radiologist (AG). ROIs were defined across all lesions in each patient for each examination separately, i.e. before initiation of chemotherapy (first pretreatment ADC map) (mean size = 57.16 cm$^3$; range = 1.46–253.25 cm$^3$) and at one (mean size = 45.13 cm$^3$; range = 1.37–247.46 cm$^3$), two (mean size = 43.40 cm$^3$; range = 1.30–231.36 cm$^3$), and six (mean size = 33.57 cm$^3$; range = 1.39–184.78 cm$^3$) weeks after therapy onset. Care was taken to exclude cavitary areas or atelectatic lung regions. Thereafter, the mean ADC of each lesion at every time point was calculated and subsequently the corresponding ADC changes relative to the pretreatment values.

**FDM Analysis.** Previous work showed that, time permitting, thresholds for fDMs should be determined directly in the tumor rather than in reference tissue to maximize their accuracy [22]. Therefore, the thresholds were calculated for each patient individually directly in the tumor tissue by statistical comparison of the two pretreatment ADC maps. Thereby, the thresholds were set to the repeatability limit of the tumor tissue in each patient determined using one-way analysis of variance (ANOVA) [14]. Beyond the significance threshold, a cluster size threshold was set at six to exclude isolated voxels which most likely correspond to false-positive results [14]. In doing so, the percentage of voxels that showed a significant increase (red voxels), a significant decrease (blue voxels) or no change (green voxels) in their ADCs at each

**Table 1.** Specific therapy, length of progression-free interval, and lesion cross section size on CT before and after treatment for each patient.

| Patient | Lesion | Specific therapy | Progression-free interval (months) | Lesion size before treatment (cm) | Lesion size after two cycles of chemotherapy (cm) |
|---|---|---|---|---|---|
| 1 | 1 | Cisplatin/Platinol | 4 | 4.4 | 1.8 |
| 2 | 1 | Carboplatin/Paraplatin+ Gemcitabine/Gemzar | * | 5.8 | 5.0 |
| 3 | 1 | Erlotinib/Tarceva | 21 | 1.9 | 0.7 |
| 4 | 1 | Carboplatin/Paraplatin+ Pemetrexed/Alimta | 12 | 3.2 | 2.9 |
| 5 | 1 | Cisplatin/Platinol+ Gemcitabine/Gemzar | 3 | 6.2 | 5.3 |
| 6 | 1 | Cisplatin/Platinol+ Pemetrexed/Alimta | 14 | 2.1 | 1.7 |
| 7 | 1 | Erlotinib/Tarceva | 10 | 2.9 | 2.7 |
|  | 2 |  |  | 2.5 | 2.1 |
| 8 | 1 | Carboplatin/Paraplatin+ Pemetrexed/Alimta | 5 | 9.3 | 7.3 |
|  | 2 |  |  | 1.4 | 0.8 |
| 9 | 1 | Cisplatin/Platinol+ Pemetrexed/Alimta | 7 | 3.5 | 2.9 |
|  | 2 |  |  | 2.8 | 1.6 |
|  | 3 |  |  | 1.9 | 1.5 |

* The patient deceased prior to tumor progression due to causes unrelated to lung cancer.

posttreatment time point relative to the pretreatment values was computed for each and every lesion in the study cohort. In this way, fDMs were generated for the intersection of each baseline ROI and the corresponding posttreatment ROI.

## Statistical Analysis

Changes in tumor diameter on CT before and after two cycles of chemotherapy were compared on a per-lesion basis using Wilcoxon signed-rank test. The mean ADC changes on a per-lesion basis and percentages of voxels with significantly increased (red voxels) and significantly decreased (blue voxels) on fDMs over time were analyzed using repeated measures ANOVA. For this analysis, the changes in tumor size on CT were first entered as covariate and second as between-subjects factor. For the latter each lesion was classified in agreement with RECIST criteria as either showing stable disease (<30% decrease in tumor size) or partial response (>30% decrease in tumor size) under anticancer treatment.

Due to the low number of patients a Kaplan-Meier survival analysis was not performed. However, to evaluate the diffusion parameters as predictive biomarkers of treatment outcome, Pearson correlation coefficients between the length of the progression-free interval and the diffusion parameters (i.e. mean ADC changes and percentages of red and blue voxels on fDMs) at the first time point after initiating treatment were calculated. In patients with multiple lesions, averaged diffusion parameters were therefore calculated on a per-patient basis as weighted means according to the size of each lesion in the patient. For this predictive analysis, data of patient 2 who died prior to tumor progression from causes unrelated to lung cancer was excluded.

Statistical analysis was performed using SPSS (IBM Corporation, Armonk, NY, USA, SPSS Statistics for Windows, Version 21.0), with p<0.05 considered to be statistically significant for each analysis.

## Results

### CT-Based Changes in Tumor Size after Two Cycles of Chemotherapy

Across the study cohort, the Wilcoxon signed-rank test showed a highly significant decrease in tumor diameter on CT (p<0.001) after two cycles of chemotherapy (mean size before therapy = 3.7 cm; range = 1.4–9.3 cm; mean size after two courses of chemotherapy = 2.8 cm; range = 0.7–7.3 cm). No patients showed an increase in tumor size after treatment.

### Diffusion Data Analysis

No violations of the assumptions of repeated measures ANOVA were observed. To this end, analysis of the residuals was performed by examining normal plots of the residuals and plots of the residuals versus the fitted values. Beyond that, Mauchly's sphericity test was computed.

**ROI Analysis of Mean ADC Changes During Therapy.** The results of the ROI analysis are summarized in Table 3. Repeated measures ANOVA revealed no significant alterations in the changes of the mean tumor ADC over time (p = 0.554). However, there was a significant dependence of the mean tumor ADC change on the change in tumor size (p = 0.011). Figure 1a shows the mean ADC change of each lesion at one, two, and six weeks after initiation of chemotherapy plotted against the reduction in tumor size on CT after two cycles of chemotherapy. To understand this dependence better, changes in tumor size were recorded as a binary variable and used as a between-subjects factor for analysis. Thereby, each lesion was classified according to RECIST criteria as either showing stable disease (<30% decrease in tumor size; n = 9) or partial response (>30% decrease in tumor size; n = 4) under chemotherapy. The relationship between size reduction and mean ADC change was still significant and revealed that the mean ADC increase was larger in lesions that showed a

**Table 2.** Overview of MRI sequence parameters.

| Sequence | Repetition time (ms) | Echo time (ms) | FOV (mm²) | Voxel size (mm²) | Slice Thickness (mm) | No. of slices | No. of signal averages | Acquisition time (s) |
|---|---|---|---|---|---|---|---|---|
| T$_1$-weighted fast SE | 796 | 26 | 280×238 | 0.8×0.8 | 6 | 30 | 1 | 23.9 |
| Dual-echo breathhold fast GE | 5.9 | 2.3/4.6 | 375×295 | 1×1 | 6 | 25 | 1 | 34.8 |
| DWI with navigator-triggered SE echo-planar imaging and SPIR* | 2174 | 62.1 | 280×233 | 2×2 | 6 | 30 | 6 | 400 |

Note: GE = gradient echo, SE = spin echo, SPIR = spectral presaturation with inversion recovery. All sequences were axial and two-dimensional.
*This sequence was performed with b-values of 100, 600, and 800 s/mm² and a parallel imaging reduction factor of 1.8. The actual repetition and scan times were longer due to navigator triggering.

large reduction in tumor size on CT compared with lesions that showed only a moderate decrease in tumor size after two cycles of chemotherapy (p = 0.045). In fact, lesions that demonstrated a large decrease in tumor size showed on average an increase in the mean ADCs across all measurement timepoints (mean at one week = 16.2%; mean at two weeks = 9.4%; mean at six weeks = 19.0%) whereas those with a moderate decrease in tumor size revealed a decrease in the mean ADCs across all measurement timepoints (mean at one week = −7.4%; mean at two weeks = −8.9%; mean at six weeks = −3.5%).

**FDM Analysis of ADC Changes with Therapy.** As a quality indicator of coregistration, Pearson's correlation coefficients between the two pretreatment ADC maps were calculated before and after coregistration. The mean correlation coefficient averaged over all patients increased from 0.74 (range = 0.56–0.93) before coregistration to 0.82 (range = 0.70–0.94) after coregistration.

The mean threshold for the fDMs of all patients beyond which a significant ADC change was deemed to have occurred was $0.64 \cdot 10^{-3}$ mm²/s (range = $0.26$–$0.89 \cdot 10^{-3}$ mm²/s). By way of example, fDMs for two patients through a single level of the lung tumors at one, two, and six weeks after initiation of chemotherapy as well as the corresponding scatterplots over the entire lesions are depicted in Figures 2 and 3. Figure 2 depicts the fDMs of the lesion in patient 1 which showed a large reduction in tumor size on CT after two cycles of chemotherapy. Large regions with significantly increased ADCs (shown in red) are observed at all timepoints after treatment began compared with pretreatment values. By contrast, Figure 3 illustrates that only minor regions with significantly increased ADCs but larger regions with significantly decreased ADCs (depicted in blue) were observed in the two lesions of patient 7 which showed only a moderate decrease in tumor size on CT.

Repeated measures ANOVA showed no significant changes in the percentage of voxels with significantly increased ADCs (red voxels) over time (p = 0.180). However, there was a significant dependence of the percentage of red voxels on the change in tumor size (p = 0.002). The percentages of voxels with significantly increased ADCs (red voxels) relative to their pretreatment values at one, two, and six weeks after initiation of chemotherapy are plotted against the reduction in tumor size on CT after two cycles of chemotherapy in Figure 1b. As before, the change in tumor size was dichotomized as a binary variable (large vs. moderate changes in tumor size on CT) for further analysis. The percentage of red voxels was significantly higher in lesions that showed a large reduction in tumor size than in those that showed only a moderate decrease in tumor size on CT after two courses of chemotherapy (p = 0.041). Finally, repeated measures ANOVA revealed neither a significant change in the percentage of voxels with significantly decreased ADCs (blue voxels) over time (p = 0.070) nor a significant relationship between the percentage of blue voxels and the change in tumor size (p = 0.181).

The pie charts in Figure 4 summarizes the results, i.e. the percentage of voxels with significantly increased ADCs compared with pretreatment values was significantly higher in lesions that showed partial response (mean at one week = 24.5%; mean at two weeks = 20.6%; mean at six weeks = 21.2%) versus lesions that only showed stable disease (mean at one week = 4.5%; mean at two weeks = 3.7%; mean at six weeks = 9.4%) on CT.

**Pearson Correlation of Diffusion Parameters and Progression-Free Interval.** Bivariate correlation did not reveal a significant relationship between the ADC change at one week after initiating treatment and the progression-free interval (r = 0.627, p = 0.096). Similarly, no significant relationships were

**Table 3.** Results of the ROI analysis of the ADCs on a per-lesion basis.

| Patient | Lesion | Mean ADC before treatment ($10^{-3}$ mm²/s) | Mean ADC change 1 week after initiation of chemotherapy ($10^{-3}$ mm²/s) | Mean ADC change 2 weeks after initiation of chemotherapy ($10^{-3}$ mm²/s) | Mean ADC change 6 weeks after initiation of chemotherapy ($10^{-3}$ mm²/s) |
|---|---|---|---|---|---|
| 1 | 1 | 1.436 | 0.293 | 0.348 | 0.298 |
| 2 | 1 | 1.348 | −0.095 | −0.073 | 0.045 |
| 3 | 1 | 1.007 | 0.789 | 0.111 | 0.328 |
| 4 | 1 | 1.341 | 0.158 | −0.223 | 0.249 |
| 5 | 1 | 1.454 | −0.006 | 0.177 | 0.022 |
| 6 | 1 | 1.702 | −0.034 | 0.046 | 0.529 |
| 7 | 1 | 1.215 | −0.316 | −0.043 | −0.255 |
|   | 2 | 1.268 | −0.273 | −0.353 | −0.136 |
| 8 | 1 | 0.998 | 0.018 | 0.046 | 0.074 |
|   | 2 | 1.286 | −0.251 | 0.010 | 0.052 |
| 9 | 1 | 1.823 | −0.331 | −0.173 | −0.411 |
|   | 2 | 1.906 | −0.275 | 0.032 | 0.353 |
|   | 3 | 1.940 | −0.105 | −0.71 | −0.755 |

found either between the percentages of the red voxels (r = 0.541, p = 0.166) or blue voxels (r = −0.506, p = 0.200) at one week after initiating treatment and the progression-free interval.

## Discussion

In patients diagnosed with locally advanced non-small cell lung cancer, treatment response to chemotherapy is usually assessed using RECIST 1.1 criteria [1] based on the reduction in the maximum axial tumor diameter on CT. RECIST remains the most widely accepted method for tumor response assessment even though this is made after the completion of chemotherapy, typically at 12 weeks after initiating treatment. However, as expensive targeted therapies are progressively introduced for the

treatment of lung cancer [23,24], there is a desire for early response and predictive biomarkers that would help to guide patient management.

The present preliminary study demonstrates that the percentage of voxels with significantly increased ADCs (red voxels) measured using fDMs may allow early identification of patients with partial response according to conventional RECIST criteria. FDMs may predict outcome of treatment as early as at one week after initiation of chemotherapy. For this reason, this ADC analysis method may allow physicians to make early adjustments to patient management so as to maximize treatment benefits and avoid side-effects from ineffective treatment. Furthermore, early treatment adaption could potentially render anticancer therapy more cost-efficient.

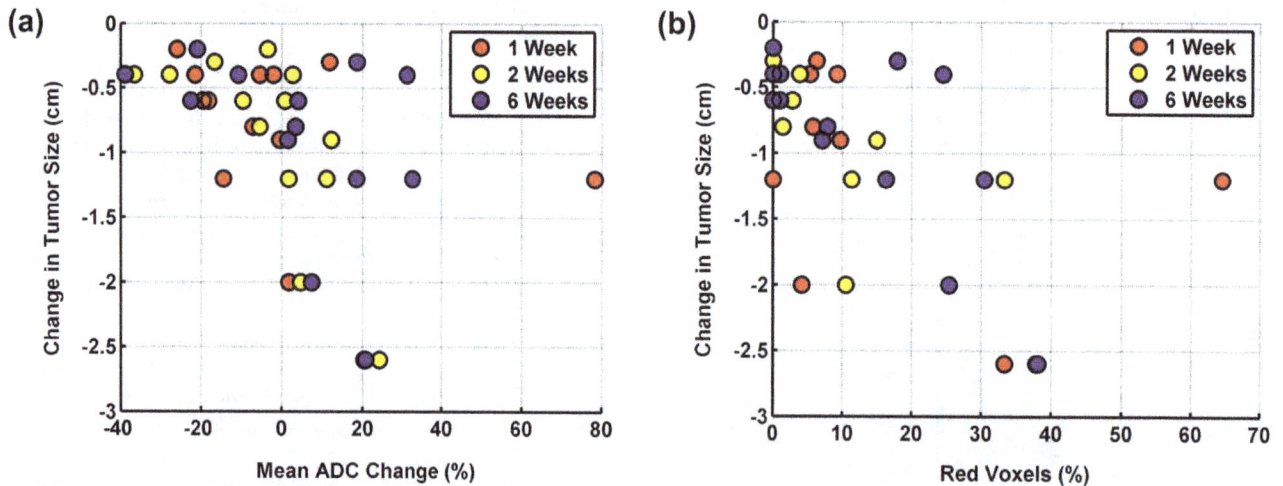

**Figure 1. Plots of the diffusion parameters against the changes in tumor volume on CT.** Plots of (a) the mean ADC change and (b) the percentage of voxels with significantly increased ADCs relative to their pretreatment values (red voxels) on fDMs in each lesion at one, two, and six weeks after initiation of chemotherapy against reduction in tumor size after two cycles of chemotherapy. Repeated measures ANOVA revealed that a large reduction in tumor size on CT was typically preceded by a large increase in the mean lesion ADC (p = 0.001) as well as a high percentage of red voxels on fDMs (p = 0.002).

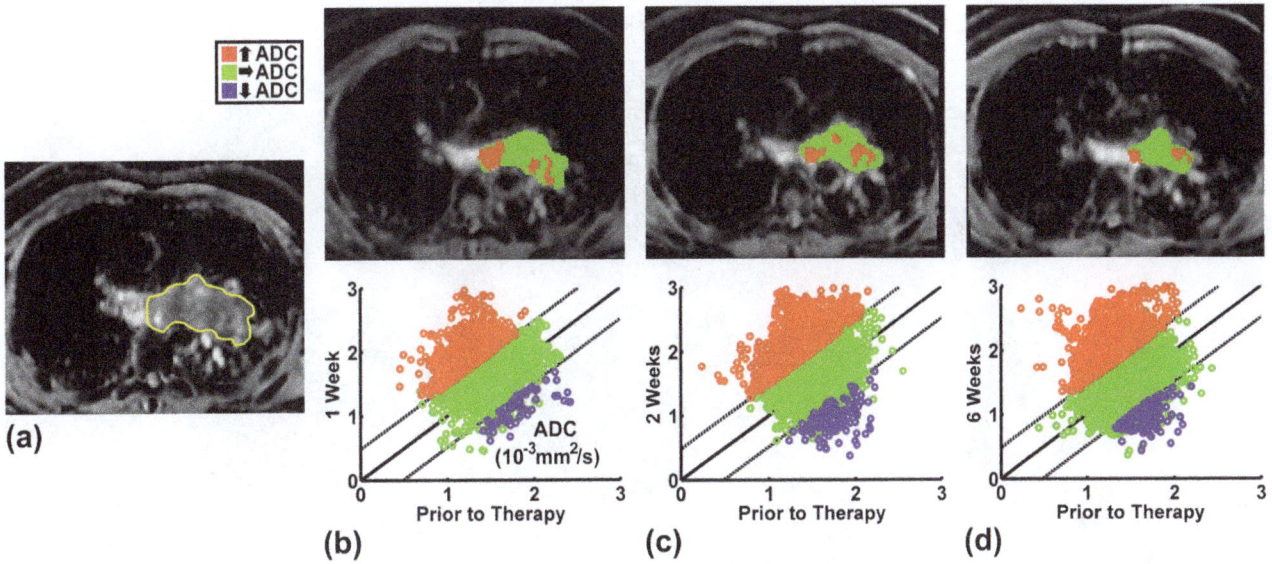

**Figure 2. FDMs of patient 1 whose lesion showed a large reduction in tumor size under chemotherapy. (a)** Pretreatment ADC map showing the ROI drawn by the radiologist and fDMs at, **(b)** one, **(c)** two, and, **(d)** six weeks after initiation of chemotherapy superimposed onto the corresponding posttreatment ADC map. The scatterplots of pretreatment versus posttreatment voxel values over the entire lesion are shown below each image. Dashed lines = threshold beyond which a significant ADC change is deemed to have occurred. Large regions within the lesion showed significantly increased ADCs (shown in red) at all time points after initiation of chemotherapy in comparison with pretreatment values. Note that there are voxels labeled with unchanged ADCs (green voxels) lying beyond the significance threshold on the scatterplots; these were isolated voxels that were excluded by the cluster size threshold.

DWI of the lungs and especially longitudinal studies in lung cancer are very challenging due to respiratory motion, the presence of susceptibility-related artifacts, and the absence of rigid landmarks that simplify image coregistration. Despite these challenges, the results of our pilot study have shown that using respiratory-triggered DWI and advanced coregistration techniques, fDM analysis in pulmonary lesions is feasible and has shown promising results. This approach may prove to be more sensitive to changes resulting from therapy compared with mean ADC changes averaged over entire lesions as it accounts for heterogeneous changes that occur within each tumor with treatment. It should be noted that respiratory triggering in some patients significantly prolonged scan time due to highly irregular breathing patterns, technical improvements are required to

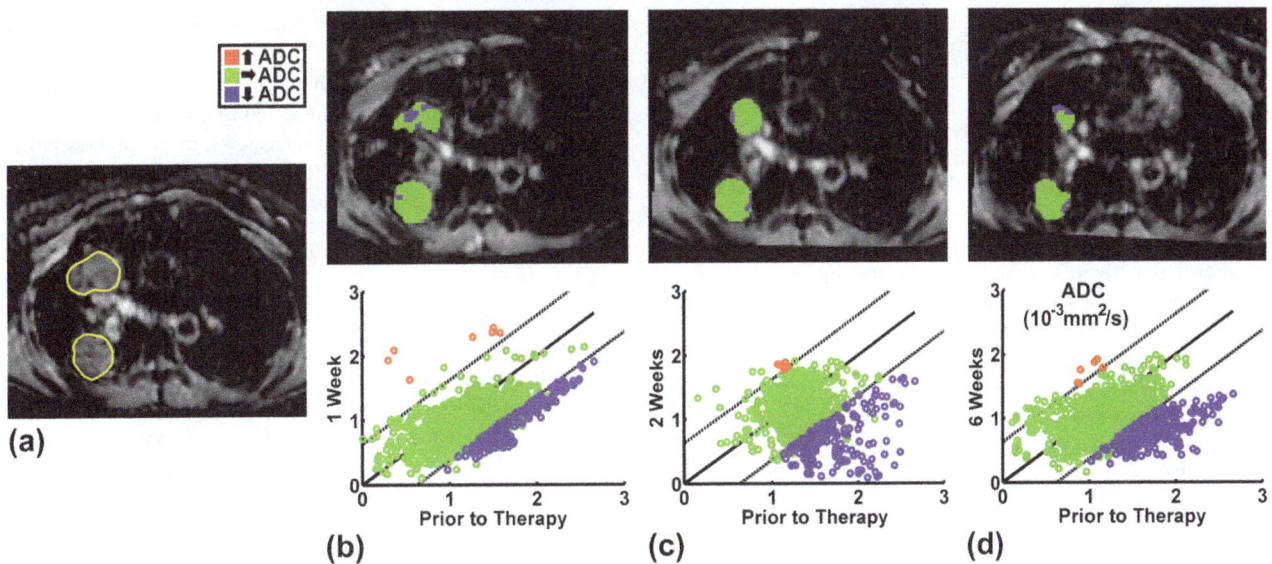

**Figure 3. FDMs of the two lesions in patient 7 which showed a moderate decrease in tumor size under chemotherapy. (a)** Pretreatment ADC map showing the ROIs circumscribing the tumors and fDMs at, **(b)** one, **(c)** two, and **(d)** six weeks after treatment onset superimposed onto the corresponding posttreatment ADC map. The scatterplots of pretreatment versus posttreatment voxel values over the entire lesions are shown below each image. Dashed lines = threshold beyond which a significant ADC change is deemed to have occurred. Few voxels feature significantly increased ADCs relative to the pretreatment values.

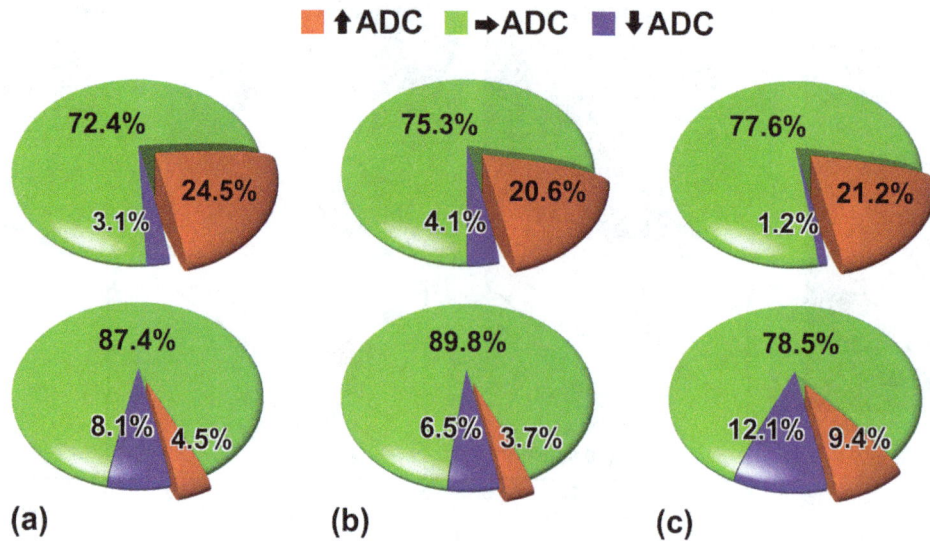

**Figure 4. Pie charts showing the percentages of voxels on fDMs that featured significantly increased (red voxels), significantly decreased (blue voxels) or unchanged (green voxels) ADCs under therapy averaged over all lesions.** The percentages at **(a)** one, **(b)** two, and **(c)** six weeks after treatment onset are depicted separately for patients that showed partial response (first row) and stable disease (second row), respectively. The percentage of voxels with significantly increased ADCs in comparison to pretreatment values was significantly higher in lesions that showed a large decrease in tumor size on CT after two cycles of chemotherapy (p = 0.041).

shorten scan time in these patients while maintaining high image quality. The total processing time amounted to approximately 20 minutes per patient, limited mostly by localization and manual definition of pulmonary lesions. Automatic or semi-automatic segmentation techniques could be utilized to alleviate the time penalty and facilitate transition into clinical practice.

Unlike previous work, which relied on applying a threshold determined from a reference tissue [14] to define the level of significant voxelwise ADC change within tumors; we determined this threshold for the fDM analysis on a per-lesion basis directly in each tumor by acquiring a second ADC map prior to chemotherapy and comparing the two baseline ADC maps by one-way ANOVA. This method should improve the reliability of the fDMs [22] and may be a key factor for fDM analysis in lung cancer and other soft tissue tumors.

Our results of the mean ADC changes on a per-lesion basis are in agreement with previously published results, which have shown that an increase in the mean ADC at three to four weeks compared with pretreatment values could predict good response in patients with non-small cell lung cancer [15]. However, our study has shown that these changes could potentially be observed as early as one week after starting treatment. In addition, the information derived from fDMs, i.e. the percentage of voxels with significantly increased ADCs (red voxels) may be a more sensitive biomarker than averaged ADC changes by accounting for heterogeneity of treatment response.

It should be noted that Yabuuchi et al. [15] reported increasing mean tumor ADC values for almost all responding tumors. Intriguingly, we found that tumors that showed <30% reduction in size after two cycles of chemotherapy were on average accompanied by a decrease in their mean ADCs across all measurement timepoints. It should be mentioned at this point that contrary to Yabuuchi et al. [15] the choice of a lower b-value of $100 \text{ mm/s}^2$ in our work should effectively diminish the influence of perfusion effects on ADC quantification [2]. Nevertheless, the biological basis for the observed decrease of the mean ADCs in lesions showing stable disease is uncertain. This may relate to the

mechanism of cell death, associated with cellular swelling and/or inflammatory infiltrates maybe even early disease progression. Nonetheless, it would be interesting to see whether these observations could be independently validated by other investigators.

There were limitations to our study. First, a relatively small number of patients was included. The reason for this was the often poor general clinical condition of the majority of stage IV lung cancer patients, which often were not able to comply with the study requisites. Furthermore, the patient population was slightly heterogeneous with respect to specific chemotherapy administered. This might influence cellular response and in turn the diffusion properties of the lesion under therapy. This may explain why significant correlations with the progression-free interval were not found. Thereby, it should be noted that bivariate correlations had to be computed on a per-patient level, in the process further diminishing the sample size. Beyond that one patient deceased prior to tumor progression and had to be secondarily excluded from the analysis. Nevertheless, it should be noted that our results showed some trend towards statistical significance and further studies with larger and more homogeneous patient cohorts are warranted. Second, for ethical reasons, no control group without systemic treatment could be included in the present study and no patient had progressive disease. In addition, it might be interesting to investigate how the results would compare to patients treated with antiangiogenic agents in addition to conventional chemotherapy. Third, in the fDM analysis, an assumption is made that tumor regression occurs from the periphery towards the center of the tumor, allowing voxelwise registration of intersecting regions of interest before and after treatment. However, the pattern of tumor regression is likely to be more complex. Nonetheless, this approach has yielded significant results, which could be further applied and tested in future studies. In spite of these limitations, to the best of our knowledge, this is the first study demonstrating the feasibility of assessing and predicting treatment response using fDMs in patients with non-small cell lung cancer.

In conclusion, the present work demonstrates that using respiratory-triggered DWI, early treatment response can be successfully determined in patients with non-small cell lung cancer using fDMs. The percentage of voxels with significantly increased ADCs (red voxels) on fDMs may allow predicting treatment response according to RECIST criteria as early as at one week after initiation of chemotherapy. Thereby, the fDM may potentially pose a more sensitive biomarker for predicting treatment response than ADCs on a per-lesion basis by accounting for spatial heterogeneity of treatment response.

## Author Contributions

Conceived and designed the experiments: CR JF MP CB DK AG. Performed the experiments: CR JF AG. Analyzed the data: CR AG. Contributed reagents/materials/analysis tools: CR MP CB AG. Contributed to the writing of the manuscript: CR JF MP CB DK AG. Designed the software used in the analysis: CR. Obtained ethics approval: AG JF. Recruited patients: CR JF MP CB AG.

## References

1. Eisenhauer EA, Therasse P, Bogaerts J, Schwartz LH, Sargent D, et al. (2009) New response evaluation criteria in solid tumours: revised RECIST guideline (version 1.1). Eur J Cancer 45: 228–247.
2. Padhani AR, Liu G, Koh DM, Chenevert TL, Thoeny HC, et al. (2009) Diffusion-weighted magnetic resonance imaging as a cancer biomarker: consensus and recommendations. Neoplasia 11: 102–125.
3. Chenevert TL, McKeever PE, Ross BD (1997) Monitoring early response of experimental brain tumors to therapy using diffusion magnetic resonance imaging. Clinical cancer research: an official journal of the American Association for Cancer Research 3: 1457–1466.
4. Lee KC, Moffat BA, Schott AF, Layman R, Ellingworth S, et al. (2007) Prospective early response imaging biomarker for neoadjuvant breast cancer chemotherapy. Clinical cancer research: an official journal of the American Association for Cancer Research 13: 443–450.
5. Yankeelov TE, Lepage M, Chakravarthy A, Broome EE, Niermann KJ, et al. (2007) Integration of quantitative DCE-MRI and ADC mapping to monitor treatment response in human breast cancer: initial results. Magn Reson Imaging 25: 1–13.
6. Woodhams R, Kakita S, Hata H, Iwabuchi K, Kuranami M, et al. (2010) Identification of residual breast carcinoma following neoadjuvant chemotherapy: diffusion-weighted imaging–comparison with contrast-enhanced MR imaging and pathologic findings. Radiology 254: 357–366.
7. Kim S, Loevner L, Quon H, Sherman E, Weinstein G, et al. (2009) Diffusion-weighted magnetic resonance imaging for predicting and detecting early response to chemoradiation therapy of squamous cell carcinomas of the head and neck. Clinical cancer research: an official journal of the American Association for Cancer Research 15: 986–994.
8. King AD, Chow KK, Yu KH, Mo FK, Yeung DK, et al. (2013) Head and neck squamous cell carcinoma: diagnostic performance of diffusion-weighted MR imaging for the prediction of treatment response. Radiology 266: 531–538.
9. Harry VN, Semple SI, Gilbert FJ, Parkin DE (2008) Diffusion-weighted magnetic resonance imaging in the early detection of response to chemoradiation in cervical cancer. Gynecol Oncol 111: 213–220.
10. Cui Y, Zhang XP, Sun YS, Tang L, Shen L (2008) Apparent diffusion coefficient: potential imaging biomarker for prediction and early detection of response to chemotherapy in hepatic metastases. Radiology 248: 894–900.
11. DeVries AF, Kremser C, Hein PA, Griebel J, Krezcy A, et al. (2003) Tumor microcirculation and diffusion predict therapy outcome for primary rectal carcinoma. International journal of radiation oncology, biology, physics 56: 958–965.
12. Dudeck O, Zeile M, Pink D, Pech M, Tunn PU, et al. (2008) Diffusion-weighted magnetic resonance imaging allows monitoring of anticancer treatment effects in patients with soft-tissue sarcomas. J Magn Reson Imaging 27: 1109–1113.
13. Lee KC, Bradley DA, Hussain M, Meyer CR, Chenevert TL, et al. (2007) A feasibility study evaluating the functional diffusion map as a predictive imaging biomarker for detection of treatment response in a patient with metastatic prostate cancer to the bone. Neoplasia 9: 1003–1011.
14. Reischauer C, Froehlich JM, Koh DM, Graf N, Padevit C, et al. (2010) Bone metastases from prostate cancer: assessing treatment response by using diffusion-weighted imaging and functional diffusion maps-initial observations. Radiology 257: 523–531.
15. Yabuuchi H, Hatakenaka M, Takayama K, Matsuo Y, Sunami S, et al. (2011) Non-small cell lung cancer: detection of early response to chemotherapy by using contrast-enhanced dynamic and diffusion-weighted MR imaging. Radiology 261: 598–604.
16. Moffat BA, Chenevert TL, Lawrence TS, Meyer CR, Johnson TD, et al. (2005) Functional diffusion map: a noninvasive MRI biomarker for early stratification of clinical brain tumor response. Proceedings of the National Academy of Sciences of the United States of America 102: 5524–5529.
17. Moffat BA, Chenevert TL, Meyer CR, McKeever PE, Hall DE, et al. (2006) The functional diffusion map: an imaging biomarker for the early prediction of cancer treatment outcome. Neoplasia 8: 259–267.
18. Hamstra DA, Chenevert TL, Moffat BA, Johnson TD, Meyer CR, et al. (2005) Evaluation of the functional diffusion map as an early biomarker of time-to-progression and overall survival in high-grade glioma. Proceedings of the National Academy of Sciences of the United States of America 102: 16759–16764.
19. Ellingson BM, Cloughesy TF, Lai A, Mischel PS, Nghiemphu PL, et al. (2011) Graded functional diffusion map-defined characteristics of apparent diffusion coefficients predict overall survival in recurrent glioblastoma treated with bevacizumab. Neuro-oncology 13: 1151–1161.
20. Netsch T, van Muiswinkel A (2004) Quantitative evaluation of image-based distortion correction in diffusion tensor imaging. IEEE Trans Med Imaging 23: 789–798.
21. Nestares O, Heeger DJ (2000) Robust multiresolution alignment of MRI brain volumes. Magn Reson Med 43: 705–715.
22. Reischauer C, Gutzeit A, Vorburger RS, Froehlich JM, Binkert CA, et al. (2012) Optimizing the functional diffusion map using Monte Carlo simulations. J Magn Reson Imaging 36: 1002–1009.
23. Stella GM, Luisetti M, Pozzi E, Comoglio PM (2013) Oncogenes in non-small-cell lung cancer: emerging connections and novel therapeutic dynamics. The lancet Respiratory medicine 1: 251–261.
24. Pirker R (2014) Novel drugs against non-small-cell lung cancer. Current opinion in oncology 26: 145–151.

# 21

# Association of Drug Transporter Expression with Mortality and Progression-Free Survival in Stage IV Head and Neck Squamous Cell Carcinoma

**Rolf Warta**[1,2,9], **Dirk Theile**[3,9], **Carolin Mogler**[4,5], **Esther Herpel**[4,5], **Niels Grabe**[6,7], **Bernd Lahrmann**[5,7], **Peter K. Plinkert**[2], **Christel Herold-Mende**[1,2], **Johanna Weiss**[3]*, **Gerhard Dyckhoff**[2]

**1** Experimental Neurosurgery Research, Department of Neurosurgery, University of Heidelberg, Heidelberg, Germany, **2** Molecular Cell Biology Group, Department of Otorhinolaryngology, Head and Neck Surgery, University of Heidelberg, Heidelberg, Germany, **3** Department of Clinical Pharmacology and Pharmacoepidemiology, University of Heidelberg, Heidelberg, Germany, **4** Tissue Bank of the National Center for Tumor Diseases (NCT), University of Heidelberg, Heidelberg, Germany, **5** Institute of Pathology, University of Heidelberg, Heidelberg, Germany, **6** Department of Medical Oncology, National Center for Tumor Diseases, University of Heidelberg, Heidelberg, Germany, **7** Hamamatsu Tissue Imaging and Analysis Center, BIOQUANT, University of Heidelberg, Heidelberg, Germany

## Abstract

Drug transporters such as P-glycoprotein (ABCB1) have been associated with chemotherapy resistance and are considered unfavorable prognostic factors for survival of cancer patients. Analyzing mRNA expression levels of a subset of drug transporters by quantitative reverse transcription polymerase chain reaction (qRT-PCR) or protein expression by tissue microarray (TMA) in tumor samples of therapy naïve stage IV head and neck squamous cell carcinoma (HNSCC) (qRT-PCR, n = 40; TMA, n = 61), this in situ study re-examined the significance of transporter expression for progression-free survival (PFS) and overall survival (OS). Data from The Cancer Genome Atlas database was used to externally validate the respective findings (n = 317). In general, HNSCC tended to lower expression of drug transporters compared to normal epithelium. High ABCB1 mRNA tumor expression was associated with both favorable progression-free survival (PFS, p = 0.0357) and overall survival (OS, p = 0.0535). Similar results were obtained for the mRNA of ABCC1 (MRP1, multidrug resistance-associated protein 1; PFS, p = 0.0183; OS, p = 0.038). In contrast, protein expression of ATP7b (copper transporter ATP7b), mRNA expression of ABCG2 (BCRP, breast cancer resistance protein), ABCC2 (MRP2), and SLC31A1 (hCTR1, human copper transporter 1) did not correlate with survival. Cluster analysis however revealed that simultaneous high expression of SLC31A1, ABCC2, and ABCG2 indicates poor survival of HNSCC patients. In conclusion, this study militates against the intuitive dogma where high expression of drug efflux transporters indicates poor survival, but demonstrates that expression of single drug transporters might indicate even improved survival. Prospectively, combined analysis of the 'transportome' should rather be performed as it likely unravels meaningful data on the impact of drug transporters on survival of patients with HNSCC.

**Editor:** Andreas-Claudius Hoffmann, West German Cancer Center, Germany

**Funding:** This project was funded by grant WE 4135/3-1 und HE 2357/2-1 from the German Research Foundation. The funders had no role in study design, data collection and analysis, decision to publish, or preparation of the manuscript.

**Competing Interests:** The authors have declared that no competing interests exist.

* Email: johanna.weiss@med.uni-heidelberg.de

⑨ These authors contributed equally to this work.

## Introduction

Chemotherapy with classical cytostatics such as antimetabolites, platinum drugs, or taxanes remains a cornerstone in the therapy of head and neck squamous cell carcinoma (HNSCC) [1]. Unresponsiveness to antineoplastic agents is frequently due to a phenomenon called multidrug-resistance (MDR) [2]. The classical MDR phenotype is mediated by ATP-binding cassette (ABC)-transporters such as P-glycoprotein (Pgp, ABCB1), breast cancer resistance protein (BCRP, ABCG2), or several multidrug-resistance-associated proteins (MRPs, ABCC family). These membrane-located proteins extrude anticancer agents or their metabolites from cells mediating drug resistance [2]. Paclitaxel, cisplatin,

and 5-fluorouracil (5-FU) are standard anti-HNSCC drugs [1], the efficacies of which are limited by several ABC-transporters at least in vitro [3–8]. In contrast to experimental studies, clinical data on the role of these proteins is less clear, although some studies for other tumor entities indeed indicated that ABC-transporters negatively influence clinical response or survival of patients suffering from tumors of the lung [9–10], the breast [11–12], the liver [13], or the kidney [14]. For HNSCC, the significance of ABC-transporters is even more uncertain. First, expression levels have been reported to range from very low [15–16] to high expression [17]. Second, impact on chemotherapy response and survival is also inconsistent. MRP1 expression in nasopharyngeal carcinomas was reported to predispose for recurrence and metastasis and to indicate poor 5-year-survival [18]. On the other hand, MRP1 was also documented not to correlate with drug sensitivity or lymph node metastasis [19]. MRP2 and Pgp expression even indicated favorable local tumor control and improved overall survival, respectively [20]. In addition to ABC-transporters such as MRP2, efficacy of cisplatin is also influenced by transporters physiologically involved in copper homeostasis. Human copper transporter 1 (hCTR1/*SLC31A1*) mediates the cellular uptake of copper, cisplatin, and oxaliplatin [21]. The P-type ATPase ATP7b (Wilson disease protein) is also associated with transport of and resistance to cisplatin in vitro, inferior clinical response to cisplatin chemotherapy, and poor survival of HNSCC patients [22–23].

We therefore determined expression levels of important drug transporters in tumor specimens of therapy-naïve patients with stage IV HNSCC using quantitative reverse transcription real-time polymerase chain reaction, tissue microarray approach, and external validation controls in order to re-examine contradictory findings by others [20]. The aim of this study was to gain a concluding overview on the significance of all these different drug transporters for progression-free and overall survival times of HNSCC patients.

## Materials and Methods

### Patients

Samples from HNSCC tumor patients and normal mucosa samples from non-cancer patients who underwent tonsillectomy were obtained from the Tissue bank of the National Center for Tumor Diseases (NCT, Heidelberg, Germany) (project no. 374). The study was approved by the institutional ethics committee and written informed consent was obtained from each patient. Clinical data of patients were assessed in an MS Access database (Microsoft, Redmond, USA). Clinical staging and follow-up data were obtained by reviewing the medical records, radiographic images and either by telephone or written correspondence. Patients included did not receive chemo- or radiotherapy prior to surgery. Patients were followed from date of first diagnosis to the end of study, whereas patients who were still alive were censored. Before further use, a vital tumor cell content $\geq 70\%$ was confirmed on hematoxylin and eosin stained sections by an experienced pathologist of the National Cancer for Tumor Diseases (NCT) Tissuebank.

### Quantification of mRNA expressions by quantitative real time reverse transcription polymerase chain reaction (qRT-PCR)

To exclude possible prognostic confounders and to analyze a rather homogeneous qRT-PCR study sample in the univariate survival analysis all included patients were in clinical stage IVa (Table 1). Drug transporter gene expression was quantified by qRT-PCR. RNA was isolated from tumor specimen using RNeasy-Kit (Qiagen, Hilden, Germany) and cDNA was synthesized with the Transcriptor First Strand cDNA Synthesis Kit (Roche Applied Science, Mannheim, Germany) according to the manufacturers' instructions. Expression of mRNA was quantified by qRT-PCR with a LightCycler 480 (Roche Applied Science, Mannheim, Germany) using the SYBR Green format with the Absolute QPCR SYBR Green Mix. Primer sequences were published previously [24]. The following genes were quantified: *ABCB1*, *ABCC1*, *ABCC2*, *ABCG2*, *SLC31A1*, and *ATP7b*. The most suitable housekeeping gene for normalization was identified using geNorm (version 3.4, Center for Medical Genetics, Ghent, Belgium) [25]. Among the housekeeping genes tested (*β2-

*microglobulin; glucose-6-phosphate dehydrogenase, G6PDH; glucuronidase β, GU; ribosomal protein L13, RPL13; hypoxanthinephosphoribosyltransferase 1, HPRT; 60S human acidic ribosomal protein P1, HUPO, GU* proved to be the most stable one for this data set. Data were evaluated by calibrator-normalized relative quantification with efficiency correction using LightCycler 480 software as published previously [26]. Results are expressed as the ratio target gene/housekeeping genes divided by the corresponding ratio of the calibrator (equivolumetric mixture of all samples). All samples were amplified in duplicate. Patient characteristics are shown in Table 1.

### Quantification of ATP7b expression by tissue microarray (TMA)

Formalin-fixed, paraffin-embedded tissue samples from 87 patients were used for TMA design (Table 2). Representative tumor regions were identified by an experienced pathologist on H&E-stained tissue sections. From all selected regions, tissue cylinders with a diameter of 0.6 mm were obtained and arrayed into a recipient block as described earlier [27]. The recipient block was subsequently cut into 5 μm sections on precleaned microscope slides (Superfrost Plus, Thermo Scientific, Braunschweig, Germany).

Prior to TMA staining specificity of primary ATP7b antibody was ensured using an isotype control (PP501P, Acris, Hiddenhausen, Germany). Proceeding staining deparaffinization was carried out by immersing slides in 100% xylol (3×3 min), followed by 90%, 80%, 70% and 50% ethanol (2×3 min each). Finally, slides were washed in distilled water (2×3 min). Antigen retrieval was performed in an autoclave at 1 bar, 125°C for 20 min using antigen retrieval buffer (DAKO, Hamburg, Germany) at pH 6.1. Incubation with primary and secondary antibodies as well as detection with Vectastain ELITE ABC Kit (Vector Laboratories, Burlingame, USA) was carried out as described [28].

Antigen expression was pre-tested in a set of HNSCC tissues to establish suitable antigen evaluation categories based on antigen expression variability. Grading scores with uniform distribution of antigen expression levels among individual grading categories were chosen for the final TMA evaluation. Slides were scanned at a 20× magnification by the Nanozoomer Digital Pathology (NDP) System (Hamamatsu Photonics, Hamamatsu, Japan) by the BIOQUANT TIGA Center of the University Heidelberg. Scanned TMAs were afterwards evaluated with the help of the NDP Viewer software (Hamamatsu Photonics, Hamamatsu, Japan). Each tumor biopsy was scored semiquantitatively on the basis of a well-established immunoreactivity scoring system (IRS) [29]. Each investigator (DT, JW) ranked a value for the expression intensity from 1 (no staining) to 4 (very strong expression) and a value describing the extent of tumor staining (1, no expression; 2, 0–24%; 3, 25–49%; 4, 50–74%, 5, 75–100%). These values were multiplied. The final score of each tumor was then calculated as the mean of these two independent evaluations. Consequently, lowest score was 1, highest score was 20.

### Data base query

The Cancer Genome Atlas (TCGA; URL: https://tcga-data.nci.nih.gov/tcga/) validation data were retrieved as level 3 normalized RNAseq gene expression files. Age, sex, clinical staging, survival times, vital status, drug and radiation treatment were annotated clinical data provided by TCGA. Only patients of clinical stage II-IVa were selected for survival analyses. Patient characteristics are shown in Table 3.

**Table 1.** Clinical characteristics of qPCR including n = 40 HNSCC patients used for correlation of protein expression with survival.

| | Mean ± SD | Range |
|---|---|---|
| **Characteristics** | | |
| Age (years) | 59±9 | 46–85 |
| OS (weeks) | 186±164 | 15–886 |
| PFS (weeks) | 167±150 | 6–670 |
| | **Frequency** | **Percent** |
| **Gender** | | |
| M | 35 | 87.5 |
| F | 5 | 12.5 |
| **Localisation** | | |
| Oropharynx | 21 | 52.5 |
| Hypopharynx | 11 | 27.5 |
| Larynx | 3 | 7.5 |
| Oral Cavity | 5 | 12.5 |
| **Therapy** | | |
| Radiation | 5 | 12.5 |
| Chemotherapy | 11 | 27.5 |
| Radio/Chemotherapy | 24 | 60.0 |
| Surgery | 40 | 100.0 |
| **Clinical stage** | | |
| I–II | 0 | 0.0 |
| III–IV | 40 | 100.0 |

**Table 2.** Clinical characteristics of TMA including n = 61 HNSCC patients used for correlation of protein expression with survival.

| | Mean ± SD | Range |
|---|---|---|
| **Characteristics** | | |
| Age (years) | 59±10 | 35–87 |
| OS (weeks) | 191±140 | 5–544 |
| PFS (weeks) | 162±143 | 5–520 |
| | **Frequency** | **Percent** |
| **Gender** | | |
| M | 51 | 85.0 |
| F | 9 | 15.0 |
| **Localisation** | | |
| Oropharynx | 29 | 47.5 |
| Hypopharynx | 15 | 24.6 |
| Larynx | 14 | 23.0 |
| Oral Cavity | 3 | 4.9 |
| **Therapy** | | |
| Radiation | 12 | 19.7 |
| Chemotherapy | 24 | 39.3 |
| Radio/Chemotherapy | 25 | 41.0 |
| Surgery | 61 | 100.0 |
| **Clinical stage** | | |
| I–II | 8 | 13.1 |
| III–IV | 53 | 86.9 |

**Table 3.** Clinical characteristics of TCGA dataset including n = 317 HNSCC patients used for correlation of RNAseq mRNA expression with survival.

|  | Mean ± SD | Range |
|---|---|---|
| **Characteristics** | | |
| Age (years) | 61±12 | 19–90 |
| OS (weeks) | 113±124 | 1–917 |
| PFS (weeks) | 98±93 | 6–561 |
|  | **Frequency** | **Percent** |
| **Gender** | | |
| M | 230 | 72.6 |
| F | 87 | 27.4 |
| **Localisation** | | |
| Oropharynx | 42 | 13.2 |
| Hypopharynx | 3 | 0.9 |
| Larynx | 77 | 24.3 |
| Oral Cavity | 195 | 61.5 |
| **Therapy** | | |
| Radiation | 39 | 12.3 |
| Chemotherapy | 0 | 0.0 |
| Radio/Chemotherapy | 72 | 22.7 |
| Surgery | 317 | 100.0 |
| **Clinical stage** | | |
| II | 70 | 22.1 |
| III | 81.00 | 25.5 |
| IV | 166.00 | 52.4 |

## Statistical analysis

Differences in drug transporter expression levels between tumor and control samples were analyzed using two-sided t-tests. RNAseq data were analyzed using Mann-Whitney U test. Probability values of $p<0.05$ were considered significant. Survival associations were calculated using a log rank test and displayed as Kaplan-Meier plots. Calculations were performed using Prism 5 statistics software (GraphPad Software, La Jolla, USA).

Heatmaps were drawn using the SUMO statistic software (http://angiogenesis.dkfz.de/oncoexpress/software/sumo/).

## Results

### mRNA expression of drug transporters in HNSCC

mRNA expression levels of a subset of drug transporters (*ABCB1*, *ABCC1*, *ABCC2*, *ABCG2*, *SLC31A1*) were determined

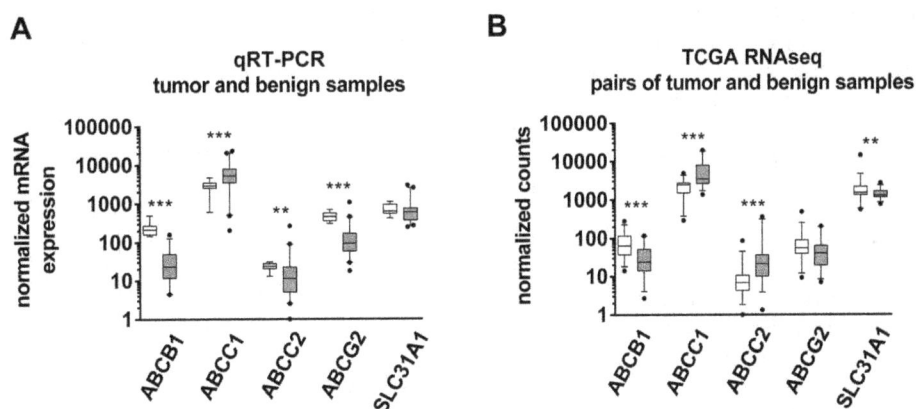

**Figure 1. mRNA expression of drug transporters in HNSCC.** (A) Determination of mRNA expression levels of drug transporters by qRT-PCR in a study sample of therapy naïve stage IVa HNSCC tumors (n = 40, grey boxes) and normal control samples (n = 14, white boxes) (relative mRNA expression normalized to the lowest value). (B) External validation by HNSCC RNAseq mRNA expression data derived from the 'The Cancer Genome Atlas' (TCGA) consortium. Comparison of normalized counts of paired tumor (n = 37, grey boxes) and adjacent noncancerous normal tissue (n = 37, white boxes). Whisker indicates 5–95 percentile; Mann-Whitney U test; **, $p<0.01$; ***, $p<0.001$.

## ABCB1

**Progression-Free Survival**

**Overall Survival**

## ABCC1

**Progression-Free Survival**

**Overall Survival**

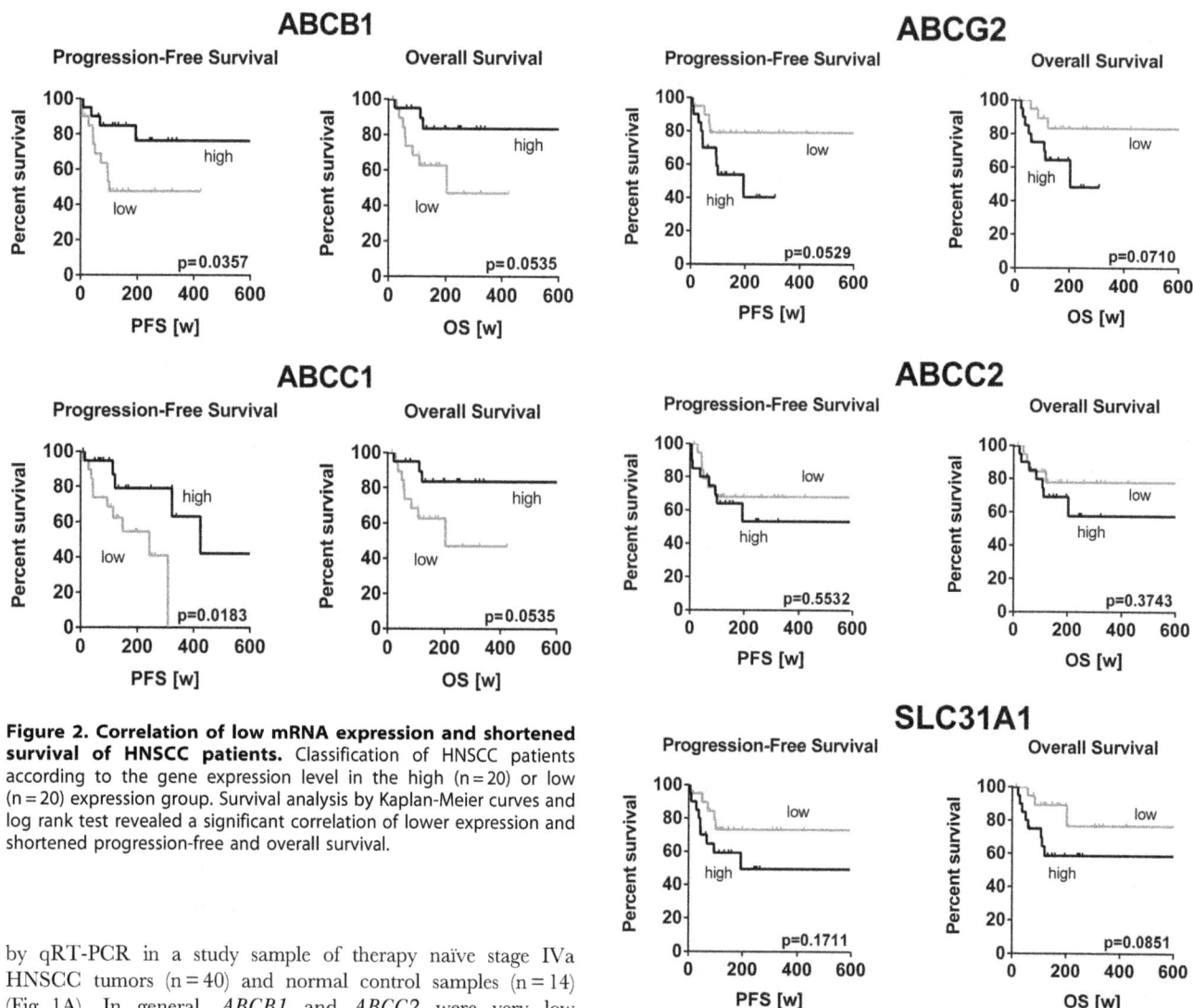

**Figure 2. Correlation of low mRNA expression and shortened survival of HNSCC patients.** Classification of HNSCC patients according to the gene expression level in the high (n = 20) or low (n = 20) expression group. Survival analysis by Kaplan-Meier curves and log rank test revealed a significant correlation of lower expression and shortened progression-free and overall survival.

## ABCG2

**Progression-Free Survival**

**Overall Survival**

## ABCC2

**Progression-Free Survival**

**Overall Survival**

## SLC31A1

**Progression-Free Survival**

**Overall Survival**

**Figure 3. Correlation of high mRNA expression and shortened survival of HNSCC patients.** Classification of HNSCC patients according to the expression level of the respective gene in high (n = 20) or low (n = 20) expression group. Survival analysis by Kaplan-Meier curves and log rank test revealed that patients with high gene expression tended to accompany a shorter progression-free and overall survival.

by qRT-PCR in a study sample of therapy naïve stage IVa HNSCC tumors (n = 40) and normal control samples (n = 14) (Fig. 1A). In general, *ABCB1* and *ABCC2* were very low expressed in HNSCC, whereas *ABCC1* was highly expressed. *ABCG2* and *SLC31A1* exhibited intermediate mRNA expression levels. Comparing tumor and normal tissues, three of the five analyzed genes showed a significant lower expression in tumors than in healthy control tissues (*ABCB1*, p<0.0001; *ABCC2*, p< 0.005; *ABCG2*, p<0.0001), whereas *ABCC1* expression was significantly up-regulated in the carcinomas (p<0.0001). These differences resulted in a 9.4-, 2.1- and 4.9-fold lower median expression of *ABCB1*, *ABCC2* and *ABCG2* in tumor samples compared to control samples, respectively. *ABCC1* exhibited a 1.8-fold higher median expression in tumor samples. *SLC31A1* expression did not differ between HNSCC and control samples.

To validate our findings in an independent dataset, we extracted RNAseq mRNA expression data from the HNSCC database derived from the TCGA consortium (Fig. 1B). *ABCB1* (p<0.0001) and *ABCG2* (not significantly) also showed lower expression in tumors, whereas *ABCC1* was also significantly (p<0.0001) higher expressed in tumors. In contrast to our study sample, *SLC31A1* expression was significantly down-regulated in the TCGA dataset of HNSCC (p = 0.0036) and *ABCC2* exhibited significantly higher expression in tumors (p = 0.0002), whereas it was significantly down-regulated in our samples.

## Impact of mRNA expression of drug transporter genes on patient survival

To analyze association of drug transporter gene expression with survival of HNSCC patients, patients were assigned into two groups differing by either higher or lower gene expression than the median of all samples. Based on this grouping the genes showed a divergent correlation with survival in the univariate log rank survival analysis.

High *ABCB1* as well as high *ABCC1* mRNA gene expression was significantly associated with longer progression free survival (p = 0.0357 and p = 0.0183, respectively) and overall survival (p = 0.0535 and p = 0.038, respectively) (Fig. 2). In contrast, high expression levels of *ABCG2*, *ABCC2* and *SLC31A1* tended to be associated with a shorter survival time of HNSCC patients (Fig. 3). However, these associations did not reach statistical significance.

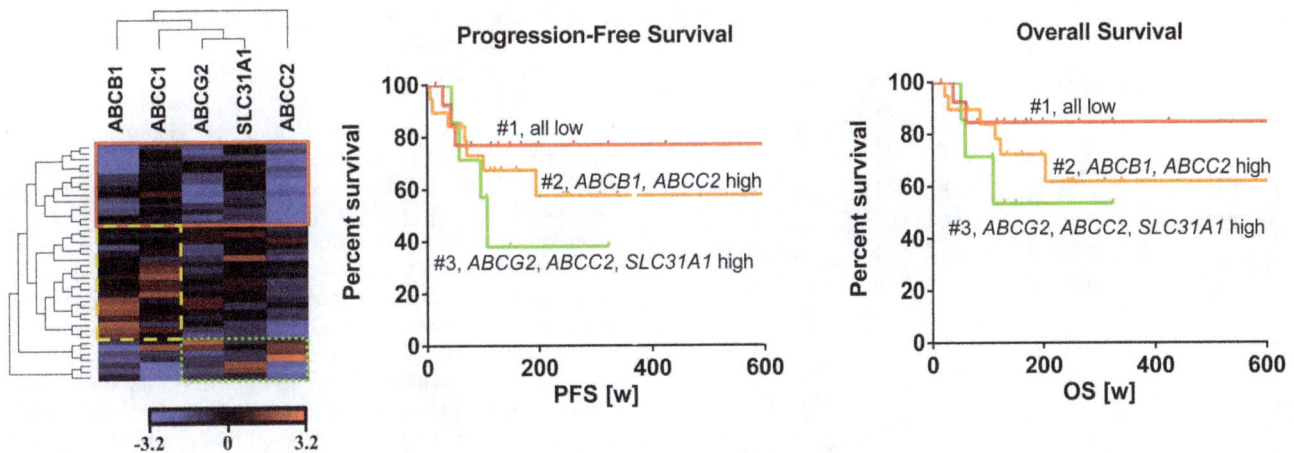

**Figure 4. Hierarchical clustering of mRNA expression and survival of HNSCC patients.** (A) Heatmap of the median normalized log2 transformed mRNA expressions hierarchically clustered with Euclidean distance matrix and complete linkage. Three distinct groups were uncovered: First group (n = 14) low expression of all drug transporters evaluated (#1, red framed), second group (n = 19) high *ABCB1* and high *ABCC1* expression (#2, yellow framed) and a third group (n = 7) showing low *ABCB1/ABCC1* expression but high levels of either *ABCG2, SLC31A1,* or *ABCC2* (#3, green framed). (B) Survival analysis by Kaplan-Meier curves and log rank test revealed that patients of group #3 (n = 7) tended to survive shorter than those of group #2 (n = 19). Best survival was seen for patients of group #1 (n = 14) who show a lower expression of drug transporters.

Because there was a substantial difference in expression levels, potential mutual exclusive up- or down-regulation of genes was analyzed through hierarchical clustering the median normalized log2 transformed mRNA expression values. The respective heatmap uncovered three distinct groups (Fig. 4): First group (n = 14) constantly exhibiting low expression of all drug transporters evaluated (#1, red framed), second group (n = 19) with both high *ABCB1* and high *ABCC1* expression (#2, yellow framed) and a third group showing low *ABCB1/ABCC1* expression but high levels of either *ABCG2, SLC31A1,* or *ABCC2* (#3, green framed). Best survival was observed for the first group with constantly low expression of all drug transporters evaluated. In contrast, lowest survival was observed for the third group of patients with tumors exhibiting high expressions of *ABCG2, SLC31A1,* and *ABCC2*. The second group (high *ABCB1* and high *ABCC1*) exhibited intermediate survival times.

## Validation of survival in the independent TCGA dataset

To challenge our findings, the publicly available TCGA HNSCC dataset containing high patient numbers of all clinical stages was again used for validation in an independent dataset. Patients with HNSCC of stage II (n = 70), stage III (n = 81) or stage IVa (n = 166) were again grouped according to our previous approach into lower or higher than the median of all samples, respectively. Consistent with our initial finding, high *ABCB1* expression significantly correlated with a better overall survival (p = 0.0003) (Fig. 5). Stratification according to clinical stage indicates significant correlation with survival within the group of stage IVa patients (p = 0.0143). In stage II and III the same trend was obvious, but it did not reach statistical significance (Fig. 5).

## ATP7b protein expression evaluated by tissue microarray

There was a high variation of ATP7b protein expression among the 61 HNSCC samples evaluated with immunoreactive scores between 1 to 19 (median 14). Grouping of these patients according to their immunoreactive score (cutoff 15) and subsequent survival analysis showed that ATP7b expression levels did not correlate with progression-free survival (p = 0.3969) or overall survival (p = 0.1405), respectively (Fig. 6). However, concordant to *ABCB1*

and *ABCC1* patients with high ATP7B protein expression tended to survive longer.

## Discussion

Identification of tissue biomarkers in biopsy specimens of HNSCC may not only select patients that may benefit from more aggressive treatment modalities but may also indicate prognosis. To date, robust clinical, molecular, or radiographic markers in HNSCC are still rare [30]. Therefore, we intended to investigate the expression of drug transporters in these tumors, because their clinical relevance is unclear so far. Besides their role as mediators of cytostatic drug resistance, ABC-transporters have also been proposed as markers of malignancy in HNSCC. In parotid mucoepidermoid carcinoma advanced grades exhibited higher Pgp expression levels than tumors of lower grades [31]. Moreover, Pgp expression has been reported to generally increase during the course of the disease [32–33]. Consequently, our samples of higher stage HNSCC were expected to also show higher expression levels of drug transporters than non-tumor controls. However, the opposite was demonstrated. *ABCB1, ABCC2,* and *ABCG2* were significantly lower expressed in tumors than in normal epithelium of tonsils. The same trend was observed for *SLC31A1* but without reaching statistical significance. *ABCC1* was the only drug transporter evaluated that was overexpressed in tumors (Fig. 1A). To validate these unexpected findings and to rule out that our observations were biased by unrelated factors, the TCGA dataset was analyzed for drug transporter expression in HNSCC and adjacent non-tumor control tissue. Because here 37 pairs of tumors and their normal counterparts of the very same patient were compared, the results are considered independent of confounders such as gender, age, or smoking status. Except *ABCC2*, the TCGA dataset generally confirmed our results by demonstrating that drug transporters such as *ABCB1* (Pgp) are highly significantly (P< 0.0001) down-regulated in HNSCC (Fig. 1B). In contrast to the intuitive dogma, such low expression seems to be associated with a malignant phenotype and advanced tumor disease. This assumption was supported by the subsequent survival analysis. HNSCC patients with low *ABCB1* expression had significantly shorter progression-free survival times and tended to die earlier (overall

## ABCB1

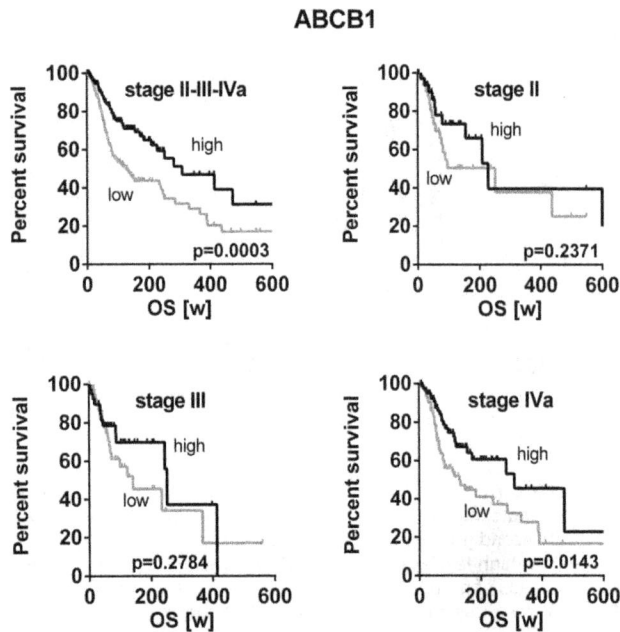

**Figure 5. Correlation of RNAseq mRNA expression and overall survival of HNSCC patients in the TCGA dataset.** Classification of stage II-III-IVa TCGA HNSCC patients according to the ABCB1 expression level in high or low. Survival analysis by Kaplan-Meier curves and log rank test of all stages together (upper left; high, n = 159; low, n = 158) or either stage II (upper right; high, n = 34; low, n = 36), stage III (lower left; high, n = 40; low, n = 41) and stage IVa (lower right; high, n = 83; low, n = 83) revealed consistently shorter survival times for patients with high ABCB1 expression, which reached significance in the whole group and the subgroup of stage IVa tumors.

survival, p = 0.0535) than patients with *ABCB1* expression higher than the median (Fig. 2). This finding was again confirmed using the TCGA dataset by demonstrating that low expression of *ABCB1* correlates with poor overall survival in HNSCC stage II - IVa while high expression of *ABCB1* rather indicates favorable survival. Stratification for tumor stages confirmed this trend and again showed that in advanced tumors (stage IVa), poor survival in association with low *ABCB1* expression (Fig. 5). Mechanistically, it is hard to understand why high expression of *ABCB1* and *ABCC1* was related to improved survival while low expressions indicated poor survival. Recently, experimental studies suggested that

overexpression of ABC-transporters leads to enhanced efflux of glutathione and diminished cellular glutathione content. When intracellular glutathione levels are low, platinum drug species are rarely complexed and thus remain pharmacologically active [34]. In consequence, increased expression of glutathione export transporters can indeed promote efficacy of platinum drugs in HNSCC and lead to a clinical benefit. This observation has been confirmed clinically in HNSCC [20]. Second, cancer is frequently accompanied by inflammatory processes in the microenvironment of the tumor, especially with advancing disease [35–36]. Secreted inflammation-associated cytokines (e.g. tumor necrosis factors, interleukines, etc) are in turn very well known to subsequently downregulate drug transporters [37]. In consequence, the observed downregulation of drug transporters in HNSCC tissue might simply be an indicator of enhanced inflammation which is typically observed in advanced stages of cancer and accompanied by poor survival [38].

In contrast to *ABCB1* and *ABCC1*, high expression of *ABCG2*, *ABCC2*, and *SLC31A1* tended to indicate poor progression-free survival and overall survival, but none of these associations reached statistical significance (Fig. 3). Due to these contradicting results, a cluster analysis was subsequently performed in order to detect dependencies or expression patterns that concertedly determine survival. Three distinct groups were identified. Best survival was observed when all drug transporters showed a reduced expression, whereas both progression-free and overall survival was shortened with coordinated high expression of *SLC31A1*, *ABCG2*, and *ABCC2* (Fig. 4). The latter two genes are known cancer-stem cell markers in HNSCC [39–40]. In consequence, it is comprehensible that patients with high expression of *ABCG2* and *ABCC2* (and thus potentially high cancer-stem cell burden) exhibit poor survival. Together, the results of the cluster analysis finally suggest that the course of the disease or survival cannot be estimated by a single drug transporter gene, but rather by the whole 'transportome' or at least the combination of certain drug transporters (e.g. cancer-stem cell marking drug transporters).

ATP7b expression was evaluated at the protein level using tissue microarray methodology (Fig. 6A). A high variation of the immunoreactive score was observed among the 61 HNSCC samples evaluated. However, survival analysis revealed that ATP7b expression does not correlate with survival times (Fig. 6B) contradicting earlier findings by others [23].

In conclusion, this study contradicts the intuitive dogma whereupon high expression of ABC-transporters such as Pgp is unfavorable for survival of HNSCC patients. In contrast,

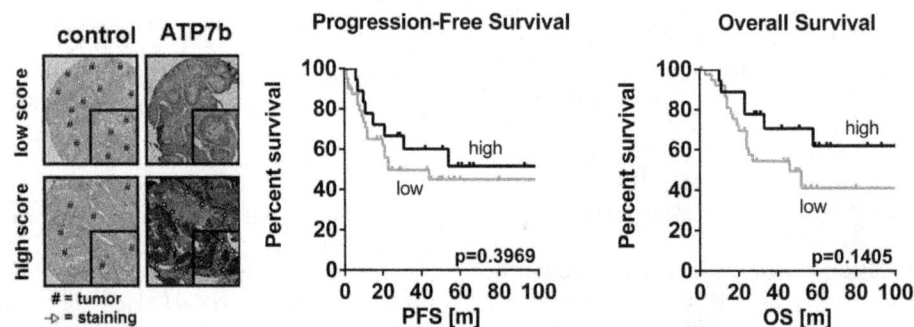

**Figure 6. Immunohistochemical staining of ATP7b protein expression in HNSCC.** Immunohistochemical staining of ATP7b protein expression in HNSCC patients (n = 61) revealed a high range of immunoreactive scores (left). Grouping of patients according to their immunoreactive scores (cutoff = 15) into low (n = 41) or high (n = 18) showed a trend towards a longer progression-free and overall survival in patients with a higher ATP7b expression (right).

overexpression of distinct drug transporters might even indicate improved survival. Cluster analysis evaluating a subset of drug transporters including cancer-stem cell markers such as *ABCG2* is suggested for further studies on the significance of drug transporters for HNSCC disease.

## References

1. Colevas AD (2006) Chemotherapy options for patients with metastatic or recurrent squamous cell carcinoma of the head and neck. J Clin Oncol 24: 2644–2652.
2. Gottesman MM, Fojo T, Bates SE (2002) Multidrug resistance in cancer: role of ATP-dependent transporters. Nat Rev Cancer 2: 48–58.
3. Kamazawa S, Kigawa J, Minagawa Y, Itamochi H, Shimada M, et al. (2000) Cellular efflux pump and interaction between cisplatin and paclitaxel in ovarian cancer cells. Oncology 59: 329–335.
4. Lagas JS, Vlaming ML, van Tellingen O, Wagenaar E, Jansen RS, et al. (2006) Multidrug resistance protein 2 is an important determinant of paclitaxel pharmacokinetics. Clin Cancer Res 12: 6125–6132.
5. Duan Z, Brakora KA, Seiden MV (2004) Inhibition of ABCB1 (MDR1) and ABCB4 (MDR3) expression by small interfering RNA and reversal of paclitaxel resistance in human ovarian cancer cells. Mol Cancer Ther 3: 833–838.
6. Pratt S, Shepard RL, Kandasamy RA, Johnston PA, Perry W, et al. (2005) The multidrug resistance protein 5 (ABCC5) confers resistance to 5-fluorouracil and transports its monophosphorylated metabolites. Mol Cancer Ther 4: 855–863.
7. Guminski AD, Balleine RL, Chiew YE, Webster LR, Tapner M, et al. (2006) MRP2 (ABCC2) and cisplatin sensitivity in hepatocytes and human ovarian carcinoma. Gynecol Oncol 100: 239–246.
8. Weaver DA, Crawford EL, Warner KA, Elkhairi F, Khuder SA, et al. (2005) ABCC5, ERCC2, XPA and XRCC1 transcript abundance levels correlate with cisplatin chemoresistance in non-small cell lung cancer cell lines. Mol Cancer 4: 18.
9. Yeh JJ, Hsu NY, Hsu WH, Tsai CH, Lin CC, et al. (2005) Comparison of chemotherapy response with P-glycoprotein, multidrug resistance-related protein-1, and lung resistance-related protein expression in untreated small cell lung cancer. Lung 183: 177–183.
10. Yoh K, Ishii G, Yokose T, Minegishi Y, Tsuta K, et al. (2004) Breast cancer resistance protein impacts clinical outcome in platinum-based chemotherapy for advanced non-small cell lung cancer. Clin Cancer Res 10: 1691–1697.
11. Surowiak P, Materna V, Matkowski R, Szczuraszek K, Kornafel J, et al. (2005) Relationship between the expression of cyclooxygenase 2 and MDR1/P-glycoprotein in invasive breast cancers and their prognostic significance. Breast Cancer Res 7: R862–70.
12. Burger H, Foekens JA, Look MP, Meijer-van Gelder ME, Klijn JG, et al. (2003) RNA expression of breast cancer resistance protein, lung resistance-related protein, multidrug resistance-associated proteins 1 and 2, and multidrug resistance gene 1 in breast cancer: correlation with chemotherapeutic response. Clin Cancer Res 9: 827–836.
13. Soini Y, Virkajärvi N, Raunio H, Pääkkö P (1996) Expression of P-glycoprotein in hepatocellular carcinoma: a potential marker of prognosis. J Clin Pathol 49: 470–473.
14. Duensing S, Dallmann I, Grosse J, Buer J, Lopez Hänninen E, et al. (1994) Immunocytochemical detection of P-glycoprotein: initial expression correlates with survival in renal cell carcinoma patients. Oncology 51: 309–313.
15. Uematsu T, Hasegawa T, Hiraoka BY, Komatsu F, Matsuura T, et al. (2001) Multidrug resistance gene 1 expression in salivary gland adenocarcinomas and oral squamous-cell carcinomas. Int J Cancer 92: 187–194.
16. Chen CL, Sheen TS, Lou IU, Huang AC (2001) Expression of multidrug resistance 1 and glutathione-S-transferase-Pi protein in nasopharyngeal carcinoma. Hum Pathol 32: 1240–1244.
17. Lo Muzio L, Staibano S, Pannone G, Mignogna MD, Serpico R, et al. (2000) The human multidrug resistance gene (MDR-1): immunocytochemical detection of its expression in oral SCC. Anticancer Res 20: 2891–2897.
18. Larbcharoensub N, Leopairat J, Sirachainan E, Narkwong L, Bhongmakapat T, et al. (2008) Association between multidrug resistance-associated protein 1 and poor prognosis in patients with nasopharyngeal carcinoma treated with radiotherapy and concurrent chemotherapy. Hum Pathol 39: 837–845.
19. Tsuzuki H, Fujieda S, Sunaga H, Sugimoto C, Tanaka N, et al. (1998) Expression of multidrug resistance-associated protein (MRP) in head and neck squamous cell carcinoma. Cancer Lett 126: 89–95.
20. van den Broek GB, Wildeman M, Rasch CR, Armstrong N, Schuuring E, et al. (2009) Molecular markers predict outcome in squamous cell carcinoma of the head and neck after concomitant cisplatin-based chemoradiation. Int J Cancer 124: 2643–2650.
21. Song IS, Savaraj N, Siddik ZH, Liu P, Wie Y, et al. (2004) Role of human copper transporter Ctr1 in the transport of platinum-based antitumor agents in cisplatin-sensitive and cisplatin-resistant cells. Mol Cancer Ther 3: 1543–1549.
22. Nakayama K, Kanzaki A, Ogawa K, Miyazaki K, Neamati N, et al. (2002) P-type adenosine triphophatase (ATP7B) as a cisplatin-based chemoresistance marker in ovarian carcinoma: comparative analysis with expression of MDR1, MRP, LRP and BCRP. Int J Cancer 101: 488–495.
23. Miyashita H, Nitta Y, Mori S, Kanzaki A, Nakayama K, et al. (2003) Expression of copper-transporting P-type adenosine triphosphatase (ATP7B) as a chemoresistance marker in human oral squamous cell carcinoma treated with cisplatin. Oral Oncol 39: 157–162.
24. Theile D, Ketabi-Kiyanvash N, Herold-Mende C, Dyckhoff G, Efferth T, et al. (2011) Evaluation of drug transporters' significance for multidrug resistance in head and neck squamous cell carcinoma. Head Neck 33: 959–968.
25. Vandesompele J, De Preter K, Pattyn F, Poppe B, Van Roy N, et al. (2002) Accurate normalization of real-time quantitative RT-PCR data by geometric averaging of multiple internal control genes. Genome Biol 3: RESEARCH0034.
26. Albermann N, Schmitz-Winnenthal FH, Z'graggen K, Volk C, Hoffmann MM, et al. (2005) Expression of the drug transporters MDR1/ABCB1, MRP1/ABCC1, MRP2/ABCC2, BCRP/ABCG2, and PXR in peripheral blood mononuclear cells and their relationship with the expression in intestine and liver. Biochem Pharmacol 70: 949–958.
27. Freier K, Bosch FX, Flechtenmacher C, Devens F, Benner A, et al. (2003) Distinct sitespecific oncoprotein overexpression in head and neck squamous cell carcinoma: a tissue microarray analysis. Anticancer Res 23: 3971–3977.
28. Karcher S, Steiner HH, Ahmadi R, Zoubaa S, Vasvari G, et al. (2006) Different angiogenic phenotypes in primary and secondary glioblastomas. Int J Cancer 118: 2182–2189.
29. Remmele W, Stegner HE (1987) Recommendation for uniform definition of an immunoreactive score (IRS) for immunohistochemical estrogen receptor detection (ER-ICA) in breast cancer tissue. Pathologe 8: 138–140.
30. Thomas GR, Nadiminti H, Regalado J (2005) Molecular predictors of clinical outcome in patients with head and neck squamous cell carcinoma. Int J Exp Pathol 86: 347–363.
31. Furusaka T1, Sasaki CT, Matsuda A, Susaki Y, Matsuda H, et al. (2013) Multidrug resistance in mucoepidermoid carcinoma of the parotid gland–immunohistochemical investigations of P-glycoprotein expression. Acta Otolaryngol 133: 552–557.
32. Ralhan R1, Narayan M, Salotra P, Shukla NK, Chauhan SS (1997) Evaluation of P-glycoprotein expression in human oral oncogenesis: correlation with clinicopathological features. Int J Cancer 72: 728–734.
33. Jain V1, Das SN, Luthra K, Shukla NK, Ralhan R (1997) Differential expression of multidrug resistance gene product, P-glycoprotein, in normal, dysplastic and malignant oral mucosa in India. Int J Cancer 74: 128–133.
34. Theile D, Grebhardt S, Haefeli WE, Weiss J (2009) Involvement of drug transporters in the synergistic action of FOLFOX combination chemotherapy. Biochem Pharmacol 78: 1366–1373.
35. Royuela M, Ricote M, Parsons MS, Garcia-Tunon I, Paniagua R, et al. (2004) Immunohistochemical analysis of the IL-6 family of cytokines and their receptors in normal, hyperplastic, and malignant human prostate. J Pathol 202: 41–49.
36. Brozek W, Bises G, Girsch T, Cross HS, Kaiser HE, et al. (2005) Differentiation dependent expression and mitogenic action of interleukin-6 in human colon carcinoma cells: relevance for tumour progression. Eur J Cancer 41: 2347–2354.
37. Morgan ET, Goralski KB, Piquette-Miller M, Renton KW, Robertson GR, et al. (2008) Regulation of drug-metabolizing enzymes and transporters in infection, inflammation, and cancer. Drug Metab Dispos 36: 205–216.
38. Rassouli A, Saliba J, Castano R, Hier M, Zeitouni AG (2013) Systemic inflammatory markers as independent prognosticators of Head and Neck Squamous cell carcinoma. Head Neck 2013.
39. Wang J, Guo LP, Chen LZ, Zeng YX, Lu SH (2007) Identification of cancer stem cell-like side population cells in human nasopharyngeal carcinoma cell line. Cancer Res 67: 3716–3724.
40. Lee SH1, Nam HJ, Kang HJ, Kwon HW, Lim YC (2013) Epigallocatechin-3-gallate attenuates head and neck cancer stem cell traits through suppression of Notch pathway. Eur J Cancer 49: 3210–3218.

## Author Contributions

Conceived and designed the experiments: DT JW RW CHM GD. Performed the experiments: DT RW. Analyzed the data: RW DT JW. Contributed reagents/materials/analysis tools: BL NG CM EH. Wrote the paper: DT JW RW CHM GD. Scientific and medical advice: PP.

# 22

# Chemo-Predictive Assay for Targeting Cancer Stem-Like Cells in Patients Affected by Brain Tumors

**Sarah E. Mathis**[1,2,9], **Anthony Alberico**[3,9], **Rounak Nande**[1,2], **Walter Neto**[1,2], **Logan Lawrence**[1,2], **Danielle R. McCallister**[1,2], **James Denvir**[1,2], **Gerrit A. Kimmey**[4], **Mark Mogul**[5], **Gerard Oakley III**[6], **Krista L. Denning**[6], **Thomas Dougherty**[6], **Jagan V. Valluri**[7], **Pier Paolo Claudio**[1,2,8]*

**1** Department of Biochemistry and Microbiology, Joan C. Edwards School of Medicine, Marshall University, Huntington, West Virginia, United States of America, **2** Translational Genomic Research Institute, Marshall University, Huntington, West Virginia, United States of America, **3** Department of Neurosurgery, Joan C. Edwards School of Medicine, Marshall University, Huntington, West Virginia, United States of America, **4** Department of Medical Oncology, St. Mary's Hospital, Huntington, West Virginia, United States of America, **5** Department of Pediatrics, Joan C. Edwards School of Medicine, Marshall University, Huntington, West Virginia, United States of America, **6** Department of Pathology, Joan C. Edwards School of Medicine, Marshall University, Huntington, West Virginia, United States of America, **7** Department of Biology, Marshall University, Huntington, West Virginia, United States of America, **8** Department of Surgery, Joan C. Edwards School of Medicine, Marshall University, Huntington, West Virginia, United States of America

## Abstract

Administration of ineffective anticancer therapy is associated with unnecessary toxicity and development of resistant clones. Cancer stem-like cells (CSLCs) resist chemotherapy, thereby causing relapse of the disease. Thus, development of a test that identifies the most effective chemotherapy management offers great promise for individualized anticancer treatments. We have developed an ex vivo chemotherapy sensitivity assay (ChemoID), which measures the sensitivity of CSLCs as well as the bulk of tumor cells to a variety of chemotherapy agents. Two patients, a 21-year old male (patient 1) and a 5-month female (patient 2), affected by anaplastic WHO grade-III ependymoma were screened using the ChemoID assay. Patient 1 was found sensitive to the combination of irinotecan and bevacizumab, which resulted in a prolonged disease progression free period of 18 months. Following recurrence, the combination of various chemotherapy drugs was tested again with the ChemoID assay. We found that benzyl isothiocyanate (BITC) greatly increased the chemosensitivity of the ependymoma cells to the combination of irinotecan and bevacizumab. After patient 1 was treated for two months with irinotecan, bevacizumab and supplements of cruciferous vegetable extracts containing BITC, we observed over 50% tumoral regression in comparison with pre-ChemoID scan as evidenced by MRI. Patient 2 was found resistant to all treatments tested and following 6 cycles of vincristine, carboplatin, cyclophosphamide, etoposide, and cisplatin in various combinations, the tumor of this patient rapidly progressed and proton beam therapy was recommended. As expected animal studies conducted with patient derived xenografts treated with ChemoID screened drugs recapitulated the clinical observation. This assay demonstrates that patients with the same histological stage and grade of cancer may vary considerably in their clinical response, suggesting that ChemoID testing which measures the sensitivity of CSLCs as well as the bulk of tumor cells to a variety of chemotherapy agents could lead to more effective and personalized anticancer treatments in the future.

**Editor:** Caterina Cinti, Institute of Clinical Physiology, c/o Toscana Life Sciences Foundation, Italy

**Funding:** The present studies were supported in part by the National Center for Advancing Translational Sciences, National Institutes of Health, through grant number UL1TR000117 from the National Center for Research Resources (NCRR), and 5P20RR020180 from the National Cancer Institute, WV-INBRE 5P20RR016477, and in part by a Marshall University Translational Award, and an award from the Marshall University Department of Neuroscience (to PPC). The content of this manuscript is solely the responsibility of the authors and does not necessarily represent the official views of NCRR and NIH. The funders had no role in study design, data collection and analysis, decision to publish, or preparation of the manuscript.

**Competing Interests:** The authors have declared that no competing interests exist.

\* Email: claudiop@marshall.edu

⑨ These authors contributed equally to this work.

## Introduction

Although ependymomas are the third most common type of brain tumor in children (following astrocytoma and medulloblastoma), they are relatively rare, with approximately 200 cases diagnosed in the US each year [1,2]. They account for 60% of all intramedullary tumors and 50% arise in the filum terminale [3].

The treatment of ependymomas can be challenging. The initial standard treatment for ependymoma is surgery often followed by radiation therapy, and chemotherapy. Although chemotherapy has been used extensively in children with ependymomas, there is little clinical evidence that chemotherapy improves survival of children with this type of tumor. Chemotherapy is often reserved for patients with residual tumor after surgery and for children younger than 3 years of age in an attempt to delay radiation therapy [4].

It is not entirely clear why there is not an improved survival with chemotherapy, but it is known that resistance to a variety of commonly used chemotherapeutic agents is common in ependymoma [5]. Therefore investigation and development of novel strategies and integrated therapies are required to find more effective treatments for this type of tumor.

Patients with the same stage and grade of cancer may vary considerably in their clinical response and toleration of chemotherapy. Ineffective anticancer therapy can result in unnecessary toxicity and the development of resistant clones. The surviving cancer cells are often more resistant to therapy. Many attempts have been made over the years to develop an *ex-vivo* anti-cancer test that could help discern the best treatment options for each individual patient while minimizing toxicity.

Animal xenograft models have shown that only a subset of cancer cells within each tumor is capable of initiating tumor growth. This capability has been shown in several types of human cancers, to include ependymomas [6]. This pool of cancer cells is operationally defined as the "Cancer Stem-Like Cell" (CSLC) subset. According to the "cancer stem-like cell" theory, tumors are a complex, growing population of abnormal cells originating from a minority of CSLCs. These cells maintain stem-like characteristics in that they proliferate very slowly and have an inherent capacity to self-renew and differentiate into phenotypically heterogeneous, aberrant progeny [7–10]. Unlike the bulk of tumor cells, CSLCs resist chemotherapy and radiation therapy and are responsible for tumor relapse and metastasis [9,10].

Some ependymomas express various markers of stemness, including CD133. In addition, relapsed tumors exhibit a gene expression signature constituted by up-regulated genes involved in the kinetochore (ASPM, KIF11) or in neural development (CD133, Wnt and Notch pathways) [11].

Targeting CSLCs in addition to the bulk of other cancer cells within a tumor is a new paradigm in cancer treatment. Our recent studies show that a Hydrodynamic Focusing Bioreactor (HFB) (Celdyne, Houston TX) selectively enriches CSLCs from cancer cell lines that can be used in a chemosensitivity assay [8]. Further, using this strategy we optimized the enrichment of CSLCs from tumor biopsies and have developed the ChemoID chemotherapy sensitivity assay, which measures the response of CSLCs and the bulk of tumor cells to chemotherapy to determine the most effective combination of anticancer drugs for malignant tumors of the nervous system.

In this study we report, for the first time, our investigation using the ChemoID assay to measure the sensitivity and resistance of CSLCs and bulk of tumor cells cultured from 2 biopsies of human ependymoma challenged with several chemotherapy agents which were also correlated to the response of animal xenografts treated with the predicted drugs and to the clinical response of the treated patients.

## Materials and Methods

### Reagents

Benzyl isothiocyanate (BITC) was purchased from Sigma Chemical Co. (St. Louis, MO). Bevacizumab (Avastin), Cisplatin, Oxaliplatin, Arabinoside-C, VP-16, Irinotecan (Camptosar, CPT-11), Busulfan, Methotrexate, were acquired as clinical grade chemotherapy agents.

### Patients

Case 1 is a 21-year-old male patient diagnosed with intradural, intramedullary, and extramedullary anaplastic diffuse spinal ependymoma, WHO grade III. Case 2 is a 5-month old female patient diagnosed with anaplastic WHO grade III ependymoma.

ChemoID assay was performed after obtaining patient's written informed consent in accordance with the ethical standards of the Helsinki Declaration (1964, amended most recently in 2008) of the World Medical Association. Any information, including illustrations, has been anonymized. Marshall University Institutional Review Board (IRB) has approved this research under the protocol #326290. Participants or guardians of participant (in case of a child participant) provided their written consent on an IRB approved informed consent form to participate in this study after being educated about the research protocol. Ethics committees/ IRB at Marshall University approved this consent procedure. For Children participants to the study, written informed consent was obtained from the next of kin, caretakers, or guardians on behalf of the minors/children enrolled in your study.

### Single Cell Suspension and Primary Cell Culture

Single-cell suspensions from the ependymoma biopsies were prepared using the gentleMACS Dissociator (Miltenyi, Auburn, CA), and C Tubes using a standardized, semi-automated protocol based on a combination of mechanical tissue disruption and incubation with a 50% solution 0.025% trypsin and Accutase (Innovative Cell Technologies, San Diego, CA). Cells were serially plated in 24-well, 12-well, 6-well, 10-cm treated dishes and cultured to subconfluence in RPMI-1640 medium supplemented with 5% irradiated, heat inactivated, defined fetal bovine serum (Thermofisher/Hyclone), and 50 U of penicillin and 5 µg of streptomycin/mL of medium (Thermofisher/Mediatech).

### Three-Dimensional Bioreactor CSLCs Culture

A hydrodynamic focusing bioreactor (HFB) (Celdyne, Houston TX) was used as previously described to selectively proliferate CD133(+) cancer stem-like cells [8]. Culture media, oxygenation, speed, temperature and $CO_2$ were kept consistently constant for ten days.

Cells were counted and $1 \times 10^6$ cells were placed in the rotating vessel set at 25 rpm with airflow set at 20%. Cells were then removed and counted again using trypan blue exclusion to determine cellular viability and cell number and plated in 96 wells for chemosensitivity testing. The cells were also incubated with florescent antibodies for phenotypic characterization [8].

### Cell Sorting

Up to $1 \times 10^7$ cells were sorted by a magnetic-activated cell sorting (MACS) system, which consists of magnetic beads conjugated to an antibody against CD133 (Miltenyi, Auburn, CA). In brief, cells were harvested using 0.25% trypsin, pelleted and labeled with CD133/1 biotin and CD133/2-PE. Cells were washed and labeled with anti-biotin magnetic beads, and then passed through a magnetic column where CD133(+) cells were retained, while unlabelled cells passed through the column. The CD133(+) retained cells were eluted from the columns after removal from the magnet. Positive and negative cells were then analyzed by FACS for purity.

### Flow Cytometry Studies

Cells were analyzed by the antigenic criteria using anti-CD34 (Milteny Biotech, Auburn, CA), -CD38 (Milteny Biotech, Auburn, CA), -CD44 (BD Bioscience, Sparks, MD), -CD117 (Milteny Biotech, Auburn, CA), -CD133/2 (prominin1) (Milteny Biotech, Auburn, CA), -Oct3/4 (BD Bioscience, Sparks, MD), and –Nanog (BD Bioscience, Sparks, MD). Briefly, cells were detached using 0.02% EDTA in PBS and pelleted (10 min at 1,000 rpm), washed in 0.1% BSA in 1X PBS at 4°C and incubated in a solution of

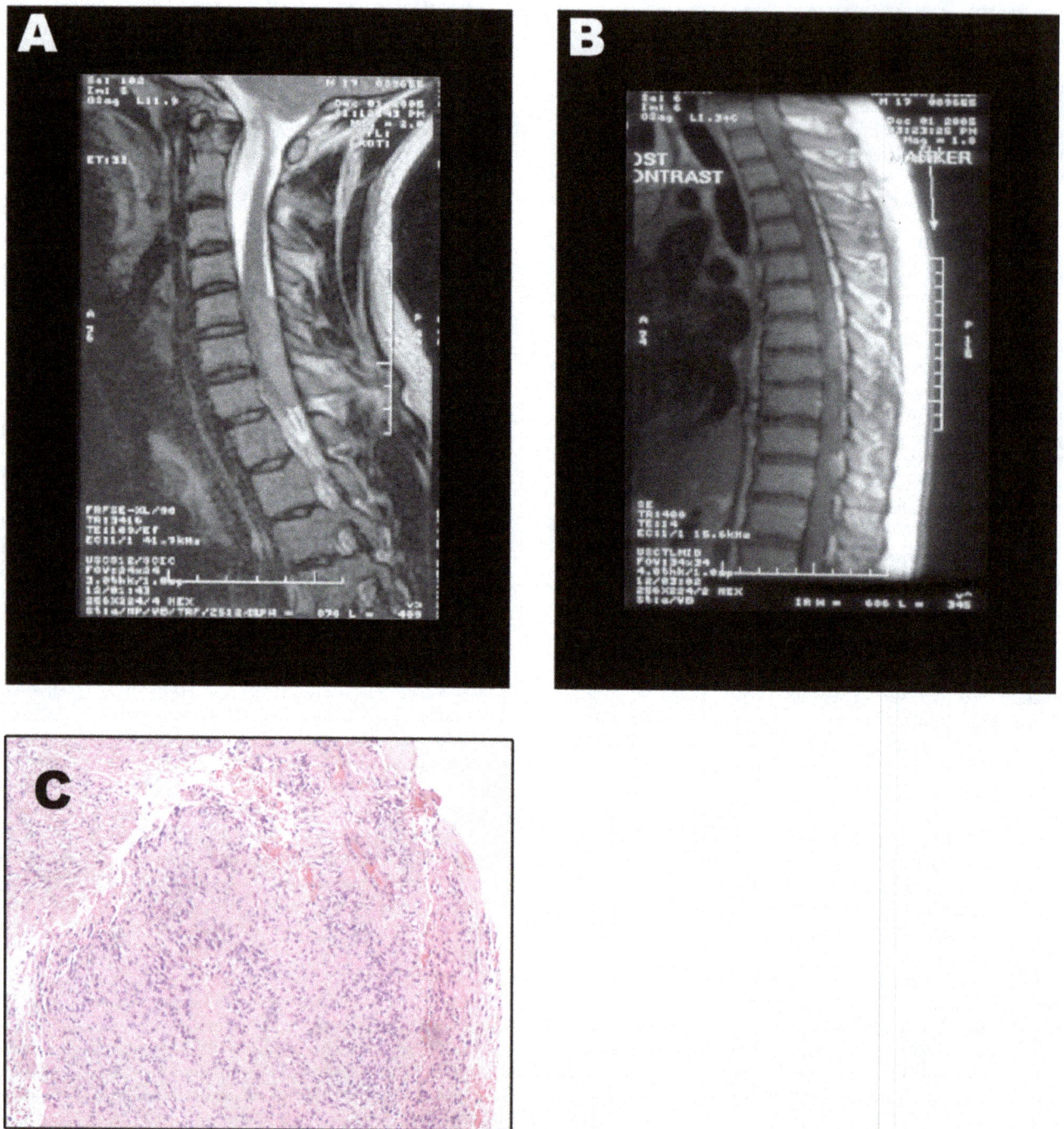

**Figure 1. MRI Images and H&E Staining of the Anaplastic Ependymoma Case at Presentation. A)** Magnetic Resonance Imaging (MRI) of the cervical spine showing the presence of an enhancing mass, which extends from mid C5 to inferior C7 (4.5 in length×1.0×2.0 in cephalocaudal and anteroposterior dimension) and causing cord compression. **B)** MRI of the thoracic spine showing an enhancing lesion at T2–3 (1.5 in length×0.6×0.6 cm in anteroposterior and transverse dimension) with several other smaller nodular masses, best seen on the T2 weighted sequence, which extended throughout the thoracic level to T11. **C)** Hematoxylin and Eosin staining of a tumor section showing an overall predominant dense cellular component, with primitive nuclear features, mitotic activity, necrosis and vascular proliferation. The presence of well formed, obvious perivascular pseudorosettes (with vasocentric pattern, perivascular nuclear-free zones, and classic thin glial processes radiating to/from the vessel wall) were found supportive of the diagnosis of intradural, extramedullary anaplastic diffuse spinal ependymoma, WHO grade III.

1 mg antibody +9 mL 0.1% BSA in 1X PBS. Cells were washed in the same solution once and were analyzed using a C6 Accuri flow cytometer (BD Biosciences, San Jose, CA).

### ChemoID Assay

Sensitivity to chemotherapy was assessed using a viability assay (WST8) on $1 \times 10^3$ cells plated in 5 replicas into 96-well plates. Briefly, equal number of bulk of tumor cells grown in monolayer and CSLCs grown in the bioreactor, were counted and seeded

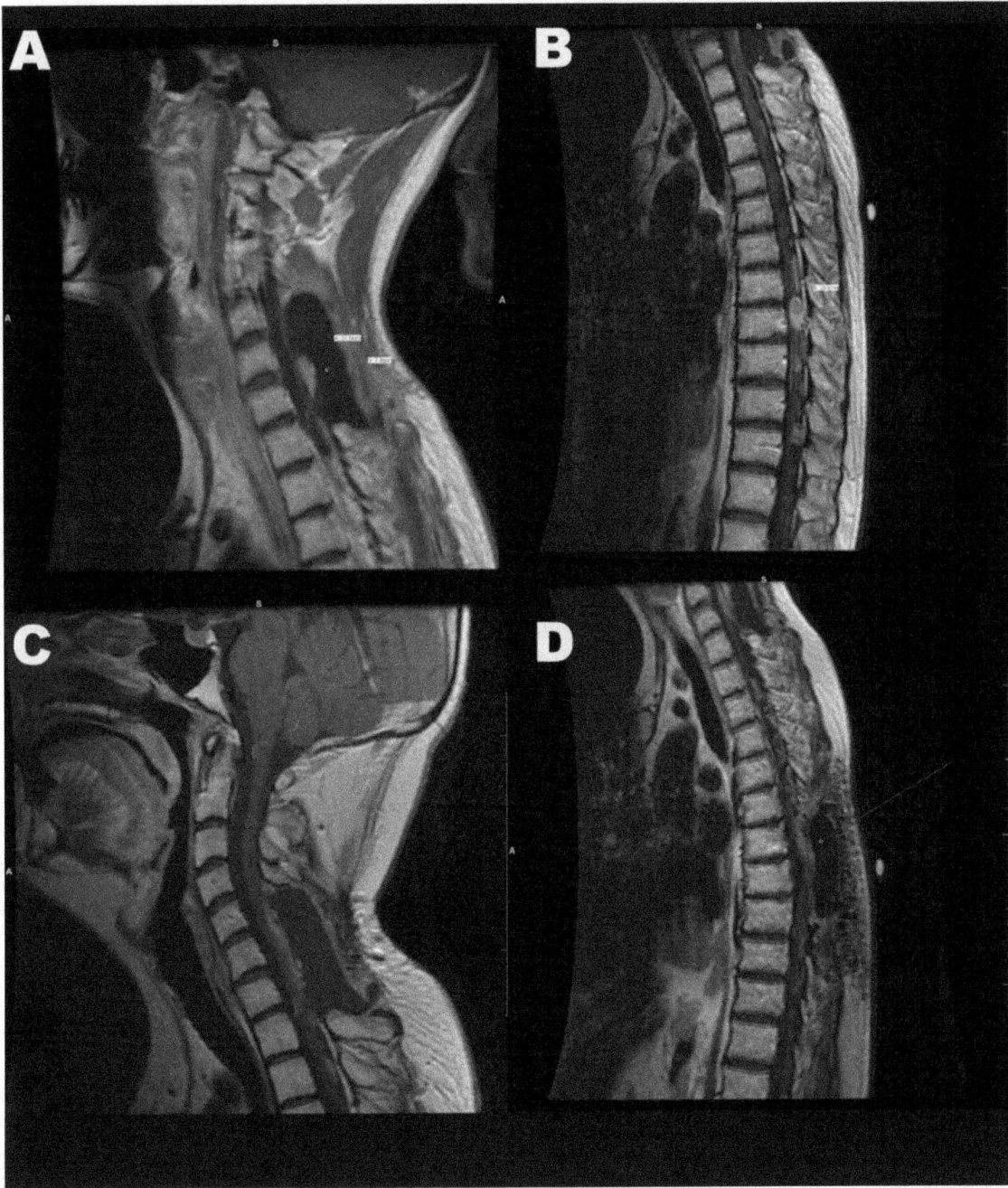

**Figure 2. MRI Images of Cervical and Thoracic Spine. A**) 2009 MRI of the cervical spine showing recurrence in the surgical area. **B**) 2009 MRI of the thoracic spine showing progression of the main lesion measuring 23.9 mm, and the appearance of several other smaller lesions. **C and D**) 2010 MRI of the cervical and thoracic spine showing tumor regression following a treatment with irinotecan and bevacizumab.

separately in 96-well dishes and incubated at 37°C for 24-hours. The cells were then challenged for a 1-hour pulse with a panel of anticancer drugs as chosen by the oncologist to mimic the average clinical chemotherapy infusion schedule.

To study the effect of BITC on chemosensitization of cancer cells to chemotherapy drugs, the cells were treated with an hour pulse 5–30 μM BITC followed by an hour of the various anticancer drugs. Each anticancer drug was tested in a range of doses including the clinically relevant dose.

A WST8 assay was performed 48-hours following chemotherapy treatment to assess cell viability as previously described [12]. A

dose response chart was developed in which samples were scored as responsive (0–30% cell survival), intermediate (30–60% cell survival), and non-responsive (60–100% cell survival).

## Limiting Dilution Tumorigenic Assay in Immune Deficient Mice

A range of $1 \times 10^2$, $1 \times 10^3$, $1 \times 10^4$, and $1 \times 10^5$ ependymoma cells from Patient 1 were injected subcutaneously in 5 athymic immunodeficient nude$^{nu/nu}$ mice per group. Briefly, an equal number of parental bulk of tumor cells grown in 2D monolayer, CD133(+) three-dimensionally grown in the hydrofocusing bioreactor, and CD133(+) MACSorted CSLCs were injected with 100 μL of matrigel in the flank of NOD-*Scid* mice and compared to the growth of CD133 negative cells for 3 months.

## Chemotherapy Animal Study

All animal studies have been conducted following approval from the Marshall University IACUC, protocol #373017. The effects of chemotherapies screened in vitro by the ChemoID assay was tested on human tumor biopsies that were xenografted in the flank of a NOD-*Scid* mouse model. $1 \times 10^{\wedge}6$ ependymoma cells were mixed to 100 μL of matrigel (BD Biosciences, San Jose, CA) injected subcutaneously in the flank of 10 athymic, NOD.Cg-Prkdc *Scid* ll2rgtm1wjl/SzJ immunodeficient mice (NOD-*Scid*)/group and were grown for 10 weeks or until 100 mm^3. Mice were randomized in different treatment and control groups and chemotherapy was administered by intraperitoneal (i.p.) injections in 200 μL as follows in a period of 4 weeks: 1) **Group #1**, Control group with primary tumor cells injected into flank and receiving i.p. sterile saline injections. **Group #2**, Experimental group injected i.p. with the least effective chemotherapy as determined by the *in vitro* ChemoID assay. **Group #3**, Experimental group injected i.p. with the most effective chemotherapy as determined by the *in vitro* ChemoID assay. **Group #4**, Experimental group injected i.p. with the second most effective chemotherapy as determined by the *in vitro* ChemoID assay. **Group #5**, Experimental group injected i.p. with the most effective combinatorial chemotherapy as determined by the *in vitro* ChemoID assay.

Chemotherapy mouse doses were calculated using a body surface area (BSA) normalization method [13] from the clinical dose and verified according to doses previously determined by a literature search.

## Euthanasia

Animals were euthanized following the current guidelines established by the latest Report of the AVMA Panel on Euthanasia using CO2 inhalation and asphyxiation followed by cervical dislocation.

## Statistical Analysis

Statistical analysis was performed using the IBM SPSS statistical software. The results for each variant in the different experimental designs represent an average of 3 different experiments. The data of 5 measurements were averaged; the coefficient of variation among these values never exceeded 10%. Mean values and standard errors were calculated for each point from the pooled normalized to control data. Statistical analysis of the significance of the results was performed with a 1-way ANOVA. *p* values of less than 0.05 were considered statistically significant.

## Results

### Patient 1 History and Selection of Chemotherapies with ChemoID Assay

A physically active 17-year-old male presented in October 2005 with paresthesia in his feet and a rather severe perceptive loss. This became progressively worse in December 2005 going up his legs with rather severe numbness in the right leg and pain in his left leg, from the mid thigh down to the mid calf medially. On examination he had no focal weakness throughout his upper and lower extremities. He had hypoalgesia with partial sensory level in the upper thoracic spine down. He also had severe proprioception loss in his feet and toes. Magnetic resonance imaging (MRI) of the cervical spine showed the presence of an abnormal enhancing mass, which extended from mid C5 to inferior C7 (4.5 in length×1.0×2.0 in cephalocaudal and anteroposterior dimension) that caused cord compression (**Figure 1A**). MRI of the thoracic spine showed an enhancing lesion at T2–3 (1.5 in length×0.6×0.6 cm in anteroposterior and transverse dimension) with several other smaller nodular masses, best seen on the T2 weighted sequence, which extended throughout the thoracic level to T11 (**Figure 1B**).

The patient received a laminectomy in December 2005 at C5, C6, and C7 with partial resection of the tumor under microscope using microsurgical techniques. Following surgery, the patient was treated with radiation and temozolomide.

Morphological analysis of the histology sections stained with Hematoxylin & Eosin showed an overall predominant dense cellular component, with primitive and pleomorphic nuclei,

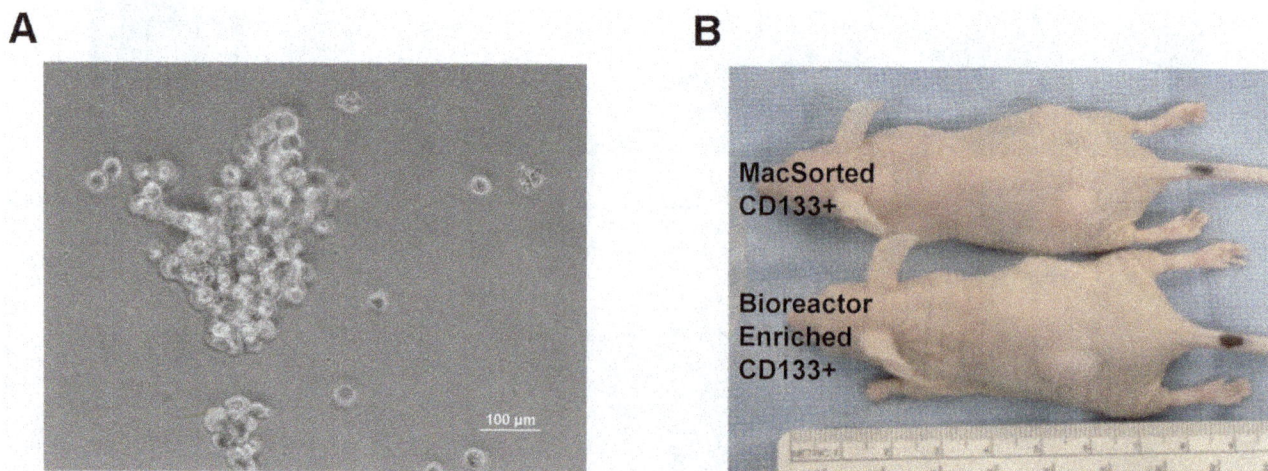

**Figure 3. CD133 (+) Cells Grown in a Hydrofocusing Bioreactor form Xenografts in nude Mice. A)** Contrast phase image of a cluster of enriched CSLCs following 7-days of culture in a hydrofocusing bioreactor. **B)** Immunodeficient nude mice (nu/nu) injected with $1 \times 10^{\wedge}2$ ependymoma cells MacSorted CD133(+) cells or CD133(+) ependymoma cells grown in the hydrofocusing bioreactor, with the aid of 100 μL of matrigel in the flank formed a tumor within 3 months compared to CD133(−) cells.

**Table 1.** Enrichment of CD133+ CSLCs using a hydrofocusing bioreactor.

| | CD133+ cells | CD133- cells |
|---|---|---|
| Day 0 | 255,000 | 245,000 |
| Day 7 | 3,748,500 | 159,036 |
| Fold | 14.7 | −1.54 |

increased mitotic rate and apoptosis, and foci with microvascular proliferation. The presence of well formed, obvious perivascular pseudorosettes (with vasocentric pattern, perivascular nuclear-free zones, and classic thin glial processes radiating to/from the vessel wall) were found to supporting the diagnosis of anaplastic diffuse spinal ependymoma, WHO grade III. **Figure 1C** shows the hematoxylin and eosin staining of a tumor section at diagnosis in 2005.

Sections of the tumor were evaluated by immunoperoxidase techniques with appropriate staining control sections. The tumor showed positive staining with antibodies to neuron specific enolase, vimentin, S-100, and GFAP. Weak staining occurred with the antibodies against actin. Focal staining occurred with antibodies to epithelial membrane antigen, cytokeratin AE1/AE3, and synaptophysin. The tumor was negative for leukocyte common antigen, desmin, and myogenin. In addition, a section stained with PAS showed a focal PAS-positive fibrillar material. Sections and tumor block were also sent to the Biopathology Center (BPC) of the Children's Oncology Group (COG) were two neuropathologists independently reviewed the case and confirmed the diagnosis of anaplastic ependymoma, WHO grade III.

Following recurrence and progression, the patient received complex chemotherapy regimen in January 2006 and March 2006 with cyclophosphamide, thalidomide, celecoxib followed by etoposide, thalidomide and celecoxib. Chemotherapy treatment was concluded in September of 2006, but in August of 2007 patient had tumor regrowth at T7–T8 for which he underwent robotic radiosurgery treatment. The patient had another debulking surgery in April of 2008, but later in December of 2008 he had progressive numbness in his legs along with back pain with MRI showing recurrence in the surgical area (**Figure 2A**) as well as the lumbar spine. He was then treated again with temozolomide, but had no response to treatment.

In March 2009 because of progression of the disease he had a thoracic laminectomy and resection of the intradural intramedullary tumor. He had severe spinal compression and began having weakness in his legs. Due to further recurrence, the patient then had another debulking surgery in July of 2009. He also received oxaliplatin and etoposide treatment in July and August 2009, but the tumor progressed even more (**Figure 2B**).

Appropriate informed consent was signed and at the time of the debulking surgery of July 2009, a sterile biopsy was taken to assess the sensitivity of the tumor cells (bulk of tumor and CSLCs) toward standard-of-care chemotherapy drugs using our ChemoID assay. The biopsy was placed in RPMI-1640 sterile media and tissue was dissociated in our laboratory into a single-cell suspension with the use of a GentleMACS tissue dissociator (Miltenyi, Aubourn, CA). The single-cell ependymoma suspension was plated in RPMI-1640 in the presence of 5% irradiated, heat inactivated, defined fetal bovine serum, streptomycin and penicillin and cells were cultured as a monolayer for 15 days. Cells were immunophenotyped by flow cytometer using antibodies against CD34, CD38, CD44, CD117, CD133, OCT3/4, and Nanog.

The ependymoma cells were found positive to OCT3/4 (2.73%), Nanog (0.95%), CD133 (49.93%), CD117 (36.81%), and CD44 (20.39%) when compared to an isotype control antibody (**Figure S1 A-E**). A double staining of CD34 and CD38 showed the presence of 1.88% of the cells CD34+/CD38+, and 78.4% CD34+/CD38- cells (**Figure S1 F**).

To expand the CSLC population of CD133+ cells from the ependymoma primary culture, the ependymoma cells were cultured as previously described [8]. $1 \times 10^6$ of the ependymoma cells from a monolayer primary culture were grown for ten days using Hydrodynamic Focusing Bioreactor (HFB) (Celdyne, Houston, TX) [8]. The ependymoma cells cultured in the bioreactor formed cell clusters (**Figure 3A**) which were expanded 14.7 fold (**Table 1**) and appeared to be 95.93% CD133 positive after 10 days of culture in the bioreactor (**Figure S1 C, enriched CSLCs**).

To verify the tumor initiating capacity of the HFB grown cells, we injected 5 immune deficient nude mice/group a range of $1 \times 10^2$, $1 \times 10^3$, $1 \times 10^4$, and $1 \times 10^5$ cells grown in the HFB (~96% CD133+) and compared their growth to an equal number of CD133(+) MACsorted cells and CD133(−) cells for 3 months. We observed that both $1 \times 10^2$ MacSorted CD133(+) cells or the CD133(+) from the bioreactor grew in all the immune deficient mice injected and formed a palpable tumor within 12 weeks (**Figure 3B**).

To perform the ChemoID assay a comparable number of cells $(1 \times 10^5)$ bulk of tumor cells grown as a 2D monolayer and CSLCs enriched in the bioreactor [8] were separately plated into 96 wells plates (n-5 replicas) and were treated for an hour with a series of anticancer drugs at a range of concentrations including the clinically relevant dosage (**Table 2**). ChemoID assay was performed using a panel of drugs comprising of cisplatin, oxaliplatin, arabinoside-C, VP-16, busulfan, methotrexate, irinotecan, and bevacizumab as chosen by the treating oncologist.

Sensitivity to chemotherapy was assessed at 48-hours by WST8 viability assay. It was categorized as follows based on the percentage of non-viable cells: responsive (0–40% cell survival), intermediate (40–70% cell survival), and non-responsive (70–100% cell survival). The WST8 assay was conducted three separate times with n-5 well replicas/drug/dose each time.

ChemoID assay showed that the ependymoma cells grown in monolayer and representing the bulk of tumor cells were sensitive to clinically relevant doses of cisplatin, irinotecan, busulfan, and a combination of irinotecan and bevacizumab in a statistically significant manner (p<0.05). Interestingly, the CSLCs were sensitive to a combination of irinotecan and bevacizumab (p< 0.05), intermediately sensitive to cisplatin, and irinotecan, but not sensitive to busulfan. On the other hand, both the CSLCs and the bulk of tumor cells were not responsive to methotrexate, oxaliplatin, arabinoside-C, and VP-16 (**Figure 4**).

Because of the lack of response to an oxaliplatin and etoposide management given in August 2009 (**Figure 2B**) (which was started prior to receiving the results from the ChemoID assay), the

**Table 2.** Clinical dose and calculated in vitro doses of the various chemotherapies.

| | Bevacizumab | Cisplatin | Oxaliplatin | Arabinoside-C | Irinotecan | Busulfan | Methotrexate | VP-16 |
|---|---|---|---|---|---|---|---|---|
| 1/10 | 0.4 µM | 0.05 mM | 0.04 mM | 1.64 mM | 0.0497 mM | 0.12 mM | 2.2 µM | 0.0339 mM |
| 1/100 | 0.04 µM | 0.005 mM | 0.004 mM | 0.164 mM | 0.0049 mM | 0.012 mM | 0.22 µM | 0.0033 mM |
| 1/1000 | 0.004 µM | 0.0005 mM | 0.0004 mM | 0.0164 mM | 0.00049 mM | 0.0012 mM | 0.0022 µM | 0.00033 mM |
| Clinical dose | 10 mg/Kg | 75 mg/m$^2$ | 80 mg/m$^2$ | 2 g/m$^2$ | 125 mg/m$^2$ | 150 mg/m$^2$ | 5 mg/m$^2$ | 100 mg/m$^2$ |
| Calculated in vitro dose equivalent to clinical dose | 4 µM | 0.5 mM | 0.4 mM | 16.44 mM | 0.497 mM | 1.22 mM | 22 µM | 0.3397 mM |

Calculated in vitro dose = [(clinical dose in mg/m$^2$×2× m$^2$)/1000J/MW of drug.

patient underwent in October 2009 a treatment with bevacizumab and irinotecan, which was administered every two weeks for 6 months. In a follow-up MRI scan in May 2010 the patient showed initial disease regression remaining free from disease progression for 18 months (**Figure 2 C and D**). This corresponded to the longest disease progression free period observed in this patient without major de-bulking surgery.

Recurrence of tumor growth after 18 months of disease free progression led us to explore novel therapeutic approaches for the treatment of this patient's cancer. In this regard, combination chemotherapy was investigated in order to identify natural compounds that may increase the clinical efficacy of anticancer drugs.

BITC has been shown in other laboratories [14,15] to increase the chemosensitivity of cancer cells. We have recently observed in our laboratory (data not shown) that benzyl isothiocyanate (BITC) increases specifically the chemosensitivity of CD133 positive cancer cells. Because the primary ependymoma cells of our patient displayed a high percentage of cells positive to CD133, we wanted to test the hypothesis that BITC could increase their chemosensitivity to irinotecan and bevacizumab. We found with the ChemoID assay that increasing concentrations of BITC ranging from 2.5 µM to 20 µM decreased the viability of CD133(+) ependymoma cells of Patient 1 from 90% to 62% in a statistically significant manner (**Figure 5A**). ChemoID assay also determined that the combination of irinotecan and a non-toxic concentration of 10 µM BITC reduced the viability of the ependymoma cells from 60% to 40% (over 40% more chemosensitive compared to non BITC treated cells) (**Figure 5 B**). Additionally, the combination of irinotecan and bevacizumab with BITC reduced even further the viability of the ependymoma cells to 30% (**Figure 5 B**). The patient was treated with irinotecan and bevacizumab, but this time with the combination of 2 capsules/day of a Triple Action Cruciferous Vegetable Extract containing high concentration of BITC (LifeExtension, http://www.lef.org), for two months. Following the combination therapy of irinotecan, bevacizumab and the supplement of cruciferous vegetables, we have observed a 4 cm regression (which corresponds to a 50% regression) of the lesions in the thoracic and the cervical area [compare **Figure 5C** (at recurrence) to **Figure 5D** (following therapy)]. Additionally, we report that the patient was able to tolerate the entire course of irinotecan and bevacizumab chemotherapy regimen with less fatigue and tolerance to cold.

The efficacy of chemotherapies screened in vitro by the ChemoID assay were tested on the ependymoma cells of Patient 1 that were xenografted in a NOD-*Scid* mouse model (**Figure 6 A and B**). Ten athymic NOD-Scid mice were injected in the flank with $1 \times 10^6$ ependymoma cells mixed to 100 µL of matrigel (BD Biosciences, San Jose, CA) and tumors were grown for 10 weeks or until 100 mm$^3$. Randomized mice were treated by weekly intraperitoneal (i.p.) injections of the different treatment arms for 4 weeks and were observed for 4 more weeks. Group #1 serving as a control received i.p. sterile saline injections. Groups #2–5 were the experimental groups, which received i.p. injections of the least effective chemotherapy, or the most effective, the second most effective, and the most effective combinatorial chemotherapy, as determined by the *in vitro* ChemoID assay.

Interestingly, the tumor xenografts in the Scid mice injected with the least effective chemotherapy as determined by the *in vitro* ChemoID assay grew faster than saline control injected mice (**Figure 6A**). As expected, we observed tumor regression in Scid mice treated with the most effective, the second most effective, and the most effective combinatorial chemotherapy as determined by the *in vitro* ChemoID assay, confirming the clinical observation

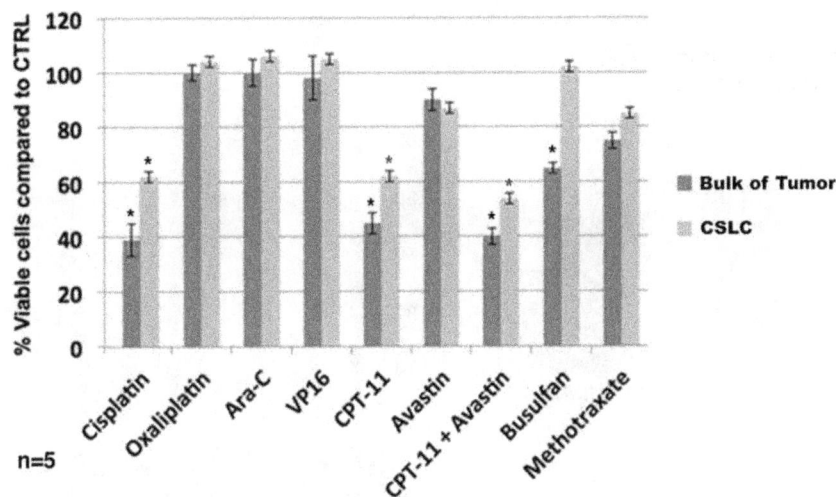

**Figure 4. Diagram of ChemoID Assay to Assess the Sensitivity to Chemotherapy of Cancer Cells or CSLCs Using a WST-8 Assay on patient 1.** $1 \times 10^3$ bulk of tumor cells or CSLCs plated in 5 replicas into 96-well plates were challenged for a 1-hour pulse with a panel of anticancer drugs indicated by the oncologist. A WST-8 assay was performed 48-hours following chemotherapy treatments to assess cell viability. Data is plotted in bar graph as responsive (0–40% cell viability), moderately responsive (40–70% cell viability), and non-responsive (70–100% cell viability). Light grey bar represent sensitivity of CSLCs to chemotherapy with respect to negative untreated control cells. Dark grey bar represent sensitivity of bulk of tumor cells to chemotherapy with respect to negative untreated control cells. Anticancer drugs tested indicated at the bottom of the diagram. Statistical analysis of the significance of the results was performed with a 1-way ANOVA. Asterisks indicate p values of less than 0.05.

that irinotecan and bevacizumab are more effective anticancer drugs in this individual patient. Mice weight was measured weekly (**Figure 6B**)

We further tested the hypothesis that mice that were failing a chemoresistant treatment could be rescued by switching them to a more sensitive treatment as determined by the *in vitro* ChemoID assay. Mice that were failing an oxaliplatin therapy regimen were taken off oxaliplatin at week 16 and were treated for 4 weeks with a combination of irinotecan and bevacizumab. As expected, mice treated with irinotecan and bevacizumab showed a regression of the xenografted tumor compared to the control mice injected with saline solution (**Figure 6C**) confirming once again the previously observed clinical data.

## Patient 2 History and ChemoID Results

Patient 2 is a 5-month-old female with an aggressive brain tumor that was surgically removed in April 2012. The tumor was diagnosed as an anaplastic ependymoma, WHO grade III with low-grade mitosis-poor areas and high cellular tissue with mitosis and high MIB-1 rate.

A biopsy from the surgically removed tumor was placed in RPMI-1640 sterile media and the tissue was dissociated in our laboratory into a single-cell suspension with the use of a GentleMACS tissue dissociator (Miltenyi, Aubourn, CA) as previously. The single-cell ependymoma suspension was plated in RPMI-1640 in the presence of 5% irradiated, heat inactivated, defined fetal bovine serum, streptomycin and penicillin and cells were cultured as a monolayer for 15 days. Cells were immunophenotyped by flow cytometer using antibodies against CD34, CD38, CD44, CD133, Nanog, and CXCR4. The ependymoma cells were found positive to Nanog (13%), CD133 (47.5%), CD44 (65.5%), and CXCR4 (89.7%) when compared to an isotype control antibody. A double staining of CD34 and CD38 showed the presence of 4.6% of the cells CD34+/CD38+, and 47.3% CD34+/CD38- cells (data not shown).

The ChemoID assay performed on the bulk of the ependymoma cells and on the CSLCs showed resistance to all of the tested chemotherapy drugs (**Figure 7**). Patient 2 received complex chemotherapy with 6 cycles of vincristine, carboplatin, cyclophosphamide, etoposide, and cisplatin in various combinations, however the tumor rapidly progressed and proton beam therapy was recommended. Because of the lack of tumor response to the various anticancer drugs and radiation therapy, the patient expired after 9 months.

## Discussion

Treatment for ependymoma is often a combinatorial approach that includes surgery, radiation therapy, and chemotherapy. Although chemotherapy has been used extensively in the treatment management of ependymomas, this therapeutic modality is often reserved for patients with residual tumor after surgery and for children younger than 3 years of age in an attempt to delay radiation therapy. Recently, the role of chemotherapy in the treatment of ependymoma has diminished because (1) chemotherapy fails to delay radiation therapy for a meaningful period of time; (2) tumors that progress during chemotherapy do not respond as well to subsequent irradiation; and (3) the combination of chemotherapy and irradiation does not improve overall survival [16].

It is not entirely clear why there is not an improved survival with chemotherapy [5], therefore investigation and development of novel strategies and integrated therapies are required to find more effective treatments for this type of tumor.

One of our patients was diagnosed with recurring undifferentiated intradural-extramedullary spinal ependymoma, WHO grade III, with a distinctive sensitivity to chemotherapy who has been followed up for 5 years following ChemoID. The second patient was also diagnosed with recurring ependymoma, WHO III but was found not sensitive to any of the chemotherapies tested and rapidly progressed.

**A**

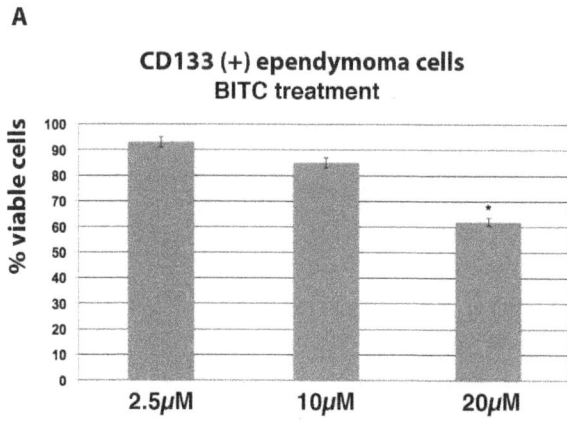

**B**

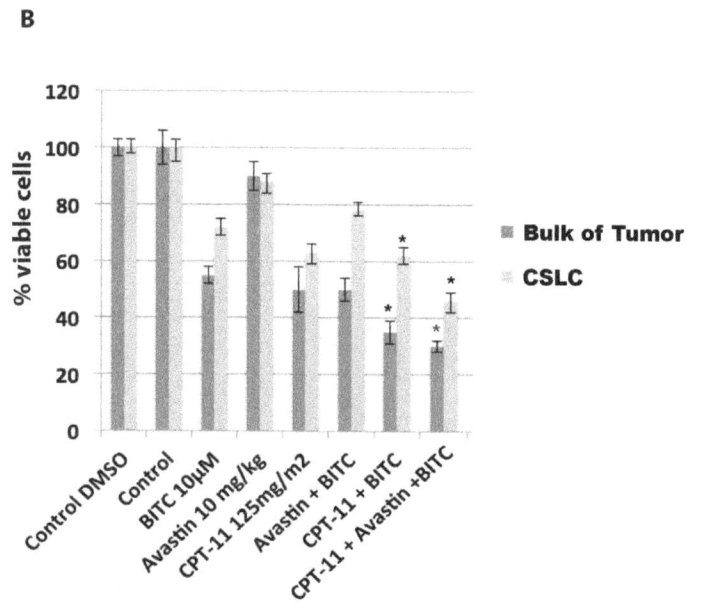

**C**

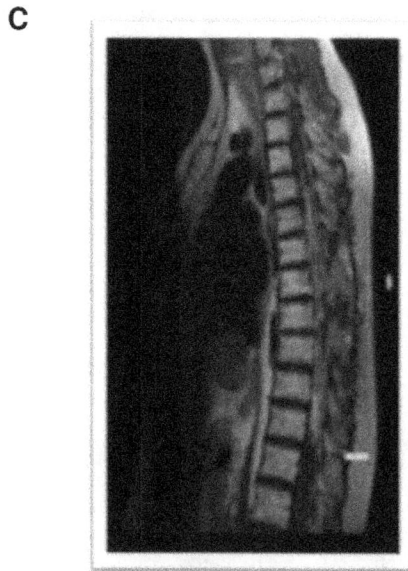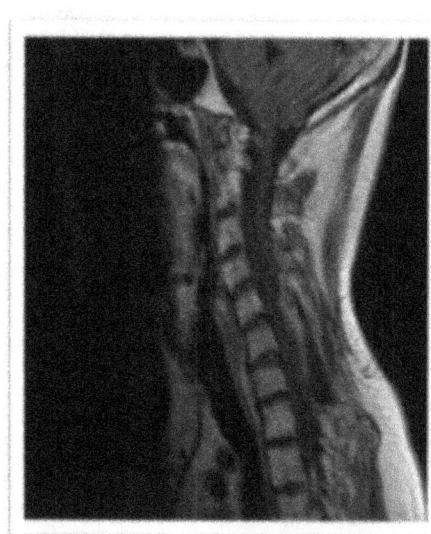

**D**

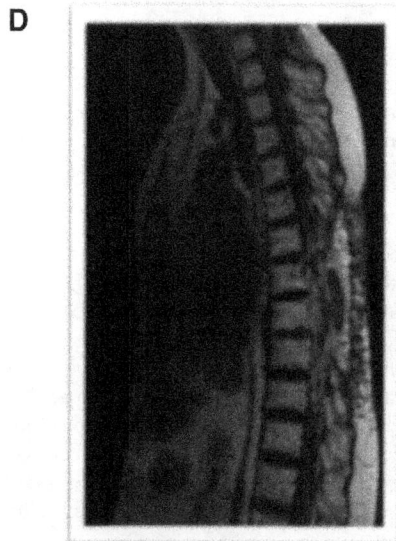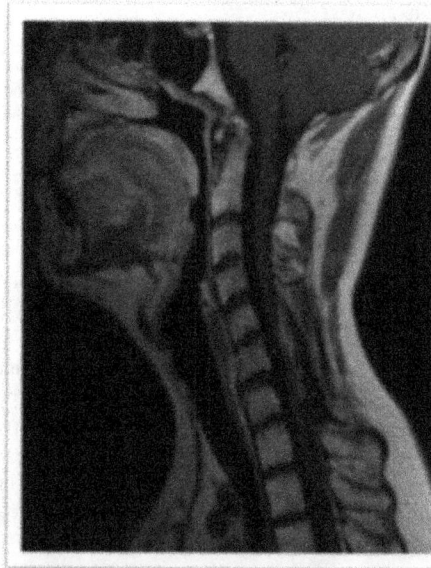

**Figure 5. Diagram of ChemoID Assay and MRI Images of Cervical and Thoracic Spine following Integrated Therapy. A**) 1×10^3 CSLCs plated in 5 replicas into 96-well plates were challenged for a 1-hour pulse with 2.5, 10, and 20 µM BITC. A WST-8 assay was performed 48-hours after treatments to assess cell viability. **B**) 1×10^3 CSLCs plated in 5 replicas into 96-well plates were challenged for a 1-hour pulse with 10 µM BITC followed by a 1-hour pulse with 0.5 mM CPT-11. A WST-8 assay was performed 48-hours following chemotherapy treatment to assess cell viability. Data is plotted in bar graph as responsive (0–40% cell viability), moderately responsive (40–70% cell viability), and non-responsive (70–100% cell viability). Light grey bar represent sensitivity of CSLCs to chemotherapy with respect to negative untreated control cells. Dark grey bar represent sensitivity of bulk of tumor cells to chemotherapy with respect to negative untreated control cells. Statistical analysis of the significance of the results was performed with a 1-way ANOVA. Asterisks indicate $p$ values of less than 0.05. **C**) 2012 MRI of the cervical and thoracic spine showing recurrence after an 18 months progression free period. **D**) 2012 MRI of the cervical spine showing marked tumor regression of the thoracic spine lesion following combined treatment with irinotecan (CPT11), bevacizumab (Avastin), and BITC supplementation.

Resistance to chemotherapy severely compromises its effectiveness. The development of resistance is a major problem for patients, researchers, and clinicians who rely on conventional cytotoxic agents for the treatment of cancer.

Despite the fact that several treatments for ependymoma are currently available, this remains a poorly treated disease [17–21]. Surgery plus postoperative radiotherapy represents the standard treatment for patients with grade III (anaplastic) ependymomas [21,22]. Additionally, surgery has been demonstrated to be associated with significant improvements in overall survival time for patients with all stages of ependymal tumors [23–27]. However, a total resection is not always achieved. Overall prognosis is improved when the entire tumor can be removed and there are no other neural axis metastasis [28]. Therefore, in cases in which the ependymoma is multifocal, metastatic, incompletely resected, or particularly aggressive; it is imperative to find the most effective alternative treatment to surgery available.

Administration of ineffective anticancer therapy is associated with unnecessary toxicity and development of resistant clones. Each time patients are treated, they have a chance of relapse and

their cancer may become more resistant to therapy. Presently used anticancer drugs have a high rate of failure and cell culture chemotherapy testing is being used to identify which drugs are more likely to be effective against a particular tumor type. Measuring the response of the tumor cells to drug exposure is valuable in any situation in which there is a choice between two or more treatments. This includes virtually all situations in cancer chemotherapy, whether the goal is cure or palliation. This kind of testing can assist in individualizing cancer therapy by providing information about the likely response of an individual patient's tumor to proposed therapy. Many attempts have been made over the years to develop an *ex-vivo* anti-cancer test that can provide clinically relevant treatment information, but all the efforts have been directed toward the bulk of tumor cells [29–35].

In the recent past, chemotherapy testing has been performed on cancer cells from patients without prior separation and enrichment of the CSLCs from the bulk of tumor cells [30,36–45].

Knowing which chemotherapy agents the patient's bulk of tumor cells as well as the CSLCs are resistant to is very important. Then, these options can be eliminated, thereby avoiding the

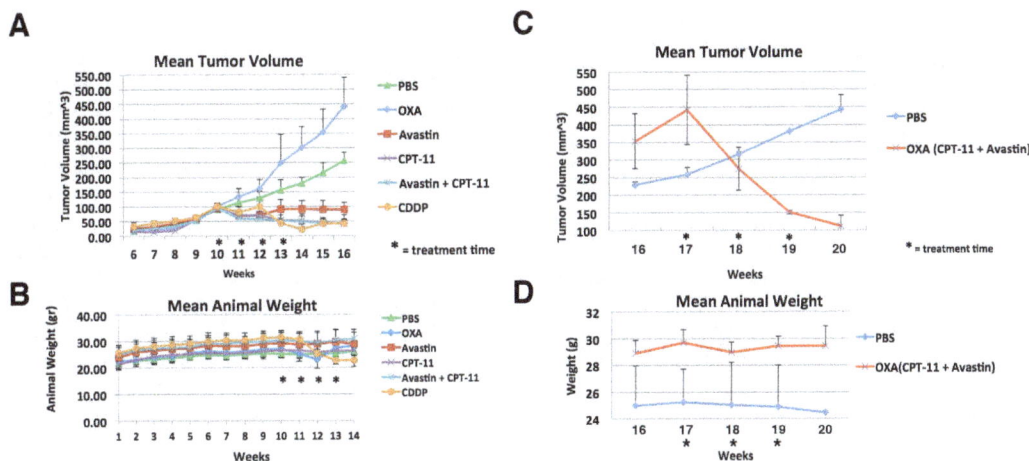

**Figure 6. Mean Tumor Volume and Mean Tumor Weight of Patient Derived Xenografts Treated with i.p. Injection of Anticancer Drugs. A**) Line diagram of the mean volumes in mm^3 (±SD) from week 6–16 of 10 patient derived xenografted tumors in NOD-Scid mice following 4 weeks of treatment with various anticancer drugs. The mean tumor volumes are indicated on the ordinate. Asterisks indicate weeks in which treatment was performed. On the right are indicated the different treatment arms. PBS: saline solution, negative control. OXA (oxaliplatin); Avastin (bevacizumab); CPT-11 (irinotecan); CDDP (cisplatin). **B**) Line diagram of the mean weight in grams (±SD) of 10 NOD-Scid mice-bearing patient derived xenografted tumors following 4 weeks of treatment with various anticancer drugs. The mean tumor weights are indicated on the ordinate. Asterisks indicate weeks in which treatment was performed. On the right are indicated the different treatment arms. PBS: saline solution is negative control. OXA (oxaliplatin); Avastin (bevacizumab); CPT-11 (irinotecan); CDDP (cisplatin). **C**) Line diagram of the mean volumes in mm^3 (±SD) from week 16 to 20 of the 10 patient derived xenografted tumors in NOD-Scid mice that failed oxaliplatin therapy (weeks 6–16 in panel A), following 3 weeks of treatment with irinotecan and bevacizumab. The mean tumor volumes are indicated on the ordinate. Asterisks indicate weeks in which treatment was performed. On the right are indicated the different treatment arms. PBS: saline solution, negative control. OXA (CPT11+Avastin): mice that failed oxaliplatin and were then treated with irinotecan and bevacizumab. **D**) Line diagram of the mean weight in grams (±SD) of the 10 NOD-Scid mice-bearing patient derived xenografted tumors following 3 weeks of treatment with irinotecan and bevacizumab. The mean tumor weights are indicated on the ordinate. Asterisks indicate weeks in which treatment was performed. On the right are indicated the different treatment arms. PBS: saline solution, negative control. OXA (CPT11+Avastin): mice that failed oxaliplatin and were then treated with irinotecan and bevacizumab.

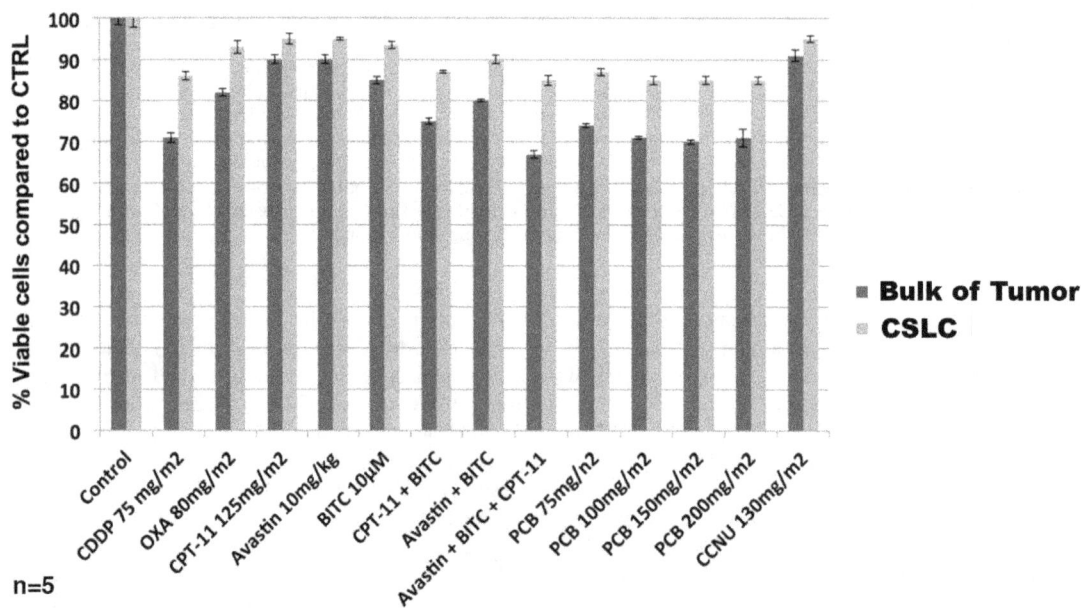

**Figure 7. Diagram of ChemoID Assay to Assess the Sensitivity to Chemotherapy of Cancer Cells or CSLCs Using a WST-8 Assay on patient 2.** $1 \times 10^3$ bulk of tumor cells or CSLCs plated in 5 replicas into 96-well plates were challenged for a 1-hour pulse with a panel of anticancer drugs indicated by the oncologist. A WST-8 assay was performed 48-hours following chemotherapy treatments to assess cell viability. Data is plotted in bar graph as responsive (0–40% cell viability), moderately responsive (40–70% cell viability), and non-responsive (70–100% cell viability). Light grey bar represent sensitivity of CSLCs to chemotherapy with respect to negative untreated control cells. Dark grey bar represent sensitivity of bulk of tumor cells to chemotherapy with respect to negative untreated control cells. Anticancer drugs tested indicated at the bottom of the diagram. Statistical analysis of the significance of the results was performed with a 1-way ANOVA. Asterisks indicate $p$ values of less than 0.05.

toxicity of ineffective agents. Choosing the most effective agent can help patients to avoid the physical, emotional, and financial costs of failed therapy and experience an increased quality of life.

ChemoID chemotherapy sensitivity assay used in this study, measures for the first time the survival of CSLCs and bulk of tumor cells cultured from human cancer biopsies following chemotherapy. The advantage of the ChemoID assay is to aid the oncologists in selecting the most appropriate chemotherapy regimen on an individual basis especially when a number of equivalent options are available. The ChemoID assay allows various available chemotherapy drugs, which are part of standard of care to be tested, for efficacy against the cancer stem cells as well as the bulk of tumors.

For patient 1 affected by a recurring anaplastic ependymoma, the ChemoID assay determined on both bulk of tumor cells and CSLCs, that the most effective treatments were either irinotecan and bevacizumab or cisplatin. Interestingly, although the entire regimen containing irinotecan and bevacizumab could not be completed, the patient showed an initial regression of the disease and remained free from disease progression for 18 months, which corresponded to the longest disease progression free period in this patient.

Following up on the recurrence after the 18 month of progression free interval observed, repeated testing was performed using the ChemoID assay on the combination of several drugs and nutritional supplements among which benzylisothiocyanate (BITC). Numerous studies have indicated that isothiocyanates (ITCs) induce robust anti-cancer effects [15,46,47]. ITCs are derived naturally from glucosinolates, which are found at high concentrations in vegetables from the Cruciferae family [14,15]. Cruciferous vegetables, which produce ITCs, include broccoli, Indian cress, cabbage, Brussel sprouts, and watercress [48]. ITCs are of interest as anticancer molecules because of their ability to

target many of the aberrant pathways associated with cancer development. However, among the numerous ITCs identified, only a few of them appear to elicit anti-carcinogenic properties [49].

Interestingly, BITC has been previously shown to increase the chemosensitivity of bulk of tumor cells [14,15], but not of CSLCs. In our laboratory we have observed that BITC can increase specifically the chemosensitivity of cells that are highly positive for CD133 (data not shown), a marker used to identify CSLCs in tumors of the nervous system. Since the primary ependymoma cells of our patient displayed a high percentage of cells positive to CD133, we tested the hypothesis that BITC could increase their chemosensitivity.

Interestingly, we demonstrated here, for the first time, that the combination of irinotecan and BITC increased the chemosensitivity of the bulk of tumor cells and of the CSLCs cultured from the ependymoma of patient 1and have observed a clinically significant regression of the lesion in the cervical area as well as regression of other lesions at the thoracic level following a combined treatment with irinotecan, bevacizumab, and BITC.

Noteworthy and as expected, we observed regression of the NOD-Scid mice xenografts treated with the most effective, the second most effective, and the most effective combinatorial chemotherapy as determined by the *in vitro* ChemoID assay. In a model of patient derived xenografts this confirms the clinical observation that irinotecan and bevacizumab are more effective anticancer drugs for this individual patient. Interestingly, the tumor xenografts in the Scid mice injected with the least effective chemotherapy as determined by the *in vitro* ChemoID assay grew faster than saline control injected mice. We do not know why the tumor xenografts in mice injected with oxaliplatin grew faster than saline control injected mice, but we speculate that because the patient was treated with oxaliplatin prior to the ChemoID assay biopsy, it had selected cellular clones that are resistant to it and that manifest a growth advantage in its presence.

Furthermore, mice that failed to oxaliplatin treatment, which mimics the clinical scenario of this particular patient, were rescued by switching them to a more sensitive treatment (irinotecan and bevacizumab) as determined by the *in vitro* ChemoID assay. As expected, in this rescue animal model the mice treated with a combination of irinotecan and bevacizumab showed a regression of the patient derived xenografted tumors compared to control mice injected with saline solution confirming once again the previously observed clinical data.

Unfortunately, the second case of ependymoma we present could not benefit from any combined therapy that was proposed indicating that although affected by the same type of tumor response to chemotherapy can be different.

This is the first report on the clinical relevance of this novel chemosensitivity assay that measures the sensitivity of bulk of tumor cells and CSLCs to chemotherapy, which has the objective to decrease unnecessary toxicity while increasing the benefit of cytotoxic therapy for patients affected by malignant tumors.

Although the ChemoID results on these two cases of ependymoma showed clinical relevance, a larger study with different histological tumor types is needed to determine the prognostic accuracy of this assay. We are currently conducting a brain and spine malignant tumor phase-I clinical trial in which we have accrued 33 patients in the past three years to study the feasibility of this new assay in predicting the most effective chemotherapy regimen to improve patients' outcomes by assessing the vulnerability to chemotherapy of the CSLCs.

## Disclosures

All research involving human participants has been approved by the authors' institutional review board, protocol #326290. Informed consent was obtained and all clinical investigation was conducted according to the principles expressed in the Declaration of Helsinki.

## References

1. Hanbali F, Fourney DR, Marmor E, Suki D, Rhines LD, et al. (2002) Spinal cord ependymoma: radical surgical resection and outcome. Neurosurgery 51: 1162–1172; discussion 1172–1164.
2. Duncan J, Hoffman H (1995) Intracranial ependymomas. In: Kaye A, Lows E, Jr. editors. Brain Tumors. Edinburgh: Churchill Livingstone. pp. 493–504.
3. Cooper IS, Craig WM, Kernohan JW (1951) Tumors of the spinal cord; primary extramedullary gliomas. Surg Gynecol Obstet 92: 183–190.
4. Bouffet E, Foreman N (1999) Chemotherapy for intracranial ependymomas. Child's nervous system: ChNS: official journal of the International Society for Pediatric Neurosurgery 15: 563–570.
5. Chou PM, Barquin N, Gonzalez-Crussi F, Ridaura Sanz C, Tomita T, et al. (1996) Ependymomas in children express the multidrug resistance gene: immunohistochemical and molecular biologic study. Pediatric pathology & laboratory medicine: journal of the Society for Pediatric Pathology, affiliated with the International Paediatric Pathology Association 16: 551–561.
6. O'Brien CA, Kreso A, Jamieson CH (2010) Cancer stem cells and self-renewal. Clin Cancer Res 16: 3113–3120.
7. Aimola P, Desiderio V, Graziano A, Claudio PP (2010) Stem cells in cancer therapy: From their role in pathogenesis to their use as therapeutic agents. Drug News Perspect 23: 175–183.
8. Kelly SE, Di Benedetto A, Greco A, Howard CM, Sollars VE, et al. (2010) Rapid selection and proliferation of CD133+ cells from cancer cell lines: chemotherapeutic implications. PLoS One 5: e10035.
9. Malik B, Nie D (2012) Cancer stem cells and resistance to chemo and radio therapy. Front Biosci (Elite Ed) 4: 2142–2149.
10. Yu Y, Ramena G, Elble RC (2012) The role of cancer stem cells in relapse of solid tumors. Front Biosci (Elite Ed) 4: 1528–1541.
11. Modena P, Buttarelli FR, Miceli R, Piccinin E, Baldi C, et al. (2012) Predictors of outcome in an AIEOP series of childhood ependymomas: a multifactorial analysis. Neuro-oncology 14: 1346–1356.
12. van Meerloo J, Kaspers GJ, Cloos J (2011) Cell sensitivity assays: the MTT assay. Methods Mol Biol 731: 237–245.

All animal work was conducted according to relevant national and international guidelines. All animal studies have been conducted following approval from the Marshall University IACUC, protocol #373017.

## Supporting Information

**Figure S1 Characterization of the Primary Ependymoma Cell Culture and of the Enriched CSLCs. *A-F)*** *Immunophenotype conducted using:* **A)** OCT3/4 antibody; Left panel: isotype antibody (bulk of tumor cells); Center panel: specific antibody (bulk of tumor cells); Right panel: specific antibody (enriched CSLCs). **B)** Nanog antibody; Left panel: isotype antibody (bulk of tumor cells); Center panel: specific antibody (bulk of tumor cells); Right panel: specific antibody (enriched CSLCs). **C)** CD133 antibody; Left panel: isotype antibody (bulk of tumor cells); Center panel: specific antibody (bulk of tumor cells); Right panel: specific antibody (enriched CSLCs). **D)** CD117 antibody; Left panel: isotype antibody (bulk of tumor cells); Center panel: specific antibody (bulk of tumor cells); Right panel: specific antibody (enriched CSLCs). **E)** CD44 antibody; Left panel: isotype antibody (bulk of tumor cells); Center panel: specific antibody (bulk of tumor cells); Right panel: specific antibody (enriched CSLCs). **F)** Double labeling with CD34 and CD38 antibodies; Panel on left: isotype antibody (bulk of tumor cells); Center panel: specific antibody (bulk of tumor cells); Panel on right: specific antibody (enriched CSLCs).

## Author Contributions

Conceived and designed the experiments: PPC JV SM. Performed the experiments: SM AA RN WN LL DM JD GK MM GO KD TD JV PPC. Analyzed the data: PPC JV GO TD JD. Contributed reagents/materials/analysis tools: PPC JV. Contributed to the writing of the manuscript: PPC JV GO JD TD.

13. Reagan-Shaw S, Nihal M, Ahmad N (2008) Dose translation from animal to human studies revisited. FASEB journal: official publication of the Federation of American Societies for Experimental Biology 22: 659–661.
14. Di Pasqua AJ, Hong C, Wu MY, McCracken E, Wang X, et al. (2010) Sensitization of non-small cell lung cancer cells to cisplatin by naturally occurring isothiocyanates. Chem Res Toxicol 23: 1307–1309.
15. Wu X, Zhou QH, Xu K (2009) Are isothiocyanates potential anti-cancer drugs? Acta Pharmacol Sin 30: 501–512.
16. Merchant TE (2002) Current management of childhood ependymoma. Oncology 16: 629–642, 644; discussion 645–626, 648.
17. Chamberlain MC, Tredway TL (2011) Adult primary intradural spinal cord tumors: a review. Curr Neurol Neurosci Rep 11: 320–328.
18. Duffau H, Gazzaz M, Kujas M, Fohanno D (2000) Primary intradural extramedullary ependymoma: case report and review of the literature. Spine (Phila Pa 1976) 25: 1993–1995.
19. McCormick PC, Post KD, Stein BM (1990) Intradural extramedullary tumors in adults. Neurosurg Clin N Am 1: 591–608.
20. Pejavar S, Polley MY, Rosenberg-Wohl S, Chennupati S, Prados MD, et al. (2012) Pediatric intracranial ependymoma: the roles of surgery, radiation and chemotherapy. J Neurooncol 106: 367–375.
21. Song KW, Shin SI, Lee JY, Kim GL, Hyun YS, et al. (2009) Surgical results of intradural extramedullary tumors. Clin Orthop Surg 1: 74–80.
22. Vandertop WP (2003) Spinal cord ependymoma: radical surgical resection and outcome. Neurosurgery 53: 246; author reply 246–247.
23. Kocak Z, Garipagaoglu M, Adli M, Uzal MC, Kurtman C (2004) Spinal cord ependymomas in adults: analysis of 15 cases. J Exp Clin Cancer Res 23: 201–206.
24. Lin YH, Huang CI, Wong TT, Chen MH, Shiau CY, et al. (2005) Treatment of spinal cord ependymomas by surgery with or without postoperative radiotherapy. J Neurooncol 71: 205–210.

25. Metellus P, Figarella-Branger D, Guyotat J, Barrie M, Giorgi R, et al. (2008) Supratentorial ependymomas: prognostic factors and outcome analysis in a retrospective series of 46 adult patients. Cancer 113: 175–185.

26. Reni M, Brandes AA, Vavassori V, Cavallo G, Casagrande F, et al. (2004) A multicenter study of the prognosis and treatment of adult brain ependymal tumors. Cancer 100: 1221–1229.

27. Reni M, Gatta G, Mazza E, Vecht C (2007) Ependymoma. Crit Rev Oncol Hematol 63: 81–89.

28. Iunes EA, Stavale JN, de Cassia Caldas Pessoa R, Ansai R, Onishi FJ, et al. (2011) Multifocal intradural extramedullary ependymoma. Case report. J Neurosurg Spine 14: 65–70.

29. Breidenbach M, Rein DT, Mallmann P, Kurbacher CM (2002) Individualized long-term chemotherapy for recurrent ovarian cancer after failing high-dose treatment. Anticancer Drugs 13: 173–176.

30. Brower SL, Fensterer JE, Bush JE (2008) The ChemoFx assay: an ex vivo chemosensitivity and resistance assay for predicting patient response to cancer chemotherapy. Methods Mol Biol 414: 57–78.

31. Kleinhans R, Brischwein M, Wang P, Becker B, Demmel F, et al. (2012) Sensor-based cell and tissue screening for personalized cancer chemotherapy. Med Biol Eng Comput 10.1007/s11517-011-0855-7.

32. Michalova E, Poprach A, Nemeckova I, Nenutil R, Valik D, et al. (2008) [Chemosensitivity prediction in tumor cells ex vivo–difficulties and limitations of the method]. Klin Onkol 21: 93–97.

33. Myatt N, Cree IA, Kurbacher CM, Foss AJ, Hungerford JL, et al. (1997) The ex vivo chemosensitivity profile of choroidal melanoma. Anticancer Drugs 8: 756–762.

34. Tsubouchi H, Takao S, Aikou T (2000) Sensitivity of human pancreatic adenocarcinoma tumor lines to chemotherapy, radiotherapy, and hyperthermia. Hum Cell 13: 203–212.

35. Wichmann G, Horn IS, Boehm A, Mozet C, Tschop K, et al. (2009) Single tissue samples from head and neck squamous cell carcinomas are representative regarding the entire tumor's chemosensitivity to cisplatin and docetaxel. Onkologie 32: 264–272.

36. Ballard KS, Tedjarati SS, Robinson WR, Homesley HD, Thurston EL (2010) Embryonal rhabdomyosarcoma: adjuvant and ex vivo assay-directed chemotherapy. Int J Gynecol Cancer 20: 561–563.

37. Gallion H, Christopherson WA, Coleman RL, DeMars L, Herzog T, et al. (2006) Progression-free interval in ovarian cancer and predictive value of an ex vivo chemoresponse assay. Int J Gynecol Cancer 16: 194–201.

38. Herzog TJ, Krivak TC, Fader AN, Coleman RL (2010) Chemosensitivity testing with ChemoFx and overall survival in primary ovarian cancer. Am J Obstet Gynecol 203: 68 e61–66.

39. Huh WK, Cibull M, Gallion HH, Gan CM, Richard S, et al. (2011) Consistency of in vitro chemoresponse assay results and population clinical response rates among women with endometrial carcinoma. Int J Gynecol Cancer 21: 494–499.

40. Ness RB, Wisniewski SR, Eng H, Christopherson W (2002) Cell viability assay for drug testing in ovarian cancer: in vitro kill versus clinical response. Anticancer Res 22: 1145–1149.

41. Ochs RL, Burholt D, Kornblith P (2005) The ChemoFx assay: an ex vivo cell culture assay for predicting anticancer drug responses. Methods Mol Med 110: 155–172.

42. Peters D, Freund J, Ochs RL (2005) Genome-wide transcriptional analysis of carboplatin response in chemosensitive and chemoresistant ovarian cancer cells. Mol Cancer Ther 4: 1605–1616.

43. Rice SD, Cassino TR, Sakhamuri L, Song N, Williams KE, et al. (2011) An in vitro chemoresponse assay defines a subset of colorectal and lung carcinomas responsive to cetuximab. Cancer Biol Ther 11: 196–203.

44. Rice SD, Heinzman JM, Brower SL, Ervin PR, Song N, et al. (2010) Analysis of chemotherapeutic response heterogeneity and drug clustering based on mechanism of action using an in vitro assay. Anticancer Res 30: 2805–2811.

45. Suchy SL, Hancher LM, Wang D, Ervin PR, Jr., Brower SL (2011) Chemoresponse assay for evaluating response to sunitinib in primary cultures of breast cancer. Cancer Biol Ther 11: 1059–1064.

46. Mi L, Hood BL, Stewart NA, Xiao Z, Govind S, et al. (2011) Identification of potential protein targets of isothiocyanates by proteomics. Chem Res Toxicol 24: 1735–1743.

47. Zhang Y (2001) Molecular mechanism of rapid cellular accumulation of anticarcinogenic isothiocyanates. Carcinogenesis 22: 425–431.

48. Kelloff GJ, Crowell JA, Steele VE, Lubet RA, Boone CW, et al. (1999) Progress in cancer chemoprevention. Ann N Y Acad Sci 889: 1–13.

49. Lamy E, Scholtes C, Herz C, Mersch-Sundermann V (2011) Pharmacokinetics and pharmacodynamics of isothiocyanates. Drug Metab Rev 43: 387–407.

# 23

# Clinicopathologic Characteristics of Typical Medullary Breast Carcinoma

**Zhaohui Chu**[1,2⑨], **Hao Lin**[1,2⑨], **Xiaohua Liang**[1,2], **Ruofan Huang**[1,2], **Qiong Zhan**[1,2], **Jingwei Jiang**[1,2], **Xinli Zhou**[1,2*]

**1** Department of Oncology, Huashan Hospital, Fudan University, Shanghai, China, 200040, **2** Department of Oncology, Shanghai Medical College, Fudan University, Shanghai, China, 200032

## Abstract

*Purpose:* This study analyzed the clinicopathologic characteristics of typical medullary breast carcinoma (TMBC) in a cohort of Chinese patients.

*Methods:* We conducted a retrospective review of clinical data including general information, pathologic results, treatment regimens, and patient survival in cases of TMBC diagnosed between February 2004 and April 2011.

*Results:* A total of 117 patients were enrolled, with a median age of 52 years (range, 28~92 years). Stage I and II disease accounted for 31.6% and 61.6% of the cases, respectively. Hormonal receptor negative disease (estrogen receptor negative, 68.4%; progestogen receptor negative, 86.3%) was more prevalent in this population. Human epidermal growth factor receptor-2 (HER-2) positivity was 20.5%, while equivocal and HER-2 negative cases represented 16.2% and 63.2% of the cohort. The triple-negative, luminal, and HER-2 overexpressing subtypes constituted 44.4%, 31.6%, and 15.4% of the cases, respectively. The various TMBC subtypes showed no differences regarding tumor size, rates of lymph node(s) metastasis, TNM staging, treatment regimens, and 2-year recurrence rates. However, patients with triple-negative disease were more likely to be younger, when compared to those with luminal disease (P = 0.002). At a median follow-up of 56 months (range, 2–112 months), the 2-year disease-free survival and overall survival rates were 99.1% and 98.2%, respectively.

*Conclusion:* Early stage disease dominated the study cohort, and at two years after surgery, recurrence was extremely low. The heterogeneity of molecular subtypes was clearly shown, and no apparent differences were found among the clinicopathologic characteristics of the triple-negative, luminal, and HER-2 overexpressing subtypes.

**Editor:** Jan P. A. Baak, Stavanger University Hospital, Norway

**Funding:** The author(s) received autonomous scientific research projects funding from Fudan University, Shanghai, China. The funders had no role in study design, data collection and analysis, decision to publish, or preparation of the manuscript.

**Competing Interests:** The authors have declared that no competing interests exist.

\* Email: xinlizhou11@gmail.com

⑨ These authors contributed equally to this work.

## Introduction

Medullary breast carcinoma (MBC) is one of the invasive breast carcinoma subtypes, which was first precisely defined by Ridolfi et al in 1977 [1]. MBC can be divided into general categories of typical medullary breast carcinoma (TMBC), and atypical medullary breast carcinoma (AMBC) based on the following five criteria: predominantly (>75%) syncytial growth pattern, microscopically completely circumscribed, moderate to marked diffuse mononuclear stromal infiltrate, absence of microglandular features and intraductal components, and moderate or marked nuclear pleomorphism [1]. A diagnosis of TMBC requires that all five of the above criteria are satisfied, while AMBC deviates slightly from TMBC, by requiring that all of the criteria except one (>75% syncytial growth pattern) are satisfied. MBC accounts for <5%of invasive breast cancers, and has a more favorable prognosis than

invasive ductal carcinoma (IDC) [1–6]. However, recent study found that 95% of the MBCs belonged to basal-like phenotype (negative for estrogen receptor (ER), progesterone receptor (PR), and human epidermal growth factor receptor-2 (HER-2)) based on a gene expression analysis [7]. This is interesting, because a previous report stated that a basal-like phenotype is associated with a worse prognosis [1]. Moreover, some studies have reported that the medullary subtype comprises up to 30%~40% of ER and PR positive tumors, as well as ~10% of HER-2 overexpressing tumors [6–13]. These findings are in contrast with the histopathological characteristics of the basal-like phenotype. In the current study, we examined the clinicopathologic characteristics of MBC in a local population, with the goal of further optimizing the treatment decisions made for Chinese patients. To reduce the heterogeneity of the study, we focused only on TMBC patients.

## Materials and Methods

### Ethics

The protocol for this study was approved by the Institutional Review Board of Huashan Hospital, Fudan University. Written informed consent was given by participants for their clinical records to be used in this study. All patient data were anonymized and de-identified in a confidential manner. The information in the data set was used exclusively for the purpose of this study, and was not shared with other individuals or organizations.

### Study Design

We conducted a retrospective review of clinical data obtained from patients diagnosed with TMBC between February 2004 and April 2011 at Huashan Hospital, Fudan University (Shanghai, China). The data inclusion criterion was that the histopathological features of the disease agreed with those described in the 2003 WHO classification for TMBC (consistent with the Ridolfi's criteria) by showing the following features: syncytial architecture in >75% of the tumor mass, a predominant and dense lymphoplasmacytic infiltrate, histological circumscription or pushing margins, high-grade nuclear atypia, and the absence of a glandular or tubular structure [14]. The pathologic changes in a typical case which satisfied these criteria are shown in Figure 1.

### Pathology analysis

ER positive (ER+) and PR positive (PR+) tumors were defined as tumors having >1% of their cells showing the appropriate nuclear staining. Hormonal receptor positive tumor was defined as one showing ER+ and/or PR+ staining, and HER-2 status was evaluated per ASCO/CAP consensus [15]. IHC staining of 3+ (uniform, intense membrane staining of >30% of invasive tumor cells) was considered as HER-2 overexpression/amplification. IHC staining of 0 or 1+ was considered to indicate a lack of HER-2 expression. Molecular subtypes were classified as luminal subtype (ER+ and/or PR+, HER-2 IHC 0~3+), HER-2 overexpressing subtype (ER- and PR-, HER-2 IHC 3+), triple-negative subtype (ER- and PR-, HER-2 IHC 0~1+), or unknown (ER- and PR-, HER-2 IHC 2+), based on guidelines established at the St. Gallen Consensus 2011 [16]. CK5/6 positivity was defined as tumors having >1% of their cells showing the appropriate cytoplasmic and/or membranous staining.

Histopathology and immunohistochemistry results were reviewed by two experienced pathologists. Disagreements were resolved by discussions with a third expert.

### Survival

Cases selected for our review had received follow-up at 3 to 6-month intervals during the first two years, 6 to 12 month intervals during the next three to five years, and annually thereafter. During these follow-up visits, patients received both a clinical examination and an imaging evaluation. Disease-free survival (DFS) was defined as the period between the first surgery and the recurrence of TMBC. Overall survival (OS) was defined as the period between the first surgery and death or last follow-up. The last follow-up for a patient in our study was conducted on July 1, 2013.

### Statistical analysis

Statistical analyses were performed using SPSS Statistics for Windows, Version 17.0. Chicago, IL: SPSS Inc. The inter-rater agreement between two pathologists was analyzed with kappa test. Differences in patient lymph node status, TNM staging, and recurrence rates among the four subtypes of TMBC were analyzed using Fisher's exact test. Differences in patient age and tumor size among the four subtypes were analyzed by Analysis of Variance. P-values for post hoc multiple comparisons were computed by LSD method. The crude survival rate was calculated using the direct method with the following equation:

$$\text{Crude survival rate} = (\text{alive at end of interval}) \div (\text{total cases})$$

## Results

### General information

A total of 117 patients diagnosed with TMBC between February 2004 and April 2011 were enrolled in this study. All patients were female, and the median age was 52 years (range, 28–92 years). The study included a slightly higher proportion of premenopausal (55.6%) than post-menopausal women (44.4%). No patient had ever received hormonal replacement treatment, and none were pregnant or lactating at the time of diagnosis. Seven patients (6.0%) reported a family history of breast cancer. All patients had initially presented with a breast lump, and were admitted after a median period of 15 days (range, 2–1460 days), during which the mass had enlarged in 11 (9.4%) patients. Pain of the mass presented in 25 patients, without correlation with menstrual cycle. Nipple discharge was found in 2 cases. A solitary mass was detected in most of the cases, while one patient presented with 2 lesions in different quadrants of ipsilateral breast; both lesions were later found to be medullary breast carcinoma. There

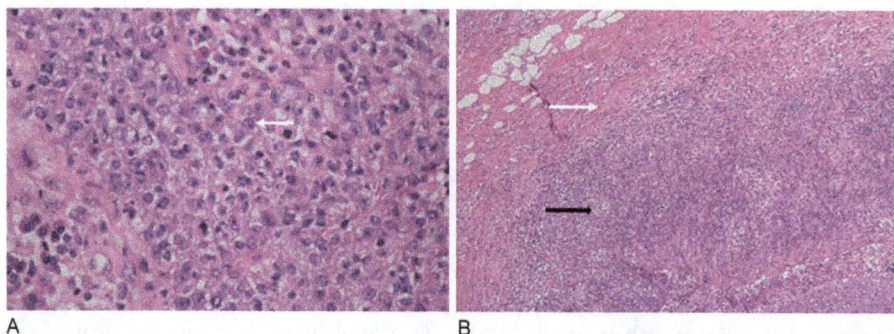

A                                    B

**Figure 1. Histopathological features of TMBC.** (A) Typical syncytial growth pattern of TMBC, with high-grade nuclear atypia (white arrow); ×400. (B) Pushing margin of TMBC (white arrow) and dense lymphoplasmacytic infiltration (black arrow); ×200.

was no difference between bilateral breasts regarding the incidence of carcinoma. One patient presented with bilateral breast cancer, and a final pathology report indicated medullary carcinoma and IDC for each side.

## Pathology

Stage I, II, and III disease accounted for 31.6%, 61.6%, and 6.8% of the cases, respectively, and the median tumor size was 2.5 cm (range, 1–7.0 cm). Thirty-one (26.5%) cases were confirmed with lymph node metastasis, as determined by axillary lymph nodes dissection. Five elderly patients with no lymph node enlargement detected before surgeries were not given axillary lymph node dissection due to their age. ER- diseases were more prevalent in the cohort, accounting for 68.4% of cases. A similar result was found regarding PR status, with 86.3% patients presenting PR- diseases. Immunohistochemistry results showed HER-2 3+ in 24 (20.5%) cases, 2+ in 19 (16.2%) cases, 1+ in 37 (31.6%) cases, and 0 in 37 (31.6%) cases. CK5/6 positivity was 55.7% (29/52) among triple-negative subtypes. The distribution of molecular subtypes is shown in Table 1. The overall concordance between the two pathologists was 96.7%, and almost perfect agreement was achieved in evaluating the molecular subtypes (kappa value of 0.817).

## Treatment arrangement

Modified radical mastectomy dominated over surgical options in the cohort, with 90 (76.9%) patients engaged in this approach. Lumpectomy and radical mastectomy contributed to only 12.8% and 10.3% of the cases, respectively. Chemotherapy regimens were assigned in accordance with NCCN guidelines for IDC treatment. With the exception of seven patients aged >75 years, all patients had received adjuvant chemotherapy. The most often used chemo regimen was a combination of epirubicin, cyclophosphamide and fluorouracil, followed by a combination of epirubicin, cyclophosphamide and paclitaxel/docetaxel. The designated regimens were administered per NCCN guidelines, and adjusted according to individual situations; they were not based on different molecular subtypes. All patients completed 6 cycles chemotherapy without serious side effects. Hormonal therapy for HR positive patients was initiated after adjuvant

chemotherapy had been completed. Patients who presented with a tumor >5 cm and/or a positive lymph node(s), and patients who underwent lumpectomy were given adjuvant radiotherapy within 6 months after surgery. Only four of the 24 patients with HER-2 3+ disease received adjuvant Herceptin therapy, which was given every three weeks. All four patients who underwent target therapy ceased treatment within 3 to 5 months due to financial reasons.

## Follow-up data

With 4 patients lost, the median follow-up time was 56 (range, 2–112) months. One patient died of heart disease 2 months after surgery, and cancer recurred in only 2 other patients, both of whom were triple-negative disease, stage IIA ($T_2N_0M_0$). DFS times for these 2 cases were 98 and 11 months, respectively. The former patient is still alive as of today (111 months survival), while the latter patient died at 24 months after surgery due to disease relapse. A total of 113 patients were followed for >2 years, and that group showed DFS and OS rates of 99.1% and 98.2%, respectively.

## Clinicopathologic presentation of different subtypes

The clinicopathologic characteristics of the different subtypes of TMBC and their prognosis are shown in Table 2. The treatments used for different TMBC subtypes are shown in Table 3. There was no apparent difference in the distribution of subtypes treated with surgery and adjuvant chemotherapy. However, adjuvant radiotherapy was used more often for the management of triple-negative subtype than for HER-2 overexpressing and luminal subtypes. The various TMBC subtypes showed no differences regarding tumor size, rates of lymph node(s) metastasis, TNM staging. However, patients with triple-negative disease were more likely to be younger, when compared to those with luminal disease (P = 0.002).

## Discussion

In this study, we detected a significantly higher rate of ER+ disease (31.6%) in TMBC patients, compared to such rates observed in Western countries. Huober et al [17] reported that only 19% of enrolled patients showed ER+ carcinoma, and a study with 3,348 MBC patients conducted in the USA [18] described

**Table 1.** Distribution of molecular subtypes in TMBC patients.

| Molecular subtypes | ER | PR | HER-2 IHC | Case(s) | Total N (%) |
|---|---|---|---|---|---|
| Luminal | + | + | 0 | 6 | 37(31.6%) |
| | + | + | 1+ | 5 | |
| | + | + | 2+ | 2 | |
| | + | + | 3+ | 3 | |
| | + | − | 0 | 4 | |
| | + | − | 1+ | 7 | |
| | + | − | 2+ | 7 | |
| | + | − | 3+ | 3 | |
| Triple-negative | − | − | 0 | 27 | 52 (44.4%) |
| | − | − | 1+ | 25 | |
| HER-2 overexpression | − | − | 3+ | 18 | 18 (15.4%) |
| Unknown | − | − | 2+ | 10 | 10 (8.5%) |

Abbreviation: TMBC, typical medullary breast cancer; ER, estrogen receptor; PR, progesterone receptor; HER-2 IHC, human epidermal growth factor receptor-2immunohistochemistry.

**Table 2.** Clinicopathologic characteristics of different molecular subtypes in TMBC patients.

| | Luminal (n = 37) | Triple-negative (n = 52) | HER-2 overexpression (n = 18) | Unknown (n = 10) | P |
|---|---|---|---|---|---|
| Age*, years (mean ± S.D.) | 57.11±13.06 | 49.56±10.34 | 53.06±10.77 | 55.50±8.95 | 0.019 |
| Tumor size, cm (mean ± S.D.) | 2.47±0.75 | 2.66±1.12 | 3.00±0.87 | 2.39±1.00 | 0.231 |
| T≤2 cm | 15 (40.5%) | 23 (44.2%) | 5 (27.8%) | 6 (60.0%) | 0.553 |
| 2<T≤5 cm | 22 (59.5%) | 28 (53.8%) | 13 (72.2%) | 4 (40.0%) | |
| T>5 cm | 0 (0.0%) | 1 (1.90%) | 0 (0.0%) | 0 (0.0%) | |
| Lymph node status, n (%) | | | | | 0.557 |
| N0 | 29 (78.4%) | 38 (73.1%) | 14 (77.8%) | 5 (50.0%) | |
| N1 | 6 (16.2%) | 9 (17.3%) | 3 (16.7%) | 4 (40.0%) | |
| N2 | 1 (2.7%) | 4 (7.7%) | 0 (0.0%) | 1 (10.0%) | |
| N3 | 1 (2.7%) | 1 (1.9%) | 1 (5.6%) | 0 (0.0%) | |
| TNM, n (%) | | | | | 0.997 |
| I | 12 (32.4%) | 17 (32.7%) | 5 (27.8%) | 3 (30.0%) | |
| IIA | 17 (45.9%) | 25 (48.1%) | 8 (44.4%) | 6 (60.0%) | |
| IIB | 5 (13.5%) | 7 (13.5%) | 3 (16.7%) | 1 (10.0%) | |
| III | 3 (8.1%) | 3 (5.8%) | 2 (11.1%) | 0 (0.0%) | |
| Recurrence in 2-year, n (%) | 0 (0.0%) | 2 (3.8%) | 0 (0.0%) | 0 (0.0%) | 0.716 |

*Difference exists between subgroups; Luminal vs. Triple-negative, MD (Mean Difference) = 7.55, P = 0.002. Luminal vs. HER-2 overexpression, MD = 4.05, P = 0.212. Luminal vs. Unknown, MD = 1.61, P = 0.689. Triple-negative vs. HER-2 overexpression, MD = −3.50, P = 0.258. Triple-negative vs. Unknown, MD = −5.94, P = 0.129. HER-2 overexpression vs. Unknown, MD = −2.44, P = 0.583.

similar low rates of ER and PR positivity (16.3% and 14%, respectively). Based on the St. Gallen International Expert Consensus of 2011, luminal subtypes should include both luminal A (ER+ and/or PR+, HER-2 +/−, and low Ki-67 index) and luminal B (ER+ and/or PR+, HER-2 +/−, and high Ki-67 index) diseases. In our analysis, luminal subtypes represented 31.6% of the TMBC cases, which was similar to results previously reported in another Chinese cohort (42%) [19]. However, these percentages were significantly higher compared to those reported in other studies, in which the MBCs were mostly triple-negative carcinomas and dominated across all the subtypes [7,20–21]. Therefore, ER status may be one of several factors contributing to the

difference in long-term survival between Eastern and Western women. MBC has been reported as a distinct subgroup of basal breast cancer, with limited myoepithelial differentiation as shown by gene expression analysis [7]. CK5/6 protein is a member of the basal/myoepithelial cytokeratin family, and is frequently detected in triple-negative invasive breast cancer (60%~72% positivity rate) [22–23]. In the current study, however, only 55% of triple-negative breast cancer cases were positive for CK5/6 protein expression. Further studies investigating other basal/myoepithelial cytokeratin proteins such as CK14, CK17, and EGFR are required to address the above difference in TMBC patients. Flucke et al [24] reported that HER-2 overexpression was more

**Table 3.** Treatment of patients with different molecular subtypes of TMBC.

| | Luminal (n = 37) | Triple-negative (n = 52) | HER-2 overexpression (n = 18) | Unknown (n = 10) |
|---|---|---|---|---|
| Surgery | | | | |
| Modified radical mastectomy | 31 (83.8%) | 37 (71.2%) | 14 (77.8%) | 8 (80.0%) |
| Radical mastectomy | 2 (5.4%) | 5 (9.6%) | 3 (16.7%) | 2 (20.0%) |
| Lumpectomy | 4 (10.8%) | 10 (19.2%) | 1 (5.6%) | 0 |
| Adjuvant chemotherapy | | | | |
| Yes | 31 (83.8%) | 52 (100.0%) | 17 (94.4%) | 10 (100.0%) |
| No | 6 (16.2%) | 0 (0%) | 1 (5.6%) | 0 |
| Adjuvant radiotherapy | | | | |
| Yes | 13 (35.1%) | 20 (38.5%) | 3 (16.7%) | 6 (60.0%) |
| No | 24 (64.9%) | 32 (61.5%) | 15 (83.3%) | 4 (40.0%) |
| Hormonal therapy | | | | |
| Yes | 37 (100.0%) | 0 (0.0%) | 0 (0.0%) | 0 (0.0%) |
| No | 0 (0.0%) | 0 (0.0%) | 0 (0.0%) | 0 (0.0%) |

prevalent in MBC than in HR negative high grade IDC (26% vs. 7%). Similarly, disease with HER-2 overexpression represented 15.4% of all TMBC cases in our study cohort, even though some cases (8.5%) had not yet been characterized by FISH. Therefore, we suggest that HER-2 amplification may be a factor contributing to the favorable prognosis of MBC.

The molecular subtype is one of the most important factors impacting the clinical outcome of breast cancer. It has been widely accepted that the triple-negative subtype and HER-2 overexpressing subtype both predict a poor clinical outcome. In this study, patients with triple-negative disease were younger at the time of diagnosis compared to patients with other subtypes. This finding correlates with our previous understanding of triple-negative cancer, and we believe that such patients should benefit from receiving standard chemotherapy and increased surveillance. The TMBC patients in our cohort were clinically managed according to NCCN guidelines for IDC, and no deviations were recommended regarding surgical treatment, adjuvant chemotherapy, hormonal therapy or adjuvant radiotherapy. No apparent difference was found in the distribution of surgery and adjuvant chemotherapy. While on the other hand, the ratio of adjuvant radiotherapy in triple-negative subtype was higher than that in HER-2 overexpressing and luminal subtypes, which may probably due to higher proportion of large tumor (>5 cm), positive lymph nodes and breast conserving therapy in the latter. However, concern still remains for the long-term survival of patients who are treated based on generally accepted guidelines used for invasive cancer, because there is no universally recognized standard of care for TMBC. Xue et al [25] reported that the 2-year DFS rates for triple-negative and HER-2 overexpressing IDC were 79% and 82%, respectively; whereas for our TMBC patients, the 2-year DFS and OS rates were 98.2% and 99.1%, respectively. Our analysis showed a more favorable prognosis for TMBC patients compared to IDC patients during a short follow-up period; however, an analysis over a long-term follow-up period still needs to be completed before general conclusions can be reached. Except for patient age, no significant differences were found regarding the clinicopathologic characteristics of given molecular subtypes, including tumor size, rates of lymph node(s) metastasis, and TNM staging. During the short follow-up period, only two relapses of triple-negative carcinoma were detected; however, it remains to be determined whether variations in molecular subtype

will affect long-term prognosis. In our cohort, the median age of patients upon entry into the study was 52 years, which was similar to the age reported for studies conducted in Europe [16]. Early stage disease was more prevalent among all patients, with 93.2% of the cases being stage I or II cancer, and this finding was similar to that in Reinfuss et al's [26] study. We also found that the probability of lymph node(s) metastasis was <30%, which was similar to results in other studies conducted in Europe and the USA [17–18]. Eisinger et al [27] reported six cases of MBC (19%) among 32 BRCA1-associated breast cancers, compared to only one MBC (0.5%) among 200 patients without a family history of breast cancer. This comparison suggests an important association between TMBC and a previous family history of breast cancer. However, in our cohort, only 6.0% of the TMBC patients had a family history of breast cancer, indicating that the correlation between TMBC and the BRCA1 mutation remains to be determined. In 2012, Chandrika et al [28] reported a case of triple-negative synchronous bilateral medullary carcinoma, and a similar result was found in one of our patients who presented with two synchronous ipsilateral breast lesions which showed triple-negative disease.

Overall, our designated TMBC patients were mostly diagnosed at early stages. Triple-negative disease was prevalent, but not dominant in the cohort, while heterogeneity was commonly presented. Whether or not molecular subtype is the most important factor affecting TMBC patients' prognosis is yet to be determined. Our evidence suggests the possibility of differences among races, and therefore, genetic analysis may be needed for Chinese TMBC patients. The short-term prognosis for patients in our cohort was favorable; nonetheless, the differences among subtypes need to be investigated in studies with a longer duration.

## Acknowledgments

Histopathology and immunohistochemistry results were reviewed by Yun Bao and Zude Xu.

## Author Contributions

Conceived and designed the experiments: ZC HL XL RH QZ JJ XZ. Performed the experiments: ZC HL XL RH QZ JJ XZ. Analyzed the data: ZC HL XL RH QZ JJ XZ. Contributed reagents/materials/analysis tools: ZC HL XL RH QZ JJ XZ. Wrote the paper: ZC HL XL RH QZ JJ XZ.

## References

1. Ridolfi RL, Rosen PP, Port A, Kinne D, Miké V (1977) Medullary carcinoma of the breast: a clinicopathologic study with 10 year follow-up. Cancer 40: 1365–1385.
2. Dendale R, Vincent-Salomon A, Mouret-Fourme E, Savignoni A, Medioni J, et al. (2003) Medullary breast carcinoma: prognostic implications of p53 expression. Int J Biol Markers 18: 99–105.
3. Reinfuss M, Stelmach A, Mitus J, Rys J, Duda K (1995) Typical medullary carcinoma of the breast: a clinical and pathological analysis of 52 cases. J Surg Oncol 60: 89–94.
4. Rakha EA, Putti TC, Abd El-Rehim DM, Paish C, Green AR, et al. (2006) Morphological and immunophenotypic analysis of breast carcinomas with basal and myoepithelial differentiation. J Pathol 208: 495–506.
5. Rapin V, Contesso G, Mouriesse H, Bertin F, Lacombe MJ, et al. (1988) Medullary breast carcinoma. A reevaluation of 95 cases of breast cancer with inflammatory stroma. Cancer 61: 2503–2510.
6. Jensen ML, Kiaer H, Andersen J, Jensen V, Melsen F (1997) Prognostic comparison of three classifications for medullary carcinomas of the breast. Histopathology 30: 523–532.
7. Bertucci F, Finetti P, Cervera N, Charafe-Jauffret E, Mamessier E, et al. (2006) Gene expression profiling shows medullary breast cancer is a subgroup of basal breast cancers. Cancer Res 66: 4636–4344.
8. Rosen PP, Lesser ML, Arroyo CD, Cranor M, Borgen P, et al. (1995) Immunohistochemical detection of HER2/neu in patients with lymph node negative breast cancer. Cancer 75: 1320–1326.
9. Foschini MP, Eusebi V (2009) Rare (new) entities of the breast and medullary carcinoma. Pathology 41: 48–56.
10. Pertschuk LP, Kim DS, Nayer K, Feldman JG, Eisenberg KB, et al. (1990) Immunocytochemical estrogen and progestin receptor assays in breast cancer with monoclonal antibodies. Cancer 66: 1663–1670.
11. Orlando L, Renne G, Rocca A, Curigliano G, Colleoni M, et al. (2005) Are all high grade breast cancers with no steroid receptor hormone expression alike? The special case of the medullary phenotype. Ann Oncol 16: 1094–1099.
12. Pedersen Ll, Zedeler K, Holck S, Schiødt T, Mouridsen HT (1995) Medullary carcinoma of the breast. Prevalence and prognostic importance of classical risk factors in breast cancer. Eur J Cancer 31A: 2289–2295.
13. Martinez SR, Beal SH, Canter RJ, Chen SL, Khatri VP, et al. (2011) Medullary carcinoma of the breast: a population-based perspective. Med Oncol 28: 738–744.
14. Tavassoli FA, Devilee P (2003) WHO classification of tumors. Pathology & genetics, tumours of the breast and female genital organs. IARC Press 2003.
15. Wolff AC, Hammond ME, Schwartz JN, Hagerty KL, Allred DC, et al. (2007) American Society of Clinical Oncology/College of American Pathologists guideline recommendations for human epidermal growth factor receptor 2 testing in breast cancer. J Clin Oncol 25: 118–145.
16. Gnant M, Harbeck N, Thomssen C (2011) St. Gallen 2011: Summary of the Consensus Discussion. Breast Care (Basel) 6: 136–141.
17. Huober J, Gelber S, Goldhirsch A, Coates AS, Viale G, et al. (2012) Prognosis of medullary breast cancer: analysis of 13 International Breast Cancer Study Group (IBCSG) trials. Ann Oncol 23: 2843–2851.

18. Martinez SR, Beal SH, Canter RJ, Chen SL, Khatri VP, et al. (2011) Medullary carcinoma of the breast: a population-based perspective. Med Oncol 28: 738–744.

19. Cao AY, He M, Huang L, Shao ZM, Di GH (2013) Clinicopathologic characteristics at diagnosis and the survival of patients with medullary breast carcinoma in China: a comparison with infiltrating ductal carcinoma-not otherwise specified. World J Surg Oncol 11: 91.

20. Jacquemier J, Padovani L, Rabayrol L, Lakhani SR, Penault-Llorca F, et al. (2005) Typical medullary breast carcinomas have a basal/myoepithelial phenotype. J Pathol 207: 260–268.

21. Vincent-Salomon A, Gruel N, Lucchesi C, MacGrogan G, Dendale R, et al. (2007) Identification of typical medullary breast carcinomas a genomic subgroup of basal-like carcinomas, a heterogeneous new molecular entity. Breast Cancer Res 24: 9.

22. Pintens S1, Neven P, Drijkoningen M, Van Belle V, Moerman P, et al. (2009) Triple negative breast cancer: a study from the point of view of basal CK5/6 and HER-1. J Clin Pathol 62: 624–628.

23. Kanapathy Pillai SK1, Tay A, Nair S, Leong CO (2012) Triple-negative breast cancer is associated with EGFR, CK5/6 and c-KIT expression in Malaysian women. BMC Clin Pathol 12: 18.

24. Flucke U, Flucke MT, Hoy L, Breuer E, Goebbels R, et al. (2010) Distinguishing medullary carcinoma of the breast from high-grade hormone receptor-negative invasive ductal carcinoma: an immunohistochemical approach. Histopathology 56: 852–859.

25. Xue C, Wang X, Peng R, Shi Y, Qin T, et al. (2012) Distribution, clinicopathologic features and survival of breast cancer subtypes in Southern China. Cancer Sci 103: 1679–1687.

26. Reinfuss M, Stelmach A, Mitus J, Rys J, Duda K (1995) Typical medullary carcinoma of the breast: a clinical and pathological analysis of 52 cases. J Surg Oncol 60: 89–94.

27. Eisinger F, Jacquemier J, Charpin C, Stoppa-Lyonnet D, Bressac-de Paillerets B, et al. (1998) Mutations at BRCA1: the medullary breast carcinoma revisited. Cancer Res 58: 1588–1592.

28. Handrika, Permi HS, Kishan Prasad HL, Mohan R, Shetty KJ, et al. (2012) Synchronous bilateral medullary carcinoma of breast: is it metastasis or second primary? J Cancer Res Ther 8: 129–131.

# 24

# Long Noncoding RNAs Expression Patterns Associated with Chemo Response to Cisplatin based Chemotherapy in Lung Squamous Cell Carcinoma Patients

**Zhibo Hou**[1,2], **Chunhua Xu**[1,2], **Haiyan Xie**[1,2], **Huae Xu**[3], **Ping Zhan**[1,2], **Like Yu**[1,2]*, **Xuefeng Fang**[4]*

**1** First Department of Respiratory Medicine, Nanjing Chest Hospital, Medicine School of Southeast University, Nanjing, Jiangsu, China, **2** Clinical Center of Nanjing Respiratory Diseases and Imaging, Nanjing, Jiangsu, China, **3** Department of Pharmacy, The First Affiliated Hospital of Nanjing Medical University, Nanjing, Jiangsu, China, **4** Department of Medical Oncology, Second Affiliated Hospital, Zhejiang University College of Medicine, Hangzhou, Zhejiang, China

## Abstract

*Background:* There is large variability among lung squamous cell carcinoma patients in response to treatment with cisplatin based chemotherapy. LncRNA is potentially a new type of predictive marker that can identify subgroups of patients who benefit from chemotherapy and it will have great value for treatment guidance.

*Methods:* Differentially expressed lncRNAs and mRNA were identified using microarray profiling of tumors with partial response (PR) vs. with progressive disease (PD) from advanced lung squamous cell carcinoma patients treated with cisplatin based chemotherapy and validated by quantitative real-time PCR (qPCR). Furthermore, the expression of AC006050.3-003 was assessed in another 60 tumor samples.

*Results:* Compared with the PD samples, 953 lncRNAs were consistently upregulated and 749 lncRNAs were downregulated consistently among the differentially expressed lncRNAs in PR samples (Fold Change≥2.0-fold, $p <0.05$). Pathway analyses showed that some classical pathways, including "Nucleotide excision repair," that participated in cisplatin chemo response were differentially expressed between PR and PD samples. Coding-non-coding gene co-expression network identified many lncRNAs, such as lncRNA AC006050.3-003, that potentially played a key role in chemo response. The expression of lncRNA AC006050.3-003 was significantly lower in PR samples compared to the PD samples in another 60 lung squamous cell carcinoma patients. Receiver operating characteristic curve analysis revealed that lncRNA AC006050.3-003 was a valuable biomarker for differentiating PR patients from PD patients with an area under the curve of 0.887 (95% confidence interval 0.779, 0.954).

*Conclusions:* LncRNAs seem to be involved in cisplatin-based chemo response and may serve as biomarkers for treatment response and candidates for therapy targets in lung squamous cell carcinoma.

**Editor:** Vinod Scaria, CSIR Institute of Genomics and Integrative Biology, India

**Funding:** This study was supported by the National Natural Science Foundation of China (No. 81101580), the Major Project of Nanjing Medical Science and Technique Development Fund (No. ZDX12013), the General Project of Nanjing Medical Science and Technology Development Fund (No. YKK13090) and Young Professional Personnel Training Fund of Nanjing Chest Hospital. The funders had no role in study design, data collection and analysis, decision to publish, or preparation of the manuscript.

**Competing Interests:** The authors have declared that no competing interests exist.

* Email: likeyunj@yeah.net (LY); xffang@zju.edu.cn (XF)

## Background

Lung cancer is a leading cause of cancer-related deaths worldwide, with non-small cell lung cancer (NSCLC) accounts for approximately 85% of all cases [1]. Most NSCLC patients are diagnosed at an advanced stage and have a 5-year survival rate of less than 20% [1]. Squamous cell carcinoma (SCC) is the second most common type of lung cancer, accounting for over 30% of NSCLC [2]. Encouraging new targeted agents have afforded benefits to lung adenocarcinoma (ADC) patients. Unfortunately, targeted agents developed for lung ADC are largely ineffective against lung SCC. Currently, the standard treatment for lung SCC remains a doublet of cisplatin plus one of the new agents other than pemetrexed [3–5]. However, there is large variability among individuals in response to treatment with cisplatin based chemotherapy [6,7]. This highlights the importance of exploring new biomarkers that can predict cisplatin-based treatment efficacy for lung SCC.

Human genome is comprised of ~1.2% protein coding genes and that ~90% of the genome is transcribed as non-coding RNA (ncRNA)[8]. The ncRNAs can be divided into two major classes: small noncoding RNAs (<200 bp), such as microRNA, and long noncoding RNAs (lncRNAs;>200 bp) according to their transcript size. lncRNAs can be classified into exonic lncRNAs, intronic lncRNAs, intergenic lncRNAs (also known as large intergenic non-coding RNAs, lincRNAs) and overlapping lncRNAs in accordance with their location relative to the protein-coding transcripts[9]. LncRNAs have been implicated in carcinogenesis and cancer progression [10–15]. lncRNAs can act as tumor oncogenes or tumor suppressors just like protein coding genes or miRNA.

Recent studies suggest that lncRNAs also play a significant role in chemotherapy sensitivity and some lncRNAs has now been associated with chemotherapy sensitivity phenotypes in cancer. The lnRNA H19 gene could induce P-glycoprotein expression and MDR1-associated drug resistance in liver cancer cells through regulation of MDR1 promoter methylation [16]. LncRNAs are differently expressed between lung ADC A549 and A549/CDDP cells, many of which could regulate cisplatin resistance through different mechanisms. LnRNAAK126698 was found to confer cisplatin resistance by targeting the Wnt pathway [17]. LncRNA HOTAIR was observed to be significantly downregulated in cisplatin-responding lung ADC tissues and contributes to cisplatin resistance of lung ADC cells via regualtion of $p21^{WAF1/CIP1}$ expression [18].

Owing to its possible effect on cisplatin resistance, we anticipated whether lncRNAs might influence tumor response to cisplatin based chemotherapy in lung SCC. The identification of lncRNAs that predict either sensitivity or resistance to cisplatin based chemotherapy is of great importance to individualized treatment of lung SCC.

In this study, we profiled lncRNA and mRNA expression in lung SCC patients having either partial response or progressive disease after cisplatin based chemotherapy. An integrative analysis combining lncRNA and mRNA changes within co-expression networks was performed to explore genes that may be related to cisplatin sensitivity in lung SCC. Several of different expressions of lncRNAs and mRNA were further validated by quantitative real-time PCR (qPCR) in lung SCC tissue samples. lncRNAs expression profiles may provide new molecular biomarkers for predicting responding to cisplatin based chemotherapy of lung SCC.

## Methods

### Patient Samples

All collected snap-frozen tissue samples used in this study were obtained by biopsy through bronchoscope or percutaneous lung biopsy under computerized tomography scan from primary sites of advanced stage lung SCC patients at Nanjing Chest Hospital and Second Affiliated Hospital of Zhejiang University College of Medicine during January 2009 and January 2013. All patients were histopathologically diagnosed by at least two independent senior pathologists. All of the tumors were unresectable and no patient underwent radiotherapy or chemotherapy prior to biopsy. Front-line chemotherapy comprised cisplatin 75 mg/m² on days 1, and gemcitabine 1000 mg/m² on days 1, 8, or docetaxel 75 mg/m2 on days 1 every 21 days for a maximum of 4 cycles. Response to therapy was defined by thoracic computerized tomography scan according to Response Evaluation Criteria In Solid Tumors (RECIST 1.1) [19]. Objective tumor response for target lesions are classed as: complete Response (CR), partial response (PR), progressive disease (PD), and stable disease (SD). In this study, PR was considered as sensitive and PD was considered as resistant. Tissue samples were obtained after patients' written informed consent under a general tissue collection protocol

approved by The Research Ethics Committee of the Nanjing Chest Hospital and The Research Ethics Committee of Second Affiliated Hospital of Zhejiang University College of Medicine.

### LncRNA microarray and Computational Analysis

**Samples.** Total RNA was extracted with TRIzol reagent (Invitrogen, Carlsbad, CA, USA) according to the manufacturer's protocol. RNA quantity and quality were measured by NanoDrop ND-1000 spectrophotometer (PeqLab, Erlangen, Germany). Total RNA integrity was assessed by Agilent 2100 Bioanalyzer (Agilent Technologies, Santa Clara, USA).

**RNA microarray.** The Arraystar Human LncRNA Array v3.0 (Arraystar, Rockville, MD) was designed for profiling both lncRNAs and protein-coding RNAs in human genome. 33,045 lncRNAs were collected from the authoritative data sources including RefSeq, UCSC Knowngenes, Ensembl and many related literatures.

### RNA labeling and array hybridization

Sample labeling and array hybridization were performed according to the Agilent One-Color Microarray-Based Gene Expression Analysis protocol (Agilent Technologies, Santa Clara, USA) with minor modifications. Briefly, mRNA was purified from total RNA after removal of rRNA using mRNA-ONLY Eukaryotic mRNA Isolation Kit (Epicentre Biotechnologies, Madison, Wisconsin, USA). Then, each sample was amplified and transcribed into fluorescent cRNA along the entire length of the transcripts without 3′ bias utilizing a random priming method. The labeled cRNAs were purified by RNeasy Mini Kit (Qiagen, Inc., Valencia, CA). The concentration and specific activity of the labeled cRNAs (pmol Cy3/μg cRNA) were measured by NanoDrop ND-1000. 1 μg of each labeled cRNA was fragmented by adding 5 μl 10 × Blocking Agent and 1 μl of 25 × Fragmentation Buffer, then heated the mixture at 60°C for 30 min, finally 25 μl 2 × GE Hybridization buffer was added to dilute the labeled cRNA. 50 μl of hybridization solution was dispensed into the gasket slide and assembled to the LncRNA expression microarray slide. The slides were incubated for 17 hours at 65°C in an Agilent Hybridization Oven. The hybridized arrays were washed, fixed and scanned with using the Agilent DNA Microarray Scanner (part number G2505C).

**Data analysis.** Agilent Feature Extraction software (version 11.0.1.1) was used to analyze acquired array images. Quantile normalization and subsequent data processing were performed with using the GeneSpring GX v11.5.1 software package (Agilent Technologies, Santa Clara, USA). After quantile normalization of the raw data, lncRNAs and mRNAs that at least 10 out of 10 samples have flags in Present or Marginal ("All Targets Value") were chosen for further data analysis. Differentially expressed lncRNAs and mRNAs with statistical significance between the two groups were identified through Volcano Plot filtering. Log fold-change means log2 value of absolute fold-change. Fold-change and $p$ value are calculated from the normalized expression. Hierarchical Clustering was performed using the Agilent GeneSpring GX software (version 11.5.1). The microarray data have been deposited in National Center for Biotechnology Information (NCBI) Gene Expression Omnibus (GEO) database and are accessible through GEO series accession number GSE59245 (http://www.ncbi.nlm.nih.gov/geo/query/acc.cgi?acc=GSE59245).

### qPCR

The expression of lncRNA or mRNA was detected by qPCR. The primers are listed as Table S1. β-actin was used as an internal control. The primers for β-actin were as follows: the forward primer 5′-AGCGAGCATCCCCCAAAGTT-3′ and the reverse primer 5′-GGGCACGAAGGCTCATCATT-3′. qPCR was performed using the SYBR Green (TaKaRa Bio Inc., Dalian, China) dye detection method on ABI PlusOne PCR instrument under default conditions: 95°C for 10 sec, and 40 cycles of 95°C for 5 s and 55°C for 31 S. Relative gene expression levels were analyzed by the $2^{-\Delta Ct}$ method, where $\Delta Ct = Ct_{target} - Ct_{\beta-actin}$ [20].

## Functional group analysis

Base on the latest KEGG (Kyoto Encyclopedia of Genes and Genomes) database (http://www.genome.jp/kegg/), we provide pathway analysis for differentially expressed mRNAs. This analysis allows us to determine the biological pathway that there is a significant enrichment of differentially expressed mRNAs. The $p$-value (EASE-score, Fisher-$P$ value or Hypergeometric-$P$ value) denotes the significance of the Pathway correlated to the conditions. The recommend $p$-value cut-off is 0.05.

## Construction of the Coding-non-coding Gene Co-expression Network

Gene co-expression network was constructed according to the specific expression lncRNAs and mRNAs [21]. The median gene expression value was used to represent the expression of the same coding gene with different transcripts. The primary lncRNA expression value was adopted with no particular processing. To normalize signal intensity of specific expression genes, we remove the subset of data that shown the differential expression of lncRNA and mRNA according to the primary lists from the microarray results. Pearson correlation coefficient (PCC) was calculated and the R value was used to compute the correlation coefficient of the PCC between lncRNAs and coding genes. LncRNAs and mRNAs with Pearson correlation coefficients not less than 0.99 were selected as significant correlation pairs to draw the co-expression network using Cytoscape. In the network, a regular hexagon node represents lncRNA, circular node represents the coding gene. A brown node represents an over-regulated lncRNA or mRNA and a blue node represents an under-regulated lncRNA or mRNA. The solid lines indicate a positive correlation and the dashed line indicates a negative correlation.

## Statistical Analysis

The GraphPad Prism 6.0 (GraphPad Software, LaJolla, CA) was used for statistical analysis. Data are expressed as the means ± SD. For a single comparison of 2 groups, Student's t test was used. Differences were considered statistically significant at $P<0.05$. A receiver operating characteristic (ROC) curve was performed by MedCalc software (version 11.4; Broekstraat, Mariakerke, Belgium).

## Results

### Differentially expressed lncRNAs

We profiled the expression of lncRNAs in tumors from patients with advanced SCC subsequently treated with cisplatin based chemotherapy. Five patients experienced PR and five patients experienced PD according to the RECIST criteria. The basic information of the ten patients was shown in Table S2. The expression profiles of lncRNAs in two groups were shown by calculating log fold change PR/PD, positive value indicates upregulation and negative value indicates downregulation. Differentially expressed lncRNAs with statistical significance were identified by a Volcano Plot filtering between PR and PD groups (Fold Change cut-off: 2.0, $P$-value<0.05). Compared with the PD samples, 953 lncRNAs were consistently upregulated, and 749

lncRNAs were downregulated consistently among the differentially expressed lncRNAs in PR samples. Hierarchical clustering analysis was used to arrange samples into groups based on their expression levels (Figure 1A). The expression levels of the 20 top ranked lncRNAs in the different samples (PR vs. PD) are listed in Table 1.

## LncRNA Classification and Subgroup Analysis

**Enhancer lncRNAs profiling.** LncRNAs with enhancer-like function are identified using GENCODE annotation of the human genes [22], [23]. The consideration of selection of lncRNAs with enhancer-like function exclude transcripts mapping to the exons and introns of annotated protein coding genes, the natural antisense transcripts, overlapping the protein coding genes and all known transcripts. Fifty-one differentially expressed enhancer-like lncRNAs and their nearby coding genes (distance, 300 kb) were showed in Table S3.

**HOX cluster profiling.** In current study, the profiling data of all probes targeting 407 discrete transcribed regions in the four human HOX loci for both lncRNAs and coding transcripts was presented in the Table S4[24]. These data suggested that 30 coding transcripts could be detected in SCC tissues with 17 of them differentially expressed. Then, about 34 lncRNAs transcribed were detected in SCC tissues and 18 of them were found differently expressed in human HOX loci.

**LincRNAs profiling.** lincRNAs are a subtype of lncRNAs, which are transcribed from intergenic regions [2]. Previous studies found that lincRNAs could regulate the expression of neighbouring genes and distant genomic sequences, thus play key roles in certain biological processes [25,26]. All probes for lincRNAs in microarray were calculated by genomic coordinates [13,27]. 405 differentially expressed lincRNAs and nearby coding gene pairs (distance <300 kb) between PR and PD groups were showed in Table S5.

## Differentially expressed mRNAs

From the mRNA expression profiling data, a total of 16,851 mRNAs were identified in the samples through microarray analysis. Compared with PD group, 1223 mRNAs were consistently upregulated, and 1947 mRNAs were consistently downregulated in PR group. The expression levels of the 20 top ranked mRNAs in the different samples (PR vs. PD) are listed in Table 2. The Hierarchical clustering analysis indicated the relationships among the mRNA expression patterns that were present in the samples (Figure 1B).

## Validation of the microarray data using qPCR

Five lncRNAs (ENST00000584612, ENST00000579363, NR_038200, ENST00000466677 and ENST00000562112) and five mRNAs (NM_020299, ENST00000171111, NM_001098517, NM_001306 and NM_001904) were randomly selected to validate the microarray consistency by using qPCR. The results demonstrated that lncRNA ENST00000584612 and ENST00000579363 were downregulated and that NR_038200, ENST00000466677 and ENST00000562112 were upregulated in the PR samples compared with PD samples (Figure 2A). For mRNA, NM_020299 and ENST00000171111 were downregulated and that NM_001098517, NM_001306 and NM_001904 were upregulated in the PR samples compared with PD samples (Figure 2B). These above qPCR results are consistent with microarray data.

## Pathway analysis

Pathway analysis indicated that 32 pathways corresponded to underregulated transcripts in PR group. Among the 32 pathways,

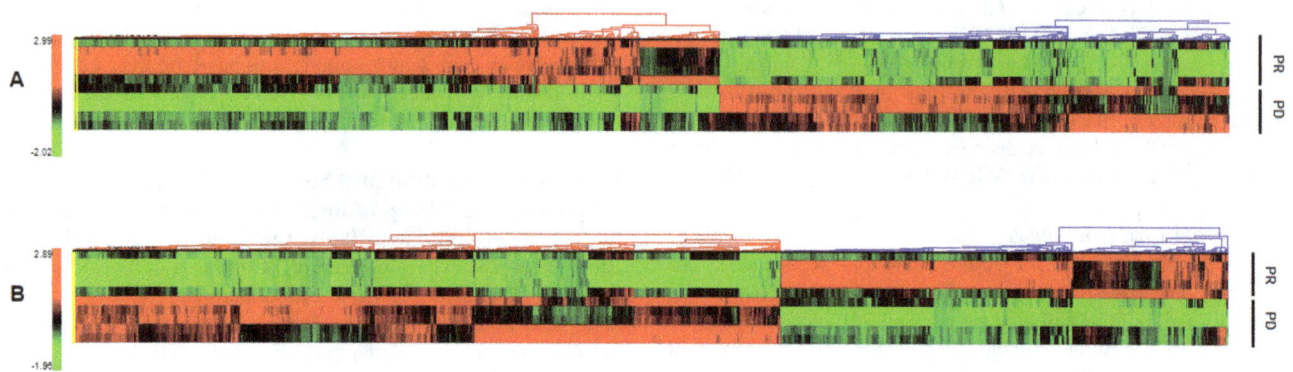

**Figure 1. Heatmaps of lncRNA and mRNA expression patterns.** RNA expression is depicted according to treatment response. (A) Hierarchical Clustering for "Differentially expressed lncRNAs". (B) Hierarchical Clustering for "Differentially expressed mRNAs". "Red" indicates high relative expression, and "green" indicates low relative expression.

we found that several enriched networks including "Nucleotide excision repair", "Glutathione metabolism", "Drug metabolism-cytochrome P450", "Metabolism of xenobiotics by cytochrome P450", "Drug metabolism-other enzymes" and "Calcium signaling pathway" were associated with chemotherapeutic drugs metabolism (Figure 3A). Of note, "Nucleotide excision repair" has been reported intensively to be correlated with cisplatin sensitivity (Figure 3B) [28,29]. Furthermore, Pathway analysis showed that 15 pathways corresponded to upregulated transcripts in PD group. One of these pathways, the gene category "Calcium signaling pathway", has been reported to be involved in the cisplatin resistance [30,31] (Figure 3A).

### Co-expression network

Coding-non-coding gene co-expression network analysis was undertaken to explore which gene played a critical role in cisplatin resistance. The more important role the gene played, the more central the gene is within the network. Co-expression network was constructed to cluster lncRNAs and coding mRNAs into phenotypically relevant modules based on the correlation analysis between the differential expressed lncRNAs and mRNAs (Figure 4). Among this co-expression network, 49 lncRNAs and 186 mRNAs composed the CNC network node. Two hundred and thirty-five network nodes made associated 1063 network pairs (700 positive correlations and 363 negative correlations) of co-expression lncRNAs and mRNAs. The results indicated that many lncRNAs such as AC006050.3, NAPSB, KRT16P2, XLOC_005280 and MI0000285 potentially play important role in the network. AC006050.3 has 3 transcripts, such as AC006050.3-001, AC006050.3-002, and AC006050.3-003. All the 3 transcripts are downregulated in PR group compared to PD group (Table 1). With co-expression network, lncRNA AC006050.3-003 (ENST00000578693) expression level correlated with many members of the NER pathway such as DDB2, POLE2 and MNAT1 (Table S6). LncRNA AC006050.3-003 might play key role in cisplatin chemo response and was selected for further study.

### Potential predictor values of AC006050.3-003

The expression of lncRNA AC006050.3-003 was next detected by qPCR in the other 60 lung SCC patients received cisplatin based chemotherapy (Figure 5A). The expression of lncRNA AC006050.3-003 was significantly lower in PR samples compared with the PD samples. These results indicated that lncRNA

AC006050.3-003 was aberrantly expressed between PC and PD patients. We next performed an analysis to identify whether lncRNA AC006050.3-003 expression could predict the effect of cisplatin chemo response. As shown in Figure 5B, ROC curve analysis revealed that lncRNA AC006050.3-003 was a valuable biomarker for differentiating PR patients from PD patients with an area under the curve (AUC) of 0.887 (95% confidence interval 0.779, 0.954). These results suggested that lower expression of lncRNA AC006050.3-003 might correlate with sensitivity to chemotherapy in lung SCC patients.

### Discussion

In the present study, we performed lncRNA expression profiling of tumor samples from patients with advanced lung SCC that showed PR or PD, following cisplatin based chemotherapy. The lncRNA profiling identified a set of differentially expressed lncRNAs that were correlated with chemotherapy response. There are 953 upregulated lncRNAs and 749 downregulated lncRNAs that were significantly differentially expressed ($\geq$2.0-fold) in PR group compared to PD group.

The qPCR results validate that expression of lncRNAs are consistent with the data of microarray. There was distinctive expression of lncRNAs between PR and PD samples. It was likely to provide potential way to distinguish PR group from PD group and provide new biomarkers to predict cisplatin sensitivity for lung SCC individualized treatment. The differentially expressed lncRNAs and nearby coding gene pairs identified here may provide novel path for better understanding of the molecular basis of cisplatin resistance in lung SCC.

The lncRNA expression microarray used in this study included five subgroups: Enhancer lncRNAs, Rinn lincRNAs, HOX cluster, lincRNAs nearby coding gene, and Enhancer lncRNAs nearby coding gene. HOX lncRNAs and the lncRNAs with enhancer-like function are two special subgroups of lncRNAs. Previous studies have shown that there is deregulation of HOX gene expression in various of cancers including lung cancer [32,33]. HOX lncRNAs are intergenic and are transcribed in the direction opposite to the HOX genes [34,35]. Many studies have reported that HOX lncRNAs are implicated in transcriptional regulation of neighboring *HOX* genes and found to involve in the occurrence and development of cancers [10,14,36,37]. For example, HOTAIR (Hox transcript antisense intergenic RNA) is significantly upregulated in NSCLC tissues, and involves in NSCLC cell proliferation and metastasis, partially via the

**Table 1.** Deregulated lncRNAs detected using microarray in 5 PR and 5 PD lung SCC patients.

| Down-regulated in PR group | | | | | Up-regulated in PR group | | | | |
|---|---|---|---|---|---|---|---|---|---|
| Genbank accession | Gene Symbol | P-value | Fold change* | FDR | Genbank accession | GeneSymbol | P-value | Fold change* | FDR |
| ENST00000583748 | AC022596.6 | 1.19E-05 | 122.41 | 0.0012 | NR_026892 | AFAP1-AS1 | 0.0001 | 142.91 | 0.0047 |
| ENST00000425692 | AC022596.6 | 4.85E-06 | 58.58 | 0.0007 | ENST00000566942 | RP11-284N8.3 | 0.0001 | 45.79 | 0.0047 |
| ENST00000584612 | KRT16P2 | 0.0043 | 56.25 | 0.0384 | ENST00000562112 | NAPSB | 0.0062 | 32.73 | 0.0458 |
| ENST00000581210 | KRT16P1 | 0.0014 | 48.55 | 0.0200 | ENST00000567369 | CTA-363E6.2 | 5.29E-07 | 19.47 | 0.0002 |
| ENST00000579062 | KRT16P2 | 0.0042 | 48.47 | 0.0381 | ENST00000579713 | RP11-403A21.2 | 2.95E-07 | 15.47 | 0.0002 |
| ENST00000395675 | FOXO3B | 0.0002 | 39.05 | 0.0056 | ENST00000565118 | ABCC6P1 | 0.0002 | 14.60 | 0.0069 |
| ENST00000446115 | RP11-439L18.3 | 0.0006 | 36.97 | 0.0121 | ENST00000450920 | SRGAP3-AS2 | 0.0040 | 13.80 | 0.0368 |
| NR_024538 | GSTM4 | 0.0003 | 29.87 | 0.0072 | TCONS_00003617 | XLOC_001406 | 0.0075 | 13.72 | 0.0509 |
| ENST00000458343 | KRT42P | 0.0015 | 29.45 | 0.0207 | ENST00000433329 | HBBP1 | 0.0006 | 12.58 | 0.0125 |
| ENST00000555300 | RP11-104E19.1 | 7.8E-07 | 28.86 | 0.0003 | uc010jub.1 | AK293020 | 0.0001 | 11.98 | 0.0044 |
| ENST00000583364 | AC015818.3 | 1.91E-07 | 28.54 | 0.0002 | ENST00000562490 | RP11-102F4.3 | 2.32E-07 | 10.89 | 0.0002 |
| ENST00000578693 | AC006050.3 | 0.0007 | 24.61 | 0.0130 | ENST00000564038 | RP11-1223D19.1 | 0.0002 | 10.67 | 0.0066 |
| ENST00000412143 | PSORS1C3 | 0.0003 | 24.57 | 0.0085 | hsa-mir-940 | MI0005762 | 0.0006 | 9.71 | 0.0115 |
| ENST00000326333 | KRT17P2 | 0.0006 | 24.09 | 0.0119 | ENST00000466677 | RP4-555L14.5 | 0.0028 | 9.27 | 0.0293 |
| ENST00000579363 | AC022596.2 | 0.0014 | 23.44 | 0.0195 | NR_024344 | LOC283174 | 0.0022 | 8.40 | 0.0261 |
| ENST00000420566 | AC006050.3 | 0.0020 | 23.12 | 0.0243 | NR_038386 | LOC728537 | 0.0001 | 7.59 | 0.0042 |
| ENST00000554221 | LINC00520 | 0.0018 | 22.79 | 0.0231 | uc022cjh.1 | IGL@ | 0.0019 | 7.11 | 0.0235 |
| ENST00000560054 | RP11-499F3.2 | 0.0056 | 22.71 | 0.0439 | uc001lku.1 | AK125699 | 3.12E-06 | 7.09 | 0.0006 |
| ENST00000577817 | AC006050.3 | 0.0011 | 21.01 | 0.0173 | NR_038200 | M1 | 0.0056 | 6.94 | 0.0440 |
| ENST00000584833 | AL353997.3 | 0.0016 | 20.29 | 0.0211 | ENST00000570700 | RP11-473M20.11 | 0.0034 | 6.86 | 0.0335 |

*Log2 (PR/PD).

**Table 2.** Deregulated mRNAs detected using microarray in 5 PR and 5 PD lung SCC patients.

| Down-regulated in PR group | | | | | Up-regulated in PR group | | | | |
|---|---|---|---|---|---|---|---|---|---|
| Genbank accession | Gene Symbol | P-value | Fold change* | FDR | Genbank accession | GeneSymbol | P-value | Fold change* | FDR |
| NM_207392 | KRTDAP | 5.97E-08 | 210.97 | 5.92E-05 | ENST0000304749 | CST1 | 0.0038 | 31.22 | 0.0244 |
| NM_003125 | SPRR1B | 9.72E-05 | 138.34 | 0.0027 | NM_001145077 | LRRC10B | 0.012 | 23.30 | 0.0480 |
| ENST00000368750 | SPRR2E | 0.0045 | 127.54 | 0.0273 | NM_001904 | CTNNB1 | 2.11E-05 | 20.46 | 0.0012 |
| ENST00000360379 | SPRR2D | 3.50E-05 | 104.87 | 0.0015 | NM_001008219 | AMY1C | 0.0041 | 19.80 | 0.0255 |
| NM_005988 | SPRR2A | 0.0051 | 93.73 | 0.0290 | NM_178452 | DNAAF1 | 0.011 | 19.07 | 0.0453 |
| NM_020299 | AKR1B10 | 0.0017 | 90.00 | 0.0149 | NM_025244 | TSGA10 | 0.0038 | 17.99 | 0.0246 |
| ENST00000368789 | LCE3E | 3.93E-05 | 86.40 | 0.0016 | NM_000699 | AMY2A | 0.0065 | 17.67 | 0.0335 |
| NM_001017418 | SPRR2B | 0.00098 | 85.02 | 0.0109 | ENST0000305904 | DYNLRB2 | 0.0099 | 17.31 | 0.0429 |
| NM_001080538 | AKR1B15 | 0.0230 | 84.25 | 0.0230 | NM_001306 | CLDN3 | 0.0072 | 16.82 | 0.0354 |
| NM_032330 | CAPNS2 | 0.0066 | 69.87 | 0.0338 | NM_001008218 | AMY1B | 0.0065 | 15.94 | 0.0335 |
| NM_182502 | TMPRSS11B | 4.28E-06 | 66.42 | 0.0005 | NM_147169 | C9orf24 | 0.012 | 15.79 | 0.0473 |
| NM_001014450 | SPRR2F | 0.0016 | 64.79 | 0.0148 | ENST0000379133 | C9orf24 | 0.011 | 15.57 | 0.0447 |
| ENST00000171111 | KEAP1 | 0.0027 | 59.87 | 0.0199 | NM_024687 | ZBBX | 0.0078 | 15.52 | 0.0371 |
| NM_002638 | PI3 | 0.0015 | 56.93 | 0.0141 | NM_152784 | CATSPERD | 0.0013 | 15.40 | 0.0128 |
| NM_012397 | SERPINB13 | 0.00059 | 50.69 | 0.0080 | NM_173554 | C10orf107 | 0.0075 | 15.16 | 0.0365 |
| NM_005218 | DEFB1 | 5.29E-07 | 47.29 | 0.0001 | NM_015668 | RGS22 | 0.0064 | 14.08 | 0.0332 |
| ENST00000368733 | S100A8 | 5.95E-05 | 46.06 | 0.0021 | NM_001935 | DPP4 | 0.0020 | 13.52 | 0.0168 |
| NM_000526 | KRT14 | 2.91E-07 | 42.90 | 0.0001 | NM_001098517 | CADM1 | 0.0004 | 13.04 | 0.0062 |
| NM_004988 | MAGEA1 | 7.86E-07 | 38.92 | 0.0002 | NM_000900 | MGP | 0.0002 | 10.71 | 0.0041 |
| NM_002639 | SERPINB5 | 0.0082 | 37.14 | 0.0385 | ENST0000288710 | CCDC164 | 0.0111 | 10.47 | 0.046 |

*Log2 (PR/PD).

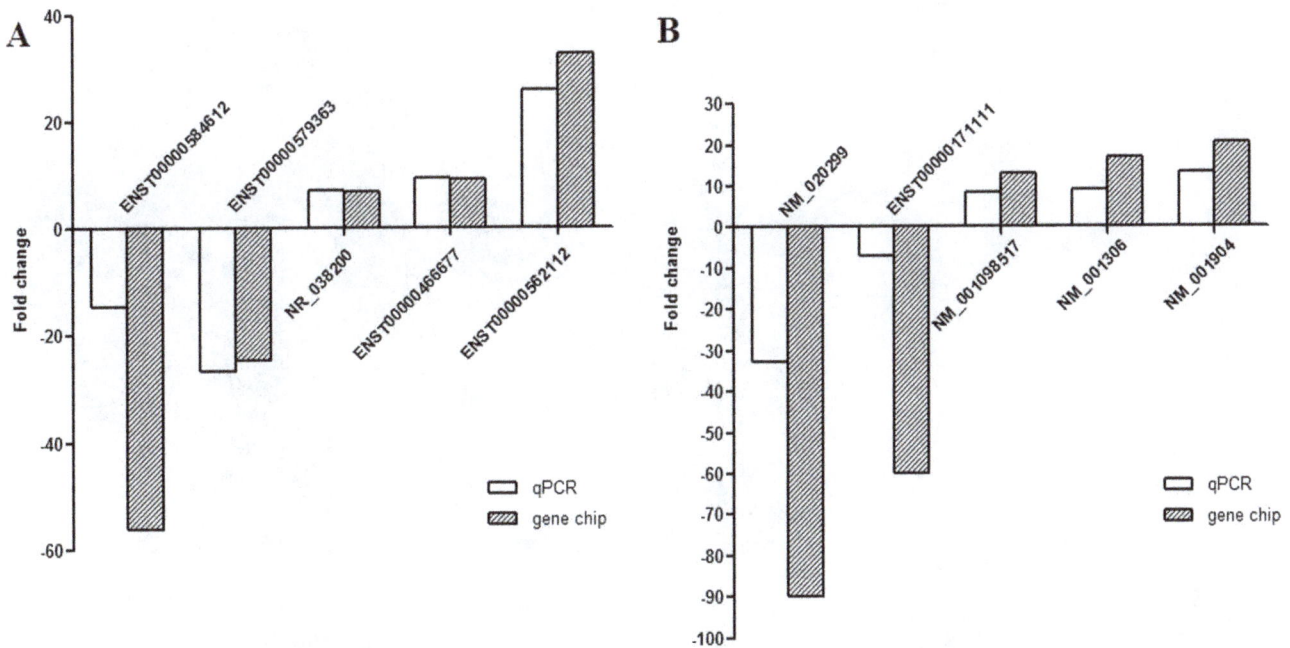

**Figure 2. Validation of microarray data by qPCR.** The differential expression of 5 lncRNAs (A) or 5 mRNAs (B) in samples of 10 patients by microarray was validated by qPCR. The relative expression level in PR samples was normalized by the PD samples. The heights of the columns in the chart represent the median fold changes (PR/PD) in expression across the patients for each of the validated lncRNAs or mRNAs. Fold changes were calculated by the $2^{-\Delta Ct}$ method. Fold changes $= \text{mean} 2^{-\Delta Ct}$ (PR)/$\text{mean} 2^{-\Delta Ct}$ (PD), where $\Delta Ct = Ct_{target} - Ct_{\beta-actin}$.

downregulation of HOXA5 [12,38]. In current study, we showed that both lncRNAs and coding transcripts transcribed of HOX loci were differentially expressed between PC and PD samples. These data suggested that differentially expressed coding tran-

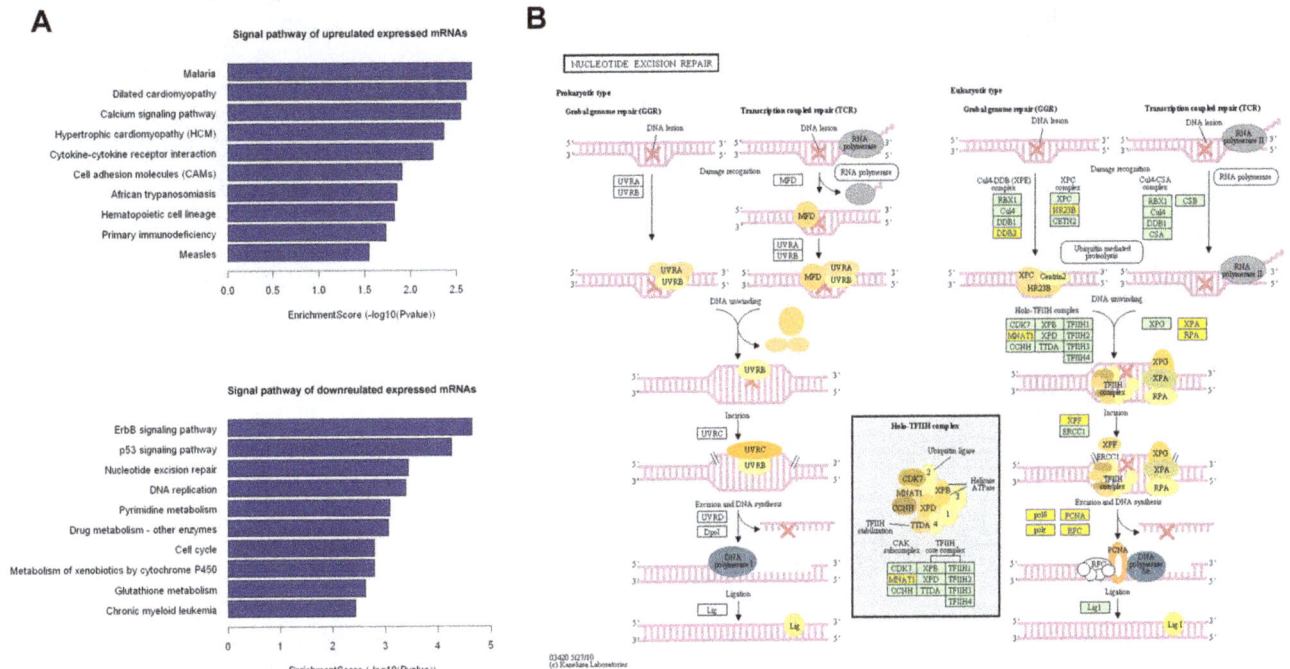

**Figure 3. Pathway analysis of the differentially expressed mRNAs.** (A) Signaling pathways of upregulated mRNAs and downregulated mRNAs. The bar plot shows the top ten Enrichment score (−log10 (P-value)) value of the significant enrichment pathway. (B) The "Nucleotide excision repair" signal pathway shows modulation in repair of nonspecific DNA damage and is associated with cisplatin sensitivity. Yellow marked nodes are associated with downregulated genes, orange marked nodes are associated with upregulated or only whole dataset genes, and green nodes have no significance.

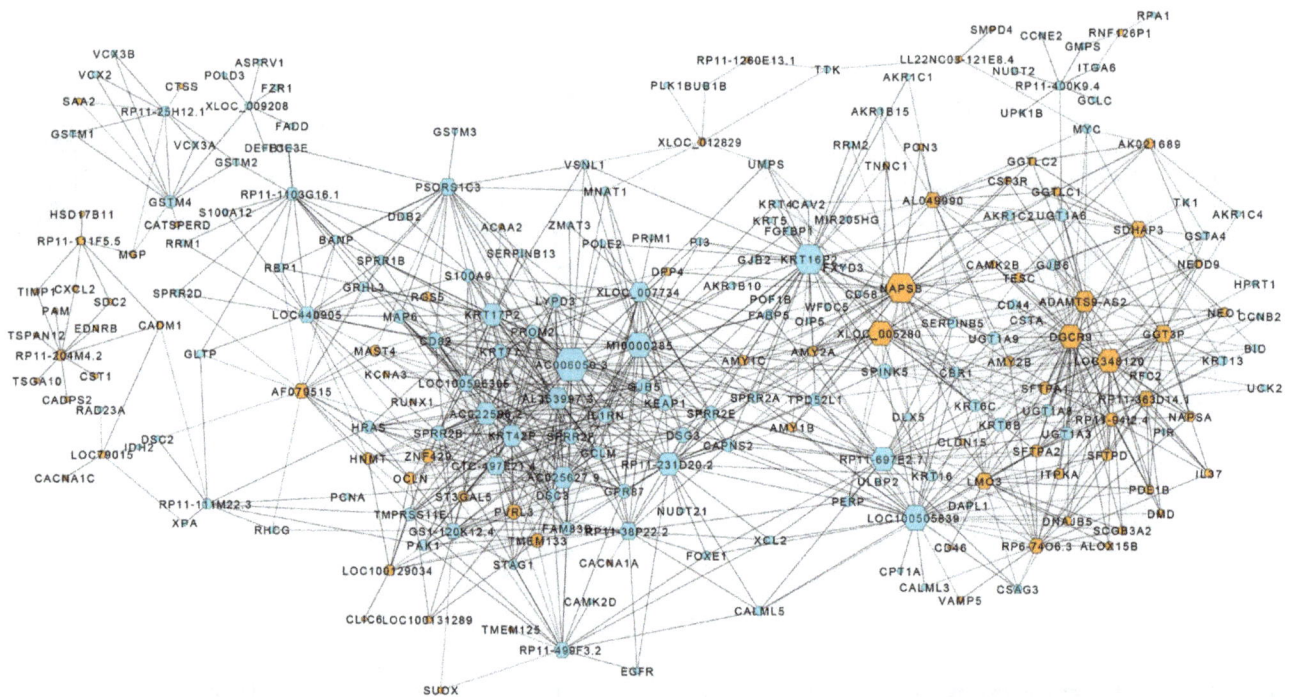

**Figure 4. LncRNA-mRNA-network was constructed based on the correlation analysis between the differential expressed lncRNAs and mRNAs.** In the network, a regular hexagon node represents lncRNA, circular node represents the mRNA. A brown node represents an upregulated lncRNA or mRNA and a blue node represents a downregulated lncRNA or mRNA.

scripts and lncRNAs transcribed of HOX loci were correlated with cisplatin chemotherapy response in lung SCC. Our microarray also displayed a portion of differentially expressed enhancer like lncRNAs. LncRNAs with an enhancer-like function were identified in various human cell lines and were involved in cellular differentiation. Depletion of a number of enhancer lncRNAs could lead to decreased expression of their neighboring protein-coding genes, such as TAL1, Snai1 and Snai2 [23]. To uncover the precise mechanism by which enhancer lncRNAs function to enhance gene expression has potential to overcome cisplatin resistance.

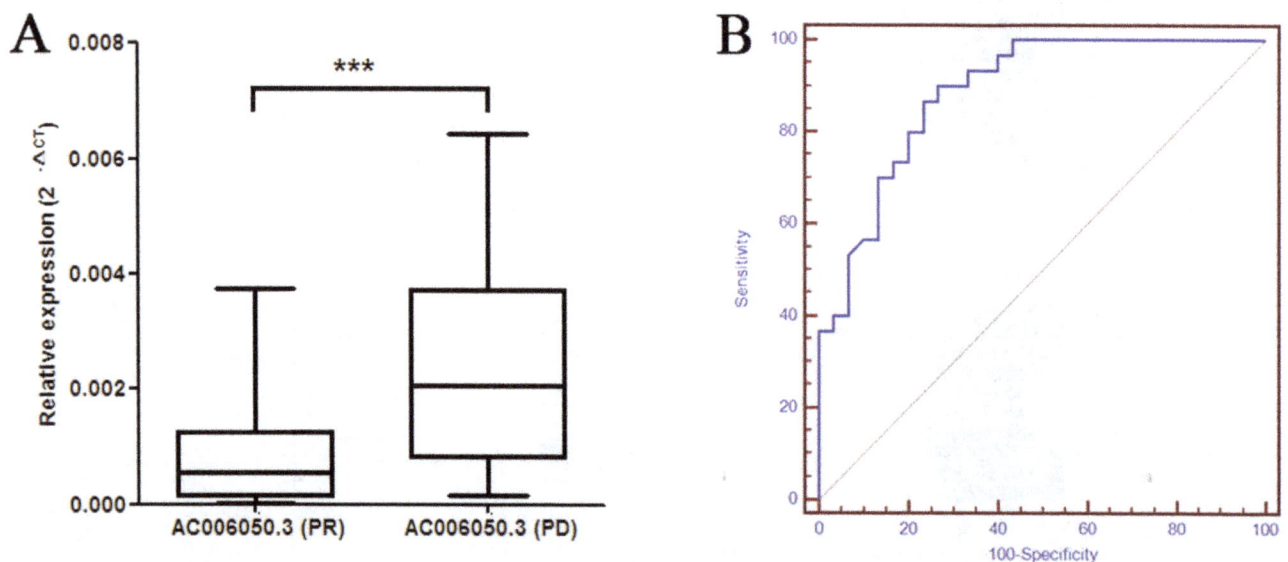

**Figure 5. The expression of lncRNA AC006050.3-003 was validated by qPCR in samples of 60 patients with lung SCC stratified according to the chemo response (PR vs. PD) following cisplatin based chemotherapy.** (A) lncRNA AC006050.3-003 was aberrantly expressed between PC and PD patients. The term $2^{-\Delta Ct}$ was used to describe the relative expression level of lncRNA ($\Delta Ct = Ct_{target} - Ct_{\beta-actin}$). ***$p <$ 0.001 for patients with PD versus patients with PR (Student's t-test). (B) ROC analysis of the ability of lncRNA AC006050.3-003 levels to discriminate between PR and PD patients with lung SCC receiving cisplatin based chemotherapy.

Simultaneously, we also identified 1,224 differentially expressed protein coding mRNAs from the same gene chip. Pathway analysis was applied to explore which particular pathways were enriched in genes controlling the distinctive features of PR group compared to PD group based on the differentially expressed mRNAs from the microarray. KEGG annotation showed that 32 pathways corresponded to downregulated transcripts and 15 pathways corresponded to upregulated transcripts. Among the pathways that corresponded to downregulated transcripts in PR group compared to PD group, "Nucleotide excision repair" and "Glutathione metabolism" pathways were previously reported correlated with cisplatin sensitivity [28,29]. Nucleotide excision repair (NER) systems are multistep enzymatic complexes involved in the repair of nonspecific DNA damage, such as cross linking, and chemical intra-/inter strand adduct formation. Cisplatin-DNA adducts is repaired primarily by the NER system [29]. Elevated glutathione may cause cisplatin resistance through inactivating cisplatin, increasing DNA repair, and decreasing cisplatin-induced oxidative stress [29]. In additional, "Drug metabolism-cytochrome P450", "Metabolism of xenobiotics by cytochrome P450", and "Drug metabolism-other enzymes" pathways are involved in drug metabolizing, affecting biotransformation of drugs. These drug metabolizing related pathways may contribute to interindividual variability in cisplatin response.

Gene co-expression networks were constructed to explore gene interactions [39,40]. Firstly, based on the different expression levels of lncRNAs and mRNAs, we calculated the Pearson correlation coefficients. Next, we chose significant correlation pairs (PCC≥0.99) to construct a co-expression network to predict the possible relationship of lncRNAs and mRNAs. The degree of gene centrality, the number of links from one gene to another, determines its relative importance within the network analysis [41]. In this study, lncRNA AC006050.3, MI0000285, KRT16P12, NAPSB, XLOC_005280 fit to these characteristics. Yang et al. profiled the differently expressed lncRNAs and mRNAs between lung ADC A549 and A549/CDDP cells. Gene co-expression network identified that lncRNAs including BX648420, ENST00000366408, and AK126698 potentially played a key role in cisplatin resistance. But we did not see the different expression of these lncRNAs in our data. NSCLC can be further divided into 3 major histological subtypes: ADC, SCC and large cell carcinoma [1]. Despite sharing many biological features, SCC and AC subtypes differ in their cell of origin, location within the lung, and growth pattern, suggesting they are distinct diseases that develop cisplatin risistance through differential molecular mechanisms.

The centrality of lncRNA AC006050.3 indicates its relative importance in the lncRNA-mRNA co-expression network. With co-expression network, we found AC006050.3-003 expression level correlated with many members of the NER pathway. So we think that lncRNA AC006050.3-003 may play important role in cisplatin chemo response in lung SCC. Its gene is located in chromosome 17: 28,894,720–28,895,457. Its transcript length is 549 nt and has 3 exsons. Whether this lncRNA is associated with cancer are unknown yet (http://asia.ensembl.org/). Based on the co-expression network analysis, lncRNA AC006050.3-003 was selected to further evaluate the predictor value in determining clinical response of lung SCC patients receiving cisplatin based chemotherapy by qPCR through additional 60 lung SCC samples. The relative level of lncRNA AC006050.3-003 was significantly reduced in the PR group compared with the PD group. The expression of lncRNA AC006050.3-003 was potential marker to distinguish the sensitivity or resistance to cisplatin based chemotherapy in patients with lung SCC.

## Conclusion

Our study showed that numerous lncRNAs and mRNAs were differently expressed between PR and PD samples in advanced lung SCC patients following cisplatin based chemotherapy. LncRNAs seem to be involved in cisplatin based chemo response and may serve as biomarkers for chemo response and candidates for therapy targets in lung SCC. However, the sample size in this study is relative small and it requires a larger data set for further confirmation. The network of lncRNA-conding RNA interactions is very complex and thus requires further study to reveal the accurately molecular mechanisms by which lncRNAs function in cisplatin chemo response.

## Supporting Information

**Table S1  Primers for qPCR.**

**Table S2  Basic medical records of ten patients.**

**Table S3  Enhancer-like lncRNAs and their nearby coding genes.**

**Table S4  HOX cluster profiling.**

**Table S5  LincRNAs and their nearby coding gene data.**

**Table S6  Pearson correlation coefficients of AC006050.3-003.**

## Acknowledgments

LncRNA microarray experiments were performed by KangChen Bio-tech (Shanghai, China). Coding-non-coding gene co-expression network analysis was analyzed by the OE Biotechnology Company (Shanghai, China).

## Author Contributions

Conceived and designed the experiments: LY XF. Performed the experiments: ZH. Analyzed the data: CX H. Xie. Contributed reagents/ materials/analysis tools: H. Xu PZ. Wrote the paper: ZH XF. Designed the software used in analysis: PZ.

## References

1. Jemal A, Bray F, Center MM, Ferlay J, Ward E, et al. (2011) Global cancer statistics. CA Cancer J Clin 61: 69–90.
2. Pikor LA, Ramnarine VR, Lam S, Lam WL (2013) Genetic alterations defining NSCLC subtypes and their therapeutic implications. Lung Cancer.
3. Crino L, Weder W, van Meerbeeck J, Felip E (2010) Early stage and locally advanced (non-metastatic) non-small-cell lung cancer: ESMO Clinical Practice Guidelines for diagnosis, treatment and follow-up. Ann Oncol 21 Suppl 5: v103–115.
4. Azzoli CG, Temin S, Giaccone G (2012) 2011 Focused Update of 2009 American Society of Clinical Oncology Clinical Practice Guideline Update on Chemotherapy for Stage IV Non-Small-Cell Lung Cancer. J Oncol Pract 8: 63–66.
5. Baggstrom MQ, Stinchcombe TE, Fried DB, Poole C, Hensing TA, et al. (2007) Third-generation chemotherapy agents in the treatment of advanced non-small cell lung cancer: a meta-analysis. J Thorac Oncol 2: 845–853.

6. Schiller JH, Harrington D, Belani CP, Langer C, Sandler A, et al. (2002) Comparison of four chemotherapy regimens for advanced non-small-cell lung cancer. N Engl J Med 346: 92–98.

7. Ardizzoni A, Boni L, Tiseo M, Fossella FV, Schiller JH, et al. (2007) Cisplatin-versus carboplatin-based chemotherapy in first-line treatment of advanced non-small-cell lung cancer: an individual patient data meta-analysis. J Natl Cancer Inst 99: 847–857.

8. Bernstein BE, Birney E, Dunham I, Green ED, Gunter C, et al. (2012) An integrated encyclopedia of DNA elements in the human genome. Nature 489: 57–74.

9. Derrien T, Johnson R, Bussotti G, Tanzer A, Djebali S, et al. (2012) The GENCODE v7 catalog of human long noncoding RNAs: analysis of their gene structure, evolution, and expression. Genome Res 22: 1775–1789.

10. Gupta RA, Shah N, Wang KC, Kim J, Horlings HM, et al. (2010) Long non-coding RNA HOTAIR reprograms chromatin state to promote cancer metastasis. Nature 464: 1071–1076.

11. Gutschner T, Diederichs S (2012) The hallmarks of cancer: a long non-coding RNA point of view. RNA Biol 9: 703–719.

12. Nakagawa T, Endo H, Yokoyama M, Abe J, Tamai K, et al. (2013) Large noncoding RNA HOTAIR enhances aggressive biological behavior and is associated with short disease-free survival in human non-small cell lung cancer. Biochem Biophys Res Commun 436: 319–324.

13. Khalil AM, Guttman M, Huarte M, Garber M, Raj A, et al. (2009) Many human large intergenic noncoding RNAs associate with chromatin-modifying complexes and affect gene expression. Proc Natl Acad Sci U S A 106: 11667–11672.

14. Kogo R, Shimamura T, Mimori K, Kawahara K, Imoto S, et al. (2011) Long noncoding RNA HOTAIR regulates polycomb-dependent chromatin modification and is associated with poor prognosis in colorectal cancers. Cancer Res 71: 6320–6326.

15. Bhan A, Mandal SS (2014) Long Noncoding RNAs: Emerging Stars in Gene Regulation, Epigenetics and Human Disease. ChemMedChem.

16. Tsang WP, Kwok TT (2007) Riboregulator H19 induction of MDR1-associated drug resistance in human hepatocellular carcinoma cells. Oncogene 26: 4877–4881.

17. Yang Y, Li H, Hou S, Hu B, Liu J, et al. (2013) The noncoding RNA expression profile and the effect of lncRNA AK126698 on cisplatin resistance in non-small-cell lung cancer cell. PLoS One 8: e65309.

18. Liu Z, Sun M, Lu K, Liu J, Zhang M, et al. (2013) The Long Noncoding RNA HOTAIR Contributes to Cisplatin Resistance of Human Lung Adenocarcinoma Cells via downregualtion of p21(WAF1/CIP1) Expression. PLoS One 8: e77293.

19. Eisenhauer EA, Therasse P, Bogaerts J, Schwartz LH, Sargent D, et al. (2009) New response evaluation criteria in solid tumours: revised RECIST guideline (version 1.1). Eur J Cancer 45: 228–247.

20. Schmittgen TD, Livak KJ (2008) Analyzing real-time PCR data by the comparative C(T) method. Nat Protoc 3: 1101–1108.

21. Liao Q, Liu C, Yuan X, Kang S, Miao R, et al. (2011) Large-scale prediction of long non-coding RNA functions in a coding-noncoding gene co-expression network. Nucleic Acids Res 39: 3864–3878.

22. Harrow J, Denoeud F, Frankish A, Reymond A, Chen CK, et al. (2006) GENCODE: producing a reference annotation for ENCODE. Genome Biol 7 Suppl 1: S4 1–9.

23. Orom UA, Derrien T, Beringer M, Gumireddy K, Gardini A, et al. (2010) Long noncoding RNAs with enhancer-like function in human cells. Cell 143: 46-58.

24. Rinn JL, Kertesz M, Wang JK, Squazzo SL, Xu X, et al. (2007) Functional demarcation of active and silent chromatin domains in human HOX loci by noncoding RNAs. Cell 129: 1311–1323.

25. Huarte M, Guttman M, Feldser D, Garber M, Koziol MJ, et al. (2010) A large intergenic noncoding RNA induced by p53 mediates global gene repression in the p53 response. Cell 142: 409–419.

26. Guttman M, Donaghey J, Carey BW, Garber M, Grenier JK, et al. (2011) lincRNAs act in the circuitry controlling pluripotency and differentiation. Nature 477: 295–300.

27. Guttman M, Amit I, Garber M, French C, Lin MF, et al. (2009) Chromatin signature reveals over a thousand highly conserved large non-coding RNAs in mammals. Nature 458: 223–227.

28. Rosell R, Taron M, Barnadas A, Scagliotti G, Sarries C, et al. (2003) Nucleotide excision repair pathways involved in Cisplatin resistance in non-small-cell lung cancer. Cancer Control 10: 297–305.

29. Stewart DJ (2007) Mechanisms of resistance to cisplatin and carboplatin. Crit Rev Oncol Hematol 63: 12-31.

30. Al-Bahlani S, Fraser M, Wong AY, Sayan BS, Bergeron R, et al. (2011) P73 regulates cisplatin-induced apoptosis in ovarian cancer cells via a calcium/calpain-dependent mechanism. Oncogene 30: 4219–4230.

31. Shang X, Lin X, Manorek G, Howell SB (2013) Claudin-3 and claudin-4 regulate sensitivity to cisplatin by controlling expression of the copper and cisplatin influx transporter CTR1. Mol Pharmacol 83: 85–94.

32. Calvo R, West J, Franklin W, Erickson P, Bemis L, et al. (2000) Altered HOX and WNT7A expression in human lung cancer. Proc Natl Acad Sci U S A 97: 12776–12781.

33. Cantile M, Cindolo L, Napodano G, Altieri V, Cillo C (2003) Hyperexpression of locus C genes in the HOX network is strongly associated in vivo with human bladder transitional cell carcinomas. Oncogene 22: 6462–6468.

34. Mainguy G, Koster J, Woltering J, Jansen H, Durston A (2007) Extensive polycistronism and antisense transcription in the mammalian Hox clusters. PLoS One 2: e356.

35. Sessa L, Breiling A, Lavorgna G, Silvestri L, Casari G, et al. (2007) Noncoding RNA synthesis and loss of Polycomb group repression accompanies the colinear activation of the human HOXA cluster. RNA 13: 223–239.

36. Li D, Feng J, Wu T, Wang Y, Sun Y, et al. (2013) Long intergenic noncoding RNA HOTAIR is overexpressed and regulates PTEN methylation in laryngeal squamous cell carcinoma. Am J Pathol 182: 64–70.

37. Yang Z, Zhou L, Wu LM, Lai MC, Xie HY, et al. (2011) Overexpression of long non-coding RNA HOTAIR predicts tumor recurrence in hepatocellular carcinoma patients following liver transplantation. Ann Surg Oncol 18: 1243–1250.

38. Liu XH, Liu ZL, Sun M, Liu J, Wang ZX, et al. (2013) The long non-coding RNA HOTAIR indicates a poor prognosis and promotes metastasis in non-small cell lung cancer. BMC Cancer 13: 464.

39. Prieto C, Risueno A, Fontanillo C, De las Rivas J (2008) Human gene coexpression landscape: confident network derived from tissue transcriptomic profiles. PLoS One 3: e3911.

40. Pujana MA, Han JD, Starita LM, Stevens KN, Tewari M, et al. (2007) Network modeling links breast cancer susceptibility and centrosome dysfunction. Nat Genet 39: 1338–1349.

41. Barabasi AL, Oltvai ZN (2004) Network biology: understanding the cell's functional organization. Nat Rev Genet 5: 101–113.

# Permissions

# List of Contributors

Jeffrey W. Martin, Susan Chilton-MacNeill and Maria Zielenska
Department of Paediatric Laboratory Medicine, Hospital for Sick Children, Toronto, Ontario, Canada,

Andre J. van Wijnen
Departments of Orthopedic Surgery and Biochemistry and Molecular Biology, Mayo Clinic, Rochester, Minnesota, United States of America

Jeremy A. Squire
Department of Pathology and Molecular Medicine, Queen's University, Kingston, Ontario, Canada, Departments of Genetics and Pathology, Faculdade de Medicina de Ribeira̅o Preto - USP, Ribeirão Preto, São Paulo, Brazil

Madhuri Koti
Department of Biomedical and Molecular Sciences, Queen's University, Kingston, Ontario, Canada

Carien H. G. Beurskens
Radboud university medical center, Department of Orthopedics, Section of Physical Therapy, Nijmegen, The Netherlands

Janine T. Hidding
Radboud university medical center, Department of Orthopedics, Section of Physical Therapy, Nijmegen, The Netherlands
Radboud university medical center, Scientific Institute for Quality of Healthcare, Nijmegen, The Netherlands

Philip J. van der Wees and Maria W. G. Nijhuis-van der Sanden
Radboud university medical center, Scientific Institute for Quality of Healthcare, Nijmegen, The Netherlands

Hanneke W. M. van Laarhoven
Academic Medical Center, Department of Medical Oncology, University of Amsterdam, Amsterdam, The Netherlands

Maria Vassilakopoulou, Huan Cheng, Jennifer Bordeaux, Veronique M. Neumeister and David L. Rimm
Yale University, School of Medicine, Department of Pathology, New Haven, Connecticut, United States of America

Taiwo Togun
Yale University, School of Public Health, Department of Biostatistics, New Haven, Connecticut, United States of America

Urania Dafni
Laboratory of Biostatistics, University of Athens School of Nursing, Athens, Greece

Mattheos Bobos
Laboratory of Molecular Oncology, Hellenic Foundation for Cancer Research, Aristotle University of Thessaloniki School of Medicine, Thessaloniki, Greece

Vassiliki Kotoula
Laboratory of Molecular Oncology, Hellenic Foundation for Cancer Research, Aristotle University of Thessaloniki School of Medicine, Thessaloniki, Greece
Department of Pathology, Aristotle University of Thessaloniki School of Medicine, Thessaloniki, Greece

George Fountzilas
Laboratory of Molecular Oncology, Hellenic Foundation for Cancer Research, Aristotle University of Thessaloniki School of Medicine, Thessaloniki, Greece
Department of Medical Oncology, "Papageorgiou" Hospital, Aristotle University of Thessaloniki School of Medicine, Thessaloniki, Greece

George Pentheroudakis
Department of Medical Oncology, Ioannina University Hospital, Ioannina, Greece

Dimosthenis V. Skarlos
Second Department of Medical Oncology, "Metropolitan" Hospital, Piraeus, Greece

Dimitrios Pectasides
Oncology Section, Second Department of Internal Medicine, "Hippokration" Hospital, Athens, Greece

Amanda Psyrri
Division of Oncology, Second Department of Internal Medicine, University of Athens School of Medicine, Attikon University Hospital, Athens, Greece

**Peipei Wang, Jiao Liu, Bin Zhang, Liang Liu and Pingping Lin**
Department of Pharmacology, Medical College of Qingdao University, Qingdao, China

**Fengmei An**
Hand Surgery Center of the Whole Army, No. 401 Hospital of Chinese People's Liberation Army, Qingdao, China

**Xingjun Zhuang**
Department of Oncology, No. 401 Hospital of Chinese People's Liberation Army, Qingdao, China

**Liyan Zhao and Mingchun Li**
Department of Pharmacy, No. 401 Hospital of Chinese People's Liberation Army, Qingdao, China

**Ruihua Mi., Qian Wang, Xudong Wei, Qingsong Yin, Lin Chen, Xinghu Zhu and Yongping Song**
Department of Hematology, Tumor Hospital of Zhengzhou University, Zhengzhou City, China

**Haiping Yang**
Department of Hematology, Tumor Hospital of Zhengzhou University, Zhengzhou City, China
Department of Hematology, First Affiliated Hospital of Henan University of Science and Technology, Zhengzhou City, China

**Jun Lin, Yi Lu and Yichen Zhu**
Department of Urology, Beijing Friendship Hospital Affiliated to Capital Medical University, Beijing, P.R China

**Qiang Zhang, Wenrui Xue, Yue Xu and Xiaopeng Hu**
Department of Urology, Beijing Chao-Yang Hospital Affiliated to Capital Medical University, Beijing, P.R China

**Minghua Yang, Pei Zeng, Yan Yu, Liangchun Yang and Lizhi Cao**
Department of Pediatrics, Xiangya Hospital, Central South University, Changsha Hunan, China,

**Daolin Tang**
Department of Infectious Diseases, Xiangya Hospital, Central South University, Changsha, Hunan, China
Department of Surgery, University of Pittsburgh Cancer Institute, Pittsburgh, Pennsylvania, United States of America

**Rui Kang**
Department of Surgery, University of Pittsburgh Cancer Institute, Pittsburgh, Pennsylvania, United States of America

**Marlinda Adham and Bambang Hermani**
Ear, Nose and Throat, University of Indonesia, Dr. Cipto Mangunkusumo hospital, Jakarta, Indonesia

**Lisnawati Rachmadi**
Anatomy-Pathology, University of Indonesia, Dr. Cipto Mangunkusumo hospital, Jakarta, Indonesia

**Soehartati Gondhowiardjo**
Radiotherapy, University of Indonesia, Dr. Cipto Mangunkusumo hospital, Jakarta, Indonesia

**Djumhana Atmakusumah**
Haematology-Medical Oncology Internal Medicine, University of Indonesia, Dr. Cipto Mangunkusumo hospital, Jakarta, Indonesia

**Djayadiman Gatot**
Medical Oncology Pediatric Department, University of Indonesia, Dr. Cipto Mangunkusumo hospital, Jakarta, Indonesia

**Sharon D. Stoker and Renske Fles**
Department of Head and Neck Oncology and Surgery, The Netherlands Cancer Institute, Amsterdam, The Netherlands

**I. Bing Tan**
Department of Head and Neck Oncology and Surgery, The Netherlands Cancer Institute, Amsterdam, The Netherlands
Ear, Nose and Throat Department, Gadjah Mada University, Yogyakarta, Indonesia
Department of Oral and Maxillofacial Surgery, Academic Medical Centre, Amsterdam, The Netherlands

**Maarten A. Wildeman**
Department of Head and Neck Oncology and Surgery, The Netherlands Cancer Institute, Amsterdam, The Netherlands
Department of Otorhinolaryngology, Academic Medical Centre, Amsterdam, The Netherlands

**Astrid E. Greijer and Jaap M. Middeldorp**
Department of Pathology, VU University Medical Center, Amsterdam, The Netherlands

**Fan Wang, Weiqi Dai, Miao Shen, Kan Chen, Ping Cheng, Yan Zhang, Chengfen Wang, Jingjing Li, Yuanyuan Zheng, Jie Lu, Jing Yang, Yingqun Zhou and Chuanyong Guo**
Department of Gastroenterology, Shanghai Tenth People's Hospital, Tongji University of Medicine, Shanghai, PR China

**Yugang Wang and Ling Xu**
Department of Gastroenterology, Shanghai Tongren Hospital, Jiaotong University of Medicine, Shanghai, PR China

**Rong Zhu**
Department of Gastroenterology, Clinical Medicine of Shanghai Tenth People's Hospital, Nanjing Medical University, Shanghai, PR China

**Huawei Zhang**
Department of Gastroenterology, The First Hospital Affiliated to Suzhou University, Suzhou, PR China

**Hyun-Kyung Jung, In-San Kim and Byung-Heon Lee**
Department of Biochemistry and Cell Biology and School of Medicine, Kyungpook National University, Daegu, Korea
BK21 Plus KNU Biomedical Convergence Program, Department of Biomedical Science, Graduate School, Kyungpook National University, Daegu, Korea

**Kai Wang**
Department of Plastic Surgery, Henan Provincial People's Hospital, Zhengzhou, Henan, China

**Min Kyu Jung**
Department of Internal Medicine, School of Medicine, Kyungpook National University, Daegu, Korea

**Kai Chen, Xiaolan Zhang, Heran Deng, Liling Zhu, Fengxi Su and Weijuan Jia**
Breast Tumor Center, Sun Yat-sen Memorial Hospital, Sun Yat-sen University, Guangzhou, P. R. China

**Xiaogeng Deng**
Department of Pediatric Surgery, Sun Yat-sen Memorial Hospital, Sun Yat-sen University, Guangzhou, P. R. China

**Anna Boltong**
Cancer Council Victoria, Melbourne, Australia

**Sanchia Aranda**
Cancer Institute NSW, Eveleigh, NSW, Australia
Department of Cancer Experiences Research, Peter MacCallum Cancer Centre, East Melbourne, Victoria, Australia
Melbourne School of Health Sciences, The University of Melbourne, Carlton, Victoria, Australia

**Karla Gough**
Department of Cancer Experiences Research, Peter MacCallum Cancer Centre, East Melbourne, Victoria, Australia

**Rochelle Wynne**
Melbourne School of Health Sciences, The University of Melbourne, Carlton, Victoria, Australia

**Russell Keast**
Centre for Physical Activity and Nutrition Research, Deakin University, Burwood, Victoria, Australia

**Prudence A. Francis**
Breast Medical Oncology, Peter MacCallum Cancer Centre, East Melbourne, Victoria, Australia

**Jacqueline Chirgwin**
Breast Medical Oncology, Eastern Health, Australia

**George L. Drusano, David Brown, Steven Fikes and Arnold Louie**
Institute for Therapeutic Innovation, College of Medicine, University of Florida, Lake Nona, Florida, United States of America

**Michael Neely, Michael Van Guilder and Alan Schumitzky**
Laboratory of Applied Pharmacokinetics, School of Medicine, University of Southern California, Los Angeles, California, United States of America

**Charles Peloquin**
Infectious Diseases PK Laboratory, College of Pharmacy, University of Florida, Gainesville, Florida, United States of America

**Alvin Ho-Kwan Cheung, Ryan Chung-Hei Pak, Oswens Siu-Hung Lo, Jensen Tung-Chung Poon and Wai Lun Law**
Department of Surgery, Li Ka Shing Faculty of Medicine, The University of Hong Kong, Hong Kong SAR, China

**Colin Siu-Chi Lam, Sunny Kit-Man Wong, Timothy Ming-Hun Wan, Lui Ng, Ariel Ka-Man Chow, Nathan Shiu-Man Cheng, Hung-Sing Li, Johnny Hon-Wai Man and Roberta Wen-Chi Pang**
Department of Surgery, Li Ka Shing Faculty of Medicine, The University of Hong Kong, Hong Kong SAR, China
Centre for Cancer Research, Li Ka Shing Faculty of Medicine, The University of Hong Kong, Hong Kong SAR, China

**Thomas Chung-Cheung Yau**
Department of Clinical Oncology, Li Ka Shing Faculty of Medicine, The University of Hong Kong, Hong Kong SAR, China

**Chun-Hua Xu, Li-Ke Yu and Ke-Ke Hao**
First Department of Respiratory Medicine and Nanjing Chest Hospital, Nanjing, Jiangsu, China,
Clinical Center of Nanjing Respiratory Diseases, Nanjing, Jiangsu, China

**Shigeto Ueda,Takashi Shigekawa, Hideki Takeuchi, Hiroshi Sano, Eiko Hirokawa, Hiroko Shimada, Akihiko Osaki and Toshiaki Saeki**
Department of Breast Oncology, International Medical Center, Saitama Medical University, Hidaka, Saitama, Japan

**Ichiei Kuji**
Department of Nuclear Medicine, International Medical Center, Saitama Medical University, Hidaka, Saitama, Japan

**Hiroaki Suzuki and Motoki Oda**
Central Research Laboratory, Hamamatsu Photonics K. K., Hamakita-ku, Hamamatsu, Japan

**Zi-Jie Long, Yuan Hu, Xu-Dong Li, Yi He, Ruo-Zhi Xiao, Zhi-Gang Fang, Dong-Ning Wang, Jia-Jun Liu, Ren-Wei Huang and Dong-Jun Lin**
Department of Hematology, Third Affiliated Hospital, Sun Yat-sen University, Sun Yat-sen Institute of Hematology, Sun Yat-sen University, Guangzhou, China

**Quentin Liu**
Department of Hematology, Third Affiliated Hospital, Sun Yat-sen University, Sun Yat-sen Institute of Hematology, Sun Yat-sen University, Guangzhou, China
Institute of Cancer Stem Cell, Dalian Medical University, Dalian, China

**Jin-Song Yan**
Department of Hematology, Second Affiliated Hospital, Dalian Medical University, Dalian, China

**Pu-Yun OuYang, Zhen Su, Jie Tang, Xiao-Wen Lan, Yan-Ping Mao and Fang-Yun Xie**
Department of Radiation Oncology, Sun Yat-sen University Cancer Center, State Key Laboratory of Oncology in South China, Collaborative Innovation Center for Cancer Medicine, Guangzhou, Guangdong, China

**Wuguo Deng**
Department of Experimental Research, Sun Yat-sen University Cancer Center, State Key Laboratory of Oncology in South China, Collaborative Innovation Center for Cancer Medicine, Guangzhou, Guangdong, China

**Seth A. Brodie and Johann C. Brandes**
Atlanta VA Medical Center, Atlanta, Georgia, United States of America
Departments of Hematology and Medical Oncology, School of Medicine, Emory University, Atlanta, Georgia, United States of America
Winship Cancer Institute, Emory University, Atlanta, Georgia, United States of America

**Shaojin You**
Atlanta VA Medical Center, Atlanta, Georgia, United States of America
Department of Pathology, School of Medicine, Emory University, Atlanta, Georgia, United States of America

**Courtney Lombardo, Ge Li, Fadlo R. Khuri and Adam Marcus**
Departments of Hematology and Medical Oncology, School of Medicine, Emory University, Atlanta, Georgia, United States of America
Winship Cancer Institute, Emory University, Atlanta, Georgia, United States of America

**Paula M. Vertino**
Department of Radiation Oncology, School of Medicine, Emory University, Atlanta, Georgia, United States of America
Winship Cancer Institute, Emory University, Atlanta, Georgia, United States of America

**Khanjan Gandhi**
Department of Human Genetics, School of Medicine, Emory University, Atlanta, Georgia, United States of America
Winship Cancer Institute, Emory University, Atlanta, Georgia, United States of America
Department of Biostatistics and Bioinformatics, Rollins School of Public Health, Atlanta, Georgia, United States of America

**Jeanne Kowalski**
Winship Cancer Institute, Emory University, Atlanta, Georgia, United States of America
Department of Biostatistics and Bioinformatics, Rollins School of Public Health, Atlanta, Georgia, United States of America

**Johannes Malte Froehlich**
Institute of Radiology and Nuclear Medicine, Clinical Research Unit, Hirslanden Hospital St. Anna, Lucerne, Switzerland

**Carolin Reischauer**
Institute of Radiology and Nuclear Medicine, Clinical Research Unit, Hirslanden Hospital St. Anna, Lucerne, Switzerland

Department of Radiology, Cantonal Hospital Winterthur, Winterthur, Switzerland
Department of Radiology, Paracelsus Medical University Salzburg, Salzburg, Austria

**Andreas Gutzeit**
Institute of Radiology and Nuclear Medicine, Clinical Research Unit, Hirslanden Hospital St. Anna, Lucerne, Switzerland
Department of Radiology, Paracelsus Medical University Salzburg, Salzburg, Austria

**Christoph Andreas Binkert**
Department of Radiology, Paracelsus Medical University Salzburg, Salzburg, Austria

**Miklos Pless**
Department of Oncology, Cantonal Hospital Winterthur, Winterthur, Switzerland

**Dow-Mu Koh**
Academic Department of Radiology, Royal Marsden NHS Foundation Trust, Sutton, Surrey, United Kingdom
CR-UK and EPSRC Cancer Imaging Centre, Institute of Cancer Research, Sutton, Surrey, United Kingdom

**Rolf Warta and Christel Herold-Mende**
Experimental Neurosurgery Research, Department of Neurosurgery, University of Heidelberg, Heidelberg, Germany,
Molecular Cell Biology Group, Department of Otorhinolaryngology, Head and Neck Surgery, University of Heidelberg, Heidelberg, Germany

**Peter K.Plinkert and Gerhard Dyckhoff**
Molecular Cell Biology Group, Department of Otorhinolaryngology, Head and Neck Surgery, University of Heidelberg, Heidelberg, Germany

**Dirk Theile and Johanna Weiss**
Department of Clinical Pharmacology and Pharmacoepidemiology, University of Heidelberg, Heidelberg, Germany

**Carolin Mogler and Esther Herpel**
Tissue Bank of the National Center for Tumor Diseases (NCT), University of Heidelberg, Heidelberg, Germany
Institute of Pathology, University of Heidelberg, Heidelberg, Germany

**Bernd Lahrmann**
Institute of Pathology, University of Heidelberg, Heidelberg, Germany
Hamamatsu Tissue Imaging and Analysis Center, BIOQUANT, University of Heidelberg, Heidelberg, Germany

**Niels Grabe**
Department of Medical Oncology, National Center for Tumor Diseases, University of Heidelberg, Heidelberg, Germany
Hamamatsu Tissue Imaging and Analysis Center, BIOQUANT, University of Heidelberg, Heidelberg, Germany

**Sarah E. Mathis, Rounak Nande, Walter Neto, Logan Lawrence, Danielle R. McCallister and James Denvir**
Department of Biochemistry and Microbiology, Joan C. Edwards School of Medicine, Marshall University, Huntington, West Virginia, United States of America
Translational Genomic Research Institute, Marshall University, Huntington, West Virginia, United States of America

**Pier Paolo Claudio**
Department of Biochemistry and Microbiology, Joan C. Edwards School of Medicine, Marshall University, Huntington, West Virginia, United States of America
Translational Genomic Research Institute, Marshall University, Huntington, West Virginia, United States of America
Department of Surgery, Joan C. Edwards School of Medicine, Marshall University, Huntington, West Virginia, United States of America

**Anthony Alberico**
Department of Neurosurgery, Joan C. Edwards School of Medicine, Marshall University, Huntington, West Virginia, United States of America

**Gerrit A. Kimmey**
Department of Medical Oncology, St. Mary's Hospital, Huntington, West Virginia, United States of America

**Mark Mogul**
Department of Pediatrics, Joan C. Edwards School of Medicine, Marshall University, Huntington, West Virginia, United States of America

**Gerard Oakley III, Krista L. Denning and Thomas Dougherty**
Department of Pathology, Joan C. Edwards School of Medicine, Marshall University, Huntington, West Virginia, United States of America
Jagan V. Valluri
Department of Biology, Marshall University, Huntington, West Virginia, United States of America

**Zhaohui Chu, Hao Lin, Xiaohua Liang, Ruofan Huang, Qiong Zhan, Jingwei Jiang and Xinli Zhou**
Department of Oncology, Huashan Hospital, Fudan University, Shanghai, China, 200040,
Department of Oncology, Shanghai Medical College, Fudan University, Shanghai, China, 200032

**Zhibo Hou, Chunhua Xu, Haiyan Xie, Ping Zhan and Like Yu**
First Department of Respiratory Medicine, Nanjing Chest Hospital, Medicine School of Southeast University, Nanjing, Jiangsu, China
Clinical Center of Nanjing Respiratory Diseases and Imaging, Nanjing, Jiangsu, China

**Huae Xu**
Department of Pharmacy, The First Affiliated Hospital of Nanjing Medical University, Nanjing, Jiangsu, China

**Xuefeng Fang**
Department of Medical Oncology, Second Affiliated Hospital, Zhejiang University College of Medicine, Hangzhou, Zhejiang, China

# Index

www.ingramcontent.com/pod-product-compliance
Lightning Source LLC
Chambersburg PA
CBHW080525200326
41458CB00012B/4339